INTERNATIONAL
HANDBOOK of
VICTIMOLOGY

T0203625

INTERNATIONAL HANDBOOK OF

VICTIMOLOGY

Edited by
Shlomo Giora Shoham
Paul Knepper
Martin Kett

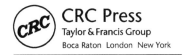

CRC Press
Taylor & Francis Group
Boca Raton London New York

CRC Press is an imprint of the
Taylor & Francis Group, an **informa** business

CRC Press
Taylor & Francis Group
6000 Broken Sound Parkway NW, Suite 300
Boca Raton, FL 33487-2742

First issued in paperback 2019

© 2010 by Taylor & Francis Group, LLC
CRC Press is an imprint of Taylor & Francis Group, an Informa business

No claim to original U.S. Government works

ISBN-13: 978-0-4200-8547-1 (hbk)
ISBN-13: 978-0-367-86429-3 (pbk)

This book contains information obtained from authentic and highly regarded sources. Reasonable efforts have been made to publish reliable data and information, but the author and publisher cannot assume responsibility for the validity of all materials or the consequences of their use. The authors and publishers have attempted to trace the copyright holders of all material reproduced in this publication and apologize to copyright holders if permission to publish in this form has not been obtained. If any copyright material has not been acknowledged please write and let us know so we may rectify in any future reprint.

Except as permitted under U.S. Copyright Law, no part of this book may be reprinted, reproduced, transmitted, or utilized in any form by any electronic, mechanical, or other means, now known or hereafter invented, including photocopying, microfilming, and recording, or in any information storage or retrieval system, without written permission from the publishers.

For permission to photocopy or use material electronically from this work, please access www.copyright.com (http://www.copyright.com/) or contact the Copyright Clearance Center, Inc. (CCC), 222 Rosewood Drive, Danvers, MA 01923, 978-750-8400. CCC is a not-for-profit organization that provides licenses and registration for a variety of users. For organizations that have been granted a photocopy license by the CCC, a separate system of payment has been arranged.

Trademark Notice: Product or corporate names may be trademarks or registered trademarks, and are used only for identification and explanation without intent to infringe.

Library of Congress Cataloging-in-Publication Data

International handbook of victimology / editors, Shlomo Giora Shoham, Paul Knepper, Martin Kett.
    p. cm.
Includes bibliographical references and index.
ISBN 978-1-4200-8547-1
    1. Victims of crimes. I. Shoham, S. Giora, 1929- II. Knepper, Paul. III. Kett, Martin.
IV. Title.

HV6250.25.I585 2010
362.88--dc22
    2009030140

Visit the Taylor & Francis Web site at
http://www.taylorandfrancis.com

and the CRC Press Web site at
http://www.crcpress.com

Table of Contents

Preface

In 1973, the First International Symposium on Victimology convened in Jerusalem. The symposium took place under the auspices of the International Society of Criminology with the support of the Hebrew University of Jerusalem, the University of Tel Aviv, and Bar Ilan University. The symposium brought together scholars across various fields from around the world; they presented papers on theoretical issues in victimology, the response to crime, victims and criminal justice, and processes of victimization. This work appeared in a five-volume collection of papers titled *Victimology: A New Focus* [1973], edited by Israel Drapkin and Emilio Viano, and has represented for some years the state of international knowledge in victimology.

After 30 years, some issues have remained important areas of interest, and new issues have emerged. Conceptions of victimhood, secondary victimization, hidden victimization, and social services for victims have remained important topics for research and theory. New topics have emerged. Restorative justice has had a major influence on theory, research, and policy in victimology. Government-sponsored crime victimization surveys, which began in the early 1970s, now represent a valuable source of information about victimization processes. Compensation and restitution schemes have operated for decades in a number of countries, and victims' rights have become enacted into law. To reflect these essential and emerging issues, we have put together the *International Handbook of Victimology*.

This handbook brings together leading scholars from around the world reflecting the state of the art in victimology. Each of these has been specifically commissioned based on recognized expertise in the field. Contributors come from Australia, Belgium, Canada, Germany, India, Ireland, Israel, Japan, Malta, the Netherlands, Portugal, Serbia, Sweden, the United Kingdom, and the United States. They bring disciplinary expertise in criminology, sociology, psychology, law, and philosophy. Some revisit the core of victimology; others present new issues at the cutting edge. Collectively, they provide an outstanding one-volume source for victimology, and we are pleased to be able to present their work.

The handbook is arranged into six sections. Section I provides an overview of theoretical and historical frameworks used in the study of victimology. The chapters examine philosophical and historical conceptions of the victim, discuss the meaning of justice for victims, and review the history of victimology as a field of study. Section II deals with advances in research methods. Chapters introduce approaches to research concerning repeat victimization, what can be learned from the International Crime Victim Survey, and the use of geographic information systems (GIS) technology in understanding victimization. Section III explains patterns of victimization. This section includes discussions of secondary victimization, drugs and alcohol in relation to victimization, victims of sex trafficking, victimization in workplaces, and issues related to tourism and victimization. Section IV concerns responses to victimization, including victims and criminal justice, victims' rights, victim support services, and fear of crime. Section V considers current issues in restorative justice. Chapters deal with victim–offender relationships, conceptions of healing, the value of apology in reparation, and the usefulness of restorative justice in transitional societies. Section VI examines victims and social divisions: hidden victimization (of women) and domestic violence, victimization in relation to disability, victimization in relation to mental health populations, and victims in relation to social services.

This handbook would not have been possible without the efforts of a number of people. To all the contributors, we would like to say that we have appreciated working with you on this project. We would like to thank Carolyn Spence and Jessica Vakili at Taylor & Francis Group for believing in the book and seeing it through to publication. We also thank Hemdat Libbi Israeli for impressive coordination, undying enthusiasm, and professional assistance in every way. Finally, we take this opportunity to dedicate this volume to the memory of Gerald Cromer. Gerald was on the staff at Bar-Ilan University. He planned to contribute a chapter to this book, but, sadly, he died several months into the project.

Shlomo G. Shoham
Tel Aviv, Israel

Paul Knepper
Sheffield, United Kingdom

Martin Kett
Tel Aviv, Israel

Editors

Shlomo G. Shoham is Professor of Law and an interdisciplinary lecturer at Faculty of Law, Tel Aviv University, and is a world-renowned criminologist who has published more than 100 books and about 1,000 articles on crime, deviance, philosophy, religion, psychology, and the human personality. Over the years, he has developed his innovative personality theory, a highly appraised new theory of personality development. In 2003, Professor Shoham was awarded the Israel Prize for research in criminology. Previously, he was awarded the Sellin-Glueck Award, the highest prize in American criminology, and recently the prestigious Emet Prize. He is the recipient of a decoration from the prime minister of France. Professor Shoham has lectured all over the world and has been a resident at the universities of Oxford, Harvard, and the Sorbonne.

Paul Knepper is Senior Lecturer, Department of Sociological Studies, University of Sheffield, and Visiting Professor, Institute of Criminology, University of Malta. His research has explored sociopolitical definitions of race, conceptual foundations of crime prevention, and historical origins of contemporary responses to crime.

Martin Kett is a self-employed technical writer and translator. He received a BSc in mathematics and statistics from Bar-Ilan University, Israel.

Contributors

Elaine Barclay
Institute for Rural Futures
University of New England
Armidale, New South Wales, Australia

Eyal Brook
The Buchmann Faculty of Law
Tel Aviv University
Tel Aviv, Israel

Michelle Butler
Queens University Belfast
Belfast, Northern Ireland

Marilyn Clark
Department of Youth and Community
    Studies
University of Malta
Msida, Malta

Cláudia Coelho
Department of Psychology
University of Minho
Braga, Portugal

Rachel Condry
Department of Sociology
University of Surrey
Guildford, United Kingdom

Sanja Ćopić
Institute for Criminological and
    Sociological Research
Victimology Society of Serbia
Belgrade, Serbia

Paul Cunningham
Lansdowne Market Research
Dublin, Ireland

Tom Daems
Research Foundation Flanders
Institute of Criminal Law
and
Department of Criminal Law and
    Criminology
Catholic University of Leuven
Leuven, Belgium

Walter S. DeKeseredy
Department of Criminology, Justice and
    Policy Studies
University of Ontario Institute of
    Technology
Oshawa, Ontario, Canada

Ana Rita Dias
Department of Psychology
University of Minho
Braga, Portugal

Jan van Dijk
International Victimology Institute
Tilburg University
Tilburg, the Netherlands

Ezzat A. Fattah
School of Criminology
Simon Fraser University
Burnaby, British Columbia, Canada

Tali Gal
Institute of Criminology
The Hebrew University of Jerusalem
Mount Scopus, Jerusalem, Israel

K. Jaishankar
Department of Criminology and Criminal
    Justice
Manonmaniam Sundaranar University
Tamil Nadu, India

Carol Jones
University of Gloucestershire
Gloucestershire, United Kingdom

John van Kesteren
International Victimology Institute
Tilburg University
Tilburg, the Netherlands

Gerd Ferdinand Kirchhoff
Tokiwa Graduate School of Victimology
Tokiwa University
Mito, Ibaraki, Japan

Paul Knepper
Department of Sociological Studies and
    Centre for Criminological Research
University of Sheffield
Sheffield, United Kingdom

Carina Ljungwald
Department of Social Work
Stockholm University
Stockholm, Sweden

Richard Lusignan
Institut Philippe-Pinel
Montréal, Quebec, Canada

Carla Machado
Department of Psychology
University of Minho
Braga, Portugal

Manuel Madriaga
Learning and Teaching Institute
Sheffield Hallam University
Sheffield, United Kingdom

Rebecca Mallett
Faculty of Development and Society
Sheffield Hallam University
Sheffield, United Kingdom

Jacques D. Marleau
Institut Philippe-Pinel
Montréal, Quebec, Canada

Rob I. Mawby
University of Gloucestershire
Gloucestershire, United Kingdom

Sanja Milivojevic
School of Social Sciences
University of Western Sydney
Sydney, New South Wales, Australia

Bernadette T. Muscat
Department of Criminology
University of California, Fresno
Fresno, California

Ken Pease
Jill Dando Institute
University College London
London, United Kingdom

Katherine R. Rossiter
School of Criminology
Simon Fraser University
Burnaby, British Columbia,
Canada

Joanna Shapland
Centre for Criminological Research
University of Sheffield
Sheffield, United Kingdom

Shlomo G. Shoham
The Buchmann Faculty of Law
Tel Aviv University
Tel Aviv, Israel

Heather Strang
Centre for Restorative Justice
Australia National University
Canberra, Australia

Rainer Strobl
Institute for Interdisciplinary Research on
    Conflict and Violence
University of Bielefeld
Bielefeld, Germany

Andromachi Tseloni
School of Social Sciences
Nottingham Trent University
Nottingham, United Kingdom

Simon N. Verdun-Jones
School of Criminology
Simon Fraser University
Burnaby, British Columbia, Canada

Sharon Warshwski-Brook
The Buchmann Faculty of Law
Tel Aviv University
Tel Aviv, Israel

Jo-Anne Wemmers
International Centre for Comparative
    Criminology
and
School of Criminology
Université de Montréal
Montréal, Quebec, Canada

Rob White
School of Sociology and Social Work
University of Tasmania
Hobart, Tasmania, Australia

Uri Yanay
Paul Baerwald School of Social Work and
    Social Welfare
The Hebrew University of Jerusalem
Mount Scopus, Jerusalem, Israel

Introduction

SHLOMO G. SHOHAM AND PAUL KNEPPER

The *International Handbook of Victimology* provides a substantive guide to emerging issues and essential topics in victimology. Individual chapters identify new topics of concern, describe current research, inform contemporary understanding, and update policy discussions. The contributors raise new questions and revisit long-standing debates to collectively present the "state of the art" in the field. The chapters are arranged into six broad categories: theoretical and historical frameworks, research methods, patterns of victimization, responses to victims, restorative justice, and victims and social divisions.

The chapters in Section I examine starting assumptions, frames of reference, and basic concepts in victimology. Rainer Strobl argues for a definition of "becoming a victim in a socially relevant sense," by which he means that the crucial condition for victim status is not suffering from wounds or experience of norm violation (as important as they are), but "being seen as a victim by others and adopting a victim role with certain rights and obligations." He offers a constructivist view of victim status premised on the belief that the realm of subjective experience and the interpretations of other persons within the victim experience can never completely be bridged by third parties. He discusses four logical possibilities for the construction of victimhood and five principles for a victimological definition of the victim. The main idea of the proposed constructivist approach, he suggests, is the need to accept the plurality of victim constructions. There are different ways to become a victim in a social relevant sense, and victims may need to adopt one form of victimhood to receive needed services and another to avoid aggression from perpetrators.

Jo-Anne Wemmers focuses on the meaning of justice for victims. She points out that justice is a multidimensional construct; it consists of informational, interactional, distributive, and procedural aspects. She reviews research concerning these aspects and observes that although these studies are very different, they suggest that procedural justice is important for victims. Victims are concerned about the quality of their interaction with authorities and the outcome of the criminal justice process in the sense of distributive or outcome fairness. A narrow focus on victims' desire for distributive or outcome justice represents an incomplete understanding of justice as a guide to policymaking. By recognizing victims' desires for informational and interactive justice, criminal justice authorities can enhance victims' judgments about the overall justice obtained. The observation that victims may substitute one kind of justice for another suggests that all these dimensions represent part of the same underlying concept. Although it does not appear that all dimensions have equal value, interactive justice may be more important than informational justice.

Ezzat A. Fattah offers a retrospective look at the development of victimology along with an overview of ideological transformations and current victim policies. Although victimology is younger than its parent discipline of criminology, it has the strength not only to become an integral part of criminology but also to reshape the entire discipline of criminology. His chapter visits essential issues, including findings of victimization surveys, conceptual differences between criminalization and victimization, policy frameworks, victims' rights, and victim support services. Based on this review, Fattah makes a plea for victimology to return to its "original scientific role, to shed its ideological mantle, and to resume its role as a scholarly discipline and as an integral part of criminology." Victimologists cannot be scientists and advocates at the same time, and if victimology is to continue to grow as a field of knowledge, victimologists must set aside political advocacy.

Gerd Ferdinand Kirchhoff presents a historical account of the development of victimology from the age of science and the Enlightenment to the emergence of positivism and interactionism in the twentieth century. Victimology represents a social science of victims, victimizations, and social reactions to these, which retains (or should retain) strong links to more general social theory. He goes on to outline the issues with which general victimology is concerned and the structure of victimology, that is, definition of the victim, victim measurement, and correlates of victimization. He looks at the victim in the criminal justice system against the larger background of social reactions to victimization. He concludes with the observation that the victim movement has engendered political action far beyond the reach of crime.

Section II of this volume presents new insights based on innovations in research technique. Andromachi Tseloni and Ken Pease take a fresh look at the connection between property crimes and repeat victimization. The extent of repeat victimization has yet to be appreciated owing to counting conventions in victimization surveys (which understate the extent) and to a central (but underappreciated) dynamic of offending, which can be seen in burglary. They set out approaches to statistical modeling of crime rates that reflect known facts of repeat victimization and make use of one of these, negative binomial modeling, to clarify risk and repeat victimization. The thrust of this analysis seeks to understand the drivers of victimization by deploying models capable of measuring risk concentration. "It is difficult to overstate the importance of this analysis," they explain, "If more generally true, it means that overall crime rates are generally responsive to rates of repeats." One of the primary goals of policies in liberal democracies is to allocate resources to need, and without understanding the concentration of victimization, this becomes impossible to achieve.

John van Kesteren and Jan van Dijk summarize key findings from the International Crime Victims Survey (ICVS). The ICVS amplifies the benefits of victimization surveys by collecting this information in a comparative, international perspective. It allows for analysis of the dynamics of actual and reported crimes, fear of crime, and satisfaction with the police across countries. Comparative victimization surveys are now recognized as an indispensable tool for benchmarking criminal policies in international settings. They have importance for research in criminology as well. Victimization surveys are useful tools for obtaining social indicators of crime and a rich source of information of direct relevance to victimology. In their chapter, van Kesteren and van Dijk review data from the most recent round of the ICVS (2004/2005) conducted in 30 countries and six cities to illustrate the potential to inform victimological studies. They compare, for example, risk assessments of victims and nonvictims and the opinions of victims and nonvictims on appropriate punishments for offenders across regions and countries.

K. Jaishankar presents the findings of a study of communal violence victimization using geographic information systems (GIS) analysis. The study looks at Coimbatore City, located in south India, to explore patterns of communal rioting during 1997–1998. Although rooted in the disharmony between Hindus and Muslims, the problem is more complex than a clash of values. The results of the GIS analysis show that victimization patterns vary with sociodemographic characteristics. The problem of communal violence is significantly related to the gender, age, and religion of the victim. The results of the study are of use to local government in charting police patrol and prevention activities. They are of use to criminology (all the patterns observed are consistent with routine activities theory) and of use to victimology in identifying directions for future research. The results suggest that crimes of communal violence tend to be more brutal and divisive than conventional crimes committed by individuals.

The chapters in Section III concern patterns of victimization. Rachel Condry examines secondary victimization. She explains the term *secondary victimization* has come to be understood in three distinct ways. Secondary victimization is said to result from victimization, or the consequences of victimization, spilling over to another party. Secondary victimization is said to refer to victims of crime when the experiences of criminal justice processes and social responses compound their feelings of victimhood, which is particularly likely for victims of rape. Finally, secondary victimization is said to be created by social reaction to a primary victim's status to the extent of leading this victim status to become central to that person's identity. She emphasizes that just as the experience and impact of victimization are mediated by social factors such as age, gender, economic standing, and ethnicity, the experience of secondary victimization varies along these lines as well. Overall, it is important to keep in mind that many more people are affected by crime than a cursory look at crime figures suggests.

Marilyn Clark discusses the links between substance abuse and offending and between substance abuse and victimization. Both issues have been the subject of research for some years, although they appear as separate issues involving discrete literatures; researchers examine substance abuse in relation to *either* offending or victimization. Clark presents both phenomena using the same conceptual framework, followed by an explanation of both phenomena within a multidisciplinary and multicultural perspective. She reviews research for Europe, the United States, and Australia concerning trends in drug and alcohol use, substance abuse in offender populations, substance abuse and victimization, and alcohol and sexual violence. Overall, this evidence supports the general observation that substance abuse, crime, and victimization are interrelated.

Sanja Milivojevic and Sanja Ćopić sort out the myths and realities surrounding victims of sex trafficking. Trafficking in people, and particularly women for sexual exploitation, has been described as "modern-day slavery" by antitrafficking campaigners. At the same time, researchers and policymakers have been criticized for buying into "trafficking hype." Based on surveys of trafficking in people within Serbia and Australia, they identify prominent vocabularies around women victims of trafficking. Specifically, they examine the language of judges, prosecutors, lawyers, nongovernmental organization (NGO) activists, scholars, and policymakers whose work involves this area. Milivojevic and Ćopić spotlight the ways in which perceptions of victim status are tied to gender and femininity. In Serbia, female victims of trafficking tend to be seen through two sharply contrasting discourses of "blaming the victim" and "ideal victim"; media representations of women trafficked for sex as well as dominant narratives of international organizations and NGOs diffuse and reinforce this duality. "It is essential," they conclude, "that the multiple identities of women trafficked for sex are acknowledged, and that women's victimization in the context of various forms of subordination and oppression is given a voice."

Richard Lusignan and Jacques D. Marleau elaborate the theme of occupational victimization. They introduce the term *socioprofessional victimization* to describe criminal victimization to which a group of individuals sharing an occupational practice is exposed. The few existing studies in this area suggest that victimization is linked to work tasks involving clients with the potential for violence and to occupations involving handling of valuables or money. Lusignan and Marleau extend this understanding to other types of workers using explanatory models from criminology, including routine activities and lifestyle models, and examine various forms of victimization involving teachers, such as robbery, assault, and burglary. By taking into account the occupations pursued within premises, it is possible to predict types of criminal activities likely to occur along a city district, street, or square. They insist that improving our knowledge of occupational behaviors will allow for more specific prevention projects tailored to risks faced by workers.

In the final chapter in this section, Rob I. Mawby, Elaine Barclay, and Carol Jones deal with the issue of tourism and victimization. Criminologists have overlooked tourism as a topic worthy of investigation partly because existing sources of data do not allow tourists to be identified as victims. Nevertheless, researching the relationship between tourism and victimization is important because it can inform practitioners in the tourism industry and contribute to theory in victimology. They review levels of risk identified in victimology and apply these to tourist victims, followed by a look at explanations of these levels of risk in relation to tourist victims. They also present four case studies to illustrate how the "average tourist" can be understood, and how risk levels can be explored for identifiable groups of tourists. Overall, they aim not only to review the literature but also to introduce criminologists to a fertile area for research that has received so little attention.

The chapters in Section IV concern responses to victimization, in particular, responses that occur in the criminal justice context. Joanna Shapland's chapter examines the responsiveness of criminal justice systems. She concentrates on the United Kingdom, which tends to publish evaluations of criminal justice delivery, and to some extent criminal justice systems on the continent, although much less information is available. Throughout Europe there has been a gradual appreciation of the effects of crime and criminal justice process on victims and of the need to amend the proceedings to meet some victims' concerns. Victim support and assistance programs exist in all countries, although the scope, coverage, and provision of services vary considerably. Shapland examines the extent of victims' interaction with criminal justice, beginning with victims' reaction to crime, subsequent progress of the case, court proceedings, and the role of victims at sentencing. She concludes, based on the experience in the United Kingdom, that although the government announced in 2002 it would put victims at the "heart of criminal justice," the level of progress has been "halting, patchy, and far from complete." The situation, as far as it can be judged, in other jurisdictions in Europe can also be characterized as one of a will to meet victims' needs, but not at the expense of significant change to the existing criminal justice institutions.

Uri Yanay and Tali Gal analyze the impact of a victims' lobby on the law-making process in Israel. They discuss the process behind enactment of the Rights of Crime Victims Law (2001). Crime had not been thought to be a problem in Israel; the needs of crime victims were believed to be met by families and friends. But, faced with the ongoing Middle East crisis, the

Knesset passed this law in response to a perception to unmet needs of victims of hostile (terrorist) acts. It occurred three years after a coalition of crime victims and other social groups had formed to put victims' rights on the public agenda, which would suggest this victims' lobby had a significant role. Yanay and Gal discuss the construction of social problems and law making, the role of crime victims in Israel before the law, the formation of the coalition for victims' rights, and the enactment of the Rights of Crime Victims Law. Their analysis reveals three actors to have been involved in the process: the state, represented by the Ministries of Justice and Finance; the crime victims' coalition; and the Knesset. They conclude that if victims' rights are to be realized, in Israel and other countries, advocates will need to continue the "push" for human rights.

Bernadette T. Muscat provides a comprehensive overview of victim services across the United States where, during the past 30 years, the victim services movement has grown from a handful of organizations to thousands. She describes the emergence of victim services, intimate partner violence services, and services for older adults. She discusses financial remedies, services for child victims, and psychological resources in regard to therapy and recovery. She considers the role of victim advocates in criminal justice proceedings and the role of victims' rights coalitions on policymaking concerning victims of crime. Despite these advances, more remains to be accomplished. There is a continued effort to secure expansion of funding for essential services, and efforts are underway to amend the U.S. Constitution to secure a victims' bill of rights.

Michelle Butler and Paul Cunningham examine the fear of crime in the Republic of Ireland. *Fear of crime* is a difficult concept to define. They explain how the concept originated in the United States and why it became an issue of public concern in Ireland. Based on their survey research, they examine fear of crime and its impact on quality of life. They point out that fear of crime varies by particular social variables, particularly gender, age, and locality, and call for further research to clarify why women are more likely to fear crime and residents of Dublin and small towns are less likely to fear crime. It is also important to investigate the role of media in influencing public perception of crime and, consequently, shaping the fear of crime and its impact on quality of life. Media portrayals may alert individuals to the need for precautionary measures but also, where these portrayals are inaccurate, contribute to an inflated perception of risk.

Section V consists of four chapters on restorative justice. In the first, Rob White engages questions about prisoner transitions from prison to community and specifically about the role of victims' rights in the course of these transitions. Specifically, he addresses three main themes: living with those we punish, supporting those who have been harmed, and the impact of crime on victims. This discussion came out of reflection about media stories concerning prisoner leave programs in Tasmania, Australia, that sensation-alized the prospect of victims running into offenders who had been released within the community. White reports on offender re-entry and prerelease programs, victims' rights in the re-entry process, and the interests of institu-tions of criminal justice. He goes on to identify the implications of prisoner transition for each group. "In the end," he concludes, "the best way to support and enhance victims' needs, interests, and rights is not to juxtapose them with those of the offender," but rather to take up the challenge of providing transitions for prisoners that "bring maximum benefit to victims, to offend-ers, and to the community as a whole."

Tom Daems critiques the conception of healing within the restorative jus-tice rationale. He points to how public debate about crime, drawing on exam-ples from the United States and Belgium, brought victims' needs to the center of attention but involved thinking about remedies in a specific way: trauma, emotional harm, and recovery. Victims' rights advocates have made frequent use of the need for "healing" in campaigns for reforms, and metaphors like that of healing do fulfill a critical function in challenging the status quo. But restorative justice advocates shifted the meaning of healing from metaphor to something "real," to an outcome to be achieved in responding to crime. This has introduced a new justification for penal interventions, a new way of looking at punishment and of evaluating criminal justice responses. In his analysis, Daems describes the increase of mental health problems in recent times on research concerning the therapeutic value of restorative justice, and how psychological restoration emerged as a goal of penal interventions.

Eyal Brook and Sharon Warshwski-Brook examine the role of apology in restorative justice encounters and, specifically, its potential to bring about emotional well-being. Research concerning victims during the past two decades reveals that what victims desire most is not material reparation but instead symbolic reparation, that is, "an apology and a sincere expression of remorse." Whereas victimology literature has not emphasized this need, the increase of the victims' movement has advanced apology as central to the process of restoration. They discuss the "healing nature" of apology and its contribution toward emotional wholeness, identify various forms of apol-ogy, and consider the benefits to offenders and victims, and they assess the reasons for the absence of apology in criminal justice proceedings. Drawing on the example of Japan, Brook and Warshwski-Brook contend that apology constitutes an important and powerful tool in everyday life, and, given its relative absence from criminal justice, urge for increased use. They conclude that "restorative justice, in which apology is a central feature, may provide a supportive framework ... for cultivating values of dialogue, empowerment, and reintegration."

Heather Strang takes a closer look at the effects of restorative justice for victims of conflict in transitional societies. Although advocates have claimed a number of benefits for restorative approaches, the only claim to have been substantiated by research is the benefit obtained by victims who are willing to meet offenders. Strang elaborates the meaning of restorative justice for victims, reviews the evidence for benefits to victims in criminal justice settings, and examines the ways in which restorative justice emerges as preferable for victims to formal criminal justice. She focuses on the issues important to victims in societies struggling in the aftermath of violent conflict with an examination of five areas of concern in "transitional justice" and reviews the results of research concerning each of these areas. What she finds is that restorative justice may do its best work in the transitional period of physical and emotional exhaustion following conflict. Restorative justice in this context recognizes the complexity and multilayered qualities of truth, prioritizes the needs of individuals, and extends to devastated communities the chance for knitting up division, estrangement, and resentment.

The chapters in Section VI, the final section of this book, concern victims in relation to social divisions. Walter S. DeKeseredy takes up violence directed at women. Violent abuse of women by male intimates constitutes a worldwide health problem, on a scale that has been described as a "war on women." DeKeseredy aims to "help give a voice to groups of women who, for the most part, suffer in silence." He pursues a definition of the phrase *violence against women* and explains why much of it remains invisible within conventional crime statistics. He explains the challenges of gathering data on male violence against female intimates and discusses two widely read theoretical paradigms. He concludes with reflection on progressive policies. Although efforts to end violence against women will be met with resistance and forms of gender inequality across societies will never disappear, it is important to engage crime prevention and control strategies that are already known to be effective. These can be coupled with other means of furthering communication about the extent and severity of violent victimization of women.

Manuel Madriaga and Rebecca Mallett seek to open up discussion about the relationship between disability and notions of criminality and victimhood. Their chapter combines insights from the discipline of disability studies with that of critical victimology. They review recent debates within disability studies around conceptualizing disability and spotlight the failure of this literature to address criminalization and victimization of disabled people. They address, in turn, the failure of victimology and criminology to take into account changing conceptions of impairment/disability. Madriaga and Mallett go on to tackle the persistence of biological normalcy or "everyday eugenics" in creating and perpetuating cultural images of disabled people. The representation of disabled people as *either* villains or victims tells much about the position of disabled people as an oppressed minority. As they point out, incorporating a "disability studies consciousness" within victimology and criminology represents a positive step toward empowering disabled people to rewrite their own definitions.

Simon N. Verdun-Jones and Katherine R. Rossiter address mental health outcomes of criminal victimization for victims. They examine several key factors, including age, gender, and psychiatric disability, which render particular groups relatively more vulnerable to victimization. In fact, those who are most vulnerable are also those who experience the greatest barriers in attempting to access support from the criminal justice and mental health systems. Following a review of the mental health outcomes of victimization, they discuss interventions for victims of crime, that is, psychological, legal, and restorative interventions. They point out that the adverse impact of victimization extends beyond primary victims to their families, their communities, and the wider public. Although many victims of crime demonstrate tremendous resilience, it is incumbent on criminal justice and mental health policymakers to provide practices and services that respond appropriately to needs of individual victims.

Carla Machado, Ana Rita Dias, and Cláudia Coelho explore wife abuse as a cultural construct. Although many researchers in victimology generally acknowledge the importance of culture in this regard, culture has seldom been translated into scientific research. They examine the awareness of the cultural dimension of wife abuse and unpack the concept of culture as a guide to research. They review theoretical perspectives about the links, including attitudinal, ecological, feminist, and multicultural approaches. Next, they provide a systematic overview of research in this area, identifying anthropological and prevalence studies. Before examining the meaning of culture in theory and research, they assess cultural competency and professional responses to victims. "Understanding [the] complex dance between structure and culture, as well as their transformations along time, is, in our perspective, the next main challenge for researchers in the area of wife abuse."

Carina Ljungwald provides a critique of crime victim legislation in Sweden. A statement promoting the interests of the *brottsoffer*, or "crime victim," is relatively recent to Swedish politics, although it is now the case that all political parties from left to right have called for increased support for crime victims. She concentrates on a 2001 amendment to the Swedish Social Services Act that introduced crime victims as a target group. This reform may, however, reflect a broader trend in social policy where provisions of the Social Services Act, such as solidarity and equality, are losing influence. The crime victim's language can be read as "part of an ideological makeover" in which the Act comes to express neoliberal values of the free market, limited government, and individual responsibility. Ljungwald offers an overview of crime victims' legislation in Sweden and related provisions in the Social Services Act. She explores trends in social policy and points to the power of the crime victim metaphor as a medium for inserting new ideology into social services delivery. She concludes with the provocative question of whether, or to what extent, a crime victim perspective should be included in social work practice.

Theoretical and Historical Frameworks

I

Becoming a Victim

1

RAINER STROBL

Contents

1.1 Introduction

At first glance we seem to know what it means to become a victim. We think of injustice or violence, of accidents or natural disasters. Although people who experience such events may regard themselves as victims, they are not necessarily seen as victims by their families, friends, or relatives, or by social institutions. For example, if a hooligan who picks a fight regularly gets injured he will most likely remain an offender in the eyes of others. On the other hand, the ascription of victim status is not always accepted by the affected individual him- or herself. This chapter deals mainly with the issue of becoming a victim in a socially relevant sense. The crucial condition for becoming a victim in this sense is not suffering from inflicted wounds or experiencing a norm violation (although these factors are certainly important) but rather being seen as a victim by others and adopting a victim role with certain rights and obligations.

Thus, becoming a victim presupposes the successful communication of a harmful experience. Overall it can be regarded as the result of an interaction or more generally of a communication process [Holstein and Miller, 1990]. Under this presumption the chapter will investigate the conditions and consequences of being recognized as a victim.

1.2 The Gap between Subjective Experience and Interpretation by Others

Describing the socially relevant identification of victimhood in terms of a communication process implies a sender and a receiver with different experiences. My assumption is that this difference between the realm of subjective experience and the interpretations of other persons and institutions is in fact a gap that can never be completely bridged. The existence of such a gap has long been ignored by traditional theory. Although Weber [1978:8–14] differentiates between understanding the sent information and the motives of the sender, he nevertheless believes that an adequate interpretation of the other's utterance is no fundamental problem. The reason is that Weber identifies the subjective meaning of the sender with the interpretation of the receiver [Schütz, 1981:34–49]. Weber would concede the existence of misunderstandings. However, his conception of the communication process resembles the classical communication model of Shannon and Weaver [1969]. As a result, misunderstandings can only be seen as technical problems of encoding and decoding the sense of a message faultlessly. From this point of view a person can in principle communicate all his or her experiences to someone else. However, the simple consideration that there are more stimuli than words and that very different experiences are subsumed under the same category shows the weakness of this assumption. In cases of severe victimization, there may not even be adequate words to express the experiences. The principal problem of a common understanding is clearly seen by Schütz [1981]. Schütz not only discusses the fundamental problem of an adequate understanding of another human but also shows the impossibility of a complete understanding of oneself. In his thorough analysis of action he differentiates between the planning of the action, the process of the action, and the reflection of the action [1981:74–83]. To determine the final meaning of what has happened, we must reflect on it after the process has ended. Thus, what has really happened to us and what we have really said or done is a contingent construction. Nevertheless, Schütz maintains the idea of an approximation to the meaning of the other's message by the way of introspection. This is a questionable theoretical position, as even the final meaning of one's own actions remains a contingent construction [Kade, 1983]. Still, it should not be denied that the common physical and psychological structure of humans provides a basis for the exchange of experiences [Merleau-Ponty, 1984:30–31].

However, taking the often traumatic experiences of severely victimized people as an example, it seems rather unlikely that such experiences can be understood adequately even if helpers or experts try hard to come close to the subjective meaning of the victim. Even the victim him- or herself might not find an adequate interpretation of what had happened. However, from a constructivist perspective, this is a general problem and not restricted to extreme experiences. In this connection Luhmann [1995:158] argues similarly to Schütz, contending that understanding is always context bound; the relevant context is first of all the background knowledge of the person involved or the background knowledge of the observer. If this is an adequate description of human communication, then becoming a victim in the sense of being recognized as such in society depends largely on the expectations of other people and institutions. Furthermore, seeing oneself as a victim can be regarded as the result of a process of reflection that is also dependent on basic cultural traditions and relevant personal experiences.

1.3 A Constructivist View of Victim Status

From a constructivist viewpoint, the successful communication of victimization, as well as the resulting recognition as a victim, largely depends on the receiver of the communication. This is a consequence of the general position that the constituting feature of an action is not intention but the interpretation of a certain behavior as the communication of information. However, successful communication in this sense only means to accept a communicative act as a starting point for further communication or action. It does not include the notion of a complete common understanding. For example, a police officer does not need to feel empathy for the victim to be able to act. For the police officer it is only necessary to perceive a norm violation in the victim's report. There are also other factors, such as informal rules and implicit knowledge, that play a role for the response to a victim's report. As these factors are discussed in Section IV, it may be sufficient to say here that general ideas about the appearance and the adequate behavior of a victim have a considerable influence.

Another important aspect of a constructivist perspective is the relativity of the image of the victim—and also of the image of the offender [e.g., Rock, 1998]. Who is conceived as a victim or as an offender depends not only on formal rules, which at least are uniform within a nation-state, but also on informal rules that vary between different cultural and subcultural units. Becoming a victim in a socially relevant sense then means the ascription of a special social status according to such rules. "Without this status a person will not be regarded as a victim and in fact will not be a victim in the social world. He or she will not get emotional support from his/her family and friends or material support from compensation schemes" [Strobl, 2004:295]. Moreover, from a constructivist perspective, even the subjective meaning of an experience is not self-evident, but rather the result of a process of reflection and interpretation. Consequently, the combination of social recognition

as a victim and self-identification as such results in four logical possibilities
for the construction of victimhood.

1. The actual victim: A person regards himself/herself as a victim and
   is also regarded as a victim by relevant others.
2. The nonvictim: A person does not regard himself/herself as a victim
   and is not regarded as a victim by relevant others.
3. The rejected victim: A person regards himself/herself as a victim but
   is not regarded as a victim by relevant others.
4. The designated victim: A person does not regard himself/herself as a
   victim but is regarded as a victim by relevant others.

The "actual victim" and the "nonvictim" are relatively unproblematic
cases, as both the person who has suffered a harmful event and those who
have learned about it categorize the event in the same way. The rules for
assigning victim status are discussed in detail below, so it is sufficient here to
point out that not being responsible for the victimization is of major importance for social recognition as a victim. In self-identification as a victim, the
subjective feeling of being in need of help may be of similar importance.
However, it may happen that a person sees himself/herself as a victim but is
denied victim status or is even ascribed offender status by important others
(rejected victim). There can be several reasons for this outcome. First, the
sufferer's personal characteristics or the circumstances of the harmful incident may disqualify him or her for the victim role [Miers, 1990:222]. Another
important reason is involvement in illegal activities, which makes a successful claim for victim status very difficult. Furthermore, the need to react to the
norm violation may lead to arbitrary justice and other forms of norm violations [Black, 1983; Fattah, 1992; Miers, 2000]. Norm-violating behavior may
also result from a strong feeling of injustice as a result of having been denied
the victim role. However, victim status can also be ascribed to a person who
does not see himself or herself in this role (designated victim). Apart from
ignorance (e.g., young children who have become victims of sexual assault)
or differences in norm and value orientation (e.g., migrants), this might also
result from a rejection of the victim role and its consequences. An extract
from a qualitative interview with a prison inmate conducted some time ago
illustrates these problems. I asked him what it means to be called a victim in
prison, and he answered:

> Then everybody offends you. Then you will not manage to fight back.
> Because if you have not beaten the person who has beaten you then you will
> not beat the others. Then a third one, a fourth one starts to beat you. Then
> you have to beat all four of them. That's why it is better to beat the first one
> at once.

The quotation shows that in some subcultures victim status will not entitle a person to sympathy and help but make him or her an object of incessant cruelty. Thus, in some social contexts self-labeling as a victim will be extremely difficult. Whether self-labeling as a victim is relatively easy, relatively hard, or nearly impossible also depends on knowledge, cultural values, attitudes, and beliefs [Burt, 1983:264–265].

But even in the relatively unproblematic cases of a congruent categorization of an event as victimization, this agreement does not necessarily mean that there is also a common understanding of what has happened. In an example from our interview material, a young man of Turkish origin felt extremely shocked because he was beaten up in a pub. However, the police seemed to regard the victimization as more or less trivial.

> Mr. A.: "I am a cautious man. That's why I am always in favor of calling the police if I don't get on with something myself. But in this case I realized that they [the police] could not help me or didn't want to help me. [...] Because not very much happened after that."

In a similar case a young man (also of Turkish origin) reacted differently after being hurt so seriously that he had to go to hospital:

> Mr. B.: "They were Englishmen, a couple of Englishmen. When they are drunk, it's a fact that people often become violent if you are drunk, everybody knows that. And of course they became more courageous. They saw us there, such a small group of kids could not do anything anyway. If I had seven big blokes stood behind me I would also have a go at them. Yes, of course I would also like to have a go at them. [...] I say, I'm not afraid of such a thing. Why should I be afraid? You know, such a thing can happen to anybody. Just because it happened to me does not mean that I don't go there anymore. I can deal with that. That I can deal with that is quite normal. Such a thing can always happen."

Both examples illustrate the constructed nature of victim status. Although the underlying events are comparable, Mr. A.'s assumption of personal invulnerability [Janoff-Bulman, 1985] was shattered, and he felt severely victimized. Unlike Mr. A., Mr. B. seemed to interpret his victimization more or less like a defeat in a sports competition. I argued before that the background knowledge has to be taken into account as context for the reconstruction of the events. In the case of Mr. A., the academic milieu where nonviolence is an important norm must be seen as the relevant background for his interpretation of the incident. In contrast, in the lifeworld of Mr. B. competition of physical strength plays a central role, and physical injuries are accepted to a certain degree. Again, for the construction of the police and other factors like the penal code are of major importance.

Because it can mean many different things to be a victim, a satisfactory communication that leads to a common understanding seems more unlikely the more different the milieus of the sender and the receiver of the communications are or the more exceptional the experiences of the victim are. In other words, if the victim belongs to a minority or if the victim has suffered from exceptional experiences, there is likely to be a communicative gap between the victim and other people. Thus, a victimized person may be not only physically and psychologically injured but also socially isolated in the sense that he or she cannot communicate important events of his or her life in such a way that they can be shared with others. Another example from our interview material may illustrate this point. It is about a woman of Turkish origin who suffered from massive violence from her husband but nevertheless always returned home.

> Mrs. C.: "I was so sick when he had beaten me. I was lying in bed because I was suffering from tonsillitis. It was Easter. It was a public holiday. It was eight o'clock in the morning. I had just come from work, I had cleaned the café. I said: 'Please don't do it.' He beat me on my legs, feet, arms. [...] He left me there because he thought I was dead. There was a dark spot, he left me there. But God gave me life, barefoot and naked. I was wearing only pajamas and a t-shirt on top. I went out. When I arrived I fainted. In the women's refuge they normally do not take you for a third time. They wanted to send me elsewhere. Then I started crying. I had no money; I did not know the language; I did not know where to go. Then I said: 'Please accommodate me only for today. Perhaps I can phone my husband tomorrow. Perhaps he will take me.' They said no."

The whole situation and the reactions of Mrs. C., including her plan to return to her violent husband, are very difficult to understand for an outside observer; the result was that she was denied accommodation in the women's refuge. In this case there is possibly also the problem of cultural misunderstanding. However, this communicative gap is a general problem when people have been severely victimized and traumatized. Janoff-Bulman [1985:18] hints at this point when she speaks about the shattered assumption of personal invulnerability, a meaningful and comprehensible world, and a positive self-perception. However, Janoff-Bulman concentrates on the psychological dimension, which is without doubt very important. My argument is that there is also a sociological dimension that results in a form of social disintegration of the victim. In this connection I use the term *integration* in the sense of participating in communication or interaction processes [Strobl, 2007]. This kind of integration remains intact as far as functional integration is concerned. The police, the courts, or the health system will continue to respond according to its program of law enforcement or medical treatment. What is threatened is social integration in the lifeworld. If the victim is no longer able to act as usual, his or her relatives and friends may first react with increasing helplessness and sometimes anger, and after awhile they may start to avoid contact with him or her.

In conclusion, I would like to emphasize that the constructivist view of victimization and victim status agrees with the statement from interpretative sociology that we can live side by side and still in very different worlds [Blumer, 1969]. I would like to add that in some cases this difference may also be a direct result of severe victimization [Haas and Lobermeier, 2005:42–43]. Thus, victimization has not only a physical and psychological impact but also a social impact, which means that communication and interaction processes of everyday life are affected. These phenomena have been addressed by traditional theory, but they have been addressed as a consequence of physical or psychological harm. From a constructivist viewpoint, the world of a severely victimized person has really changed, and it may be difficult or even impossible for him or her to bridge the gap between this new lifeworld and the everyday routines of his or her relatives, friends, and colleagues. In this respect becoming a victim can mean to be thrown into a realm of reality where a common understanding of exceptional and in most cases terrible experiences is not possible.

1.4 Expectations of the Victim and Conditions for Assigning Victim Status

I have shown above that severe victimization is likely to go along with a form of disintegration from normal communication and interaction processes. This inability to take part in any aspect of normal life can be regarded as structurally equivalent to a disease. For that reason Parsons' analysis of the sick role [1968:428–479] can be applied at least to severe victimizations. One important aspect of the sick role is the release from normal role obligations, combined with a number of new obligations. In the case of a severely injured or traumatized person there will almost certainly be an overlap between the sick role and the victim role as both include some release from normal role obligations and responsibilities. Generally, the victim—like the sick person—is regarded as being guiltlessly in an adverse situation. As the ascription of guilt constitutes offender status, it tends to destroy victim status. In classical victimology Mendelsohn [1956] even created a typology based on the question of guilt. In this typology the "ideal" victim is completely innocent. An example would be a baby beaten to death. Then there are several nuances of guilt like the victim with little guilt, the provoking victim, and so on. This typology has been heavily criticized in scientific debate because of the value judgments it involves. However, in everyday life such judgments play an important role for the assignment of victim status.

With respect to the duties of the victim and the sick, there are some differences in content but striking structural similarities. First, being a victim is—like being sick—regarded as something undesirable that has to be overcome sooner or later. The victim is not expected to stay in bed, but he or she is expected to behave rationally in society's terms. This includes not following possible feelings of hatred or longing for revenge. To the contrary, the victim is expected to choose the law as the decisive frame of reference even if the law does not correspond with his or her personal feelings. The existence of a legal system in the sense of a generally accepted normative frame of reference implies that only certain incidents are socially recognized as victimization. In this connection a person who has experienced some other form of victimization is expected to refrain from any action. For example, for some traditionally oriented people with a rural Turkish background it is a massive norm violation if their children reject an arranged marriage. Possible sanctions can go as far as killing the child [Strobl and Lobermeier, 2007]. However, defiance of an arranged marriage is not recognized as victimization in modern Western society, and any action by the parents to force their children into such a marriage will thus be illegal. Furthermore, it is expected that the victim of a norm violation will refrain from immediate satisfaction of his or her needs to help with the prosecution of the offender. For example, it is expected that a raped woman should not follow the immediate and natural need to wash but go to a medical examination first. In this connection cooperation with the police and other institutions is a central element of the victim role. The victim is expected to put self-interest last and to accept costs (e.g., time) and trouble (e.g., embarrassing questioning) to meet the requirements of the police and the justice system.

Like the sick person, the victim is seen as being in need of professional services because neither the victim nor their relatives or friends are entitled to any kind of autonomous law enforcement. Therefore, the socially defined situation of the victim is characterized by helplessness and professional incompetence. There is emotional engagement on the part of the victim's social environment but also an expectation that the victim will fulfill his or her duties, overcome the trauma, and resume former life after a certain time. If the victim is not able or willing to meet these demands, there is a high chance that the emotional support of the social environment will fade.

Hence it is obvious that there are social expectations regarding the character and the behavior of the victim. In this connection the ideal victim is completely innocent and cooperates perfectly with the police and the court. On a theoretical level the role of the victim can be described as (1) universalistic, insofar as the victim should choose the law as his or her frame of reference; (2) functionally specific, in the sense that the social expectations affect only particular situations; (3) affectively neutral, because the victim is not allowed to take the law into his or her own hands; and (4) collectively oriented, where the victim is expected to put self-interest last and accept costs (e.g., time) and trouble (e.g., embarrassing questioning) to meet the requirements of the police and the justice system [Parsons, 1968:428–479]. In victimological literature several descriptions of such an ideal victim can be found [Mendelsohn, 1956; Schneider, 1975; Christie, 1986; Kiefl and Lamnek, 1986; Fattah, 1991]. The gist of these descriptions is that the ideal victim is a weak person of flawless character and behavior. Some illustrative cases of ideal victimhood:

- The ideal victim has been physically attacked by a powerful stranger even though he or she has done everything to prevent such a situation. Furthermore, the ideal victim cannot be blamed for provoking the offender in any way or for being in the wrong place at the wrong time or for having done objectionable things.
- The ideal victim makes a report to the police without hesitation and ensures that the evidence of the offense is not lost. He or she reports everything to the police even if this is psychologically difficult and distressing.

The ideal victim construction is widely disseminated by the media and plays an important role in the constant staging of good and evil [Elias, 1986:233; McShane and Williams, 1992:267; Viano, 1992]. However, the construction of the ideal victim influences not only public opinion but also the law. In this connection, it is interesting to note that German victim compensation law allows compensation only to victims of violence who have satisfactorily cooperated with the police and who have not been involved in any reprehensible activities [Tampe, 1992:188–189]. Fattah [2003] also argues that especially those persons who are in a marginal social position have both a high risk of being victimized and also difficulties in being recognized as victims. An example is the situation of victimized asylum seekers in Germany, where there were many brutal attacks against asylum seekers, especially in the early 1990s. At the same time there was a fervent political debate about misuse of the right of asylum that led to a perception of asylum seekers as spongers and troublemakers and contaminated the victim status of attacked persons from this group. Instead, they were seen as members of a troublesome outgroup and were often refused efficient forms of help and support.

It is important to remember that these victims from marginalized groups fulfill the formal condition for an ascription of victim status: They have suffered from grave violations of the law. What prevents effective help is that they do not correspond to the widespread image of the ideal victim. Thus, the victim status can be spoiled by doubts concerning appropriate behavior or the character of the victim. The underlying process that may lead to such a result is the communication of the victimization. Adopting

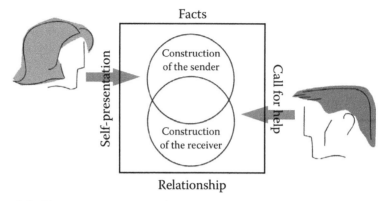

Figure 1.1 The communication of victimization.

the communication model by Schulz von Thun [1981] allows us to detect important factors for the success or failure of such a communication (see Figure 1.1).

First, it should be pointed out again that the victim cannot transfuse his or her experiences (or rather the subjective reconstruction of these experiences) to someone else. Another person will develop his or her own construction of the incident in which the image of the ideal victim often plays an important role. According to the communication model in Figure 1.1 there are four aspects that influence this construction and thence the assignment or refusal of victim status. What can be called the actual *facts* of the victimization represent an important factor. For a successful communication it is important that the listener comes to the conclusion that a "real" case of victimization has occurred. This does not necessarily mean a shared understanding of what has happened. For a successful communication in the sense of triggering a relevant reaction it is sufficient if the victim's report or other evidence gives the receiver of the communication a clear idea that victimization has occurred. Apart from the formal criteria of a norm violation Strobl [1998] shows that the importance of the norm, the seriousness of the injuries, and the amount of financial loss influence the assignment of victim status. However, people from different milieus or different cultural backgrounds may differ considerably regarding the importance of a violated norm, the seriousness of an injury, or a financial loss. For example, a financial loss of 500 euros is something very different for an unemployed worker than it is for a millionaire, and controversial caricatures of Mohammed are something very different for a deeply religious Muslim than for an atheist or a Christian.

Second, in every face-to-face communication there is also some form of *self-presentation*. In this connection it has already been stressed that the kind of impression that the victim makes on the receiver of the communication plays an important role for the assignment of victim status. Strobl's

[1998] data show that generally persons who make the impression of being shy, weak, and vulnerable have better chances of being considered as victims than persons who seem to be aggressive, strong, or powerful. Similar findings are reported by Vrij and Fischer [1997]. Generally, anything that relativizes the picture of the ideal victim with flawless character and behavior can be an obstacle for the assignment of victim status. Again, the impression that the victim wants to make can be different from the impression that the observer gains.

A third obstacle for assigning victim status can result from the *relationship* between different groups in society. With respect to the reactions of the police and the justice system it is important that the victim is perceived as a member of the ingroup of law-abiding people. Those who belong to an unaccepted outgroup are likely to be seen as offenders rather than as victims. As physical appearance (e.g., skin color or hairstyle) can play a major role in this kind of categorization, the victim's influence on the outcome is sometimes restricted. In this context Winkel [1991] demonstrated in several experiments that culturally determined nonverbal behavior of people with a migration background is often misunderstood by autochthonous police officers and interpreted as a sign of a guilty conscience.

Fourth, it is important that the representatives of society are able to *understand* the victim's call for help and get an idea about the kind of help the victim needs. Language skills and the victim's ability to communicate his or her experience convincingly play an important role. Equally important is the ability of the victim to put him- or herself in the position of the listener. If they are able to talk in the language of officials from the police and justice system their chances of adequate help will considerably increase. Thus, a victim who can provide accurate information and state his or her needs clearly has better chances of being helped than a victim who only utters a diffuse cry for help.

1.5 Coping with Victimization

The gap between the perspective of the victim and the perspective of other people or institutions is also highly relevant for the issue of coping. As being a victim is normally something undesirable, the victim will try to improve his or her unsatisfactory current condition and is also expected to do so. Generally, there are two major ways to overcome an adverse "actual state" and to reach the "desired state"; namely, through a problem-centered solution modifying the actual state, which constitutes the problem (proactive coping), or through a reaction-centered solution or internal adaptation modifying the desired state (of internal perception and evaluation structures) that has been making the actual state a problem (accommodative coping) [Brandtstädter and Greve, 1994; Greve and Strobl, 2004]. A third option is avoidance, although this cannot be seen as coping in the sense of solving or resolving a problem [e.g., Haan, 1977; Vaillant, 2000; Greve and Strobl, 2004].

The victim's actual coping reaction is dependent on various factors such as subjective perception and interpretation of the event, individual values and beliefs, and expectations placed on the social environment:

> Coping [...] is a process that does not occur in isolation but in social contexts with specific values and norms. Alongside the social evaluation of certain reactions as being desirable or undesirable, the social framing of reality always leads to a preselection of what is at all conceivable and can be chosen as an action option by the individual. [Greve and Strobl, 2004:204]

Thus, there are always different constructions of an event, and there are probably competing views about the appropriate coping reaction. Expectations concerning the desirability and appropriateness of a coping reaction ultimately refer to the problem of ensuring the usual way of functioning. In other words, the question is how the continuity and connectivity of the normal way of acting can be guaranteed. Thus, refusal or inability to react to victimization in the expected way can have severe consequences. For example, in an ethnographic study of a small Turkish village Schiffauer [1987:48] describes how a farmer and his son who were unable to respond aggressively to victimization lost face and were ultimately excluded from the community. From the perspective of the villagers the inappropriate reaction to the victimization was itself a norm violation. Thus, the reactions of the village community can be seen as a form of proactive coping to re-establish a violated norm.

In modern societies specialized social systems like the police or the justice system are of particular importance for any evaluation of the victim's coping reaction. From the perspective of these systems, reactions that violate formal norms appear not only inappropriate but also unlawful. To overcome such an unsatisfactory actual state a system has to react, that is, it shows coping reactions itself. For example, unauthorized punishment of a fraud will be prosecuted by the justice system. From the perspective of the individual the picture is similar. Certain reactions by the police or justice system to a victimization (e.g., dropping charges) can be regarded as a violation of personal norms that requires a coping strategy. For example, victims can choose a proactive form of coping and take legal action themselves, or they might prefer an accommodative way of coping and simply give up the expectation that the offender has to be punished. Victims can more or less anticipate the responses of important social systems or persons to their coping reactions, and this knowledge will influence the coping strategy. In this connection there is the difficulty that individuals (and also organizations) are typically integrated in heterogeneous social contexts in modern functionally differentiated societies [Scott, 1987; Luhmann, 1995], and there are often very different conceptions about adequate and inadequate coping strategies in these contexts. For example, in a violent conflict with fans from an opposing football team a person may well find that friends, colleagues, family, the police, the local pub, and so forth hold very heterogeneous and, in some circumstances, incompatible views about an appropriate reaction. Thus, finding an ideal coping strategy that guarantees at least the normal functioning of a person or of a social system is a multidimensional problem. From the perspective of sociological systems theory there are three important issues in this connection: stability, temporality, and reflexivity [Greve and Strobl, 2004:202]. Stability refers to the continuity and consistency of communication and action; temporality has to be seen in connection with connectivity and acceptance; and reflexivity refers to recognition and positive evaluation. Consequently, coping means first to re-establish the stability of a person or of a social system. For example, regaining trust and the usual certainties of everyday life is an important aspect here. Second, it is important to act and communicate in a way that is at least accepted in important social contexts. Therefore, it is important for a traumatized person to overcome terrible experiences to be able to participate in everyday life [Orth, 2000]. The third important aspect is regaining self-esteem and a positive self-perception. In this general and abstract form, coping can also be regarded as a solution for the general problem of social integration. Stability requires participation or functional integration, and connectivity (i.e., being able to communicate and act in an accepted way) presupposes a minimum of normative integration, that is, the ability to conform to the normative expectations of others. If both forms of integration are ensured, positive reactions to a person's identity concepts are very likely, which assures a positive self-perception [e.g., Strobl and Kühnel, 2000:59–60].

For this form of successful coping it is important that there is no backlash from people or institutions in the victim's social context that undoes the success. Problematic reactions to the victim's experiences are generally known as secondary victimization. This form of victimization can now be understood in the context of coping. In fact, hearing from a victim about terrible experiences or dealing with an upset or traumatized person is a difficult situation even for an uninvolved observer, one with which he or she has to cope. This coping reaction can in an adverse case constitute new victimization, that is, it can violate both subjective norms and values and legal norms.

The discussion above shows that victimization has to be conceived as a process rather than as an isolated incident. This is obvious in violent social contexts where the offender of today might be the victim of tomorrow and vice versa [Black, 1983; Fattah, 1992; Miers, 2000]. But even when the injured person approximates the image of the ideal victim he or she might answer an experienced wrong in a way that provokes new negative reactions. Thus, the question of becoming a victim in a socially relevant sense is also a question of the punctuation of events in the process of actions and coping reactions.

1.6 A Victimological Construction of the Victim

Thus far we have not distinguished systematically between different forms of victimization. In fact, with respect to the forms of coping with disturbing or traumatic incidents there are many parallels between victims of accidents, natural disasters, and crime. Therefore, Beniamin Mendelsohn argued for a victimology that deals with all kinds of victimization [Ziegenhagen, 1977:9–10; Mendelsohn, 1982; Elias, 1986:24–25]. However, this concept proved to be too broad for the establishment of an independent research tradition [Kirchhoff and Sessar, 1979]. As a consequence, since Hans von Hentig [1967], empirical research and theoretical debate in victimology have generally taken penal law as the frame of reference to determine the borders of the research field. This "solution" is unsatisfactory as it prevents the blind spots of penal law from becoming a topic for victimological research. The advantage of every independent new perspective and of every new construction is that they elucidate some of the blind spots that are an inevitable byproduct of every construction (while accepting others). The major blind spots of penal law result from the constructed nature of the legal system. As laws are human-made, who will become a victim and who will become an offender in a socially relevant sense is ultimately a decision of the legislator. This decision is influenced by the cultural standards and value preferences of powerful social groups [Sellin, 1938; Sack, 1978; Becker, 1981; Quinney, 1982; Lamnek, 1988]. As a consequence, there may be considerable disagreement about the definition and importance of offenses and victimizations in a society. Social, ethnic, and religious minorities especially may hold different convictions in some areas. The controversy about the Mohammed caricatures (already mentioned above) is a good example of the phenomenon that there are always people who cannot accept the legal classification of their experiences. In some cases, like the legal treatment of homosexuality, the law has changed considerably in many countries, and as a consequence the respective constructions of victims and offenders have changed as well.

1.7 Criteria for a Victimological Concept of the Victim

If the consequences of victimization are to play a major role in victimology, it is important to widen the perspective for the subjective meaning of a wide range of subjective experiences. Consequently, we argue in favor of a broad victim concept [Greve, Strobl, and Wetzels, 1994, 1997; Strobl, 2004]. However, a victimological construction of the victim that is able to offer new insights should try to reproduce neither official nor subjective victim constructions. Instead, it should shed new light on the whole process of victimization so that certain phenomena like norm violations in response to victimization can be better understood and new or more adequate solutions be found where conventional theorizing has led to a dead end. However, if this form of independence from legal definitions is not to result in an arbitrary construction, definite principles for the victimological definition of victimization and the resulting construction of the victim have to be determined. We suggest five principles [Greve et al., 1994, 1997; Strobl, 2004]:

1. *Identifiable single event.* If we start from the very wide range of experiences that people may call victimization, we will probably learn that some people feel victimized by general forms of inequality or injustice. They may see themselves as victims of a xenophobic mood, of globalization, of climate change, and so on. Although this is certainly an interesting area for sociological or psychological inquiry, it is definitely too broad for victimological research. Therefore, we propose to include only identifiable single events in the definition of victimization. As a consequence, a person must name a concrete incident (e.g., a xenophobic insult) to be regarded as a victim.
2. *Negative evaluation.* It is obvious that victimization is something negative (even though positive changes like a lottery prize may also have irritating consequences and will require substantial coping reactions). Victimization should be restricted to events that cause an unsatisfactory actual state.
3. *Uncontrollable event.* It is also clear that someone who has caused the unsatisfactory actual state him- or herself should not be called a victim (although certain forms of self-destructive behavior could suggest such a classification). We would rather use medical categories in this latter connection. Generally, assigning the victim role to a person means absolving him or her of responsibility, which precludes self-inflicted suffering.
4. *Attribution to a personal or social offender.* Thus far our definition still includes victims of traffic accidents, natural disasters, and so on. Is there any good theoretical reason to make a distinction between victimizations caused by humans and victimizations caused by nature? Is a further restriction of the field of victimological research and debate justifiable? One important distinction between human actors and physical objects and animals is that the former are free to act in another, not victimizing way, whereas the latter are governed by laws of nature. This difference is connected with the

sociological distinction between cognitive and normative expectations [Luhmann, 1995]. A characteristic of cognitive expectations
is the willingness to learn. For example, if we expect that there will
be no earthquakes in a certain area and there is an earthquake any-
way we usually change our expectations, that is, if we attribute the
causes of a negative uncontrollable event to nature we are willing to
adjust our expectations to our experiences. For that reason a violation of cognitive expectations demands an accommodative coping
style. In contrast, normative expectations (or norms) are normally
connected with a refusal to learn [Strobl, 1998:11]. Even when persons are robbed they usually keep their expectation that other people will respect their property. As they are not willing to change
their expectations (the desired state), it is necessary to change
the problematic actual state (the actual behavior of the offender).
Besides, as we assume that a social actor can behave differently and
is thus responsible for what he or she did, such a change seems possible and plausible. Therefore, a violation of normative expectations
demands sanctions and suggests a proactive coping style [see also
Bayley, 1991:56]. In this connection it has to be mentioned that people can start to learn that their normative expectations are no longer
valid. In this case a norm will vanish [Strobl, 2004]. For that reason
Merton [1968] used the term *innovation* for a norm violation. The
discussion shows that negative uncontrollable events that are attributed to personal or social offenders have important characteristics
that justify an independent field of theoretical debate and empirical
research.

5. *Violation of a socially shared norm.* A victimological construction
of the victim has to bear in mind that the violation of purely idiosyncratic normative expectations that nobody shares will not lead to
recognition as a victim or to an assignment of victim status. For that
reason it should be different from a purely psychological approach
and should concentrate on the violation of socially shared norms.
However, if group norms are taken into account for the definition
and evaluation of victimization, the construction is still considerably
broader than the legal approach. For example, in a very traditional
Turkish or Pakistani context the community may well accept that a
father regards himself as the victim of the disrespectfulness of his
daughter who refuses to agree to an arranged marriage. Thus, his
coping reactions and the reactions of the community can be analyzed as reactions to victimization.

The proposed definition results in a victim concept that is different from
both legal and subjective constructions. As it refers to any socially shared

norms, it can help to understand processes of norm violation, victimization, and norm enforcement within the frame of reference of subcultures. Thus, the definition can shed new light on victimizations and also on norm violations if they can be conceived as reactions to victimizations. Consequently, it can guide research into context-sensitive victimological research. This research can adequately deal with questions like problematic reactions to victimizations or lack of sympathy for some victims.

Although we consider this definition to be a good starting point for scientific victimological research, it might be too broad for practical purposes, such as counseling and professional help. Freedom from value judgments, especially, would lead to an arbitrary offer of help. Therefore, for practical purposes it will be necessary to introduce additional criteria that refer to widely accepted normative standards like human rights or fundamental laws. Otherwise, a robber who has become the victim of betrayal according to the standards of his gang would have to be treated equally to the person he robbed.

1.8 Direct and Indirect Victimization

There is yet another important issue to address. Thus far our discussion has focused on the case where a person is victimized him- or herself. However, a person can also suffer seriously when a negative, uncontrollable event occurs not to him- or herself but to a member of his or her family, to a relative, or to a close friend. Parents who have lost a child in a crime feel intensely victimized [Riggs and Kilpatrick, 1990; Boers, 1991]. Because these indirect victims have experienced the victimization in a mediated way, Strobl [2004] speaks of mediated victimization. In such a case the offender probably had no intention to harm the indirect victim. However, there is another kind of indirect victimization where the underlying motive of the offender is directed not only against the directly victimized person but also against all members of a certain social category. This form of indirect victimization, which is often a problem for discriminated minorities, can be called *collective victimization* [Strobl, 2004]. Such an incident often puts persons who belong to a certain social category in fear of direct victimization and may thus seriously reduce their quality of life. One example is so-called hate crimes, which are regarded as especially grave in many countries for that reason. However, the example of hate crimes also makes it clear that indirect victims have very unequal chances of being recognized as victims in society. Whereas it is, for example, common to ascribe victim status to family members of homicide victims, it is rather unusual to do so in the case of members of a minority group who have not been direct victims of hate crimes. In this connection prejudices existing in parts of the general population can effectively prevent members of discriminated minorities from being regarded as victims [Ray and Smith, 2001; Perry, 2003; Strobl et al., 2005]. The aforementioned situation in Germany in the early 1990s is a good example of this problem. During that time there was an increased prevalence of attacks against asylum seekers, and there were also xenophobic arson attacks that alarmed the Turkish minority. Many asylum seekers and many Turkish men and women felt collectively victimized when they heard about these incidents, and some even left Germany. However, during the period there were media reports about offenders from these groups that contradicted the image of the ideal victim with flawless character and behavior. As a consequence, the label attached to all persons associated with these groups was rather "offender" than "victim."

Another important aspect for the ascription of victim status is the motive of the offender. In the staging of the battle between good and evil, the wickedness of the offender highlights the innocence of the victim. This is especially effective in direct victimization of a person (personal victimization). However, it sometimes happens that a person is harmed by an offender accidentally. Perhaps the aggression was originally directed against someone else or a person was in the wrong place at the wrong time. Such victimizations can be called *vicarious victimizations* [Strobl, 2004]. An inhumane military expression in cases of war is *collateral damage*. It is important to note that the impression of a wicked offender is relativized in these cases. As a consequence, the ascription of victim status in the discussed sense can be impeded. Thus, civilians who are wounded or killed in war are seen as victims of fate rather than as victims of social offenders. In fact, in such a situation the expectation of physical inviolability may have to be given up if nobody can successfully enforce such a norm.

1.9 Implications for Victimological Research and Counseling

According to the outlined constructivist approach there are always different constructions of the victim, none of which is true or false in an absolute sense. They just highlight different aspects of subjective experiences and collective classifications, and their relevance is limited to a specific issue. The victim's idiosyncratic constructions and reconstructions may be of great relevance for explaining subjective well-being and behavior. However, to become socially relevant such experiences have to be communicated in a form that can be understood by others. To become a victim for the police and the justice system it is first important that a person can communicate his or her experiences in a way that is in accordance with the criteria of penal law. As Kürzinger [1978] shows based on 100 participant observations, underprivileged people especially often have considerable problems in communicating their experiences in such a way:

> Hardly anywhere is the inability of people with low social status to formulate "correctly" and to assert their own wishes more obvious than in the process of reporting to the police. [Kürzinger, 1978:211]

To ensure adequate support for severely victimized persons from low social classes or with a migration background, victim aid organizations should try to assist them in expressing the impact of the norm violation, asking for specific help or specific actions, or presenting themselves adequately. Victim aid organizations should also turn to the other side of the communication process and sensitize police and judicial officers to the special communication problems of migrants and underprivileged persons.

However, the reasons for these problems are beyond the scope of the legal victim construction. That is why I propose a considerably broader victimological perspective. As victimization often has a prehistory and always has consequences in terms of coping reactions of the victim and responses of people in his or her social context, the focus should be on a process rather than on a single incident. Suffering a norm violation is an important event in this process, but it does not automatically lead to the ascription of victim status. Real or supposed character faults, problematic behavior, or incomprehensible communication can contaminate the image as a victim. Furthermore, what is regarded as a relevant norm violation depends on the social context. From this point of view, victimological research should not restrict itself to conventional society and its institutions but also focus on subgroups and subcultures and investigate under which conditions victim status is ascribed in these social systems. This relativity of victim definitions is a consequence of the proposed constructivist approach. Its advantage is an independent victimological perspective that can also explain several forms of deviant behavior as reactions to norm violations. As discussed above, some reactions that are defined as deviant from the perspective of the social majority are normal or even demanded in some subcultural communities [Black, 1983; Fattah, 1992]. Thus, for victimological research one crucial question is: "Who becomes a victim in a certain social context?" [Strobl, 2004:309].

This proposed perspective also has its blind spot. Freedom from value judgment is adequate for scientific research but not for victim assistance and counseling. For practical purposes the main problem is that under a value-free approach there is no substantiated criterion for differentiating between different kinds of victims. Thus, a counselor would be unable to treat a rowdy youth who is regarded according to the normative standards of his gang as the victim of a police informer differently from the victim of a violent attack [e.g., Bayley, 1991]. Therefore, counseling needs a construction of the victim that includes accepted value standards. The simplest solution would be the adoption of legal norms as a frame of reference. However, the disadvantage of this solution would be a bias toward the normative worldview of the dominant social groups, which is especially problematic in all kinds of dictatorships. But there are also more general problems for counselors. One major problem facing the individual when selecting a certain coping strategy is that the social environment can be irritated by his or her behavior and then react, in turn, with its own coping strategies. An example is the situation of one of our Turkish interviewees who got divorced from her husband because she could not stand his violence any longer. However, a divorced woman has very low social status in a traditional Turkish community, and she was treated more or less as an outcast after her divorce. She had successfully coped with one problem, but as a consequence she had a new problem that seemed even bigger to her. Analysis of such cases shows that it is not possible to calculate the costs of a coping strategy beforehand. The decisive reason is the impossibility of reliably predicting other people's reactions. As a consequence, counselors should give up the idea that there is one ideal solution. What is best for the victim will in many cases turn out to be the result of a longer process. In this process a counselor must be able to show alternatives, and these alternatives have to be formulated based on a certain value system. Human rights can serve as a general framework in this connection, but more concrete ethics are needed in victim assistance.

Finally, for some purposes a construction that concentrates solely on victims of norm violations might not be useful. This will probably be the case when the focus lies in psychological coping processes that are in many respects similar for victims of crime, accidents, and natural disasters.

In conclusion, I would like to emphasize that the main idea of the proposed constructivist approach is to accept a plurality of victim constructions. None of them is true or false in an absolute sense; instead, each has to be regarded as functional or dysfunctional in respect of a specific purpose. Thus, there are different ways to become a victim in a socially relevant sense. Sometimes a person has to appear as weak and innocent to be entitled to help, but in other contexts the demonstration of weakness might provoke aggression. Victimological research needs a theoretical framework and a victim concept that can deal with this plurality and describe the phenomena from an independent point of view. Under this condition it will be possible to generate a different kind of knowledge—not better than the knowledge of victims, counselors, police officers, or lawyers but possibly capable of showing alternatives where existing knowledge has led to a dead end.

References

Bayley, J. E. 1991. The concept of victimhood. In *To be a victim: Encounters with crime and injustice*, ed. D. Sank and D. I. Caplan, 53–62. New York: Plenum.

Becker, H. S. 1981. *Außenseiter: Zur soziologie abweichenden verhaltens*. Frankfurt am Main: Fischer.

Black, D. 1983. Crime as social control. *American Sociological Review* 48:34–45.

Blumer, H. 1969. *Symbolic interactionism: Perspective and method*. Englewood Cliffs, NJ: Prentice Hall.

Boers, K. 1991. *Kriminalitätsfurcht*. Pfaffenweiler: Centaurus.

Brandtstädter, J. and W. Greve. 1994. The aging self: Stabilizing and protective processes. *Developmental Review* 14:52–80.

Burt, M. R. 1983. A conceptual framework for victimological research. *Victimology: An International Journal* 8:261–69.

Christie, N. 1986. The ideal victim. In *From crime policy to victim policy: Reorienting the justice system*, ed. E. A. Fattah, 17–30. New York: St. Martin's.

Elias, R. 1986. *The politics of victimization: Victims, victimology and human rights*. New York and Oxford: Oxford University Press.

Fattah, E. A. 1991. *Understanding criminal victimization: An introduction to theoretical victimology*. Scarborough, ON: Prentice Hall.

_____. 1992. *Victimization as antecedent to offending: The revolving and interchangeable roles of victim and victimizer*. President's faculty lecture series. Simon Fraser University, Halpern Centre.

_____. 2003. Violence against the socially expendable. In *International handbook of violence research*, ed. W. Heitmeyer and J. Hagan, 767–83. Dordrecht: Kluwer Academic.

Greve, W. and R. Strobl. 2004. Social and individual coping with threats: Outlines of an interdisciplinary approach. *Review of General Psychology* 8:194–207.

Greve, W., R. Strobl, and P. Wetzels. 1994. Das Opfer kriminellen Handelns—Flüchtig und nicht zu fassen: Konzeptuelle Probleme und methodische Implikationen eines sozialwissenschaftlichen Opferbegriffs. *KFN Forschungsberichte* No. 33. Hannover: KFN.

_____. 1997. Opferzeugen in der empirisch-viktimologischen Forschung. In *Psychologie der Zeugenaussage: Ergebnisse der rechtspsychologischen Forschung*, ed. L. Greuel, T. Fabian, and M. Stadler, 247–60. Weinheim: Beltz-PVU.

Haan, N. 1977. *Coping and defending*. New York: Academic.

Haas, U. I. and O. Lobermeier. 2005. *Bürgerschaftliches engagement in der Opferhilfe*. Baden-Baden: Nomos.

Hentig, H. von. 1967. *The criminal and his victim*. First published 1948. N.P: Archon Books.

Holstein, J. A. and G. Miller. 1990. Rethinking victimization: An interactional approach to victimology. *Symbolic Interaction* 13:103–22.

Janoff-Bulman, R. 1985. The aftermath of victimization: Rebuilding shattered assumptions. In *Trauma and its wake: The study and treatment of post-traumatic stress disorder*, ed. C. R. Figley, 15–35. New York: Brunner and Mazel.

Kade, S. 1983. *Methoden des fremdverstehens: Ein zugang zu theorie und praxis des fremdverstehens*. Bad Heilbrunn: Klinkhardt.

Kiefl, W. and S. Lamnek. 1986. *Soziologie des opfers: Theorie, methoden und empirie der viktimologie*. Munich: Fink.

Kirchhoff, F. and K. Sessar. 1979. Einführung. In *Das verbrechensopfer*, ed. F. Kirchhoff and K. Sessar, 3–12. Bochum: Studienverlag Brockmeyer.

Kürzinger, J. 1978. *Private strafanzeige und polizeiliche reaktion.* Berlin: Duncker und Humblot.

Lamnek, S. 1988. *Theorien abweichenden Verhaltens.* Munich: Fink.

Luhmann, N. 1995. *Social systems.* Stanford, CA: Stanford University Press.

McShane, M. D. and F. P. Williams. 1992. Radical victimology: A critique of the concept of victim in traditional victimology. *Crime and Delinquency* 38: 258–71.

Mendelsohn, B. 1956. Une nouvelle branche de la science bio-psycho-sociale—la victimologie. *Revue Internationale de Criminologie et de Police Technique* 10:95–109.

_____. 1982. Sozio-analytische einführung in allgemeine viktimologische und kriminologische forschungsperspektiven. In *Das Verbrechensopfer in der Strafrechtspflege*, ed. H. J. Schneider, 60–66. Berlin and New York: De Gruyter.

Merleau-Ponty, M. 1984. *Die prosa der welt.* Munich: Fink.

Merton, R. K. 1968. *Social theory and social structure.* Enlarged edition. New York: Free.

Miers, D. 1990. Positivist victimology: A critique; Part 2: Critical victimology. *International Review of Victimology* 1:219–30.

_____. 2000. Taking the law into their own hands: Victims as offenders. In *Integrating a victim perspective within criminal justice*, ed. A. Crawford and J. Goodey, 77–95. Aldershot: Ashgate.

Orth, U. 2000. Strafgerechtigkeit und bewältigung krimineller viktimisierung: Eine untersuchung zu den folgen des strafverfahrens bei opfern von gewalttaten. PhD diss., Trier University.

Parsons, T. 1968. *The social system.* New York: The Free Press.

Perry, B. 2003. Where do we go from here? Researching hate crime. *Internet Journal of Criminology* 1–59. http://www.internetjournalofcriminology.com (accessed October 14, 2003).

Quinney, R. 1982. Die ideologie des rechts: Über eine radikale alternative zum legalen zwang; In *Seminar abweichendes verhalten I: Die selektiven normen der gesellschaft*, 2nd ed., ed. K. Lüderssen and F. Sack, 80–125. Frankfurt am Main: Suhrkamp.

Ray, R. and D. Smith. 2001. Racist offenders and the politics of "hate crime". *Law and Critique* 12:203–21.

Riggs, D. S. and D. G. Kilpatrick. 1990. Families and friends: Indirect victimization by crime. In *Victims of crime: Problems, policies and programs*, ed. A. J. Lurigio, W. G. Skogan, and R. C. Davis, 120–38. Newbury Park, CA and London: Sage.

Rock, P. 1998. Murderers, victims and "survivors": The social construction of deviance. *The British Journal of Criminology* 38:185–200.

Sack, F. 1978. Probleme der kriminalsoziologie. In *Handbuch der empirischen sozialforschung, band 12. Wahlverhalten, vorurteile, kriminalität*, 2nd ed., ed. R. König, 192–492. Stuttgart: Enke.

Schiffauer, W. 1987. *Die bauern von subay: Das leben in einem türkischen dorf.* Stuttgart: Klett-Cotta.

Schneider, H. J. 1975. *Viktimologie: Wissenschaft vom verbrechensopfer.* Tübingen: Mohr.

Schulz von Thun, F. 1981. *Miteinander Reden 1: Störungen und Erklärungen: Allgemeine Psychologie der Kommunikation.* Reinbek bei Hamburg: Rowohlt.

Schütz, A. 1981. *Der sinnhafte aufbau der sozialen welt: Eine einleitung in die verstehende soziologie,* 2nd ed. Frankfurt am Main: Suhrkamp.

Scott, W. R. 1987. *Organizations: Rational, national and open systems,* 2nd ed. London: Prentice-Hall.

Sellin, T. 1938. *Culture, conflict and crime.* New York: Social Science Research Council.

Shannon, C. E. and W. Weaver. 1969. *The mathematical theory of communication.* Urbana: University of Illinois Press.

Strobl, R. 1998. *Soziale folgen der opfererfahrungen ethnischer minderheiten.* Baden-Baden: Nomos.

_____. 2004. Constructing the victim: Theoretical reflections and empirical examples. *International Review of Victimology* 11:295–311.

_____. 2007. Social integration and inclusion. In *The Blackwell encyclopedia of sociology,* ed. G. Ritzer, 4429–32. Oxford: Blackwell.

Strobl, R., J. Klemm, and S. Würtz. 2005. Preventing hate crimes—Experiences from two East German towns. *The British Journal of Criminology* 45:634–46.

Strobl, R. and W. Kühnel. 2000. *Dazugehörig und ausgegrenzt: Analysen zu integrationschancen junger aussiedler.* Weinheim and Munich: Juventa.

Strobl, R. and O. Lobermeier. 2007. Zwangsverheiratung: Risikofaktoren und ansatzpunkte zur intervention. In *Bundesministerium für Familie,* ed. F. Senioren und J. Senioren, 27–71. Baden-Baden: Nomos.

Tampe, E. 1992. *Verbrechensopfer: Schutz, beratung, unterstützung.* Stuttgart: Boorberg.

Vaillant, G. E. 2000. Adaptive mental mechanisms: Their role in a positive psychology. *American Psychologist* 55:89–98.

Viano, E. C. 1992. The news media and crime victims: The right to know versus the right to privacy. In *Critical issues in victimology: International perspectives,* ed. E. C. Viano, 24–34. New York: Springer.

Vrij, D. and C. Fischer. 1997. The role of display of emotions and ethnicity in judgments of rape victims. *International Review of Victimology* 4:255–65.

Weber, M. 1978. *Economy and society: An outline of interpretive sociology,* ed. G. Roth and C. Wittich. Berkeley: University of California Press.

Winkel, F. W. 1991. Interaction between the police and minority group members: Victimization through the incorrect interpretation of nonverbal behavior. *International Review of Victimology* 2:15–27.

Ziegenhagen, E. A. 1977. *Victims, crime, and social control.* New York: Praeger.

The Meaning of Justice for Victims

2

JO-ANNE WEMMERS

Contents

In the 1970s criminologists discovered victims, the forgotten party in the criminal justice system. This was followed in the 1980s by the introduction of measures meant to include victims in the criminal justice process. In recent years, a body of research has emerged on the meaning of justice for victims. Inspired largely by the work of Lind and Tyler on procedural justice, researchers have examined victims' perceptions of fairness in the conventional criminal justice. More recently, justice theory has been applied in the area of restorative justice. The research shows that justice means more to victims than punishment of the offender. How a particular outcome is reached is also important. In essence, it is not enough that justice be done; justice must be seen to be done.

This chapter looks at the research literature on fairness and considers its implications for victim policy.

2.1 Introduction

In the 1970s, victims emerged as the forgotten party in the criminal justice system. Victims were considered witnesses to a crime against the State and that essentially defined their role in the criminal justice system. Still today, in common law, or adversarial criminal justice systems, the trial is based on two parties: the State versus the accused. These two parties, both armed with the law to protect them, battle it out before a judge. The victim is not a party to the trial.

The victim is a witness to a crime and can be called to testify before the court. However, as cases are often plea-bargained and thus never go to trial, victims are often excluded from the criminal justice process. Moreover, when there is a trial and the victim is called to testify, victims often complain about being treated like a suspect [Burgess and Holstrom, 1975; Lees, 1997; Lievore, 2005]. Of all the different stages of the criminal justice process, cross-examination by the defense is often particularly difficult for victims [Herman, 2002]. Excluded from the proceedings, victims are often left feeling frustrated with the criminal justice system and without a sense that justice has been done. Insensitive reactions by criminal justice authorities can lead to secondary victimization [Symonds, 1980; Maguire, 1991].

The 1980s saw the emergence of new services for victims that were meant to improve the treatment of crime victims in the criminal justice system. For example, in 1985, the General Assembly the of the United Nations (UN) adopted the *Declaration of Basic Principles of Justice for Victims of Crime and Abuse of Power*, which contains a list of recommendations for Member States aimed at improving access to justice and the fair treatment of victims. However, despite efforts, the implementation of victims' rights proved to be difficult. The UN Declaration is a nonbinding document and, although many countries have introduced Bills of Rights for victims, these are often unenforceable rights that are left to the discretion of criminal justice authorities [Wemmers, 2003]. In 1995, 10 years after the adoption of the UN Declaration, the UN undertook an evaluation of the implementation of the Declaration. The evaluation had one of the worst response rates for any UN survey. The results showed that the implementation of the UN Declaration was far from optimal [Groenhuijsen, 1999]. A more extensive study was conducted on the implementation of the 1985 Recommendations of the Council of Europe (R 85/11) on the position of the victim in the framework of criminal law and procedure. The researchers found that not one of the 22 countries included in the study had implemented the recommendations fully [Brienen and Hoegen, 2000].

Arguably, the victims' movement has been less successful in introducing procedural rights for victims than in influencing the sentencing of offenders [Roach, 1999; Garland, 2001]. In the past 20 years victims have been regularly used to support punitive measures. In the United States, laws restricting the rights of convicted offenders are passed and named for victims. An example is Megan's Law, which made mandatory the public registration of sex offenders in California [Garland, 2001]. Another example is the introduction of the victim impact statement (VIS). VIS provides victims with an opportunity at sentencing to express to the court how they were impacted by the crime. It can be a written statement by the victim, or the victim can choose to read his or her statement aloud before the court. Unlike testifying where victims are limited to answering questions, the VIS allows victims to say what they feel is important. In Canada, victims can also make a VIS at parole hearings. The VIS provides victims with an opportunity to influence decisions made by the court or the parole board regarding the sentencing of the offender. It was only with the introduction of the VIS that the word *victim* finally appeared in the Canadian criminal code [Laurin and Viens, 1996]. Thus, although procedural rights for victims may be weak, victims have made considerable inroads with regard to punishment [Roach, 1999].

This focus on punishment has been reinforced by the proponents of "just deserts" [Von Hirsch, 1985; Ashworth and Von Hirsch, 1998]. Just deserts emphasizes fairness in terms of proportionality and equality in sentencing and has fueled the public discourse on punishments [Garland, 2001]. Ironically, some of the strongest opponents of victim participation in the criminal justice system are proponents of just deserts, like Andrew Ashworth [1993, 2000]. The inclusion of victims in the criminal justice system feeds concerns among some legal experts that they will upset the balance of justice, and their desire for revenge will lead to harsher punishments [Roach, 1999; Ashworth, 2000]. While just deserts emphasizes the harm caused to the victim and society, it focuses on objective rather than subjective harm. Inclusion of victims and their subjective experiences risks introducing ambiguity into sentencing and therefore threatens the delicate balance between crime and punishment. Concern for fairness and the rights of the accused is used as an argument to justify the exclusion of the victim [Roach, 1999].

Hence fairness has been used to justify victims' exclusion from the criminal justice process, as well as their inclusion in the criminal justice discourse on sanctions. Both sides base their argument on victims' apparent concern for punishment. This begs the question: What does justice mean to victims? In this chapter we will examine the meaning of justice for victims and, in particular, the relative importance of outcomes and procedures for victims' justice judgments. Following a review of the literature on fairness, the implications for victim policy will be addressed.

2.2 Fairness

Since the 1960s, social psychologists have asked the question, what is justice? The early literature in this area focused on the fairness of outcomes or distributive justice [Homans, 1961; Adams, 1965; Walster, Walster, and Berscheid, 1973; Deutsch, 1975]. Distributive justice refers to people's moral

evaluation and actions in response to the allocation of rewards and punishments [Austin and Tobias, 1984]. It is promoted when outcomes are consistent
with certain implicit norms for the allocation or distribution of resources,
such as equality (everyone gets the same outcome) or need. In other words,
victims' fairness judgments are presumed to be based on the outcomes or
sentences imposed on offenders.

In the 1970s, however, Thibaut and Walker introduced the concept of
procedural justice. They argued that of importance were not only outcomes
but also how one arrived at the outcome [Thibaut and Walker, 1975]. More
recently, Van den Bos and his colleagues [Van den Bos, Lind, and Wilke, 2001;
Van den Bos and Lind, 2002] demonstrated that, although both procedural
and distributive justice are important, what comes first matters. Typically,
people receive procedural information before they know the outcome. When
procedural information precedes outcome information, it has a stronger
impact on the individual's overall fairness judgment than distributive
justice.

Lind and Van den Bos [2002; Van den Bos and Lind, 2002] have tried to
explain why fairness matters to people. They argue that fairness is all about
the management of uncertainty: When people are confronted with uncertainty in their environment, they turn to their impressions of fair treatment
to help them decide how to react. In other words, fairness becomes especially
important when people are faced with uncertainty.

Crime victims are confronted with a great deal of uncertainty following
their victimization. Victimization may cause victims to question their basic
beliefs about the world [Lerner, 1980]. Victims are often uncertain about the
criminal justice process: What will happen with their case, and what will be
their role [Baril et al., 1983; Shapland, Wilmore, and Duff, 1985; Shapland
and Hall, 2007]? Victims are often surprised to learn that they have no formal
control over the criminal justice process [Shapland et al., 1985]. People tend to
experience distress when their expectations regarding choice or participation
in a decision are disconfirmed [Austin and Tobias, 1984]. According to Lind
and Van den Bos [2002], uncertainty is increased in situations where people
feel that they are not in control. Victims may also be uncertain and fearful
about the reaction by their offender, who, they may fear, might seek revenge.
Because they are confronted with a great deal of distress and uncertainty,
fairness may be particularly important to crime victims.

2.2.1 Determinants of Procedural Justice

In the early studies on procedural justice Thibaut and Walker [1975] identified
two determinants of procedural justice: process control and decision control.
Process control refers to whether and to what extent parties are able to present information throughout the decision-making procedure. Later, this was

referred to as voice [Folger, 1977], and since then, voice has been identified as one of the most stable findings in procedural justice research [Van den Bos, 1996]. Decision control refers to whether parties have control over the outcome. In other words, do they have the power to accept or refuse decisions made by a third party (veto power)? Hence when parties are allowed to have input, they view the procedure as fair. Based on this model, restorative justice programs such as victim–offender mediation, which allows victims to present their views and gives them veto power over any offer made by the offender, would be viewed as fair.

Later, Tyler and Lind [1992] developed what they called the relational model of procedural justice. In their view procedural justice has a normative value instead of an instrumental value. This means that procedural justice is not just a means to an end but also has a value in itself. They emphasize the quality of the interactions between individuals and organizations like the criminal justice system. Departing from Thibaut and Walker's original theory, neither process control nor decision control is included in Tyler and Lind's model. They identify three determinants of procedural justice: trust, standing, and neutrality. Trust is directed at the individual's concern about an authority's intentions (e.g., is the authority trying to do right?). Standing is defined in terms of being treated with dignity and respect and showing respect for the rights of the individual. When people are treated with dignity and respect, they feel like valued members of society and feel good about themselves. Neutrality refers to honesty, the absence of bias, and making informed decisions based on the facts of the case. People want authorities, such as the police and judges, to be impartial and free from any bias. Based on this model, victims' procedural justice judgments will be based on the quality of the interaction with authorities, regardless of whether they feel that they had any power over the outcome.

While Tyler and Lind's relational model is based on empirical research, none of their research dealt explicitly with crime victims. Wemmers [1996], however, examined the meaning of fairness for victims of crime in the conventional criminal justice system and used procedural justice as the theoretical framework. Testing the relational model, Wemmers found that a two-factor model best fit the data for victims. The two factors that emerged from the victims' data are neutrality and respect. Neutrality is based on victims' perceptions that authorities were impartial, were honest, and made informed decisions based on the facts of the case. Respect refers to the quality of the interpersonal treatment of crime victims by criminal justice authorities. It includes whether victims were treated in a friendly manner, whether they were given an opportunity to express themselves (voice), and whether authorities showed an interest in the victim and took their concerns into consideration. These findings suggest that the quality of the interaction between victims and criminal justice authorities is essential for victims' procedural justice judgments.

Elsewhere, Tyler [1997, 2000] has identified another set of determinants of procedural justice. As in the relational model, Tyler [2000] identifies neutrality and trust as important determinants of procedural justice. However, to emphasize the quality of the interaction, standing is now replaced by two separate factors, namely, participation and respect. Participation is a derivative of voice or process control, first identified by Thibaut and Walker [1975]. According to Tyler, "people feel more fairly treated when they are given an opportunity to make arguments about what should be done to resolve a problem or conflict" [2000:121]. Placing special emphasis on participation, Tyler suggests that when parties are given an active role they will feel that the procedure was just. Respect focuses on the interpersonal treatment of parties by authorities [Tyler, 1997]. When people are treated with dignity and respect, they are more likely to feel that they have been treated fairly. Based on this model, the active role given to victims in restorative justice programs (i.e., victim–offender mediation), together with the respectful treatment by project workers, would enhance their perceptions of fairness.

More recently, Tyler [2003] has identified trust as a factor that is separate from but closely intertwined with procedural justice. Similarly, Van den Bos and Lind [2002] argue that the trustworthiness of authorities is separate from procedural justice. They view trustworthiness as a factor contributing to uncertainty. When people have information about the trustworthiness of an authority, they are faced with less uncertainty, and procedural justice is less salient. Tyler uses the term *motive-based trust* to reflect the perceived motives of the decision makers and whether they appear to be acting in good faith. Procedural justice judgments, Tyler argues, are based on the quality of decision making and the quality of the treatment by authorities. The quality of decision making reflects the neutrality of the decision maker (absence of bias, neutrality). The second determinant, quality of the treatment, is essentially whether the individual was treated with dignity and respect. This two-factor model resembles the model by Wemmers [1996] presented above. Tyler emphasizes the importance of the quality of the interpersonal treatment for procedural justice judgments.

2.2.2 Interactional Justice

This notion of procedural justice, however, has come under fire with the introduction of interactional justice. First introduced by Bies and Moag in 1986, interactional justice refers to people's sensitivity to "the quality of interpersonal treatment they receive during the enactment of organizational procedures" [ibid.:44]. According to Bies [1986], interactional justice is separate from procedural justice as it represents the enactment of procedures rather than the development of procedures themselves. Greenberg [1993] points out that interpersonal aspects of justice are not limited to procedures and include distributions as well, which once again suggests that interactional justice is not the same as procedural justice.

Greenberg [1993] developed a taxonomy of justice classes in which he identifies two categories of justice (procedural and distributive) and two focal determinants (structural and social). This gives rise to four classes of justice: systemic justice, information justice, configural justice, and interpersonal justice. Systemic justice refers to the formal rules and procedures, such as the right to have input or voice in the decision-making process; for example, rules that allow victims to make a VIS or request compensation from the accused, or rules that exclude victim participation in criminal justice procedures. Informational justice refers to the social determinants of procedural justice such as the open sharing of information and the use of explanations regarding procedures. For example, a public prosecutor who takes the time to explain to the victim what will happen in the trial and why would score high on informational justice. Configural justice refers to how the outcomes are structured. Outcomes may be structured to conform to social norms (e.g., equity, equality, need) or to promote certain goals (e.g., promoting peace, reducing conflict). Greenberg reserves the term *interpersonal justice* for the social aspects of distributive justice. It is about showing concern for individuals regarding the distributive outcomes they received; for example, showing concern for the plight of the victim. Apologies, according to Greenberg, are a tactic for enhancing interpersonal justice and as such should be included in it as well.

In his study on the dimensionality of justice, Colquitt [2003] presents support for Greenberg's contention that justice judgments are made up of four distinct factors. Colquitt contends that justice judgments are made up of distributive, procedural, interpersonal, and informational justice. Greenberg's concept of systemic and configural justice essentially corresponds with Colquitt's operationalization of procedural and distributive justice. Based on factor analysis, Colquitt claims that a four-factor structure of justice fits that better than a two-factor (procedural and distributive justice) or three-factor (procedural, distributive, and interpersonal justice) solution.

However, careful inspection of the correlations between the dimensions that are reported by Colquitt reveals that they do not follow the expected pattern. In Greenberg's classification, systemic and informational justice are two faces of procedural justice, whereas configural and interpersonal justice are two dimensions of distributive justice. Therefore, one would expect the two types of distributive justice to be more strongly correlated with one another than with the two types of procedural justice and vice versa. Instead, in both of the studies reported by Colquitt, informational justice is more strongly correlated with distributive (or configural) justice ($r = .36$) than interpersonal justice ($r = .14$). Moreover, the correlation between procedural and informational justice is very high ($r = .74$), which raises the question of whether these are two separate concepts. Hence Colquitt's findings are not unambiguous.

Others, however, reject the notion of interactional justice and view interpersonal treatment as part of procedural justice [Tyler and Bies, 1990; Brockner et al., 1994; Tyler, 2003]. Blader and Tyler [2003] argue for a two-factor model of procedural justice that is based on the quality of the interpersonal treatment and the quality of the decision making.

The above studies illustrate that there remains considerable conceptual uncertainty regarding the dimensionality of social justice judgments. We do not know whether how people are treated is one concept (procedural justice), two (procedural and informational justice), or three (procedural, informational, and interpersonal). What is clear, however, is that in addition to the actual outcomes that people achieve, such matters as how they are treated, the information that they are given, and the rules governing procedures (e.g., neutrality, consistency) are also important. In the following section we will examine the research on victims to understand what justice means to victims.

2.3 Research on Victims' Justice Judgments

2.3.1 Informational Justice

A key element of victim policy has been information and notification. Information refers to informing victims about procedures and services, whereas notification refers to keeping victims informed or notified of the developments in their case. Since the 1980s, countless studies have shown that victims often complain about the lack of information provided to them [Baril et al., 1983; Shapland et al., 1985; Strang, 2002; Brickman, 2003; Wemmers and Cyr, 2006; Shapland and Hall, 2007]. However, research on the impact of information on victims' justice judgments is scant.

One exception is a study by Wemmers [1996] that studied the experiences of 435 victims as their cases proceeded through the Dutch criminal justice system. She found that although most victims wanted to be notified of the developments in their case, most victims were not actually notified by authorities. When victim notification was examined in relation to victims' justice judgments, victims who wanted notification and received it were more likely to feel that they had been treated fairly by authorities than victims who wanted to be notified but were not. Hence in accordance with the theory on procedural justice discussed above, these findings seem to suggest that information is an important element of victims' fairness judgments.

Similarly, Carr, Logio, and Maier [2003] found that information was a key determinant of victims' evaluations of their experience with the criminal justice system. In this particular study, 272 victims were followed as their cases proceeded through the juvenile justice system in Philadelphia. The authors conclude that overall, victims want to be treated fairly and informed about their case.

2.3.2 Interactional Justice

The importance of interactional variables is illustrated by Wemmers's [1996] finding that victims tend to judge the police more favorably even though in objective terms they are no better at informing victims than the prosecution. Although 26% of the victims were notified by the police and 24% of the victims were notified by the prosecution, 79% of victims felt that the police had treated them fairly, whereas only 19% of victims felt this way about the prosecution. Thus, despite similar treatment, victims judged their treatment by the police as fairer than that by the public prosecution. One very important difference, however, is that most victims in this study had face-to-face contact with the police, and they rarely had any personal contact with the public prosecutor. In other words, when victims interacted with an authority, this contributed to their fairness evaluations and seemed to compensate for the failure by police to notify the victim. Because there was no personal interaction with the public prosecution, victims' evaluations of how fairly they were treated by the prosecutor were strongly linked to the information that the prosecutor's office shared with victims.

Similar results are reported by Carr et al. (2003), who found that notification did impact victims' evaluations of their contact with the District Attorney (DA) but not their evaluations of the police. As in the Dutch study, here too victims' contact with the DA's office was largely in relation to notification. The authors go on to conclude that what matters most for victims, despite legislation on VIS or the characteristics of the crime or of the victim, is positive interaction with criminal justice personnel. The authors identify two stages in the criminal justice process: The first stage is when the victim reports the crime to the police. This is a relatively short stage; however, it is one that is vividly recalled by most victims. The second stage is longer and occurs after the immediate aftermath of the crime, when the case has been received by the public prosecutor's office, and continues until the conclusion of the case. It is at this longer, second stage that timely and pertinent notification is important for victims.

In contrast, Orth [2002] examined outcome satisfaction, procedural justice, and interactional justice among 137 German victims of violent crimes. The victims in this study were involved in trials on average three years earlier. Procedural justice was based on six items: (1) whether the victim felt that the judge felt that his or her primary duty was to administer justice; (2) whether the judge had sufficient information on which to base his or her decision; (3) whether the criminal investigation had been conducted well enough; (4) whether the victims felt that their interests were sufficiently taken into account at the trial; (5) whether, compared with the offender, the victim had too few rights; and (6) whether the victims felt that they had sufficient opportunities to present their point of view and demands. This operationalization of procedural justice closely resembles what Blader and Tyler [2003] refer to as the quality of decision making. Orth's operationalization of interactional justice essentially corresponds with what Greenberg [1993] refers to as interpersonal justice. It is made up of three items: (1) whether the judge has prejudices toward the victim; (2) whether the judge insinuated that the victim was partially to blame for the crime; and (3) whether the judge treated the victim with respect and politeness. This conceptualization of interactional justice closely resembles what Blader and Tyler [2003] refer to as the quality of the treatment.

Orth finds that satisfaction with the outcome and procedural justice predict secondary victimization. Interactional justice was not found to predict secondary victimization. The latter finding is somewhat surprising given the importance placed on interactional justice in the literature. This raises the question to what extent did the victims in this study interact with the judge? After all, victims are the "forgotten party," and as a result they are often not informed of court dates, and unless they have to testify, they may not know that a hearing will take place [Brienen and Hoegen, 2000]. Victims who do not attend court may not be able to indicate how they were treated by the judge. Unfortunately, the author does not address this question.

2.3.3 Distributive Justice

Orth's [2002] study does, however, illustrate that both outcomes and procedural justice are important for victims. The findings show that victims' satisfaction with the outcome means more than just the severity of sentencing. Orth reaches a similar conclusion based on another study in which he examined the punishment goals of 174 victims of rape and nonsexual assault [Orth, 2003]. The author examined a variety of goals, including just deserts, and found that victims pursue diverse punishment goals. Victims gave the highest support to instrumental goals, namely, deterrence for the offender and the security of the victim and society. Just deserts and revenge received less support from the victims in this study. These results suggest that victims are not only interested in punishment.

Research on justice in organizational settings suggests that victims' reactions in terms of revenge, resentment, and forgiveness are in part influenced by the perceived fairness of procedures. Based on written interviews with 129 employees regarding victimization in their workplace, the authors conclude that how people respond to harm and wrongdoing is not just a function of individual factors or traits and that victims' perceptions regarding the fairness of procedures and thus the ability of the organization to ensure that justice will be served is critical in shaping victims' responses to harm. When people perceived procedures as fair, they were less likely to seek revenge. Brockner et al. [1994] report similar findings regarding layoff victims. Fair procedures have a moderating effect on victims' reactions, including their desire for revenge, or inclination to forgiveness or reconciliation.

2.3.4 Procedural Justice

In recent years there has been considerable work done on restorative justice as alternatives to the conventional criminal justice process. An interesting feature of restorative justice programs such as conferencing or mediation, which bring victims and their offenders together to discuss the crime and try to come to an agreement on how the crime should be responded to, is the role that they give to victims. Unlike the conventional criminal justice system, which shuts out victims, restorative justice programs allow victims to participate in the decision-making process and give them control over the outcome. In other words, they provide victims with considerable process and decision control, both key features of procedural justice.

Evidence of the importance of procedural justice among victims who participated in conferencing is reported by Strang [2002]. Based on interviews with 116 Australian victims who participated in conferencing, Strang reports strong perceptions of fairness by these victims. Procedural justice was measured indirectly, and conference victims were asked about five different facets of procedural justice: impartiality, ethicality, absence of bias, control over the process, and correctability. Unfortunately, although the study compares conferencing with conventional criminal justice, the author does not have procedural justice data on court victims. And although she does claim that court victims were "effectively excluded from any part of the processing of their cases" [ibid.:129], she does not examine how their exclusion impacted their procedural justice judgments.

The meaning of procedural justice for victims was the focus of a Canadian study with 54 victims who were invited to participate in a victim–offender mediation program for young offenders [Wemmers and Cyr, 2006]. Procedural justice was assessed using the direct method: Victims were asked how fair the procedures were and how fairly they had been treated. The authors found that most (71%) victims felt that the procedures were fair. Only 26% felt that they were unfair. The most important determinant of procedural justice was voice. This factor consisted of two items: (1) to be heard; and (2) to not feel hindered in making demands. This factor explained 81% of the variance in victims' procedural justice judgments. A second determinant of procedural justice was trust. This factor was based on two variables: whether the victim felt understood by the mediator and whether the victim had faith in the mediator. Together, trust and voice were able to explain 88% of the variance in victims' procedural justice judgments. The authors conclude that victims' procedural justice judgments have more to do with consultation with and recognition of victims in the process than about giving victims decision control. Indeed, when victims in this study were asked how much control they felt that victims should have in criminal justice procedures, they replied that victims should be consulted but that they should not be given decision-making power over the outcome [Wemmers and Cyr, 2004].

2.4 Discussion: Implications

Although the studies presented here are all very different, they suggest that procedural justice is important for crime victims. Victims seem to be concerned about the quality of their interactions with authorities and the quality of the decisions made by authorities. The interaction between victims and authorities, and especially the police, is an important aspect of victims' justice judgments. In the absence of interpersonal contact or in addition to it, information and notification are critical and nourish victims' procedural justice judgments. It informs victims of the decisions made and shows recognition of their interest in the case. Knowing what is happening in their case can give victims confidence that their case is being dealt with properly by authorities.

Outcomes or distributive justice is only one facet of fairness. Victims' satisfaction with the outcome of their case is distinct from the severity of punishment [Orth, 2002, 2003]. Focusing exclusively on outcomes provides an incomplete understanding of justice. What comes first matters, and if victims are excluded from the process and only receive information about the outcome that their offender received, they will use that information to form their justice judgments. The finding that when victims have little faith in the ability of the system to provide justice they are more likely to want revenge [Aquino et al., 2006] raises the question whether the exclusion of victims from the criminal justice process does not foster a desire for revenge and punitiveness? If victims have information about the process and the outcome, if they are regularly notified of what actions authorities are taking, then they will have more information available to them on which they can base their justice judgments. In other words, criminal justice authorities can enhance victims' justice judgments by providing them with informational and interactional justice.

Justice is a multidimensional concept. It consists of distributive or outcome fairness and procedural justice. What is not clear is whether interactional and informational justice are part of procedural justice or whether they are distinct dimensions of justice. What is clear, however, is that in addition to formal procedures, people's interactions with authorities, including any information that they receive from authorities, are also important. The research with crime victims shows that they are sensitive to these different dimensions of justice and that they are meaningful to them.

While justice judgments may have different dimensions, the finding that victims will substitute one type of fairness information for another suggests that they are all part of the same underlying concept. As we have already noted, victims will base their justice judgments on whatever information is available to them, and what comes first matters. If they only have information about the outcome and not the procedure, then they will base their fairness evaluations on that. Also, if victims do not have interpersonal contact with an authority but did receive written information, then they will base their judgments on that [Wemmers, 1996; Carr et al., 2003].

Do all four dimensions have equal value? Interpersonal interactions with authorities—interactional justice—may be more important for victims' justice judgments than informational justice. Victims tend to judge the police favorably, regardless of the fact that, in terms of information, the police treat victims no better than the public prosecutor [Wemmers, 1996]. This could mean that interpersonal contact has a stronger bearing on victims' justice judgments than information. However, it may also be that the contact with the police is more important because it comes first [Van den Bos et al., 2001; Van den Bos and Lind, 2002]. Further research is needed to understand how these dimensions of fairness affect one another.

The implications of fairness research for victim policy are significant. To begin with, the overall importance of interpersonal contact and information may mean that administrative measures such as VIS will be ineffective. Carr et al. [2003] argue that although rights are important, rights such as preparing a VIS may matter less to victims than the provision of basic information. Sanders et al. [2001] argue that VIS do not and cannot work because victims seek interpersonal contact with authorities. Victims desire to participate in the process is not about giving them decision control: Victims do not want decision-making power, and they value neutral and unbiased procedures [Shapland et al., 1985; Wemmers and Cry, 2004]. Their desire to participate is normative: It reflects recognition of their interest in the case. In other words, to satisfy victims' sense of justice, there needs to be more emphasis placed on notification and consultation without giving control to victims and compromising the neutrality of procedures.

Second, by including victims in the criminal justice process through consultation and notification, authorities can make the criminal justice system less punitive. By informing and consulting with victims, authorities can enhance victims' confidence in the criminal justice system [Wemmers, 1996] and thereby reduce victims' desire for revenge [Aquino et al., 2006]. Shutting victims out of the criminal justice process and undermining their faith in the ability of the criminal justice system to provide justice may make victims more punitive, as they feel the need to take matters into their own hands to ensure justice.

However, if victims were included in the process through notification and consultation, they might be more inclined to forgive and seek reconciliation. Hence, contrary to the concerns of many legal theorists [Ashworth, 1993, 2000; Roach, 1999], the inclusion of victims in the criminal justice process would not lead to a more punitive system but a less punitive one. However, this means that victims need to be included throughout the criminal justice process and not be shut out until the sentencing stage.

In conclusion, fairness is not a reason to exclude victims from the criminal justice system but a reason to include them. Understanding the meaning of justice for victims may encourage lawmakers to create legal procedures that will be accepted by victims and the public while being consistent with human rights requirements. This would lead to a more humane justice system where both victims and defendants would be treated as subjects of the law and not as objects, a legal system in which victims would see justice being done.

References

Adams, J. S. 1965. Inequity in social exchange. In *Advances in social psychology*, vol. 2, ed. L. Berkowitz, 267–99. New York: Academic Press.

Aquino, K., T. M. Tripp, and R. J. Bies. 2006. Getting even or moving on? Power, procedural justice and types of offense as predictors of revenge, forgiveness, reconciliation, and avoidance in organizations. *Journal of Applied Psychology* 91(3):653–68.

Ashworth, A. 1993. Victim impact statements and sentencing. *Criminal Law Review* 39:498–509.

_____. 2000. Victims' rights, defendants' rights and criminal procedure. In *Integrating a victim perspective within criminal justice*, ed. A. Crawford and J. Goodey, 185–206. Aldershot: Darmouth.

Ashworth, A. and A. Von Hirsch. 1998. Desert and the three R's. In *Principled sentencing: Readings on theory and policy*, 2nd ed., ed. A. Von Hirsch and A. Ashworth, 331–35. Oxford: Hart.

Austin, W. and J. M. Tobias. 1984. Legal justice and the psychology of conflict resolution. In *The sense of injustice: Social psychological perspectives*, ed. R. Folger, 227–74. New York: Plenum.

Baril, M., S. Durand, M. M. Cousineau, and S. Gravel. 1983. *Mais nous, les témoins....* Montréal: École de criminologie, Université de Montréal.

Brienen, M. and E. Hoegen. 2000. *Victims of crime in 22 European criminal justice systems*. Nijmegen: Wolf Legal.

Brockner, J., M. Konovsky, R. Cooper-Schneider, R. Folger, M. Christopher, and R. J. Bies. 1994. Interactive effects of procedural justice and outcome negativity on victims and survivors of job loss. *Academy of Management Journal* 37(2):397–409.

Burgess, A. and L. Holstrom. 1975. Rape: The victim and the criminal justice system. In *Victimology: A new focus*, ed. I. Drapkin and E. Viano, 21–30. Lexington, MA: Lexington Books.

Carr, P. J., K. A. Logio, and S. Maier. 2003. Keep me informed: What matters for victims as they navigate the juvenile criminal justice system in Philadelphia. *International Review of Victimology* 10:117–36.

Colquitt, J. A. 2001. On the dimensionality of organization justice: A construct validation of a measure. *Journal of Applied Psychology* 86(1):386–400.

Deutsch, M. 1975. Equity, equality, and need: What determines which value will be used as the basis for distributive justice? *Journal of Social Issues* 31:137–49.

Folger, R. 1977. Distributive and procedural justice: Combined impact of "voice" and improvement of experienced inequity. *Journal of Personality and Social Psychology* 35:108–19.

Garland, D. 2001. *The culture of control: Crime and social order in contemporary society*. Chicago: University of Chicago Press.

Groenhuijsen, M. 1999. Victims' rights in the criminal justice system: A call for more comprehensive implementation theory. In *Caring for victims of crime*, ed. J. J. M. van Dijk, R. van Kaam, and J. Wemmers, 85–114. Monsey, NY: Criminal Justice Press.

Herman, J. L. 2003. The mental health of crime victims: Impact of legal intervention. *Journal of Traumatic Stress* 16(2):159–66.

Homans, G. C. 1961. *Social behaviour: Its elementary forms*. London: Routledge and Kegan Paul.

Laurin, C. and C. Viens, 1996. La place de la victime dans le système de justice pénale. In *Question d'équité: L'aide aux victimes d'actes criminals*, ed. J. Coiteux, P. Campeau, M. Clarkson, and M. M. Cousineau, 109–34. Montréal: Association québécoise plaidoyer-victimes.

Lees, S. 1997. Carnal knowledge: *Rape on trial*. Harmondsworth: Penguin.

Lievore, D. 2005. *No longer silent: A study of women's help-seeking decisions and services responses to sexual assault*. Report prepared by the Australian Institute of Criminology, Canberra: Commonwealth of Australia.

Lind, E. A. and K. Van den Bos. 2002. When fairness works: Toward a general theory of uncertainty management. *Research in Organizational Behavior* 24:181–223.

Maguire, M. 1991. The needs and rights of victims of crime. In *Crime and justice: A review of the research*, ed. M. Tonry, 363–433. Chicago: University of Chicago Press.

Roach, K. 1999. *Due process and victims' rights*. Toronto: University of Toronto Press.

Sanders, A., C. Hoyle, R. Morgan, and E. Cape. 2001. Victim impact statements: Don't work, can't work. *Criminal Law Review* June:447–58.

Shapland, J. and M. Hall. 2007. What do we know about the effects of crime on victims? *International Review of Victimology* 14:175–217.

Shapland, J., J. Wilmore, and P. Duff. 1985. *Victims in the criminal justice system*. Aldershot: Gower.

Strang, H. 2002. *Repair or revenge: Victims and restorative justice*. Oxford: Clarendon.

Symonds, M. 1980. The second injury. *Evaluation and Change* 20:36–38.

Thibaut, J. and L. Walker. 1975. *Procedural justice: A psychological analysis*. Hillsdale, NJ: Wiley.

Tyler, T. 1997. Citizen discontent with legal procedures: A social science perspective on civil procedure reform. *The American Journal of Comparative Law* 45:871–903.

———. 2000. Social justice: Outcome and procedure. *International Journal of Psychology* 35(2):117–25.

———. 2003. Procedural justice, legitimacy and the effective rule of law. In *Crime and justice: A review of research*, vol. 30, ed. M. Tonry, 257–83. Chicago: University of Chicago Press.

Tyler, T. and E. A. Lind. 1992. A relational model of authority in groups. In *Advances in experimental social psychology*, vol. 25, ed. M. P. Zanna, 115–91. San Diego: Academic Press.

Van den Bos, K. 1996. Procedural justice and conflict. PhD diss., Rijksuniversiteit Leiden.

Van den Bos, K. and E. A. Lind. 2002. Uncertainty management by means of fairness judgements. *Advances in Experimental Social Psychology* 34:1–59.

Van den Bos, K., E. A. Lind, and H. Wilke. 2001. The psychology of procedural and distributive justice viewed from the perspective of fairness heuristic theory. In *Justice in the workplace: From theory to practice*, vol. 2., ed. R. Cropanzano, 49–66. Mahwah, NJ: Lawrence Erlbaum.

Von Hirsch, A. 1985. *Past or future crimes: Deservedness and dangerousness in sentencing criminals*. New Brunswick, NJ: Rutgers University Press.

Walster, E., G. W. Walster, and E. Berscheid. 1973. New directions in equity research. *Journal of Personality and Social Psychology* 25(2):151–76.

Wemmers, J. M. 1996. *Victims in the criminal justice system*. Amsterdam: Kugler.

_____. 2003. *Introduction à la victimologie*. Montreal: Les presses de l'université de Montréal.

_____. 2004. How much control are victims looking for? *International Review of Victimology* 11:1–16.

Wemmers, J. M. and K. Cyr. 2006. What fairness means to crime victims: A social psychological perspective on victim-offender mediation. *Applied Psychology in Criminal Justice* 2(2):102–28.

The Evolution of a Young, Promising Discipline

3

Sixty Years of Victimology, a Retrospective and Prospective Look

EZZAT A. FATTAH

Contents

Foreword

In 2008, victimology turned 60 years old! The birth of this exciting branch of criminology is usually traced to the 1948 publication of Hans von Hentig's seminal work, *The Criminal and His Victim* [see Fattah, 1967a&b]. As one of the oldest, perhaps *the* oldest, pioneers in victimology [Viano, 1976] still alive, having published articles pertaining to this nascent discipline as early as 1966 [Fattah, 1966] and having devoted a large part of my scholarly output during the past 40 years to this young discipline, I believe the best contribution I can make to this victimology handbook is to revisit the issues I raised over the years, the questions I asked, and the criticisms I made, and to trace the evolution of victimology in the last half century.

3.1 Introduction

3.1.1 The Emergence of Victimology: A Brief History

Although the emergence and development of victimology make a fascinating story, surprisingly no comprehensive history of the discipline has been written. There are also no systematic assessments of its present state or its likely future evolvement. The reasons for this are not clear. It could well be that the strong applied orientation that has dominated victimology in the past three decades has obscured the need for such important historical and theoretical analyses [Fattah, 2000:21].

Victimology is much younger than its parent discipline: criminology. It is difficult to explain how criminology's need to thoroughly study the victims of crime, a need that today may appear obvious, even axiomatic, has escaped the attention of criminologists for more than a century. But it is not rare for social scientists to miss the obvious. As Rock [1994:11] points out:

> Even criminology and the sociology of deviance—disciplines concentrated most squarely on the analysis of crime, criminals and criminal justice—tended somehow to obliterate the victim for a very long while, failing to see what, in retrospect, should probably have been evident all along. Such omissions occur continually. They are an ineluctable part of any discipline, a consequence of the truth marked by Burke when he said that "a way of seeing is always a way of not seeing." The price of organizing, specializing and accumulating knowledge about any area is a systematic neglect of the other matters thrown out of focus and beyond the margins. Precisely because criminology is an empirically-driven discipline, it has tended to ignore those things that do not bear the name of crime, criminals and criminal justice.

Sixty years after the publication of von Hentig's [1948] book it hardly needs affirming that victimology is neither a fad nor a fashion. It is a scientific reality that has imposed itself, a field of study that emerged to fill a serious gap in the scholarly knowledge of the crime phenomenon. But like its mother discipline, the development of victimology has not followed the same path in every part of the world, and as with any other discipline, it is more advanced in some countries than in others. Although there are some similarities in the way victimology took off and moved ahead, there are also significant qualitative and even quantitative differences. Although victim legislation is developed in some countries, it is nonexistent in most. Victim assistance programs have flourished in some societies but are still unheard of in many parts of the world. Victimization surveys have been conducted on a regular basis in some places and are conspicuously absent in others. Victimological therapy is being encouraged and practiced in some cultures but is frowned on in others. Courses and seminars in victimology have been in existence for several decades in some universities but have been totally lacking in others. Such huge differences, however, should not make it impossible to provide a more or less unified picture of the discipline's evolution or an insightful analysis of its current state and its future developments. Nevertheless, as with all global and concise overviews, selections and generalizations are inevitable and oversimplifications are unavoidable [Fattah, 2000a:21–22].

3.1.2 The *Raison d'Être* of Victimology

The *raison d'être* of victimology is rather simple. It is the duet frame of most crimes, the fact that the majority of conventional criminal acts involve an offender and a victim, and that the motives for criminal behavior do not develop in a vacuum [von Hentig, 1948]. The motivation to perpetrate a victimizing act comes into being through needs, urges, and drives. It emerges from contacts, communications, interactions, attitudes, and counterattitudes. Not infrequently, the prospective victim is involved consciously or unconsciously in the motivational process and in the process of mental reasoning and rationalization the victimizer engages in before the commission of the crime [Fattah, 1976, 1991a]. In most instances victims are not chosen at random, and in many cases the motives for the criminal act develop around a specific and nonexchangeable victim. Therefore, an examination of victim characteristics, of the place the victim occupies, and the role the victim plays in these dynamic processes is essential to understanding why the crime was committed in a given situation, at a given moment, and why a particular target was chosen. This explains why "offender target selection," although neglected, is an important and a promising research area in victimology.

For all those reasons, the study of crime victims has become an integral part of criminology. Not only this, but victimology also has the potential of reshaping the entire field of criminology. It may very well be the long-awaited paradigm shift that criminology badly needs, given the failure of its traditional paradigms, namely, the search for the causes of crime, deterrence, rehabilitation, treatment, just deserts, etc. [Fattah, 2000a]. Unfortunately, this ambitious goal remains an unfulfilled promise.

3.1.3 Two Important Developments in Victimology

There can hardly be any doubt about the two most important and most significant developments in victimology in the past 50 years: (1) the advent of victimization surveys and the wealth of data they yielded on crime victims and on criminal victimization; and (2) the ideological transformation of victimology and the political, social, and legal changes that followed this transformation. Both developments will be reviewed in this chapter.

The chapter is divided into four parts: Part 3.2 reviews the scholarly and theoretical advances in victimology. Part 3.3 analyzes the ideological transformation of victimology and contrasts the position of the "new" victimologists with that of criminologists on a number of issues. Part 3.4 critically analyzes some aspects of recent victim policy. Part 3.5 critically examines and assesses certain victimological programs and services aimed at assisting the victims of crime.

3.2 Victimology: The Scholarly Discipline

3.2.1 Theoretical and Research Advances in Victimology

Theoretical victimology is a scholarly attempt to convert criminology into a dynamic, holistic discipline, to shift the focus of research from the one-dimensional study of criminals' traits and attributes to situational and interpersonal dynamics. Its point of departure is that victimizing behavior is dynamic behavior that cannot be adequately explained by the static etiological theories that have dominated criminology for more than a century. Crime needs to be explained by a dynamic approach where the offender, the act, and the victim are inseparable elements of a total situation that conditions the dialectic of the victimizing behavior [Fattah, 1976, 1991a, 1997a]. Victimology seeks the genesis of victimization not in the characteristics and background of the victimizer, as traditional criminology did, but in a complex model of total interactions. It places a great deal of emphasis on situational factors, on victim–offender relationships and interactions, and the role all of them play in actualizing or triggering criminal behavior. Whereas traditional criminology viewed criminal behavior as simply the product of the offender's traits and personality, victimology sees it as the outcome of a long or brief interaction with the victim. It considers unscientific and futile any attempt to treat the act of victimization as an isolated gesture, to dissociate it from the dynamic forces that have prepared, influenced, conditioned, or determined its commission or from the motivational and situational processes that were vital to its conception. Victimology insists that in most cases crime is not an action but a reaction (or even an overreaction) to external and environmental stimuli. Some of these stimuli emanate from the victim. Therefore, the victim is an important, often an integral, element of the criminogenic environment and of the victimogenic situation.

3.2.2 The Need for Victimology

Although those were the premises that guided the earlier studies in victimology, it soon became apparent that the study of victims is both needed and useful for many other purposes as well. Not only is it necessary to establish the frequency and the patterns of victimization, but it also sheds light on other issues such as proneness to victimization, fear of victimization, responses to victimization, consequences and impact of victimization, and so forth. Such knowledge provides a solid scholarly foundation for "applied victimology," which is mainly concerned with aiding and assisting victims, alleviating the negative consequences of the victimizing act, preventing its reoccurrence, and helping victims overcome the traumatic effects of victimization. A thorough knowledge of victims of crime is also essential to the formulation of a rational criminal policy, to the evaluation of crime prevention strategies, and for taking social action aimed at protecting vulnerable targets, increasing safety and security, and improving the quality of life. By studying victims, victimology seeks other types of information that are of great value to lawmakers and to society. The victim has a strong impact on criminal justice decisions, particularly those of the police and the courts. In the vast majority of cases, it is the victim who decides whether to mobilize the criminal justice system by reporting or not reporting the victimization to the authorities. Not only this, but the characteristics, attitudes, and behavior of the victim and the victim's relationship to the offender also have a significant bearing on the decision of the police to proceed in a formal or informal way as well as the decision of the prosecutor to lay or not to lay charges. Victim-related factors can have a major impact on the final outcome and on the sanction meted out by the court. Thus, victimology can lead to a better understanding of the functioning of the criminal justice system and to improving the decision-making process. A better understanding of the role victims currently play in the criminal justice process is necessary to enhancing victim involvement, as well as to establishing or improving the modalities of such involvement.

Research in victimology tries to discover why certain individuals or groups of individuals are more frequently victimized than others, and why certain targets are repeatedly victimized, and to find sound empirically based explanations for the differential risks and rates of victimization. By studying victims' characteristics and by analyzing their behavior, victimology attempts to establish whether there exists a certain proneness to criminal victimization—whether there are given predispositions or specific behaviors that enhance the risks and chances of criminal victimization—that is responsible for, or conducive to, becoming a victim.

3.2.3 An Unanswered Question: Who Is the Victim?

3.2.3.1 The Social Construction and Deconstruction of Victims
Although the word *victim* is one of the staples of the criminological language, and although it was used to coin the term *victimology*, its real criminological meaning remains unclear, and its utility remains in doubt. Just what does the term, as used in criminology and victimology, mean? Is it a label, a

stereotype? Is it a state, a condition? Is it meant to assign a status, a role, to the one so described? Is it a self-perception, a social construction, an expression of sympathy, a legal qualification, a juridical designation [Fattah, 1994e:83, 1997b:257]?

Quinney [1972] suggested that the "victim" is nothing but a social construction. He pointed out that we all deal in a conventional wisdom that influences our perception of the world around us and that this wisdom defines for us just who the victim is in any situation, which also means that alternative victims can be constructed.

In every society, there is a continuous process of constructing and deconstructing victims. The witches who were burned at the stake for being criminal and dangerous are now defined as victims of witch hunts. Not very long ago, women beaten (or even raped) by their husbands, as well as children subjected to acts of violence in the process of upbringing, were neither defined as victims nor assigned victim status. As social attitudes changed, both groups were seen as legitimate candidates for the status of victim. When the age of consent to sexual practices was set at 21 or 18 years, those under that age were defined and treated as victims. When the age was lowered to 14, teenagers between 14 and 18 or 21 years were deconstructed as victims.

In recent years, the general tendency among victimologists has been to broaden the notion of victimization, to define it too widely and too loosely, and to apply the victim label to a wide variety of individuals and groups (see Part 3.3). In the process, victims were constructed and created and included persons who neither define nor perceive themselves as victims. The discrepancy between the self-perception and the external label is well illustrated in Boutellier's [1993] study of prostitutes in Holland. He notes that external observers tend to view the relationship of a prostitute to her pimp as one of exploitation and victimization. No one cares to see whether this diagnostic label, imposed from without, is shared by the prostitute herself, whether *she* defines and perceives herself as a victim. Boutellier contrasted the "structuralist" and "subjectivist" views of prostitution. The structuralist (one may say the ideological) view argues that prostitution, by definition, is sexual violence, one of the ways in which men oppress women. The subjectivist position, on the other hand, takes as its point of departure the experiences of the women involved. In this perspective, prostitution is seen as a legitimate form of labor freely chosen by thousands of women. Hence the change in terminology from the pejorative term *prostitute* to the neutral term *sex trade worker.* Boutellier pointed out that in the Netherlands, women are no longer seen as just victims of sexuality. Prostitutes are viewed as able to decide their own lives, as having freely chosen their occupation. He hastens to add that this does not necessarily mean that there are no situations where women are forced into prostitution. But, generally speaking, prostitutes in the Netherlands are no longer viewed or defined as victims.

What this example shows is that victimization is not an objective reality but is rather a personal, subjective, and essentially relative experience. Victimization defined according to the normative standards, a specific ideology, or the law may not be defined as such by those who are involved. Inversely, people may define and perceive themselves as victims, although what they suffered does not fit the legal definition of criminal victimization. The discrepancy is well described by Bilsky and Wetzels [1992:5–6]:

> Obviously, individual thresholds come into play that reflect the ability and readiness to tolerate distressing or harmful events without feeling victimized. The harmfulness of an event, the probability of its occurrence, and the personal vulnerability as perceived by the afflicted person may differ significantly from a bystander's point of view. Consequently, categorization of an incidence may fall apart and people may consider themselves victims of crime although this judgment neither fits the perception of others nor bears legal examination.

Bilsky and Wetzels further add that there are cases in which people have definitely been victimized according to normative (legal) standards, although they do not understand their situation this way. The discrepancy in judgment can be attributed to different reasons, depending on the respective situation [ibid.:6].

Not only are victimization experiences perceived, defined, and lived differently within the same culture, but they vary widely across cultures [Fattah, 1993b]. This creates a serious methodological hurdle for victimization surveys, particularly international or transcultural surveys [Fattah, 1993b].

3.2.4 Victimization Surveys and Their Findings

3.2.4.1 Some Conceptual and Methodological Problems

One of the most notable advances in criminology and victimology in the past 50 years is the advent of victimization surveys. The word *victimization* became part of the criminological lexicon in the 1960s. In 1964, the Finnish criminologist Inkeri Anttila published an article in *Excerpta Criminologica* titled "The Criminological Significance of Unregistered Criminality." In it she suggested that it would be possible by means of surveys to establish how many individuals in a given period were victimized and how many reported their victimization to the police. Following up on this original idea, Biderman and Reiss [1967] suggested to the U.S. President's Commission on Law Enforcement and Administration of Justice a pilot survey designed according to Professor Anttila's suggestion. That survey was the beginning of what has since become a standard measurement tool in criminology. The first large-scale victimization survey was carried out in the United States in 1965 for the same Commission [Ennis, 1967]. The findings of this pioneering survey were an eye opener, as they showed that the volume of unreported crime revealed by the survey was far beyond expectations and previous estimates. The survey yielded rates of victimization, even serious types of victimization, that were far higher than those reported annually in the FBI Uniform Crime Reports.

In their quest for standardized measures, victimization surveys usually use legally defined offenses. But because victimization is a personal, subjective, and relative experience, the feeling of being victimized does not always coincide with the legal definition of victimization (see above). Therefore, it is not clear what exactly victimization surveys are trying to measure. Is their objective to measure those criminal victimizations that meet the legal criteria set by the criminal code, or are they meant to measure the subjective victimizations experienced by the respondents? These, needless to say, are two different realities. In other words, are the surveys designed to measure crime or victimization? The titles *crime survey* and *victimization survey* continue to be used interchangeably [for a more detailed discussion of the problems of victimization surveys, see Fattah, 1997a:103–111].

Rape is a good case in point because of the enormous gap that may exist between the legal definition and the subjective experience of the female, as well as because the sexual act can be experienced in very different ways by different women.

Another major problem is that definitions and experiences of victimization greatly vary from one society to another and from one culture to another [Fattah, 1993b]. Several types of victimization are culturally constructed. This is particularly the case in the areas of sexuality, child labor, child abuse, and neglect, to mention a few. Even serious acts of violence may NOT in some cultures be defined or experienced as victimization. This is the case, for example, of many rites of passage and initiation rituals in non-industrial societies, as well as the common practice of hazing in Western societies, common in colleges, sports, the army, and the navy [Fattah, 1993b]. International Crime Surveys, which collect standardized victimization data from a number of countries for comparative purposes, are particularly prone to the problem of the cultural relativity of victimization.

3.2.4.2 *Major Findings of Victimization Surveys*
Despite some unresolved conceptual and methodological problems, victimization surveys have greatly enhanced our knowledge of victims and victimization. Probably the major contribution of victimization surveys, over and above the attempt to measure the volume of certain types of crime, is to have revealed that victims of crime do not constitute an unbiased cross-section of the general population and that victimization is not evenly distributed within society. They showed that victimization is clustered within certain

groups and certain areas and revealed that there is much greater affinity between offenders and victims than is commonly believed [Fattah, 1989a, 1991a, 1992c). Criminological studies in Europe, the United States, Canada, and Australia have always shown that offenders involved in the types of crimes usually covered by victimization surveys are disproportionately male, young, urban residents, of lower socioeconomic status, unemployed (and not in school), unmarried, and, in the United States, black. Victimization surveys reveal that victims disproportionately share those characteristics and confirm that the demographic profiles of crime victims and of convicted criminals are strikingly similar [Gottfredson, 1984]. Although these findings may have come as a surprise to some when first released, they are both logical and understandable. It seems rather obvious that the frequency with which some individuals become involved in violence-prone situations is bound to affect both their chances of using violence and of being recipients of violence, of attacking and being attacked, of injuring and being injured, of killing and being killed. Who will be the victim and who will be legally considered the offender depends often on chance factors rather than deliberate action, planning, or intent. Thus, victim/offender roles are not necessarily antagonistic or incompatible but are frequently complementary and interchangeable [Fattah, 1994b]. This situation is particularly true of brawls, quarrels, disputes, and altercations. In many instances, dangerousness and vulnerability may be regarded as the two sides of the same coin. They often coexist because many of the factors that contribute to dangerousness may create or enhance a state of vulnerability. One such factor is alcohol consumption, which may act simultaneously as a criminogenic and as a victimogenic factor, enhancing the potentiality of violent behavior in one party and of violent victimization in the other [see Fattah and Raic, 1970].

3.2.4.3 The Similarities between the Victim and Offender Populations

That victim and offender populations are homogeneous populations who share similar characteristics is undoubtedly a result of the social and geographical proximity of victims and victimizers. Proximity and accessibility, for example, are important factors in family violence. Crimes of violence, particularly those not motivated by sex or financial gain, are interpersonal crimes or crimes of relationships. Because the motives for the violence do not develop in a vacuum [von Hentig, 1948], it is understandable that these crimes are often committed between people who know each other, who interact with one another, and who are bound by family, friendship, or business ties. The typical contexts in which criminal homicide, attempted murder, or assault occur are domestic fights, family disputes, quarrels between nonstrangers, or other altercations where insult, abuse, or jealousy are present. The interpersonal and the intraracial character of crimes of violence,

particularly criminal homicide, are well documented in many studies conducted in different cultures [Svalastoga, 1956; Wolfgang, 1958; Driver, 1961].
The notions of social and geographical proximity apply to many property
offenses as well. Brantingham and Brantingham [1984] point to a well-es-
tablished distance decay pattern in human spatial behavior. They explain
that people interact more with people and things that are close to their home
location than with people or things that are far away and that interactions
decrease as distance increases (distance decay). They further note that some
of this decrease in activity as distance increases is the result of the "costs" of
overcoming distance. According to the Brantinghams [1984:345]:

> Crimes generally occur close to the home of the criminal. The operational
> definition of close varies by offence, but the distance decay gradient is evident
> in all offences. . . . Generally, violent offences have a high concentration close
> to home, with many assaults and murders actually occurring in the home.
> The search pattern is a little broader for property offences, but these are still
> clustered close to home.

While sociodemographic characteristics are strong determinants of
risks and rates of victimization, research also suggests that delinquency is
one of the most important variables influencing the probability of becoming a victim. Empirical evidence shows that criminals are more frequently
victimized than noncriminals and indicates that victims of violent crime
themselves have considerable criminal involvement [Statistics Canada, 1991;
Friday, 1995; Fattah, 1997a]. The evidence also suggests that marginal groups
are more involved in crime and more often victimized than nonmarginal
groups. Typical examples of those prone to victimization are persons implicated in illicit activities or those who have opted for a deviant lifestyle: gang
members, drug pushers, drug addicts, prostitutes, pimps, persons involved
in illegal gambling, loan sharks, and so forth [Fattah, 2003b].

3.3 The Ideological Transformation of Victimology

The ideological transformation of victimology, in the past 30 years or so,
from a scholarly branch of criminology into an advocacy movement and a
political lobby brought about a dramatic and profound change, particularly
in policy and practice. The metamorphosis of victimology resulted in two
groups with opposed ideals, different agendas, and divergent philosophies.
In one camp were those scholars and researchers, a small minority one has to
admit, who remained faithful to the original conception of victimology as a
branch of criminology. In the other camp were the feminists, the therapists,
the social workers, as well as the social and political activists who defined

their mission as improving the lot of crime victims and obtaining justice for those who are victimized. Both groups spoke a different language and were operating at a different wavelength. The late Donald Cressey [1992:57] called them the humanists and the scientists, thus:

> Victimology is characterized by a clash between two equally desirable orientations to human suffering—the humanistic and the scientific. . . . The humanists' work tends to be deprecated because it is considered propagandistic rather than scientific, and the scientists' work tends to be deprecated because it is not sufficiently oriented to social action.

The original victimology, theoretical as it was, was meant to broaden the scope of criminology, to fill an obvious gap in criminological research and theory, and to transform criminology from a static, one-sided discipline into a dynamic, tri-dimensional science of criminal behavior with a holistic approach encompassing the offender, the victim, and the situation [Fattah, 1973, 1976, 1979, 1989a, 1991a, 1992c). This is why victimology was widely regarded, and for good reason, as a branch of criminology, or rather as *"the other side of criminology."*

The new applied/activist victimology, on the other hand, has little, if anything, in common with criminology. Its concepts, its criminal policies, its penal philosophy, and its general outlook are not only different from but also, in many respects, they are the antithesis, the opposite pole of those of criminology. In fact, the contrast between the two streams is so pronounced that it does not seem unfair to brand this activist victimology as "anticriminology." As this is a rather serious charge, it needs to be carefully explained, documented, and sustained. To do so, I will contrast, at some length, some criminological concepts with those of the "new" victimology and will examine some of the main tenets of the criminal policy and the penal philosophy, as well as the vision and general outlook, of both.

3.3.1 Conceptual Differences

3.3.1.1 *Criminalization/Victimization*

One way of comparing criminology and the new victimology is to contrast the views on, and the approach to, central concepts such as criminalization and victimization. Criminologists, whether liberal, radical, or critical, advocate a narrow definition of what crime is and a restrictive inventory of the behaviors that ought to be criminalized. The new victimologists argue for an extremely broad, even encompassing definition of victimization.

Criminologists maintain that because the criminal law has a monopoly on the use of force and because of the drastic punishments it prescribes, it should be used very sparingly and only as a last resort (*ultima ratio*) when no other means of control are available or are adequate for dealing with the problematic behavior in question. Over the years, criminologists have consequently voiced bitter criticism of the inflationary policy of criminalization and have forcefully argued for a drastically limited inventory of criminalized behaviors. They always defended the view that the category "crime" should be reserved only for the most serious, the most harmful, and the most dangerous types of antisocial behaviors, in other words, to acts whose antisocial character is very pronounced [see Fattah, 1997a].

The new victimologists' approach and views are different. Their tendency has been to define victimization too loosely and too broadly to the extent that the concept no longer has any specificity or concreteness. As a result, the term *victimization* has become almost synonymous with the notions of pain and suffering. The new victimologists endeavored to bring under the generic heading *victimization* every conceivable form of injury, loss, harm, pain, or suffering. They spared no effort in their search for new types and new forms of victimization and neatly classified them into different categories: primary victimization, secondary victimization, tertiary victimization; direct victimization, indirect victimization; personal victimization, vicarious victimization; and so forth.

To them, existing criminal code definitions of criminalized behaviors were far too narrow, so they resorted to elastic, stretchable, all-embracing terms such as *abuse*. When all the possible subcategories of abuse—physical, mental, psychological, sexual, and financial—were identified and exhausted, a new category of victimization was added: neglect. Soon it was realized that abuse and neglect are perpetrated not only by others but also by those who suffer, hence two new subcategories were added to the list: self-abuse and self-neglect. New laws were enacted to mandate the reporting of child (and elderly) abuse and to punish those who fail to report. Telephone lines were set up to enable anonymous callers to report suspected abuse, and registers were established to list the names and addresses of alleged abusers. Getting the name of someone on the register was much too easy; getting the same name off the list was quasi-impossible. Worse still, most of those whose names were on the register did not even know that they were [see Fattah, 1994a].

3.3.1.2 White Collar Crime/Conventional Crime

Criminologists and the new victimologists also differ in their focus and their emphasis. Ever since Edwin Sutherland published his original work on *White Collar Crime* [1949], criminologists have been trying to empirically demonstrate that the harm—deaths, injuries, losses, damage to the economy and the environment—caused by white collar crime, corporate crime, business crime, and other crimes by the powerful far exceeds the harm resulting from conventional crimes and crimes of the powerless. To overcome public apathy and politicians' indifference, there were valiant attempts to sensitize them to the depredations of crime in the suites as opposed to those of crime in the streets. Criminologists' aim was to shift the focus of attention and policy from those offenses that unduly create fear and anxiety in members of the general public to those crimes whose incidence is less visible and whose danger is more subtle but whose harmful consequences are more far reaching and much longer lasting [Fattah, 1980a, 1989c, 1992a&b].

In contrast, the new victimologists have been extremely selective in the types of crime they denounce and the groups of victims whose cause they champion. They chose to focus their attention and to concentrate their political efforts and action on traditional crime and its victims, on crimes that cause individual harm rather than the ones that cause collective harm. As a result, victims of white collar crime and its depredations have been once again relegated to the shadow, to the background.

The total disproportion between the section devoted to victims of abuse of power and the one on victims of conventional crime in the United Nations' [1985] *Declaration of Basic Principles of Justice for Victims of Crime and Abuse of Power* is a clear indication of where the focus of the new victimologists lie.

3.3.1.3 Moral Entrepreneurship/Ideological Entrepreneurship

Criminologists, particularly in the 1960s and the 1970s, were very critical (and also suspicious) of those whom Becker [1962] called the "moral entrepreneurs." They denounced moral crusaders who try to impose their religious and moral convictions on others and who, in the process, advocate the use of the criminal law and its sanctions as instruments of intimidation to force others to adhere to their rigid standards of morality and to adopt the lifestyles the crusaders judge to be the only appropriate ones.

In the new victimology, "ideological entrepreneurship" not only is accepted but also is a widely practiced form of advocacy. All criminologists and victimologists are expected to subscribe to the new ideology and to join the political action on behalf of crime victims. Those who refuse to share the ideological views of the new victimologists are belittled, ridiculed, and accused of being pro-offenders and antivictims.

The focal point of the new ideology is the pain and suffering victims of crime go through. The direct outcome of this rather emotional stand is that the cause and the interests of crime victims are defended and pursued in an unsubtle, unsophisticated, and rather indiscriminate manner.

Although the new victim ideology has replaced the old morality that was the mobilizing force of the moral entrepreneurs, it is still possible to find traces of the latter in some of the types of victimization that are denounced with religious fervor by the new victimologists, for example, sexually motivated acts with children. A state of moral panic [Jenkins, 1992; Fattah, 1994a] is created around those deviant activities, and the outrage and indignation are transmitted to the media and the public, generating demands for harsher sanctions and more severe penalties.

3.3.1.4 Stereotyping

Criminologists, particularly in the 1960s and the 1970s (see for example D. Chapman's book [1968] *Sociology and the Stereotype of the Criminal* and Sarbin's [1979] article *The Myth of the Criminal Type*), were anxious to fight the popular, but inaccurate, stereotype of the criminal. They promoted the view that the vast majority of criminals are normal and criticized their portrayal as sick, mad, or bad. New criminological approaches, such as "the rational choice perspective" [Cornish and Clarke, 1986], continued to de-emphasize the alleged differences between criminals and noncriminals, differences that are often exaggerated and amplified by the causal theories that stress offenders' psychopathology. Cornish and Clarke [1986], for example, are critical of the popular trend to overpathologize crime and criminals, and they affirm that much of criminal activity is essentially nonpathological, mundane, commonplace, and opportunistic. The Japanese criminologist Hiroshi Tsutomi [1991:14] went as far as claiming that "people commit crimes not because they are pathological or wicked, but because they are normal." Even proponents of the biological approach to crime causation, like Deborah Denno [1990:108], had to admit that "the most striking about the comparisons between criminals and their controls are their similarities, not their differences."

The position of the new victimology is the opposite. Not only does it perpetuate the false dichotomy between offenders and victims and the popular stereotypes of both, but it also reinforces the predator–prey model of criminal victimization and the normative distinction between the active aggressor and the passive sufferer. The new victimologists' portrayal of offenders and victims follows closely the mental images the general public holds of them, depicting them as distinct and neatly classifying them as the guilty and the innocent, the good and the evil.

For obvious reasons activist victimology deliberately denies, minimizes, or de-emphasizes the homogeneity, the affinities, the similarities, and the substantial overlap between the victim and offender populations. It implies, to use David Miers's [1989] words, "that there is a qualitative disjunction between victims and offenders," an implication that is in clear contradiction to the available empirical evidence (see also Reiss [1981]; Singer [1981]; Fattah [1989a, 1991a, 1992c]).

There is little doubt that the empirical evidence, showing the homogeneity and the overlap between the victim and offender populations, makes activist victimologists uncomfortable because it is at odds with their basic message, namely, that the victims, to use Gilbert Geis's words, "are good people done in by those who are bad" [1990].

By using the horror story syndrome and by capitalizing on atypical and unusual cases to gain sympathy for the victims' plight and to highlight the pain and suffering they go through, activist victimologists, wittingly or unwittingly, contribute to conservative politicians' revival of the old "monster" image of criminals and cater to the punitive attitudes of the general public.

3.3.1.5 Labeling

The victim designation is a label and a debasing one. However, although the label *criminal* has been widely criticized in criminology [Schur, 1971; Shoham and Rahav, 1982], the use of the label *victim* seems to generate few, if any, objections or criticism. Labeling theorists have decried the stigma, degradation, and stereotyping attached to the criminal label and have cautioned against the danger of the person so labeled identifying with the label. They insist on the deviance-amplifying functions of labeling. To highlight the danger of victim labeling, I coined the term *The Mark of Abel* [Fattah, 1999:195–197].

The dramatization of evil, described so well by Frank Tannenbaum in his 1938 book, *Crime and the Community*, in cases of criminal labeling, applies perfectly to victim labeling. To illustrate this, the word *criminal* in the following original passage [ibid.:19–20] has been replaced by the word *victim*:

> The first dramatization of "evil" which separates the child out of his group for specialized treatment plays a greater role in making the (victim) than perhaps any other experience. It cannot be too often emphasized that for the child the whole situation has become different. He now lives in a different world. He has been tagged. A new and hitherto nonexistent environment has been precipitated out for him. The process of making the (victim), therefore, is a process of tagging, defining, identifying, segregating, describing, emphasizing, making conscious and self-conscious, it becomes a way of stimulating, suggesting, emphasizing, and evolving to the very traits that are complained of.

The new victimologists, on the other hand, seem all too willing, even anxious, to use the victim label in a wide variety of contexts and to apply it to a wide variety of individuals and groups. One negative consequence of the present indiscriminate use of the label is to perpetuate the popular stereotypes of the crime protagonists and to reinforce the notion that criminals and victims are as different as night and day. The readiness with which the label is currently applied ignores the complementarity and the interchangeability of the roles of victim and victimizer. It overlooks the fact that today's victims may be the offenders of tomorrow and that yesterday's offenders may be the victims of today [Fattah, 1994b].

In their zeal to heighten public awareness of the pain and suffering of the victims and to highlight the negative effects of victimization, activist victimologists often contribute—sometimes advertently, other times inadvertently—to eternalizing the victim status and condition [Fattah, 1999a]. Contrary to criminology, where the conventional wisdom is to help the offender shed the negative criminal label, a popular motto in the new politicized victimology appears to be "once a victim, always a victim." Measures, supposedly designed to help the victim, such as appearance before parole boards, betray insensitivity to the fact that bringing the victim back to the parole hearing years and years after the victimization can only foster the victim status, serve as a reminder of the past, and bring back the memories of victimization.

3.3.2 Policy Differences

It does not take long, when the criminal policies of criminologists and the new victimologists are examined and compared, to realize that they are dissimilar and in many instances are diametrically opposed.

3.3.2.1 Intervention/Nonintervention

Criminologists in general and labeling theorists in particular are strongly opposed to the State's interventionist policies and deplore the significant increase in the intrusive powers and measures of the State and its agents, namely, the police. They favor a minimally interventionist, nonintrusive, and nonstigmatizing approach. Edwin Schur's book [1973], *Radical Non-Intervention*, in which he called for a hands-off approach to juvenile delinquents, is one of many that appeared in the 1960s and 1970s to highlight the disastrous effects of intervention and to outline the advantages of the proposed change.

The three major elements of the proposed criminal policy at that time were often described as the three Ds: decriminalization/depenalization, diversion, and decarceration. The first D, decriminalization and depenalization, was prompted by the urgent and pressing need to modernize the archaic criminal codes, to redraw the boundaries of the criminal law, and to narrow the frontiers of criminalization. Criminologists called for the decriminalization or depenalization of a wide variety of behaviors that did not cause serious or tangible harm to others. Many of those criminal offenses were included in what are now obsolete and anachronistic criminal codes (most of which were enacted in the nineteenth century) for historical, religious, or moral reasons that reflected the thinking and mentality of past centuries. Some government commissions or task forces in the Scandinavian countries went as far as demanding or recommending that minor forms of theft (such as shoplifting) and fraud (such as bad checks) be decriminalized or depenalized. In Sweden, for example, it was suggested that minor property offenses (e.g., petty thefts through shoplifting in self-service stores) should lie outside the criminal law and be dealt with by measures other than punishment. It was held to be unreasonable that society should use its already hard-pressed criminal justice resources to hunt down shoplifters when the firms in question deliberately make crime easy and draw humans into a criminal risk zone [Aspelin et al., 1975].

The second D, diversion, became a very popular concept and a very fashionable trend in the late 1960s and early 1970s. It was a logical outcome of hidden delinquency studies suggesting that those who are formally processed within the criminal justice system and who are officially labeled run a higher risk of recidivating and developing a criminal career than those who are not. The labeling perspective, popular at the time, stressed the dangers of the label and the negative consequences of stigmatization and suggested as a remedy that a large number of offenders (e.g., in particular young offenders, petty offenders, and first timers) be diverted from the criminal justice system.

The third D, decarceration, focused on the extensive and indiscriminate use of imprisonment as punishment. Criminologists used findings from a wide array of studies demonstrating the nefarious effects of incarceration (particularly long-term confinement), the dismal failure of imprisonment as a deterrent or as an instrument of special prevention, the disruptive consequences for the inmates' families, and so forth. Pointing to these results, criminologists suggested that the use of imprisonment be severely restricted, that alternatives to incarceration be expanded, that prison sentences be shortened substantially, and that the criteria and eligibility for early release be broadened. Typical of the books outlining criminology's views on imprisonment was Scull's book, *Decarceration* [1977].

Criminologists were calling not only for a moratorium on prison construction and the phasing out of existing ones but also for a retrenchment of the criminal justice system in general [Jobson, 1977]. They believed that the system is ineffective, overexpanded, overextended, overburdened, and overused. They were convinced that it does more harm than good and that the less it is used, the better it is for offenders, for the system itself, and for society at large. Some criminologists, like Louk Hulsman [1982], went as far as calling for the total abolition of the system. Others, like Keith Jobson [1977], suggested that it be dismantled. Nils Christie [1977] accused the system of stealing the conflicts from their owners and made a plea to have the conflicts returned to those to whom they belong, to the parties involved.

To summarize, one may say that criminologists were able to demonstrate the serious limitations and shortcomings of the criminal justice system, as well as its awful inadequacy as a social problem solver. They showed, evidence in hand, that the criminal justice system is neither the most appropriate nor the most effective vehicle for dealing with society's ills and headaches whether they have to do with drugs, prostitution, gambling, wife beating, child battering, and elder abuse, to name a few.

The stand of victim advocates on the issue of State powers, the intrusion of the criminal law, and the punitive practices of the criminal justice system is startlingly different. For obvious reasons, decriminalization or depenalization is not on the new victimologists' agenda. If anything, it is the reverse. In fact, as a result of their efforts and their pressure many new offenses have been created. The demands for retributive justice for the victims, epitomized in the report of the *U.S. President's Task Force on Victims of Crime* [1982], are also incompatible with practices such as diversion or decarceration. They added to the burden of the justice system and contributed to the increase in the use of imprisonment and in the length of incarceration. This change was brought about by either legislative change or change in judicial practices and has pushed the prison populations in many countries to new records. Of course, it would be unfair to blame the new victimology for the record incarceration rates or for the present overcrowding of prisons, a large part of which can be traced to drug offenses. It is undeniable, however, that the demands for retribution symbolized in the rhetorical cry "justice for victims" have contributed to a general punitive climate and have played in the hands of conservative politicians who were anxious to use the victims as pawns in their law-and-order policy.

Victim advocates also have a very different view from that of criminologists regarding the role and the effectiveness of the criminal justice system. They favor expansion, not retrenchment. For example, as a result of the incessant demands that family violence in its various forms be treated the same way as violence between strangers and that the guilty male be automatically arrested (zero tolerance), there has been a shift from the criminal justice system as a last resort to the criminal justice system as the first resort. According to Lorraine Berzins [1990], the criminal justice system was being called on more than any other institution to deal with violence in the home. Ironically, this is so when research [Berk et al., 1992; Hirschel et al., 1992; Pate and Hamilton, 1992; Sherman and Smith, 1992] indicates that arrest is no more effective in deterring subsequent violence than alternative methods, such as advising and possibly separating the couple or issuing a citation to the offender.

There is little doubt that many of the policies advocated by the new victimologists are policies of intrusion and exclusion. Scheingold et al. [1992, 1994] point out that victim advocates support the kind of intrusive state and exclusionary policies that criminology rejects. They warn against the obvious threats to freedom that enhancing the power of the State can pose. Scheingold et al. are critical of the new victimologists' policy process for being driven by extreme and atypical events and insist that such process, even in strictly instrumental terms, is worrisome. They echo Al Reiss's [1981:225] statement that a serious mismatch between problem and policy could easily develop insofar as misconceptions and exaggerations are driving policy decisions.

They equally reiterate Reiss' warning that victim advocacy tends to build idiosyncratically on the public's reaction to extreme crimes.

The intrusive measures advocated by victim advocates are not limited to the area of family conflicts; they extend to other areas as well. One example is that of offender registration and community notification when someone is released from prison or when someone is placed in a halfway house. But there are many, many others.

Child abuse has become the new pretext that allows professionals to inspect, punish, and regulate the poor [Chase, 1976:5]. The enormous power and broad discretion now invested in social workers and child workers as a result of current hysteria about the problem lend themselves easily to all kinds of abuse [Wexler, 1985]. Kendrick [1988] quotes estimates indicating that in the United States more than half a million families each year are investigated for allegations that turn out to be unfounded. The social and psychological consequences are, as he points out, horrendous.

Child abuse is also an area that illustrates well how inflation can permeate the area of criminal legislation. The number of laws that were passed with the aim of detecting, investigating, punishing, and preventing child abuse is truly staggering. It is reported, for example, that New York considered no fewer than 43 bills, whereas California looked at 100 [Wexler, 1985]. The sweeping provisions and the low standards of proof required under the new bills are largely responsible for what has been described by one commentator as "an invasion of latter day child savers who sometimes destroy children in order to save them" [ibid.:20].

Child abuse legislation is just one example of activist victimologists' attempts to extend the power of the State, the ambit of the criminal law, to widen the net of social control and to bring more and more groups under the umbrella of State control agencies.

3.3.2.2 Legal Safeguards

One of the major preoccupations of Beccaria and the legal scholars of the Classical School was to protect the individual against those in power, to guard those brought before the courts against the despotism and excesses of the judges and against the vagaries and arbitrariness of the justice system. They waged a battle for the recognition, establishment, and entrenchment of human rights and freedoms, and for the introduction of legal safeguards in criminal procedures. Over the years, the established legal safeguards became one of the main features of democratic justice systems, distinguishing them from those in totalitarian or authoritarian regimes. The motto of democratic justice became "It is better to acquit a hundred guilty persons than to convict a single innocent one."

In their effort to tilt the scales of justice in favor of crime victims, victim advocates targeted many of the traditional safeguards for abolition and created a false contest between the rights of offenders and the rights of victims [Karmen, 1990; Elias, 1992a; Fattah, 1992b; Henderson, 1992]. They claimed that much concern has been shown for the "rights of criminals" and not enough for the plight of the innocent people they harm. Consequently, they demanded that the rights of victims be restored at the expense of offenders' rights [Karmen, 1990]. Summarizing the demands of victims' advocates, Karmen [1990:331] writes:

> To restore some semblance of balance to the scales of justice, which have been tipped in favor of criminals, some of the "anti-victim" opportunities and privileges offenders have accumulated must be stripped away. According to this analysis, victims need rights to counterbalance, match, or even "trump" the rights of criminals. In this context, reform means reversing previous court decisions and legal trends, shifting the balance of power away from wrongdoers and toward injured parties.

The report of the 1982 *President's Task Force on Victims of Crime* in the United States and its recommendations can be read as a damning indictment of many of the legal safeguards that the American justice system established over the years to protect against the conviction of the innocent and to uphold the rights and freedoms so deeply cherished in a democracy [Fattah, 1992b]. One of the main recommendations of the report is the abolition of the exclusionary rule, something which President Reagan had advocated as a major step in the fight against crime. The exclusionary rule, which stipulates that illegally obtained evidence cannot be used in court to secure a conviction of an accused in a criminal case, is used predominantly in drug cases. One has to wonder about the benefits that victims would gain by having it abolished! In fact, its abolition in California following the "yes" vote on Proposition 8 (*The Victims' Bill of Rights*) has worked not for, but against, victims, particularly victims of rape, by making it possible for defense lawyers to have the victims examined by psychiatrists or to question the victim about sexual activity she had engaged in shortly before the alleged rape [Paltrow, 1982].

Another recommendation of the *U.S. President's Task Force on Victims of Crime* was to impose severe restrictions on the right to be released on bail, a right that is derived directly from the presumption of innocence.

To the consternation of many, victim advocates' fight to have some of the traditional legal safeguards abolished has been successful. For example, rules of evidence used to require that the testimony of alleged rape victims be corroborated to protect against false accusations. Surprisingly, almost all American states have relieved the prosecution of the burden of providing corroboration of the rape accusation [Feher, 1992].

Not only this, but in some cases, such as cases of child abuse, the burden of proof has almost been reversed. Noting that child sexual abuse is a crime that will often leave no physical evidence even when it has occurred, Feher [1992:22] draws attention to the inherent danger in doing away with the corroboration requirement, thus:

> In the context of an *actual* occurrence of abuse, the repeal of this rule (corroboration) would appear beneficial. But in the context of a man on trial for accusations which are the product of the interviewing process, the result is that one more procedural safeguard to incorrect convictions has been removed.

In addition to eliminating the corroboration requirement, some jurisdictions have introduced new rules that severely inhibit the defendant's ability to cross-examine the child witness. Other changes include permitting a videotaped statement or live testimony through closed-circuit television instead of the normal under-oath deposition followed by cross-examination [Fattah, 1992b].

Another important change has been the introduction of the so-called *rape shield laws*, which prohibit the use of either reputation or opinion evidence of an alleged rape victim's past sexual behavior, thus restricting the circumstances in which and the extent to which the defendant in a rape case may present this type of evidence to the jury [Anonymous, 1988]. In 1991, the Supreme Court of Canada, in a 7–2 ruling, declared the rape shield provision of the Canadian criminal code to be unconstitutional because it potentially could lead to the conviction of innocent defendants [Fattah, 1992b].

To summarize, one can fairly say that many of the procedural changes introduced at the demand of the new victimologists do not meet the evidentiary standards required by the fundamental principle of due process.

3.3.2.3 *Differences in Penal Philosophy*

The penal philosophy of the new victimology differs markedly from the philosophy that dominated criminological thinking since the early days of criminology, since the era of Beccaria and the Classical School. With very few exceptions, criminologists have preached a humane penal philosophy and have pleaded for mildness and less punishment. As a result of this humanitarian philosophy, cruel and unusual punishments were abolished in most countries of the Western world. Politicians, legislators, and policymakers were constantly reminded that it is the certainty, not the severity, of punishment that is essential for effective deterrence. Once corporal punishments and bodily mutilations were abolished, and once the death penalty was abolished or severely restricted, criminologists directed their efforts to the prisons. Several publications advocated a society without prisons [Menninger, 1966; Mitford, 1971; Nagel, 1973; Mathiesen, 1974; Prison Research Education Action Project, 1976; Sommer, 1976]. Associations were formed, and national and international meetings were organized to discuss the best strategies for bringing about an end to imprisonment (*National Moratorium on Prison Construction, Prison Research Education Action Project*).

In line with their view that incarceration should be sparingly used, and only when everything else has failed, criminologists favored all means and programs of early release, conditional or unconditional. Parole was seen not only as an effective means of reducing the prison population and the costs of incarceration but also as an instrument of rehabilitation and social reintegration facilitating the transition from confinement to total freedom. The words *rehabilitation, resocialization,* and *social reintegration* occupied a prominent place in the vocabulary of criminology in the twentieth century and until three or four decades ago were generally viewed as the primary goals of an enlightened penal philosophy. Although it is true that rehabilitation lost favor with criminologists in recent years, particularly after Martinson's much publicized statement that nothing works [1974], they never abandoned the belief that social reintegration is the most effective way of reducing the rate of recidivism and of preventing future criminal behavior.

Few would challenge or dispute the claim that the new victimologists are in favor of a *crime control model* and are not fans of the treatment/rehabilitation/reintegration model. As Scheingold [1992:8–9] points out in his discussion of the state of Washington's *Sexual Predator Legislation*, victim advocates oppose reintegration measures because:

> They believe that sexual criminals, especially the worst of them, sexual predators, are driven by their compulsions, and thus are bound to reoffend. They want to keep them permanently out of circulation. What they liked about the (new) civil commitment provision for sexual predators was not that it provided treatment but that, because treatment would not work, predators, perhaps without exceptions, would remain incarcerated for the rest of their lives.

It has already been pointed out that the new victimologists are very selective in the types of crimes and types of criminals they fight against. One group that is targeted for their wrath is that of sexual abusers, and they have succeeded in creating a state of moral panic [Jenkins, 1992] surrounding sexual abuse of children. The religious fervor with which the perpetrators have been (and are being) pursued and prosecuted (sometimes for offenses committed decades earlier) has led some [McNeill, 1987; Moore, 1987; Kendrick, 1988; Repo, 1992] to liken the prosecution of present-day child abusers to the persecution of witches (and lepers) in past centuries. What is rather ironical is that the urge to punish, which seems to motivate most of the prosecutions, has blinded the crusaders to the potential trauma victims can suffer as a result of reliving events that had taken place in their early childhood [Fattah, 1992b].

But the demands of punishment and deterrence are not limited, by any means, to sexual offenses and sexual predators. They cover other behaviors as well. These range from harassment to discrimination, from drunken driving to nonpayment of alimony. Such demands and the pressure tactics used to have them met have been moving the criminal law and the criminal justice system into a punitive, retributive direction. The right of allocution, victim impact statements, and victim involvement in parole hearings are all designed, as Ranish and Shicor [1992] point out, to intimidate judges and parole board members and to influence them in one policy direction: toward harsher punishment or denial of parole. The punitive intentions of victim advocates are even more evident in the calls for restrictions on release on bail, the elimination of the exclusionary rule, the abolition of parole, and so forth. Clearly, the primary objective of all these items on the agenda of the new victimology is not to help, assist, ensure justice for crime victims, or to alleviate their suffering, but simply to reverse the humanitarian trend of the 1950s and the 1960s [Fattah, 1992a, b, e]. Even the terminology used, such as the popular phrase "the scales of justice have been tipped in favor of the offender and need to be rebalanced to ensure justice for the victim," betrays the real intentions and the background motives.

In fact, the motives are not at all hidden. For example, President Reagan's *Task Force on Crime Victims* [1982], echoing their master's voice, went to great length to explain that offenders are not being punished enough but are being "pampered" by the criminal justice system. The following example is typical of the attitude and the reasoning that permeate the report [1982:11]:

> The judge sentences your attacker to three years in prison, less than one year for every hour he kept you in pain and terror. That seems very lenient to you. Only later do you discover that he will probably serve less than half of his actual sentence in prison because of good-time and work-time credits that are given to him immediately. The man who broke into your home, threatened to slit your throat with a knife, and raped, beat, and robbed you will be out of custody in less than eighteen months. . . . The defendant's every right has been protected, and now he serves his time in a public facility, receiving education at public expense. In a few months his sentence will have run. Victims receive sentences too: their sentences may be life long.

In addition to calling for longer prison sentences, victim advocates have called for additional penalties, for example, *victim fine surcharge*.

The insistence on punishment betrays an unwarranted and misplaced faith in the efficacy of penal sanctions as a means of reducing the recidivism of violent and sex offenders. This is paradoxical because these offenders in general seem to be among the least deterrable categories, and many of them are in desperate need of treatment because of sexual, social, or mental inadequacies.

3.3.3 Outlook

Last but not least, criminologists and activist victimologists also differ in their general outlook. The outlook of the former is optimistic, whereas that of the latter is overly pessimistic. Criminologists have a tendency to stress the positive and to seize on any encouraging sign in offenders and law breakers. The new victimologists focus not only on everything that is negative in those who offend but also on the terrible impact that victimization has had on the victims and their lives.

Since the time of Beccaria, criminologists adopted and propagated Rousseau's view that humans are good by nature. Despite the discouraging results of evaluative studies of treatment and rehabilitation programs, they continue to show faith in offenders' ability to learn and to change their behavior. The new victimologists tend to emphasize what is bad in humans: the evil, the wickedness, the madness, the sickness. They have a dim view of the chances of rehabilitation. For them, offenders, whether violent or nonviolent, whether guilty of violence against the person, of sex crimes, or property crime, are bound to repeat their offenses, and nothing could protect future victims and the community against their predatory behavior except segregation and incarceration [Fattah, 2003a:17–18].

The difference in outlook clearly manifests itself in two documents: the presentence report (the criminological document) and the victim impact statement (the victimological document). The first looks at the future, highlights the positive, and outlines what could possibly be achieved. The second looks at the past, stresses the negative, and documents the victim's failure to recover from, or to cope with, the consequences of victimization [Fattah, 2003a:17–18].

3.4 Victim Policy

3.4.1 The Rediscovery of Crime Victims

One intriguing question that has always baffled me is this: Why did it take so long for society to recognize the plight of crime victims, to acknowledge their desperate need for assistance, and for the State to come to their rescue by setting up programs aimed at helping and compensating them? The question is even more perplexing when examined in the social and political contexts of welfare states like Canada and the Scandinavian countries. How, and why, is it that in those countries—countries that became a world model of caring and sharing, helping and assisting almost every type of disenfranchised group—no attention was given to the needs of crime victims? How is it that crime victims were among the very last groups to benefit from the generous assistance of the welfare state and the plethora of aid programs that the State provided?

In societies where there are only two social classes—the rich and the poor—neglect of crime victims is understandable. Victims of violence are predominantly the poor, victimized either by the wealthy and the powerful or by other have-nots. Their victimization does not generate any outcry or raise much concern. The neglect is also understandable in countries like the United States, where blacks, until very recently, were a poor, oppressed, and exploited minority. As the majority of violent crimes were committed by blacks against other blacks, their plight did not stir much sympathy or empathy among members of the dominant white majority. No attempt was made to heal their wounds or to provide them with some redress.

But to those who live in a caring, sharing society, who experienced firsthand the benevolence of the welfare state, it is hard to understand how the plight of those unfortunate enough to be victimized by crime could have been overlooked or ignored for as long as it was! Commenting on the centuries-long lack of recognition, as well as the absence of aid and assistance to crime victims, Gil Geis [1990:255] writes:

> Their condition for centuries aroused little comment or interest. Suddenly, they were "discovered," and afterwards it was unclear how their obvious neglect could have so long gone without attention and remedy. . . . Until a few decades ago, the plight of large numbers of crime victims in virtually all parts of the world was abominable. They were mugged, raped, their homes invaded, their handbags or wallets stolen. If that were not both bad and sad enough, they were double victimized, first by the criminal offenders and then by the authorities. Police officers and prosecutors all too often had been hardened into cynicism from having dealt with too many crimes for too long, and they had come to forget that for most of us, victimization is rare, often a unique and novel experience. Further frustrated by their inability to do much about such offenses as burglary and car theft—those in which nobody saw and could describe the perpetrator—the authorities often were abrupt and dismissive in the face of victim despair. . . . These were the ills; it became the aim of the victim's movement to rectify them.

In recent years, great strides have been made in the field of victim assistance and victim services. Having been ignored for centuries, and after decades of horrendous suffering and utter neglect, which led to them being described as the "orphans of social and criminal justice" [Amernic, 1984], they suddenly became the darlings of both legislators and policymakers. The rediscovery of crime victims, spearheaded by the feminist movement, a movement that championed the cause of victims of rape, sexual assault, and the cause of battered women, generated a great deal of empathy and sympathy for a largely forgotten and neglected group [Fattah, 1991b, 1997b, 2000a&b]. As a result, the past 30 years or so saw the creation and extremely rapid expansion of victim services in many parts of the world. Victim assistance programs, totally nonexistent three or four decades ago, have mushroomed all over the globe from Australia in the south to England and the Scandinavian countries in the north, from South America to Asia, and from the large islands of Japan to the relatively small Canary Islands. The development has been nothing but phenomenal. In fact, in the late 1980s, Davis and Henley [1990:157] estimated the number of victim service programs in the United States to be in excess of 5,000, whereas 20 years earlier there had been none! [Fattah, 2003a:18–19]

Despite the great strides that have been made in the field of victim assistance and despite the continuing efforts to improve the sad lot of crime victims, the road ahead remains a long and treacherous one. A great deal more needs to be accomplished, and a lot of improvements can, and should, be made. Past mistakes are to be avoided. Precious lessons need to be learned. Reforms to the legislation and changes to the practice ought to be introduced. Criticism is the key to reform, and reform is the key to progress and evolution. An analytical critique of the policies of victim assistance is overdue. Victim assistance and victim services developed rapidly in most countries, and there were lots of politics involved. Because the services were desperately needed and because they are a worthy humanitarian and social endeavor, serving an eminently just cause, they were not subjected to many critical evaluations or empirical investigation. It would certainly be pretentious to try to offer here a comprehensive critique of victim assistance and victim services, although I have published a number of papers dealing with various aspects of those services [Fattah, 1989a, 1992b&c, 1997b, 1999a, 2000a&b&c, 2001a].

3.4.2 The Thorny Issue of Victims' Rights[*]

If we are to put aside the ideological and political rhetoric that has permeated the debates on victim rights in countries such as the United States and Canada, and if we are to examine and discuss the issue in a nonrhetorical, nonpartisan, dispassionate manner, then we first have to ask what rights do crime victims want and are entitled to, and second, who are the victims whose rights we are claiming or defending?

What rights are demanded for victims? Are they formal legal rights, or is the talk simply about specific social and humanitarian considerations that need to be given to crime victims? Victim advocates have focused on legal rights, thus neglecting what may be far more important for the victim. In my humble personal view, the most important right of crime victims is the right to be protected against future victimization, yet this is a social not a legal right, and it rarely, if ever, figures on the victims' rights agenda. Legal rights are derived, most of the time, from a specific legal status. Property rights are derived from ownership, civil rights from citizenship, marital rights from

[*] This section is based mainly on Fattah [2001b].

the status of being a spouse, parental rights from the status of being a parent, and so forth. One of the biggest hurdles in the fight for victims' rights is that at present, and as unbelievable as this may seem, crime victims in most jurisdictions have no legal status. As will be seen later, in modern societies the legal process is between the defendant and the State. It excludes the victim. Kelly [1987:81] points out that "victims have no independent status, no standing in court, no right to choose counsel, no right to appeal, no control in the prosecution of their case or voice in its disposition."

Another difficulty in claiming victims' rights is the ambiguity of the victim qualification. This is because the concept of victim is not easy to define. It is a loose, elastic, and relative concept (see Part 1). Who is the victim? As simple as this question may seem, it is not easy to answer. In homicide, for example, is the victim the person who is killed and who no longer suffers, or is it the members of the family who will be grief-stricken for the rest of their lives? When a very young child is sexually molested, who is the victim? Is it the child who does not understand or realize that he/she was victimized, or is it the parents who will forever live with the memory? When a married woman is raped, is she the only victim, or are her husband and children also victims? The crime, any crime, does not victimize only one person. There are direct victims and indirect victims; actual victims and virtual victims; manifest and latent victims; primary, secondary, and even tertiary victims. Who should be given legal status? Who should be awarded legal rights? Who should qualify for state aid and state compensation? Are all rights being claimed for crime victims of equal importance, or are some more important than others? Is it possible to establish a hierarchy of victims' rights according to how vital they are to victims' survival, well-being, and thirst for justice?

It has always surprised me that what are touted as victims' rights are in reality nothing more than basic principles that should unequivocally govern the operations of a criminal justice system in a civilized democratic society. When I hear the claim that crime victims should have the right to be treated with dignity and respect, I ask myself isn't the criminal justice system supposed to treat everyone with dignity and respect whether they are victims or offenders, complainants, witnesses, or defendants, and whether they are citizens or immigrants, male or female, young or old? Do we need legislation to force those in the justice system to show consideration, sensitivity, and compassion to the users of the system in whatever capacity this use may be? When I read that crime victims should be protected against intimidation I wonder aren't we all supposed to be protected by law and by the justice agents against intimidation of any kind? To me, this right does nothing but state the obvious. The same could be said of the other "rights" that are being solicited for crime victims, for example, the right to be informed, to be present, to be heard, to be consulted before important decisions in their case are made, and to be advised of the progress and the final disposition of their case.

These are basic principles that apply to all those who are involved as is the principle of speedy disposition, or the principle that in a caring society the state should come to the rescue of those who suffer by awarding them fair and adequate compensation. Restitution to the victim by the party who caused the death, injury, harm, or loss is a principle of justice; it is the same principle that governs civil litigation.

As can be seen from above, the question of which rights victims should have is problematic. Equally problematic is the question of which victims. Public perceptions and social views of who is a victim do not always coincide with legal definitions. The examples are many, but one will probably suffice. We may view prostitutes as victims of society, of their family environment, of their pimps (see Part 1). But the law, which often treats them not as victims but as criminals, does not define them as such. Crime victims are a very heterogeneous population, and they suffer victimizations of all kinds and varieties. Surely, we can all agree that different victims have different needs according to their sociodemographic characteristics, psychological makeup, social network, and ability to cope. Their needs also differ according to the type of victimization they have been subjected to (e.g., violent, sexual, material). But can we agree whether all victims should have the same rights and should receive the same treatment? Contrary to the notion of needs, which by their very nature are as diverse as the population concerned, the concept of rights opens the gate to a flood of endless questions. Are all victims equal? Do they all have the same rights, or do certain victims have more rights than others? Are certain categories of victims more worthy of rights than others? Are there different classes of victims? Are there good victims and bad victims, innocent victims and guilty victims, clean victims and dirty-hand victims? Does increased vulnerability generate more rights? If so, what other victim characteristics should also lead to increased rights? Do victims of intentional criminal acts have more rights than victims of negligence, recklessness, or imprudence, or victims of accidents? Do victims of rape and sexual assaults have more rights than victims whose assault and injuries were not sexually motivated? Do victims of terrorism, torture, or kidnapping have more rights than other victims, and if so, why? Some years ago in France, a law was passed to provide preferential treatment to victims of so-called terrorist attacks (*attentats*). If the answer to any of these questions is negative, one has to ask whether, in practice, all victims are treated in an equal manner. One has to ask whether all victims are perceived in the same way, whether they receive equal consideration from the police, prosecutors, judges, and victim compensation boards. Is equality among victims a right worth fighting for?

Unfortunately, advocates of victims' rights have been very selective in their endeavors and have not campaigned equally on behalf of all crime victims. According to Frank Weed [1995:45]:

The crimes that constitute official crime statistics do not always represent the crimes that are of central concern for the victim rights movement. The major crimes that are central to the victims' movement are murder, rape, domestic violence, child sexual abuse, abducted children, elder abuse, and drunk driving.

This listing by Frank Weed makes it clear that the rights of the vast majority of crime victims have not been a primary concern of those advocating victims' rights and have not figured prominently on their agenda. It also shows that in the final analysis, and despite our vehement denials, we do create different classes of victims and do consider certain victims to be worthier than others [Fattah, 2001b:83–86].

3.4.3 Selectivity, Inequality, and Discrimination in the Treatment of Crime Victims*

3.4.3.1 Worthless, Deserving, Disposable, and Socially Expendable Victims

To anyone who values equality and abhors discrimination, the differential reaction to, as well as the differential treatment of, certain victims of violence is nothing less than shocking! The prevalent attitude that violent victimization of certain individuals or groups should be of no concern to us because those who are victimized simply got what they deserve or have brought it on themselves is a dangerous, uncaring, and, in many respects, inhumane attitude. The shocking apathy or indifference to the pain and suffering, to the injury, and even death of some fellow citizens because they supposedly "deserved" what they got is in sharp contrast to the strong emotions of pity, empathy, and compassion felt and exhibited toward those whom we define, according to our moral and ideological beliefs, as "innocent victims." In many instances, more sympathy is shown at the victimization of an animal, be it a cat, a dog, or whatever, than is shown toward those who are judged to be "unworthy" or "expendable" victims! As if the past misbehavior of those victims, as horrible as it may be, is a ground for depriving them of the quality of being human. I find it perplexing, even revolting, that the humanitarianism that guides our actions toward our fellow citizens who are victimized by violence or crime is not extended to those whom we define, using dubious moral standards, as "social trash" or "social junk" [Fattah, 2003a]. In a chapter I wrote for *The International Handbook of Violence Research*, I coined the term *socially expendable victims* [2003a] to describe those groups who are considered culturally, socially, and politically to be expendable.

---

* This section is based mainly on Fattah [2003a, b].

Members of such groups could be rightly described as "culturally legitimate targets." Not infrequently, lethal violence against some of those who are socially burdensome, unneeded, or worthless is welcomed as one way of ridding society of certain unwanted elements. Lesser forms of violence against the others are encouraged, condoned, or simply ignored. The outright relief or the startling indifference that often greets the violence against them is in sharp contrast to the outrage and demands for punishment that greets violent acts directed at the "valued" groups of society. The reaction of the authorities and the general public to the victimization of these "devalued" citizens is simply appalling. There is no outpour of sympathy. No one seems sorry for the victim. There is no outcry of indignation, and little (if anything) is done to find, pursue, and bring to justice those who are responsible for the victimization. The few offenders who are occasionally caught are often treated with great leniency by the courts [Fattah, 1997a:160].

Members of those expendable groups (and they are fairly numerous) may be described as *social junk*, to use a term coined by Steven Spitzer [1975] to refer to those members of society who do not play an important role in the system of capitalist production. The proneness of those groups to violence is often the outcome of a complex interaction between their personal attributes and social attitudes. Certain attributes of those individuals (e.g., deviant lifestyle, old age, unproductivity, physical or mental handicap) render them easy prey to various forms of violence, whereas the negative attitudes toward them invite or facilitate their victimization. This makes them popular and easy targets, not only for violence perpetrated by individuals and groups but also for institutional violence as well. A single example will suffice to illustrate the extreme vulnerability of those expendable groups. As unbelievable as it may seem, shocking eugenic practices persisted in some Canadian provinces (such as Alberta and British Columbia) way into the 1960s. Mentally handicapped persons (and those who were misdiagnosed as such) were institutionalized and involuntarily sterilized. These insidious practices came to light only some years ago when a number of victims filed civil suits against the government seeking compensation.

The idea that certain groups in society are expendable, and may (or should) therefore be disposed of, may seem both shocking and far-fetched. To designate groups of fellow citizens as *social trash* or *social refuse* may seem offensive. However, this is precisely how certain individuals and certain groups are defined by the culture, and by the economic and political systems, and how they are viewed by the general public or by the dominant groups in society. The death penalty is one example of state violence against one of these expendable groups. The killing of newborn babies, particularly girls, in preindustrialized societies is one of the oldest forms of violence against the socially unneeded. But the killing of the aged, the infirm, the deformed, the severely disabled, and the mentally handicapped is still a common practice in some remote and tribal communities. The killing is sometimes motivated by egoistic considerations (ridding the community of unwanted, unneeded, unproductive, and burdensome members) and other times by altruistic motives where it is used as a form of euthanasia or mercy killing aimed at putting an end to the pain and suffering of the victims. Over the years, with social evolution, killing gave way in certain circumstances to lesser and more subtle forms of violence. The definition of the socially unwanted/unneeded also underwent certain changes, although unproductivity remained an important criterion for determining who is socially expendable. The belief that certain groups are expendable is not limited to a given society, a specific culture, or a certain political or economic system. In totalitarian societies such attitude applies to dissidents, to troublemakers, to those perceived as a threat to the regime, and so forth. In capitalist societies it applies to those who live on the fringes of society and to those who are socially unproductive. Often, it makes little difference whether their lack of productivity is involuntary, the result of advanced age (ageism), mental or physical handicap, or is believed to be voluntary as in the case of vagrants, hobos, beggars, tramps, drug addicts, and alcoholics. In a society dominated by the protestant work ethic, where the greatest emphasis is put on productivity, being unproductive, be it a personal choice or the result of an unwanted condition, becomes a social handicap. Unproductive citizens are viewed not only as noncontributing members but also as a burden, as "parasites," as people living off the sweat and hard work of others [Fattah, 2003a, b].

How much does society care about the prevalent victimization of inmates in penal institutions whether at the hands of other inmates or prison guards? How much victim assistance and how many victim services are available to those who are victimized behind bars? Does the fact that they committed a crime for which they are being punished negate their rights as victims or allow the society that put them in prison to deny them the victim status? Is it not shocking that some victim compensation schemes explicitly exclude inmates of penal institutions who are violently victimized (e.g., the *Compensation Act* of New South Wales, Australia)?

Who cares about the victims of police brutality and unlawful police actions, such as illegal arrest, search, and seizure? Who cares about victims of abuse of power, or victims who become sick, injured, or even die as a result of corporate wrongdoing or white collar crime? What assistance programs and what services are available to those victims?

Are drug addicts, alcoholics, criminals, and sex trade workers, when victimized, treated in the same manner by the police and other social services as other victims? Hatty [1989] contends that the discriminatory attitude toward violence against prostitutes is especially obvious in instances in which prostitutes are killed. In such cases, prostitutes are often portrayed as expendable objects, and their deaths are considered less worthy of attention than those of nonprostitutes. In support of her contention, Hatty quotes Sir Michael Havers, the Attorney General of Britain at the time of the killings perpetrated by Peter Sutcliffe, known as "the Yorkshire Ripper." Commenting on Sutcliffe's victims, the Attorney General publicly declared: "Some were prostitutes, but perhaps the saddest part of this case is that some were not." In other words, if you are a prostitute your killing is not as tragic or as attention-worthy as that of another woman!

One can also wonder how many homosexuals, drug addicts, alcoholics, gang members, or members of minority groups decide to endure their victimization in silence, rather than report it and risk a secondary victimization at the hands of the agents of the criminal justice system who are supposedly there to protect them?

3.4.4 Creating a Normative Hierarchy of Victims

What is distressing but true is that society, the agents of the criminal justice system, and, to a certain extent, those involved in victim assistance and victim services have created a normative hierarchy of victims. As a result, they impute to those who are victimized superiority or inferiority based on their own moral judgments and their personal beliefs about the worth of the victim. They create moral categories of victims: guilty victims and innocent victims, good victims and bad victims, worthy victims and unworthy victims, deserving victims and undeserving victims. In any other field, such moral and ideological distinctions would have been a serious cause for consternation and condemnation. One can imagine what the reaction would be were the members of another helping profession (be it medicine, nursing, psychology, or psychiatry) engaged in similar value judgments and discriminatory practices based on their personal assessments of who deserves and who does not deserve to be treated or helped! Can we imagine any of those helping professions coming to the rescue of some and ignoring others because they deem the survival of the former to be more important than the survival of the latter, or because the former are considered more worthy of treatment and assistance than the latter? Is it too naïve or too idealistic to believe that pity, empathy, compassion, and commiseration are not emotions to be dispensed selectively according to the victim's race, color, religion, social class, occupation, behavior, or lifestyle? Humaneness and humanitarianism are indivisible. To be humane and to show kindness to some victims while being inhumane and showing apathy, indifference, and lack of compassion to other victims seems to be a serious contradiction [Fattah, 1986]. However, those prejudicial and discriminatory attitudes toward different types of victims are extremely widespread. How much sympathy or empathy is felt for gang members victimized by rival gangs, for members of organized crime liquidated in gangland slayings? One has to admit that despite utterances to the contrary, society does condone or even encourage acts of violence against certain individuals or against members of certain groups because they are deemed responsible for what befalls them.

The marginalization of certain groups—either by reason of their attributes or lifestyle—contributes to their isolation and thus promotes their victimization. Members of those groups become defined as culturally *legitimate victims* (a term coined by Weiss and Borges [1973]), whose victimization is perceived as justifiable or insufficiently reprehensible to warrant condemnation or even indignation. They are explicitly or implicitly designated as "fair game," as appropriate targets for violent (and nonviolent) victimization.

Another way by which society encourages or promotes violence against members of those groups is to make them appear culpable, guilty, or blameworthy in some manner, and thus deserving to be victimized. By demonizing certain groups, by attributing to them a host of negative qualities, by denouncing some of their traits or behaviors, by questioning their loyalty, by depreciating their worth, by devaluating their status, their role, and their contribution, and by degrading, debasing, and vilifying them, society turns them into outcasts, whose containment, elimination, or extermination is appropriate and desirable. Instead of evoking the normal feelings of pity and sympathy when victimized, their victimization is met with a sense of relief and contentment.

3.4.5 Impact of Social Prejudices on Victim Policy and on Service Delivery to Crime Victims

The concept of social expendability describes a specific social attitude toward less fortunate members of society who, for one reason or another, are seen as dangerous, culpable, burdensome, troublesome, unproductive, worthless, unwanted, and hence disposable. What is rather ironical, when talking about victim assistance and victim services, is the tendency to forget that the vast majority of victims of violence do in fact belong to those demonized, marginalized, and ostracized groups. They are the ones who suffer the greatest burden of violent victimization, but they are also the ones who benefit the least from the services and programs made available to crime victims. The reasons for this tragic situation are many: lack of accessibility, lack of willingness to interact with and to use state-operated or -funded programs, etc. To add insult to injury, those in charge of those services often shun the few members of those marginalized groups who are desperate enough to seek help from victim services. Why? Because they do not fit the typical stereotype or the normal profile of crime victim!

As victim services mirror the views and attitudes of the larger society they are bound to share the prejudices and biases of the society in which they operate. One bias that is prevalent in our societies is a false dichotomy between victims and offenders. The two groups are erroneously viewed as mutually exclusive and antagonistic populations, as different as black and white, as night and day. In the eyes of the ordinary citizen, offenders and victims represent guilt and innocence, evil versus good, cunning, skillful, and uncontrolled predators victimizing helpless and unsuspecting individuals, hungry wolves preying on defenseless lambs. These popular perceptions are, and have always been, influenced by the biblical story of Cain and Abel. As popular as those perceptions are, they are in stark contrast to the empirical reality of the revolving and interchangeable roles of victim and victimizer [Fattah, 1994b]. In dealing with victims and offenders, we are always inclined to look only at the current incident, the crime that has been committed, and to ignore or disregard anything else. We tend to forget about the social histories of the parties involved, as if it is totally irrelevant that today's offenders are yesterday's victims and today's victims are tomorrow's offenders. To define the parties solely in function of the current incident is to take a very myopic view of crime. The current incident is merely a snapshot in the life of the offender. Most of the time it is the outcome of a long victimization history; it is merely the most recent reaction to their previous victimization.

The popular, yet erroneous, predator-prey model of criminal victimization—the active aggressor and the passive sufferer—is sharply contradicted by empirical facts and the findings of victimological research. Susan Smith [1986:98], for example, reports that:

> Empirical research is increasingly gnawing away at the concept of mutually exclusive offender and victim populations, showing it to be a figment of political imagination and a sop to social conscience. . . . In some instances, therefore, it may be most appropriate to analyze crime as a form of social interaction arising out of specific social contexts in which the distinction between offender and victim is not always conceptually helpful. This is particularly true of direct contact crimes against the person.

In view of the ever-growing body of research findings, it seems futile to deny, minimize, or de-emphasize the substantial homogeneity, the affinity, the similarities, and the overlap between the victim and offender populations [Reiss, 1981; Singer, 1981; Smith, 1986; Fattah, 1991a].

3.5 Victimology: The Practice

3.5.1 Victim Support and Victim Services: The Balance Sheet

To remedy the situation of neglect that existed for centuries, to do justice to the victims, and to alleviate their plight, many changes were introduced in the past four decades. Victim compensation schemes, victim assistance programs, and other victim services have been in existence for more than a quarter of a century. The time has come to examine the balance sheet, to assess the effectiveness and success of those initiatives, and to evaluate the impact they have had on improving the sad lot of crime victims. To what extent have they achieved their avowed goals, their enunciated objectives? Have they been successful in doing what they were supposed to do, and with good results?

Unfortunately, most evaluations of victim programs, victim services, and other victim initiatives, rather than highlighting positive achievements, generally point to a negative balance sheet. For political and ideological reasons, the new policies and initiatives, despite the great fanfare that accompanied their introduction, targeted only a few categories of victims. The vast majority of crime victims remained without help, assistance, care, or compensation.

The conclusions of the experts who have studied the programs and services are definitely discouraging and hardly inspire much confidence in the programs or much optimism about their future. State compensation programs for crime victims, introduced in the mid-1960s, created a great deal of expectations that were never met. The programs were described as political palliatives [Burns, 1980], political placebos [Chappell, 1972], and "Band-Aid" measures, even as a symbolic humanitarian gesture.

Victim support, writes Maguire and Pointing [1988], remains essentially a grassroots, low-budget enterprise that relies on the goodwill and hard work of volunteers. Shapland et al. [1985] maintain that the major projects aimed at fulfilling victims' needs were set up without regard to, or even investigation into, victims' expressed needs. Rock [1990] insists that victims' interests were never the motivating or mobilizing force behind the new initiatives to help victims. Mawby and Gill [1987:228] detected a right-wing, law-and-order focus among victim support scheme volunteers. They expressed concerns that crime victims might become "the victims of political expediency." Elias [1992] affirms that victims' services really serve official needs, not victims' needs.

3.5.2 State Compensation for Crime Victims: The Quest for Universality*

To remedy the problem of selectivity, inequality, and discrimination in the treatment of victims of crime, I have, over the years, repeatedly proposed a universal state insurance system for crime victims similar to traffic accident insurance, labor accident insurance, unemployment insurance, etc., but the idea was always summarily rejected as a utopian dream. Therefore, although almost all other risks are covered in the welfare state by some form of

---

* This section is based mainly on Fattah [1999a].

insurance, the risk of becoming a victim of crime is not. This leads in practice to flagrant injustices. In Canada, for example, if someone is killed, injured, or disabled as a result of a car accident, plane crash, ski lift mishap, medical malpractice, or pharmaceutical error, he or she (or heirs) can receive millions of dollars in compensation. If the death or injury resulted from a criminal act, the maximum award available from the criminal injuries compensation scheme can be as low as $20,000. Because state compensation schemes are strictly and explicitly limited to victims of violent or sex crimes, the vast majority of victims receive no compensation whatsoever for the losses they have suffered. In the United States, Karmen [1996:332] reports that the rate of compensation in a particular state in a given year, calculated as the proportion of crimes actually compensated, compared to all reported crimes that are potentially eligible for compensation was as low as 1% in Michigan and averaged out at 19%. Add to this the fact that most victims of property crime, who are usually excluded from state compensation schemes, do not have and cannot afford private insurance. Their plight becomes evident when keeping in mind that in four of five cases of those property crimes, the culprit is neither identified nor caught. The few who are arrested, charged, and convicted are, more often than not, poor or so insolvent that nothing can be obtained from them through a civil judgment. To add insult to injury, in most countries, the collection of criminal fines continues to have priority over the payment of civil damages or of restitution/compensation orders [Fattah, 1999a].

Victims of violence for whom the schemes were designed in the first place do not fare much better. The conditions of eligibility for state compensation are such that only a small fraction does qualify. In almost all systems, eligibility is contingent on reporting the offense to the police and the victims' willingness to cooperate with the criminal justice system. Moreover, many schemes have a means test ensuring that compensation is given only to the poorest of the poor. Most exclude violence among family members, whereas a good part of all violence occurs in domestic settings! Most schemes also exclude (or drastically reduce the awards to) victims who provoked or otherwise contributed to their own victimization. One sure way of making the majority of victims of violence ineligible for state compensation is to set a high minimum limit for compensation below which victims do not qualify. In the United Kingdom, for example, the lower limit was set at £1,000, despite the recommendations made by victims groups to remove it. The burden of proof is on the victim, and it is easy to imagine how difficult it can be to prove that the injury resulted from a criminal attack when the attacker has run away and there are no witnesses. With the exception of sexual victimization, most schemes do not provide funds to compensate the victim's emotional pain and suffering [Fattah, 1999a].

It is not surprising that many victims are deterred from applying by the lengthy bureaucratic procedures and the investigative process. According to Maguire and Shapland [1997] compensation procedures in the Netherlands are very bureaucratic, require the participation of lawyers, and ensure delays of more than two years before awards are made. The findings of van Dijk [1989] affirm that the great dissatisfaction with the operation of the schemes is such that victim support associations are not recommending them to victims. More distressing still is that many victims are simply unaware of the existence of the schemes. As in many jurisdictions, the budget is determined in advance and cannot be exceeded; the more applications the program receives, the lower are the awards. Because the schemes are poorly funded in the first place, successful applicants usually receive ridiculously low amounts as compensation for their victimization. Therefore, it is easy to understand why in some countries there is a deliberate attempt not to publicize those state compensation schemes [Fattah, 1999a].

Smith and Hillenbrand [1997] examined three ways that victims may be repaid for the financial harm inflicted on them: restitution, victim–offender reconciliation programs, and compensation. They found that only a small minority of victims benefit from these programs. Among the reasons they give for this sad reality is the lack of awareness about the programs, the inability or unwillingness of defendants to pay restitution, an insufficiency of state funds to compensate victims, and limits on which victims are eligible for compensation.

If this brief description of state compensation schemes to victims of crime is accurate, and I believe it is, then it is fair to say that their primary function is not really to financially help victims or alleviate their distress but to assuage society's conscience and appease the guilt we feel about the plight of the victims. The sad conclusion that state compensation is not really meant to serve the interests of crime victims is supported by Rock's [1990] revelations about the history and politics of victim compensation in England and Wales. Having traced and analyzed the history of state compensation programs to victims of violence, Rock concluded [1990:408]:

> Criminal injuries compensation was supposed to mollify the reactionary victim-vigilante, and reparation was a device to divert offenders from custody. In both instances, victims were the creatures of penal imperatives, invested with the characters needed to get on with the business of reforming prisons. Compensation and reparation did not have much of a foundation in the declared or observed requirements of victims themselves: they were bestowed on victims in order to achieve particular ends.

The same observation was made by Törnudd [1996]. He reports that the Finnish State Committee, which, in 1972, proposed a law granting victims the right to demand compensation from state funds, was explicitly motivated in its proposal by "the need to lessen the aggressive feelings of the general public towards offenders" [Törnudd:127].

Despite the lip service that politicians pay to crime victims, several governments have decided in recent years to transfer the financial burden of victim compensation to offenders through a levy called a *victim fine surcharge*. This surcharge is imposed on those who are sentenced to a fine, even when the sentence is for so-called victimless crimes [Fattah, 1999a, 2000a].

3.5.3 The Dangers of Victim Therapy

In my keynote address to the Ninth International Symposium on Victimology [Amsterdam, 1997], I drew attention to the huge expansion of therapeutic interventions with crime victims. I highlighted some of the actual and potential dangers of victim therapy [Fattah, 1999a]. One of the biggest fads at the time was the highly questionable and extremely dangerous psychological notion of so-called *repressed memory syndrome* [Loftus and Ketcham, 1991, 1994]. Another danger I drew attention to is the psychological trauma resulting from the overzealous criminal justice intervention with children suspected of having been sexually abused [Eberle and Eberle, 1993]. To buttress my criticism of therapeutic interventions, I emphasized the potential healing functions of self-blame. In an attempt to illustrate the stigmatizing and traumatizing effects of victim labeling, I used the concept of the *Mark of Abel*.

3.5.3.1 *The Mark of Abel**

Crime victims, regardless of the type of victimization they suffer, need different types of support and varying kinds of assistance. They need practical services such as fixing the lock, replacing the window, or driving the kids to school. They need information and advice, particularly on how to avoid future victimization. They might need referral to other services or legal assistance. They need a great deal of emotional support. None of these types of services is problematic, and the more of them are available to the victim after the event, the better. It is the other kind of well-intentioned support—counseling, therapy, and treatment—that can pose real problems and that may produce negative and undesirable side effects.

Luckily enough, while preparing my keynote address for the Amsterdam symposium, I came across the July 1997 issue of the *Harvard Mental Health Letter* published by the reputable Harvard Medical School. It contained a brief article by Dr. Robert A. Hahn [1997] that included a statement that bears great relevance to the discipline of victimology and the field of victim

---

* This section is based on Fattah [1999a:195–200].

assistance. Speaking of harmful effects, using the Latin word *nocebo*, Hahn wrote [ibid.:8]:

> Nocebo effects are different in different cultures because societies teach their members which illnesses exist, which symptoms indicate the illnesses, how they are acquired, and how they are treated. These categories may promote as well as describe illness; causing the pathologies they are meant to heal.

Reading Hahn's statement immediately brought to my mind some of the dangers I outlined in the early history of the victim movement [Fattah, 1986, 1992e]. I wondered then, as I do now, whether the outpouring of sympathy for crime victims was doing more harm than good, and whether it was hurting victims rather than facilitating and speeding their recovery. The amplification of the negative effects of victimization and the pathologizing of the normal reactions it evokes might have been done with the best of intentions. But by doing so, victim advocates portrayed and communicated to crime victims (actual and potential) a specific pattern of suffering that almost forces them to feel and behave in a certain manner. Victims feel compelled to conform to this pattern of suffering because otherwise they might not be, or be seen as, normal or typical victims. Thus, by trying hard to highlight the intense suffering some victims might go through and to draw attention to their plight, and by trying to help them cope with the negative effects of victimization, victim advocates might inadvertently create undue suffering.

A good illustration of the dangers is the moving story of a 25-year-old woman from Nova Scotia, Canada, who as a child had been a victim of incest and who as a grown-up mother was denied custody of her 5-year-old son, allegedly because she has not received psychological therapy to deal with her childhood victimization. The woman's words as she was interviewed by the Canadian Press [*Globe and Mail*, 1997:A3] are very telling. They illustrate what I mean when saying that we force victims into specific patterns of suffering, inculcating in their minds that they cannot cope on their own and that their recovery hinges on getting the appropriate psychological or psychiatric treatment. Here is what the victim said:

> They are classifying me as this person who can't get anywhere in life because this happened, that no one can overcome something that terrible. But they don't know me. I didn't give up on life because this happened to me. It made me the person I am now.

Then she added:

> I don't believe I need help, okay? Not at the present time. Maybe when I am 50, it might bother me, or even when I am 29. But right now my life is going in a positive direction, and it's not something that even affects me.

One cannot help but say, "Good for you!" But one then wonders how many other victims gave up on life because they believed what they were told: that the trauma of victimization lasts a lifetime, that they will forever suffer from what they endured in their early childhood. There is an important lesson to be learned from the experience of the Nova Scotia victim. It tells us to exercise a great deal of caution before labeling victims with the *mark of Abel* [Fattah, 1999a].

3.5.4 Potential Nocebo Effects of Intervention

Telling victims of incest, rape, sexual assault, or other types of victimization that the effects are disastrous, nefarious, too serious, too traumatic, long-lasting, and telling them that they cannot cope on their own without the help of psychiatrists, psychologists, sex therapists, and social workers can easily become a self-fulfilling prophecy. It can delay the process of natural healing and the process of self-recovery. It can be particularly damaging in the case of impressionable young children. For example, in many cases of incest or child sexual abuse, the children are too young to understand the wrongfulness of the behavior or to realize the seriousness of what happened. It is the parents, the child welfare workers, the therapists, and the criminal justice personnel (e.g., police, prosecutors) who, through their questions, attitudes, and behavior, communicate to the child that something really awful has been done to them. By so doing, these professionals can themselves create what may be a long-lasting trauma. In other words, the help and assistance they try to give the child victim can produce more trauma than the trauma of the victimization itself [Fattah, 1994a, 1999a, 2001a].

Surprisingly, the message victims often get from those trying to help them is the opposite of the one usually offered by physicians and psychiatrists to their patients. In their attempts to aid and hasten a patient's recovery, those well-trained professionals usually take a reassuring stance, trying to minimize the seriousness of the ailment while emphasizing the potential for recovery. They try to foster in the patient an aura of optimism rather than distress, pessimism, or despair. This positive, supportive attitude is in sharp contrast to the one exhibited *vis-à-vis* crime victims [Fattah, 1999a].

Even seemingly innocent, harmless slogans such as "justice for victims" or "victims deserve better" may prove detrimental to victims' interests and well-being. Such slogans are invariably interpreted as a call for more and harsher punishment for the victimizers. As such, they tend to create among victims expectations that may not be easily fulfilled, such as the promise of severe sanctions—death, long prison sentences, denial of parole—which too often cannot be met in practice. This is a sure recipe for producing angry, bitter, resentful, and frustrated victims. Fomenting victims' vindictiveness and hailing revenge as the ultimate goal of justice inevitably leave a host of unhappy, unsatisfied victims who feel betrayed whenever the goal has not been attained and every time punishment falls short of their heightened expectations. Those who knowingly or unwittingly fuel the vindictiveness of victims might be doing them a disservice because this emotion does not facilitate closure and delays the healing process [Fattah, 1999a].

Well-intentioned assistance practices may also hurt crime victims in other ways. There is a widespread, yet misguided, belief that every well-intentioned reform is bound to yield good results and should therefore be enthusiastically (and unquestioningly) endorsed. Social scientists know better. They are fully aware of the potentially disastrous consequences of doing good. Those who want examples need only look at the noble attempts to assimilate North America's first nations, and the Aborigines in Australia, to save their souls and secure them a place in heaven. Criminologists are painfully aware of the countless intervention programs and techniques aimed at treating, helping, and rehabilitating young offenders that produce the opposite results, intensifying delinquent activities and prolonging a delinquent career. The field of victim assistance is no different. Intervention with victims (victim therapy), although widely regarded as being in their best interest and as necessary, beneficial, and commendable, can also have adverse, unanticipated ill effects. This is perhaps the saddest aspect of victim support, the possibility that those who genuinely try to help victims may inadvertently hurt them. No discussion of victim assistance and services would be complete without pointing out the dangers inherent in such assistance [Fattah, 1999a].

3.6 Conclusion

Science and partisanship are incompatible. They do not go hand in hand. Once researchers take sides or become advocates they lose their neutrality, their objectivity, and their credibility. This is a fundamental principle that should be seriously considered by those well-intentioned criminologists and victimologists who have adopted the cause of crime victims and who claim to speak on their behalf. It flies in the face of those victim advocates who try incessantly to separate victimology from criminology and to create a political and ideological enterprise that has nothing to do with science [Fattah, 2008].

The future of victimology will depend on its ability to return to its original scientific role, to shed its ideological mantle, and to resume its role as a scholarly discipline and as an integral part of criminology. It is the need to separate research from action and science from activism that dictates that victimology be separated from victim policy. To restore the neutrality of victimology and to regain and maintain its scientific integrity, it has to detach itself from politics and ideology. It was precisely the need to affirm the non normative and nonideological character of criminology that led some of the most distinguished criminologists of the twentieth century, such as Thorsten Sellin [1938] and Hermann Mannheim [1965], to name a few, to call for divorcing criminal policy from criminology.

As early as 1938, Sellin suggested that the term *criminology* be used to designate only the body of *scientific* knowledge and the deliberate pursuit of such knowledge. He then proposed that the technical use of knowledge in the treatment and prevention of crime be separate. As he could not find a suitable term to designate this field, he hinted that it may be called *crimino-technology*.

Three decades later, Hermann Mannheim [1965:13] suggested that criminal policy be treated as a discipline apart rather than as an integral part of criminology. Affirming the nonnormative character of criminology, Mannheim believed it is preferable that questions of what ought to be done to reform the criminal law and the penal system be treated as a separate discipline based on the factual findings of the criminologist and the penologist. Criminology, he insisted, should remain a non-policymaking discipline that regards the "ends" as beyond its province. Mannheim hastened to add that this does not prevent the criminologist from advocating a certain measure of legal and administrative penal reform, but he or she has to do so as a politician or an ordinary citizen and voter rather than in the capacity of criminologist.

In line with their thinking I suggest that the term *victimology* be used only to designate the body of scientific knowledge related to victims and the pursuit of such knowledge. The advice Mannheim [1965] offered to criminologists applies equally to victimology. Victimology should remain a scholarly, scientific endeavor, a non-policymaking discipline that regards the "ends" as beyond its province. I would also hasten to add that the wisdom of such advice was never as evident as it is today.

A fact that is often ignored or overlooked in the social sciences is that the pursuit of knowledge and the practical application or implementation of that knowledge are two different, distinct, and separate endeavors. The pursuit of knowledge for knowledge's sake, as in anthropology, archeology, or history, is a laudable and worthwhile exercise, whether the knowledge has or does not have any practical applications. It is a more valuable pursuit because it is neutral and does not carry with it the danger that the acquired knowledge may be misused or deformed when applied [Fattah, 2008].

Dedication

I dedicate this chapter to my dear colleagues and fellow victimologists, Professor Tony Peters (Leuven) and Professor Marc S. Groenhuijsen (Tilburg).

References

Amernic, J. 1984. *Victims: The orphans of justice.* Toronto: McClelland and Stewart.

Anttila, I. 1964. The criminological significance of unregistered criminality. *Excerpta Criminologica* 4:411.

Aspelin, E., N. Bishop, H. Thornstedt, and P. Tornudd. 1975. *Some developments in Nordic criminal policy.* Stockholm: Scandinavian Research Council for Criminology.

Bass, E. and L. Davis. 1988. *The courage to heal: A guide for women survivors of child sexual abuse,* 3rd ed. New York: HarperCollins.

Becker, H. 1963. *Outsiders.* London: Free Press of Glencoe.

Berk, R. A., A. Campbell, R. Klap, and B. Western. 1992. The deterrent effect of arrest: A Bayesian analysis of four field experiments. *American Sociological Review* 57:698–708.

Berzins, L. 1990. Wife assault and the criminal justice system. *Vis a Vis* 8(2):1.

Biderman, A. D. 1967. Survey of population samples for estimating crime incidence. *The Annals of the American Academy of Political and Social Science* 374:16–33.

Biderman, A. D. and A. J. Reiss, Jr. 1967. On exploring the dark figure of crime. *The Annals of the American Academy of Political and Social Science* 374:1–15.

Bilsky, W. and P. Wetzels. 1992. Victimization and crime: Normative and individual standards of evaluation. *International Annals of Criminology* 32(1/2): 135–52.

Bisson, J. I. and M. P. Deahl. 1994. Psychological debriefing and prevention of posttraumatic stress—more research is needed. *British Journal of Psychiatry* (165):717–20.

Boutellier, J. C. J. 1993. *Solidariteit en Slachtofferschap: De morele betekenis van criminaliteit in een postmoderne cultur.* Nijmegen: SUN.

Brantingham, P. J. and P. L. Brantingham. 1984. *Patterns in crime.* New York: Macmillan.

Burns, P. 1980. *Criminal injuries compensation: Social remedy or political palliative for victims of crime.* Toronto: Butterworths.

Canada. 1992. Canadian Homicide Statistics 1991. Ottawa: *Juristat.* Published by Statistics Canada.

Carlier, I. V. E., R. D. Lamberts, B. P. R., Gersons, and A. J. Van Uchelen. 1995. *Het lange-termijn effect van debriefen: Een Vervolgonderzoek bij de Amsterdamse Politie Naar Aanleiding van de Bijlmerramp.* Amsterdam, NETH: Academic Medical Centre, University of Amsterdam.

Chapman, D. 1968. *Sociology and the stereotype of the criminal.* London: Tavistock.

Chappell, D. 1972. Providing for the victim of crime: political placebos or progressive programs? *Adelaide Law Review* (4):294–306.

Chase, N. F. 1976. *A child is being beaten.* New York: McGraw-Hill.

Christie, N. 1977. Conflicts as property. *British Journal of Criminology* 17(1):1–17.

Cornish, D. B. and R. V. Clarke. 1986. *The reasoning criminal: Rational choice perspective on offending.* New York: Springer Verlag.

Cozijn, C. 1984. *Schadefonds Geweldsmisdrijven.* The Hague: Dutch Ministry of Justice.

Cressey, D. R. 1985. Research implications of conflicting conceptions of victimology. In *International action and study of victims*, ed. Z. P. Separovic, 43–54. Zagreb: University of Zagreb. Reprinted in 1992 In *Towards a Critical Victimology*, ed. E. A. Fattah. London: Macmillan.

Crews, F., H. P. Blum, M. Cavell, M. Eagle, and F. Crews. 1995. *The memory wars: Freud's legacy in dispute*. New York: New York Review Books.

Davis, R. 1987. Studying the effects of services for victims in crisis. *Crime & Delinquency* 33(4):520–31.

Davis, R. C. and M. Henley. 1990. Victim service programs. In *Victims of crime, problems, policies and programs*, ed. A. J. Lurigio, W. S. Skogan, and R. C. Davis, 157–71. Newbury Park, CA: Sage.

Denno, D. W. 1990. *Biology and violence: From birth to adulthood*. Cambridge: Cambridge University Press.

Doerner, W. 1978. A quasi-experimental analysis of selected victim compensation programs. *Canadian Journal of Criminology* 20(3):239–51.

Driver, E. 1961. Interaction and criminal homicide in India. *Social Forces* 40:153–58.

Eberle, P. and S. Eberle. 1993. *The abuse of innocence: The McMartin pre-school trial*. Buffalo, NY: Prometheus Books.

Elias, R. 1983a. *Victims of the system: Crime victims and compensation in American politics and criminal justice*. New Brunswick, NJ: Transaction Books.

_____. 1983b. The symbolic politics of victim compensation. *Victimology* 8(1–2): 213–24.

_____. 1992a. Which victim movement? The politics of victim policy. In *Towards a critical victimology*, ed. E. A. Fattah, 74–99. London and New York: Macmillan and St. Martin's.

_____. 1992b. Community control, criminal justice and victim services. In *Towards a critical victimology*, ed. E. A Fattah, 372–97. London and New York: Macmillan and St. Martin's.

_____. 1994. Has victimology outlived its usefulness? *The Journal of Human Justice* 6(Autumn):4–25.

Ennis, P. H. 1967. *Criminal victimization in the United States: A report of a national survey*. Washington, DC: U.S. Government Printing Office.

Fattah, E. A. 1966. Quelques problemes poses a la justice penale par la victimologie. *Annales Internationales de Criminologie* 5(2):335–61.

_____. 1967a. La Victimologie: Qu'est-elle et quel est son avenir? (premiere partie). *Revue Internationale de Criminologie et de Police Technique*. 21(2): 113–24.

_____. 1967b. La Victimologie: Qu'est-elle et quel est son avenir? (suite et fin). *Revue Internationale de Criminologie et de Police Technique*. 21(3):192–202.

_____. 1973. Le rôle de la victime dans le passage a l'acte. *Revue Internationale de Criminologie et de Police Technique*. 36(2):173–88.

_____. 1976. The use of the victim as an agent of self-legitimization: Towards a dynamic explanation of criminal behaviour. In *Victims and society*, ed. E. C. Viano, 105–29. Washington, DC: Visage.

_____. 1978. Moving to the right: A return to punishment? *Crime and Justice* 6(2):79–92.

_____. 1979. Some recent theoretical developments in victimology. *Victimology: An International Journal* 4:198–213.

_____. 1980a. *Crime and the abuse of power: Offences and offenders beyond the reach of the law*. Final General Report Published in English and French by the International Society of Criminology, International Association of Penal Law, International Society for Social Defense, and the International Penal and Penitentiary Foundation, Milan, Italy, 70–92.

_____. 1980b. Victimologie: Tendances recentes. *Criminologie* 13(1):6–36.

_____. 1984. Victims' response to confrontational victimization: A neglected aspect of victim research. *Crime and Delinquency* 30(1):75–89.

_____. 1986. On some visible and hidden dangers of victim movements. In *From crime policy to victim policy*, ed. E. A. Fattah, 1–14. London: Macmillan.

_____. 1989a. Victims and victimology: The facts and the rhetoric. *International Review of Victimology* 1(1):1–21.

_____. 1989b. The child as victim: Victimological aspects of child abuse. In *The plight of crime victims in modern society*, ed. E. A. Fattah, 175–209. London: Macmillan.

_____. 1989c. Victims of abuse of power: The David/Goliath syndrome. In *The plight of crime victims in modern society*, ed. E. A. Fattah, 25–69. London: Macmillan.

_____. 1991a. *Understanding criminal victimization*. Scarborough, Ontario: Prentice Hall.

_____. 1991b. From crime policy to victim policy—The need for a fundamental policy change. *International Annals of Criminology* 29:1&2.

_____. 1992a. *Towards a critical victimology*. London and New York: Macmillan and St. Martin's.

_____. 1992b. The need for a critical victimology. In *Towards a critical victimology*, ed. E. A. Fattah, 3–26. London and New York: Macmillan and St. Martin's.

_____. 1992c. Victims and victimology: The facts and the rhetoric. In *Towards a critical victimology*, ed. E. A. Fattah, 29–56. London and New York: Macmillan and St. Martin's.

_____. 1992d. The UN declaration of basic principles of justice for victims of crime and abuse of power: A constructive critique. In *Towards a critical victimology*, ed. E. A. Fattah, 401–24. London and New York: Macmillan and St. Martin's.

_____. 1992e. *The positives and negatives of the victim movement: A critical assessment*. Paper presented at the 4th Symposium on Violence and Aggression, Saskatoon.

_____. 1993a. Research on fear of crime: Some common conceptual and measurement problems, In *Fear of crime and criminal victimization*, ed. W. Bilsky, C. Pfeiffer, and P. Wetzeis, 45–70. Stuttgart: Ferdinand Enke Verlag.

_____. 1993b. La relativite culturelle de la victimisation. *Criminologie* 26(2):121–36.

_____. 1993c. Doing unto others: The revolving roles of victim and victimizer. *Simon Fraser University Alumni Journal* 11(1):12–15.

_____. 1993d. The rational choice/opportunity perspective as a vehicle for integrating criminological and victimological theories. In *Advances in criminological theory*, vol. 5, ed. R. V. Clarke and M. Felson, 225–58. New Brunswick: Transaction.

_____. 1994a. The criminalization of social problems: Child abuse as a case study. In *Mental health law and practice through the life cycle*, ed. S. N. Verdun-Jones and M. Layton, 7–15. Burnaby: Simon Fraser University.

_____. 1994b. The interchangeable roles of victim and victimizer. Second Inkeri Anttila's Honour Lecture. Helsinki, Finland: HEUNI. Translated into Spanish and published in *Cuadernos de Criminologia* (Chile) 1997, 7:23–53.

_____. 1994c. La victimologie au carrefour: Entre la science et l'ideologie. *Présentations à la Société Royale du Canada* 47:159–72.

_____. 1994d. Some recent theoretical developments in victimology. In *Victimology*, ed. P. Rock, 285–300. Dartmouth: Aldershot.

_____. 1994e. Victimology: Some problematic concepts, unjustified criticism and popular misconceptions. In *International Debates of Victimology*, ed. G. F. Kirchhoff, E. Kosovski, and H. J. Schneider, 82–103. Mönchengladbach: WSV.

_____. 1995. La victimologie au carrefour: Entre la science et l'ideologie. *Revue Internationale de Criminologie et de Police Technique* 2:131–39.

_____. 1997a. *Criminology: Past, present and future—a critical overview.* London and New York: Macmillan and St. Martin's.

_____. 1997b. Toward a victim policy aimed at healing not suffering. In *Victims of Crime*, 2nd ed., ed. R. C. Davis, A. J. Lurigio, and W. G. Skogan, 257–72. Thousand Oaks, CA: Sage.

_____. 1999a. From a handful of dollars to tea and sympathy: The sad history of victim assistance. In *Caring for crime victims: Selected proceedings of the 9th international symposium on victimology*, ed. J. J. M. Van Dijk, R. G. H. Van Kaam, and J. Wemmers, 187–206. Monsey, NY: Criminal Justice Press.

_____. 1999b. Moving against the tide—Academics' duty to challenge, defy and contradict. Lecture given on the occasion of receiving The Nora and Ted Sterling Prize in Support of Controversy. Vancouver, October 19, 1999.

_____. 2000a. Victimology: Past, present and future. *Criminologie* 33(1):17–46.

_____. 2000b. Victim assistance in Canada. *Resource Material Series* 56:48–59. Fuchu/Tokyo: UNAFEI.

_____. 2000c. Victimology today: Recent theoretical and applied developments. *Resource Material Series* 56:60–70. Fuchu/Tokyo: UNAFEI.

_____. 2001a. Does victimology need deontology? Ethical conundrums in a young discipline. Proceedings of the 10th International Symposium on Victimology. In *Beyond boundaries: Research and action for the third millennium*, ed. A. Gaudreault and I. Waller, 129–54. Montréal: Association Québécoise Plaidoyer-Victimes. Translated into Spanish and published in *Cuadernos de Criminologia* (Chile) 1997, 11:53–76.

_____. 2001b. Victims rights: Past, present and future. A global view. In *Oeuvre de justice et des victims*, ed. R. Cario and D. Salas, vol. 1, 81–108. Paris: L'Harmattan.

_____. 2001c. Preventing repeat victimization as the ultimate goal of victim services. *International Annals of Criminology* 38(1/2):113–33.

_____. 2003a. Selectivity, inequality and discrimination in the treatment of victims of crime. In *Våldets offer—Vårt ansvar*, ed. G. Nordborg and A. Sigfridsson, 16–36. Stockholm, Sweden: Brottsoffermyndigheten.

_____. 2003b. Violence against the socially expendable. In *International handbook on violence research*, ed. W. Heitmeyer and J. Hagan, 767–83. London: Kluwer Academic.

_____. 2004a. Gearing justice action to victim satisfaction. Contrasting two justice philosophies: Retribution and redress. In *Crime, victims and justice—Essays on principles and practice*, ed. H. Kaptein and M. Malsch, 16–30. Burlington, VT: Ashgate.

_____. 2004b. Positions savantes et ideologiques sur le role de la victime et sa contribution a la genese du crime. In *La victime est-elle coupable? Collection Sciences Criminelles (Les Controverses)*, ed. R. Cario and P. Mbanzoulou, 23–41. Paris: L'Harmattan.

_____. 2006. Le sentiment d'insecurite et la victimisation criminelle dans une perspective de victimologie comparée. In *Une criminologie de la tradition a l'innovation. En hommage à Georges Kellens*, ed. M. Born, F. Kéfer, and A. Lemaître, 89–106. Bruxelles: De Boeck & Larcier.

_____. 2008. The future of criminology as a social science and academic discipline: Reflections on criminology's unholy alliance with criminal policy and on current attempts to divorce victimology from criminology. *International Annals of Criminology* 45:135–70.

Fattah, E. A. and A. Raic. 1970. L'Alcool en tant que facteur victimogène. *Toxicomanies* 3(2):143–73.

Feher, T. L. 1992. The alleged molestation victim. The rules of evidence and the constitution: should children really be seen and not heard? In *Towards a critical victimology*, ed. E. A. Fattah, 260–91. London: Macmillan.

Flynn, E. E. 1982. Theory development in victimology: An assessment of recent programs and of continuing challenges. In *The victim in international perspective*, ed. H. J. Schneider, 96–104. Berlin: De Gruyter.

Friday, P. 1995. *Personal communication to the author.*

Frieze, I. S., M. S. Greenberg, and S. Hymer. 1987. Describing the crime victim: Psychological reactions to victimization. *Professional Psychology, Research and Practice* 18(4):299–315.

Gallaway, B. and J. Hudson. 1981. *Perspectives on crime victims.* St. Louis, MO: C. V. Mosby.

Geis, G. 1990. Crime victims: Practices and prospects. In *Victims of crime: Problems, policies and programs*, ed. A. J. Lurigio, W. G. Skogan, and R. C. Davis, 251–68. Newbury Park, CA: Sage.

Globe and Mail. 1997. Incest victims can't escape past. *Canadian Press Release*, July 7, A3.

Gottfredson, M. R. 1984. *Victims of crime: The dimensions of risk.* Home Office Research and Planning Unit Report No. 81. London: HMSO.

Hahn, R. A. 1997. What is a nocebo? *The Harvard Mental Health Letter* 14(1):8.

Hatty, S. 1989. Violence against prostitute women, *Australian Journal of Social Issues* 24(4):235–48.

Henderson, L. N. 1985. The wrongs of victims' rights. *Stanford Law Review* 37. Reprinted 1992, In *Towards a critical victimology*, ed. E. A. Fattah, 100–192. London and New York: Macmillan and St. Martin's.

Hirschel, J. D., I. W. Hutchison, C. W. Dean, and A. M. Mills. 1992. Review essay on the law enforcement response to spouse abuse. *The Justice Quarterly* 9: 247–83.

Hirschel, J. D., I. W. Hutchison, and C. W. Dean. 1992. The failure of arrest to deter abuse. *Journal of Research in Crime and Delinquency* 29(1):7–33.

Hoyle, C., R. Morgan, and A. Sanders. 1999. The victim's charter—An evaluation of pilot projects. *Home Office Research Findings*, No. 107. London: Research, Development and Statistics Directorate.

Hulsman, L. 1986. Critical criminology and the concept of crime. In *Abolitionism: Towards a nonrepressive approach to crime*, ed. H. Bianchi and R. Van Swaaningen. Amsterdam: Free University Press. Printed in *Contemporary Crises* 10(1):63–80.

Jobson, K. B. 1977. Dismantling the system. *Canadian Journal of Criminology* 19(3):254–72.

Karmen, A. 1990. *Crime victims: An introduction to victimology*, 2nd ed. Monterey, CA: Brooks/Cole.

_____. 1996. *Crime victims: An introduction to victimology*, 3rd ed. Belmont, CA: Wadsworth.

Kelly, D. P. 1987. Victims. *The Wayne Law Review* 34(1):69–86.

Kelly, D. P. and E. Erez. 1997. Victim participation in the criminal justice system, In *Victims of crime*, 2nd ed., ed. R. C. Davis, A. J. Lurigio, and W. G. Skogan, 231–44. Thousand Oaks, CA: Sage.

Kendrick, M. 1988. *Anatomy of a nightmare—The failure of society in dealing with child sexual abuse*. Toronto: Macmillan of Canada.

Kennedy, L. W. and V. F. Sacco. 1998. *Crime victims in context*. Los Angeles: Roxbury.

Kilpatrick, D. G. and R. K. Otto. 1987. Constitutionally guaranteed participation in criminal justice proceedings for victims—Potential effects of psychological functioning. *The Wayne Law Review* 34(1):7–28.

Laframboise, D. 1998. Society's unspoken family violence—What is a man married to an abusive wife to do if he has children? *National Post* November 9:A14.

Lamborn, L. L. 1987. Victim participation in the criminal justice process: The proposals for a constitutional amendment. *The Wayne Law Review* 34(1):125–220.

_____. 1994. The constitutionalization of victims' rights in the United States: The rationale. In *International debates of victimology*, ed. G. F. Kirchhoff, E. Kosovski, and H. J. Schneider, 280–97. Monchengladbach: World Society of Victimology.

Loftus, E. and K. Ketcham. 1991. *Witness for the defense: The accused, the eyewitness, and the expert who puts memory on trial*. New York: St. Martin's.

_____. 1994. *The myth of repressed memory: False memories and allegations of sexual abuse*. New York: St. Martin's.

Lurigio, A. J. and P. A. Resick. 1990. Healing the psychological wounds of criminal victimization: Predicting postcrime distress and recovery. In *Victims of crime: Problems, policies and programs*, ed. A. J. Lurigio, R. C. Davis, and W. G. Skogan, 50–68. Newbury Park, CA: Sage.

Maguire, M. and J. Pointing. 1988. *Victims of crime—A new deal?* Milton Keynes, UK: Open University Press.

Maguire, M. and J. Shapland. 1997. Provision for victims in an international context. In *Victims of crime*, 2nd ed., ed. R. C. Davis, A. J. Lurigio, and W. G. Skogan, 211–28. Newbury Park, CA: Sage.

Mannheim, H. 1965. *Comparative criminology*. London: Routledge and Kegan, Paul.

Martinson, R. 1974. What works: Questions and answers about prison reform. *The Public Interest* Spring:22–54.

Mathiesen, T. 1974. *The politics of abolition*. Oxford: Martin Robertson.

Mawby, R. I. and M. L. Gill. 1987. *Crime victims: Needs, services and the voluntary sector*. London: Tavistock.

Menninger, K. 1966. *The crime of punishment*. New York: Viking.

Michaelsson, J. and A. Wergens. 2001. *Repairing the irreparable: State compensation to crime victims in the European Union*. Umeå, Stockholm: Brottsoffermyndigheten, Regeringskansliet, Swedish Ministry of Justice.

Miers, D. 1978. *Response to victimization*. Oxford: Milton Trading Estate.

_____. 1989. Positivist victimology: A critique. *International Review of Victimology* 1:3–22.

_____. 1990. *Compensation for criminal injuries.* London: Butterworths.

Mitford, J. 1974. *Kind and usual punishment. The prison business.* New York: Vintage.

Moore, R. L. 1987. *The formation of a persecuting society.* Oxford: Basil, Blackwell.

Mullens, A. 1992. Interview with Elizabeth Loftus. *The Vancouver Sun,* November 28, A.

Nagel, W. 1977. On behalf of a moratorium on prison construction. *Crime and Delinquency* 23(2):154–71.

Ofshe, R. and E. Watters. 1995. Making monsters. In *Fraud and fallible judgment: Varieties of deception in the social and behavioral sciences,* ed. N. J. Pallone and J. Hennessy, 109–34. New Brunswick, NJ: Transaction Books.

Paltrow, S. J. 1982. Opposite effects: New anti-crime law in California is helping some accused felons. *The Wall Street Journal* November 26, A.

Pate, A. M. and E. E. Hamilton. 1992. Formal and informal deterrents to domestic violence: The Dade County spouse assault experiment. *American Sociological Review* 57:691–97.

Paterson, A. 1996. Preventing re-victimization: The South Australian experience. In *International victimology—Selected papers from the 8th international symposium,* ed. C. Sumner, M. Israel, M. O'Connell, and R. Sarre, 227–31. Canberra: Australian Institute of Criminology.

Prison Research Education Action Project. 1976. *Instead of prison: A handbook for abolitionists.* New York: Prison Research Education Action Project.

Quinney, R. 1972. Who is the victim? *Criminology* 10(3):314–23.

Ranish, D. R. and D. Shicor. 1992. The victim's role in the penal process: Recent developments in California. In *Towards a critical victimology,* ed. E. A. Fattah, 227–37. London: Macmillan.

Reiss, A. Jr. 1981. Foreword: Towards a revitalization of theory and research on victimization by crime. *The Journal of Criminal Law and Criminology* 72(2):704–10.

Repo, M. 1992. Fairytales of abuse make for nightmare. *The Globe and Mail* July 28, A17.

Rock, P. 1990. *Helping crime victims: The Home Office and the rise of victim support in England and Wales.* Oxford: Clarendon.

_____. 1994. *Victimology.* Aldershot: Dartmouth.

Rosenbaum, D. P. 1980. *Victim blame as a strategy for coping with criminal victimization. An analysis of victim. Community and police reactions.* Ann Arbor, MI: University Microfilms International.

Sarbin, T. R. 1969. The myth of the criminal type. Paper read at Russell House, University of California.

Scheingold, S. A., T. Olson, and J. Pershing. 1992. Republican criminology and victim advocacy. Paper presented at the American Society of Criminology, New Orleans, LA.

_____. 1994. Sexual violence, victim advocacy and republican criminology: Washington state's community protection act. *Law and Society Review* 28(4):729.

Scull, A. 1976. *Decarceration: Community treatment and the deviant: A radical view.* Englewood Cliffs, NJ: Prentice Hall.

Schur, E. M. 1969. *Our criminal society.* Englewood Cliffs, NJ: Prentice Hall.

_____. 1971. *Labeling deviant behavior: Its sociological implications.* New York: HarperCollins.

_____. 1973. *Radical non-intervention: Rethinking the delinquency problem.* Englewood Cliffs, NJ: Prentice Hall.

Sellin, T. 1938. *Culture conflict and crime.* New York: Social Science Research Council.

Shapland, J., J. Willmore, and P. Duff. 1985. *Victims in the criminal justice system.* Aldershot, UK: Gower.

Sherman, L. W., D. A. Smith, J. E. Achmidt, and D. P. Rogan. 1992. Crime, punishment and stake in conformity: Legal and informal control of domestic violence. *American Sociological Review* 57:680–90.

Shoham, S. G. and G. Rahav. 1982. *The mark of Cain: The stigma theory of crime and social deviance.* St. Lucia, Qld: University of Queensland Press.

Showalter, E. 1997. *Histories: Hysterical epidemics and modern culture.* New York: Columbia University Press.

Singer, S. 1981. Homogeneous victim-offender populations: A review and some research implications. *Journal of Criminal Law and Criminology* 72:779–88.

Smith, B. E. and S. W. Hillenbrand. 1997. Making victims whole again—Restitution, VORP, and compensation. In *Victims of Crime,* 2nd ed., ed. R. C. Davis, A. J. Lurigio, and W. S. Skogan, 245–56. London: Sage.

Smith, S. J. 1986. *Crime, space and society.* Cambridge: Cambridge University Press.

Sommer, R. 1976. *The end of imprisonment.* New York: Oxford University Press.

Spitzer, S. 1975. Towards a Marxian theory of deviance. *Social Problems* 22:638–51.

Statistics Canada. 2000. *Canadian Survey of Family Violence.* Catalogue No. 85–224. Ottawa: Statistics Canada.

Sutherland, E. H. 1949. *White collar crime.* New York: Dryden.

Svalastoga, K. 1956. Homicide and social contact in Denmark. *American Journal of Sociology* 62:37–41.

Sweden. 1978. The criminal injuries compensation act. *SFS:* 413.

Tannenbaum, F. 1938. *Crime and the community.* New York: Ginn.

Tornudd, P. 1996. *Facts, values and visions—Essays in criminology and crime policy.* Helsinki, Finland: National Research Institute of Legal Policy.

Tsutomi, H. 1991. Reformulating Cloward and Ohlin's differential opportunity theory into rational choice perspective: Occupational orientation of Japanese institutionalized delinquents. Paper presented at the ASC meeting, San Francisco.

United Nations. 1985. *Declaration of Basic Principles of Justice for Victims of Crime and Abuse of Power.* New York: United Nations Department of Public Information.

United States of America. 1982. *President's Task Force on Victims of Crime: Report.* Washington, DC: Government Printing Office.

_____. 1996. *The Justice for Victims of Terrorism Act.* Washington, DC: Government Printing Office.

Van Dijk, J. J. M. 1989. Recent developments in the criminal policies concerning victims in the Netherlands. In *Changing victim policy: The United Nations victim declaration and recent developments in Europe.* Helsinki, Finland: Helsinki Institute for Crime Prevention and Control.

Vancouver Sun. 1997. October 10, AI4.

Viano, E. 1976. Pioneers in victimology: Ezzat A. Fattah. *Victimology: An International Journal* 1(2):198–202.

Villmoure, E. and V. V. Neto. 1987. *Victim appearances at sentencing hearings under the California victims' bill of rights.* Washington, DC: U.S. Dept. of Justice.

Von Hentig, H. 1948. *The criminal and his victim.* New Haven, CT: Yale University Press.

Weed, F. J. 1995. *Certainty of justice—Reform in the crime victim movement.* New York: Aldine de Gruyter.

Weis, K. and S. Borges. 1973. Victimology and rape: The case of the legitimate victim. *Issues in Criminology* 8(2):71–115.

Welling, S. N. 1988. Victims in the criminal process: A utilitarian analysis of victim participation in the charging decision. *Arizona Law Review* 30:85.

Wergens, A. 1999. *Crime victims in the European Union: A survey of legislation and support to crime victims in the fifteen member states of the European Union.* Umeå, Stockholm: Brottsoffermyndigheten (Crime Victim Compensation and Support Authority), Regeringskansliet, Swedish Ministry of Justice.

Wexler, R. 1985. Invasion of the child savers—No one is safe in the war against abuse. *The Progressive* September:19–22.

Wolfgang, M. E. 1957. Victim-precipitated criminal homicide. *Journal of Criminal Law, Criminology and Police Science* 48(1):1–11.

_____. 1958. *Patterns in criminal homicide.* Philadelphia: University of Pennsylvania Press.

History and a Theoretical Structure of Victimology

4

GERD FERDINAND KIRCHHOFF

Contents

4.1 Introduction

The reader finds here a historical journey that contributes to the knowledge where victimology stands today. Vessel, maps, and route of the journey are selected from a European, rather than an Asian, point of view [e.g., Ohta, 2007:1–7]. This remark is necessary: Often authors write as if they live in one-world culture and one-world science. They often write as if regional differences or differences in socialization no longer exist, as if differences in sociocultural definitions have vanished. The approach chosen here is nevertheless not provincial because European thoughts have been influential in the field worldwide. A scientist with an African or Asian background probably will use different elements to construct the history of the field. In most regions of the world, there still is to be constructed a "history of the victim" starting with a collection of reports of how victims fared at a certain time in that particular society, let alone a history of the whole field covering victims, victimizations, and social responses to both. Examples for early studies in this sense are Botsman [2005] and Agostino [2005].

Victimology as a social science of victims, victimizations, and reactions toward these is not a stand-alone field. It has—and hopefully maintains—strong bonds to social theory in general. These bonds are like bridges from an island to the mainland in an ocean of activism to improve situations of need for victims. The spectacular development in victim assistance and therapy, especially in the United States and some European countries, has been a vital motor for the science but does not dominate it. Nor can victimology be isolated. Isolation means lack of orientation. The connection especially to social theory is vital if the field does not want to appear as the fig leaf for victim-oriented social action. Research contributions often do not put themselves *expressis verbis* into a historical or scientific context. But such a positioning appears to be useful. It makes the field strong because it shows on whose shoulders the authors stand. Without such positioning, victimology can easily be hijacked or co-opted by other fields. In teaching, European professors seem to concentrate often on the history of their subject and not so much on its theoretical system [Saponaro, 2005 and personal communication]. Scientists do not want to omit important contributions of those who dealt with similar topics previously. But omissions are necessary. If we want to say everything at once, we often produce nothing but noise.

Lucio Fontana (1899–1968), an Argentinian/Italian painter, sculptor, and theorist, from 1958 created objects consisting of slashes on a painted canvas; for example, a white canvas is cut over the distance of roughly half its diagonal (*Monochrome in White*, Museum Abteiberg, Moenchengladbach). The cut into the monochrome canvas demonstrates nothing but one cut, selected by the artist out of a universe of possible ways to treat (cut) a painted surface. As interpreted in the framework of linguistics: Before communication starts, there is a universe of possible beginnings of communication. Communication begins with making a difference: The French philosopher and sociologist Jean-François Lyotard (1924–1998) observes that every "phrase" in operation (i.e., by connecting the "phrase" to other "phrases") produces a *différend*, like the cut into a canvas [Lyotard, 1983, 2002]. Selection is unavoidable—the process of communication, starting with the cut into a universe of possibilities, leads necessarily to silencing. It creates *victims*, according to the French author. The operative unavoidability of the *différend*—in the context of the next connection, other possibilities are produced to be silenced again in the next sequence—is a root for the historical self-definition as "postmodern" [Luhmann and Fuchs, 1998:10]. Every communication produces an operation (a *différend*), just as every system coproduces something that is "environment"—an outside world, something that is clearly not included in the system. This is a kind of silencing. The risk is embedded already in the selection of this point of departure, exactly this point among the many other possibilities. Sociologists today know that description of society describes implicitly what society excludes and what is sentenced to be silenced. From Marx to Lyotard—so Fuchs and Luhmann—this happened under the viewpoint of "victimology" [ibid.:20]: The excluded became defined as class or is in other ways discovered as human and reclaimed for the further analysis of society.

Exactly that happened with victimology. Science, especially sociology, law, and criminology, had overlooked the victim. Law was more concerned with crime and punishment; generally sociology was more concerned about explaining society by structures, functions, or deviance than paying attention to victims. Even the science of history still seems to be concerned about actors and winners, whereas victims—those who are the necessary part of the gains and victories—are excluded. Criminology had forgotten to include victim issues. Law science had banned the victim into the civil law arena of reparation for damage where it was object of dogmatic jurisprudence. Or it co-opted the victim to serve as witness in criminal law. Still, in 1977, Nils Christie [1977] could describe how the victim was deprived of autonomy by lawyers, psychologists, economists, psychiatrists, and criminologists. That was to change.

Victimologists reclaimed the overlooked and silenced victim as focus of the social analysis. Victims were positioned in the center of scientific social analysis. Without any doubts, standing on the shoulders of criminology, the field developed into its own science. Sessar [1986, 1987] rightly observed that victimology at that time "lived from the neglect of the victim" in other sciences.

The word *victim* can be used in a juristic, medical, psychological, and historical context. As a word alone, it does not make much sense. It is the interconnectedness of the concept with other concepts, the "phrases" of Lyotard, that creates the essence of this science. Bassiouni maintains that victims of crime and abuse of power are persons whose basic human rights have been violated [Bassiouni, 1988:9]. He places the victim into a human rights context, like the contemporary victimologists following Neuman [1994a&b, 1995], Elias [1986, 1993, 1996], and Separovic [1985, 1988, 1989].Of course, we can put the victim into other contexts like a psychotherapeutic; a legal with the subcontext of civil, criminal, and administrative law; or a theological-spiritual context. In addition, as a modern science, victimology is not purely theoretical but applicable. Therefore, some observers wrongly equate victimology and victim assistance [Fattah, 1992, 2000]. Fattah contributed convincingly to the development of victimology but blamed it as serving a law and order–oriented conservative repressive criminal policy.

This all makes it very difficult to construct a history of this field [Walklate, 1998:2]. For constructivists, it is self-understood that such history does not exist "out there." Outside of our constructions, it is not existent; it must be constructed. It shows us why and in what context victimology rose to the point where it is now. From Kuhn [1962, 1970:28, 212–20] we know in essence all scientific work is nothing but a special construction of reality.

We cannot state from a certain moment onward, there exists "victimology"—this is the hour of its birth. From the sociology of social movements it is known that new problematic topics are first discussed in private circles or "publics" and then in wider ones [Blumer, 1951, 1971; Mauss, 1975; Kirchhoff, 1991, 2007]. The discussion here deals with victims, victimization, and abuse of power. Victims and "supporters" claim injustices in increasingly wider circles. When people of influence react—negatively or positively—then the discussion leaves the private room and becomes public. We take notice of the influence of the backdrop, the leading contextual philosophical ideologies, and of their intentions. We will have to deal with early documents of victimological interests and with precursors of victimology before we will deal with victimology and its structure.

4.2 The Historical Development of Victimology

4.2.1 Early Documents of Victimological Interest

Such a historical journey starts usually in ancient times, preferably in Mesopotamian cultures, the cradle of European culture. But they are important for non-Western cultures as well. Clearly, the development worldwide has been often in response to Western culture (e.g., Botsman [2005:5ff]). The following explanations draw from Kirchhoff [1994, 2007].

In ancient acephalous societies [Weitekamp, 1999:79], the loss of people was regarded as severe damage to the community. That is plausible. As cuneiform writing was deciphered, more and more ancient codes were found. The most ancient code that we are aware of today, that of Ur-Nammu (ca. 2100–2050 BC), prescribed, besides the death penalty and imprisonment (e.g., nr. 3), restitution (e.g., nr. 9) to be paid by the offender to the victim. This code already recognizes especially vulnerable groups, orphans and widows, who needed special protection against the rich and powerful. It is wrong to say that these oldest codes focus mainly on the victim, that they reflect what can be called "The Golden Age of the Victim." They do not use rules for restitution as sole means of social control.

About 400 years later, the Codex of King Hammurabi (CH; ca. 1750 BC) was created [Kind, 1997]. This king prided himself as the "shepherd of the oppressed and of the slaves," who cared "that the strong should not harm the weak." In this code, legal consequences depend on an important condition: "If the offender is caught" (e.g., CH Rule 22, robbery)—reminding us that sanctions depend on the simple fact that the offender is "available." In one exception, the code rules what has to happen if that is not the case: The authorities (representatives of the central power? of the temple?) were liable for loss incurred by robbery—this, Rule 27, is often seen as a precursor of state compensation laws.

The phrase Golden Age of the Victim [Schafer, 1976:5–15] is to be used with care. In those ancient periods, it was already clear that controlling crime meant good governance by the king. These laws do not give a clear direction from restitution to harsher repression. In the Code of Ur-Nammu, we already find rules for taking an eye (nr. 18), for cutting off a foot (nr. 17), and for severing the nose; these were considered forms of restitution.

This clear direction is missing as well in the old Hebrew laws. In the second Book of Moses (Exodus, chapters 21 and 22, partly revised in chapter 23) we find different sanctions for different cases, as shown in Table 4.1.

Table 4.1 Sanctions for Various Cases of Crime

Norm	Principle	Case	Sanction
21:22	Restitution when victims demand so	Negligent causing end of pregnancy	Husband of woman determines the amount to which offender will be sentenced
21:23–25	Limitation of retribution	Mirror punishment: "eye for an eye"	The same what offender did
21:29, 30	Retribution or—if victim demands so—restitution	Lack of supervision over dangerous animal leads to death	Animal and owner shall die, but owner can pay restitution instead
21:18, 19	Limited restitution	Severe assault in the course of a fight	Victim can get restitution for treatment costs and loss of income
22:2–4	Penal damage restitution	Breaking and entering	Restitution in double value of stolen goods; if this is impossible, victim can enslave the offender
21:15–17	Retribution	Cursing and hitting against parents, stealing a free man for enslavement	Death

This unsystematic listing reminds us of the older cuneiform laws, reflecting the flexibility of formal systems of social control and the general aim to accommodate the interests of the victim. Naturally, in the center of what we would call today the *social control of crime*, there were the victims: If they did not want to bear the loss without any recompense, they must "bring" the offender to justice. But given the absence of effective law enforcement by special social institutions, this task was perhaps more a curse than a blessing. The doctrine of the Golden Age of the Victim appears to overlook such dark shadows.

It is remarkable that victimological texts do not mention a document of high interest that tells us how people interpreted victimization in a nonscientific, spiritual way. The biblical book of Job [see Hitzig, 1874] is poetry about the justice of the divine government of the world, exemplified by the victimization of the main character, Job, whose victimizations are described as an outcome of a contract of divine forces. It is a good example how people constructed victimization in a prescientific manner.

Historical researchers have easier access to the development of Germanic tribal law. We know from Germanic tribal laws that the possibility existed of a bereaved family not demanding the execution of a murderer (that was counterproductive in a time when communities could not afford to lose a member) but rather of restitution. The conflict between the offender and victim('s family) could be, and often was, solved not by killing (which was prone to provoke chains of blood feud murders). The preferred method for dealing with conflict was *Urfehde* (other versions of the word are *Urphed*, *Urphede*, *Urpfedt*, and *Unfehde*), a formal mutual oath between the offender and victim (or the bereaved family) stipulating that peace would henceforth prevail. Breach of the oath was deemed perjury, punishable by cutting off the tongue or the arm that was lifted to swear the oath. This served the purposes of the offender and the victim—both were forced to discontinue violence and to keep peace in the future (so-called *Streiturfehde*). *Urfehde* contracts were very often used in medieval times [Modestin, 2001]. Peace could be achieved by the offender in offering certain restitutive actions. *Urfehde* was used as a punishment of banishment, usually with the obligation never to return to the area for which it was sworn. Later, prison administrations used to let the convicts undergo *Urfehde* before they were given the "farewell," a severe beating before release. This is a typical procedure—institutions that originally served to protect the interest of victims and offenders are occupied with the formal agencies of social control. The original purpose—to establish peace between the parties of a conflict, such as a crime—is lost in this co-optation process. Until now, we have dealt with a time where magic thinking prevailed.

4.2.2 Introduction to the Scientific Context

In the context of victimology, when was the first time victimhood became an issue of scientific thinking?

Usually, textbooks of victimology refer to Hans von Hentig and Beniamin Mendelsohn as the founding fathers of victimology [Morosawa, 2002:52; Rock, 2005]. Hans von Hentig is the famous author of an early pioneering scientific contribution. Beniamin Mendelsohn's presentation in Bucharest in 1947 is said to have been the first time where the term *victimology* was used and a new science was designated [all references to Mendelsohn in Hoffmann, 1992]. The term first saw print in Wertham [1949:259] more as a byproduct. Clearly, the topic is older.

If we use the term *scientific* today, we have in mind the connotations of the twenty-first century. Scholarly writing in the eighteenth century surely was different. The arsenal of science—the scholarly methodology—did not include the same tools we have today. Nevertheless, it would be utterly unfair to deny scholarship to those who do not have "our" methodological equipment.

4.2.3 Victim Issues in the Era of Enlightenment

The reference for the following discussions on Cesare Beccaria is a collection of papers published in 1788 [Anonymous] and 1784 [Roessig] in Breslau, Austria, in German, comprising three volumes. Volumes 1 and 2 were edited anonymously, and volume 3 was edited by Karl Gottlob Roessig.

The first volume contains a translation (by an unknown German) of *De delitti i delle peine*, annotated by Ferdinand Hummel (1722–1781) of Leipzig University, an experienced high court judge in a criminal justice system very similar to that with which Beccaria was familiar. Beccaria's text is illustrated by Hummel's own thoughts, well informed about the reality of criminal law in his time. The first volume also contains the famous *Commentary of Voltaire* [pp. 207–273], followed by several letters of Jean Le Rond d'Alembert (1717–1783), the principal collaborator of Voltaire in the *Encyclopedia* (that is, the first collection of human knowledge not censored by the Roman Catholic church—the famous *Encyclopédie, ou dictionnaire raisonné des sciences, des art, et des métiers*, published by Diderot and Jean Le Rond D'Alembert). Letters of d'Alembert to a certain Brother Frisio, obviously an enlightened Italian priest, indicate a vivid exchange on the new philosophy between enlightened persons of different countries. From these letters we know that d'Alembert gave "many good philosophers" (translation by the author) access to Beccaria's Italian text—obviously to the second edition. In the book, we find two additional documents: philosophical letters [pp. 273–292] by Franz Zacchiroli (under whose name most of the minor contributions to the collection are referenced). It contains short unattributed news—reports on the Calas and Sirven scandals [p. 293ff], which fueled the oppositional enthusiasm of the European intellectuals and served as a pretext for extended propaganda for the new enlightened way, against the "ancient regime." We find new detailed reports on how the Italian text of Beccaria's book came into the hands of the Encyclopedists, who in return pressed for the French translation of the book, which they regarded as the apex of enlightened philosophical thinking, a book written "as a very appropriate defence of … unfortunate victims" [Voltaire in Anonymous (ed.), 1788 Vol. I:300, translation by the author].

The second volume of the collection was *Of Crimes and Punishments: Counterarguments and Many Other Things*. In the voice of Cesare Beccaria, a defense is written against accusations of a religious zealot who obviously published an "Anti-Beccaria" treatise. It is a defense against the accusation that Beccaria was an enemy of the feudal system. The second part refutes the allegation that Beccaria was an enemy of religion [pp. 1–86]. Further—mainly anonymous—expert statements on the dogmatic content of Beccaria's book are printed [pp. 87–202], especially on Beccaria's opposition to the death penalty. We find supportive expertise by the famous scholar Carl von Sonnenfels (1733–1817).

The third volume was edited by Karl Gottlob Roessig. This publication includes a text by Ferdinand Hommel, edited by Karl Roessing (his son-in-law). We know Hommel already as the author of commentaries in the text in the first volume of anonymously edited papers. Hommel points out the systemic victimization of unwed mothers. Hommel, whose text is proof that Beccaria had a deep influence on the thinking elite of his time, emphasizes several times that Beccaria obviously brought into a convincing form what others—including Hommel himself—had published already.

Beccaria lived during the "Enlightenment." For the first time in European history, philosophers and political scientists insisted that rationality should be the ruling principle of explanation, abolishing any magical spiritual interpretation of the world. Rationality was the only accepted basis for scientific thinking. In opposition to that, the church, in alliance with the feudal nobility, for transparent reasons, maintained that the only ruling principle of explanation was the "Will of God," of which they deemed themselves the administrators.

Enlightened philosophers proclaimed the "contract social": The state was created by contracts of free people with the aim to serve the greatest happiness of all. Beccaria [Anonymous, 1788 Vol. I:10 §2] believed that laws are the conditions by which free and independent humans united themselves into a society; people could not enjoy liberty if everyone was in war with everyone. People sacrificed a part of their rights to enjoy the others in peace and security. The sum of these sacrificed parts of their human rights is the material out of which the government is made (all translations and paraphrases are the author's).

Excessive exercise of power (not limited by consent) is abuse of power and creates victims. Moreover, it justifies the overthrow of government. This theory proved dynamite, underpinning the right to resist and abolish abusive authority. It was immediately regarded as a danger to the ruling classes and their power—and Beccaria rightly was afraid to become a martyr to the truth.

What did Beccaria say that was so dangerous? He challenged his readers to think independently, for themselves. Dare to have your own ideas! Dare to know—and do not rely on what others tell you to believe! Usually people follow authorities—not so the enlightened man; he does not accept any authority, but rather reason instead. All ideas are to be rejected if they are not logical in construction and useful in application, useful for the well-being of all (Jeremy Bentham—commonly called the father of utilitarianism—published his books at a time when Beccaria had already been translated into all European languages). Rational, reasonable thinking is the only measure against which ideas are to be evaluated.

For such rational thinkers, power must be exercised usefully—that is, to promote the greatest well-being of the citizens. "Therefore every act of power is tyrannical which infringes without necessity on the rights of people." Such was the enlightened credo of Beccaria: "Reasonable laws enhance the good of all. They serve the interest of all. Unreasonable laws are biased and they favour: they give all possible power to a small part of the population while leaving all the misery and all suffering to the other person" (translation by the author).

Who are these other persons? The people in misery, the suffering people? Today, we call them victims. Beccaria's topic is primarily abuse of power, not victims. He looked at real relationships between the ruler and ruled, at the tyrannical use of criminal law:

> (People) realize the horrors of cruel punishment and torture. Should not the world rulers instead of being caught in traditional opinions, wake up by the cries of the oppressed which have been sacrificed regularly to the shameful lack of knowledge and to the cold emotionless indifference of the rich and the powerful?

Surely, this text deals with oppressed victims of the ruling classes, of the ignorance and the self-interest of those in power. Rereading Beccaria's original text, we find a clear engagement on the side of the victims, the powerless. On one occasion, he gave them a voice when characterizing the ruling laws:

> Argh, these laws are nothing but a covering blanket for power, nothing but sophisticated performances of an adventurous justice. They are nothing

but a conspiracy of the powerful to slaughter us with increased certainty as victimized animals on the altar of an insatiable goddess named lust for power. [Beccariain Anonymous (ed.), 1788 Vol. I:83 §16; all translations of Beccaria above and in ensuring sections are by the author]

Certainly it would be overstated to call Beccaria an early victimologist. He discussed the victim with the scientific means of his time—rational thought to achieve useful results and intellectual freedom.

4.2.4 Victims in the Classical School

Excessive punishment means abuse of power by the state also involves victimization. How can we limit the power of the state? How can we protect the victim and—because we all are threatened to be victimized by such a state—how can we protect ourselves? The answer of the Classical School: Respect the human rights of defendants, avoiding their victimization. Tame the inhuman powers of criminal procedure! Prohibit torture and the death penalty! The remedy is seen in introducing offender rights, thus limiting the power of the state!

The Classical School had made its ideological decisions about free will as a rational backdrop of behavior. On this basis, the continental European system of criminal justice developed. These systems co-opted the victims: It was self-understood that victims sought revenge, and because they could no longer do that themselves, the state acted. That was enough—the state apparently did not have to care for the victim in any particular way. Both state and victim were assumed to have the same interest: punishing the offender. Victims (as witnesses) have nothing but a subsidiary role in these systems.

4.2.5 Victims in the Positivist School

The result is the absolute school of criminal law: Punishment is justified alone and exclusively by the principle of avenging wrong. Other purposes are not valid. The offender decided to commit the crime. That was his or her guilt and the sole justification of punishment. The absolute school of criminal law, as well as its dogmatic fixation on free will and retribution of guilt, becomes the favorite whipping boy of a new way of thinking.

In the meantime a scientific revolution had taken place, a change of paradigms occurred: Positivism became the "new" direction in the philosophy of science and is still today extremely important for sciences generally. Positivism in the nineteenth century elevated the natural sciences to the model of a serious science. This school was founded by the French philosopher and social reformer Auguste Comte (1798–1857), who also coined the term *sociology*.

Positivism declares natural (empirical) sciences to be the sole source of true knowledge. It rejects the cognitive value of philosophical study, as well as theoretical speculation as a means of obtaining knowledge. Positivism declared false and senseless all those problems that could not be verified by experience. It claimed to be a fundamentally new, nonmetaphysical, and therefore "positive" philosophy, modeled on empirical sciences and providing a sound methodology.

In the light of these new ideas, the previous revolution, that of the Classical School, seemed conservative—and with it the leading authorities in law, administration, state, and philosophy as well, not to mention the priests and ministers and their organizations. They saw in positivism the enemy incarnate.

In the history of the victim, the Italian School of Positivism became very important. This school represented the "modern" way of constructing the criminal and criminal justice. Three Italian scientists are the famous representatives of this school: Cesare Lombroso, the socialist physician who introduced the positivist method into criminology, and the somewhat younger scholars Enrico Ferri and Rafaele Garofalo. Here we concentrate on Ferri and Garofalo.

Enrico Ferri (1856–1929), an Italian lawyer and disciple of Lombroso, published in 1884 his *Sociologia Criminale*. He opposed the Classical School and its unproven reliance on free will and retribution of guilt. The retributive actions of the past must be substituted by crime prevention and by "positive" reactions. An important new goal of justice must be "indemnification of the victim."

Indemnification takes two routes: One is the indemnification by the offender (termed nowadays as *restitution*). The other is the indemnification by the state (termed *compensation*).

The Classical School saw reparation of damage as a civil law obligation and punishment as a criminal law obligation—two completely different spheres. But in the view of empirical reality, the classical way of thinking paid "lip service without consequence." In Ferri's essay of 1895 (Ferri, trans. Zimmermann) we read that reparation appears in three forms: (1) as an obligation of the criminal to the injured party, that is, the civil law consequence; (2) as an alternative to imprisonment for slight offenses committed by nonhabitual criminals, that is, restitution as a criminal sanction in its own right; and (3) as a social function of the state on behalf of the injured person, but also—and no less important—in the indirect interests of social defense.

Ferri and the Positivists believe that just as everyone who commits a crime is responsible to the state, so too must victims of crime must be indemnified for the crimes they suffered. The state also must indemnify individuals because it has not prevented their victimization.

Italy in the period under consideration had already had a public fund financed by fines. This fund was used to compensate people who had been wrongfully sentenced, who were victims of the justice system. Ferri proposed to widen the scope of compensation to include victims of crime; thus, compensation would be part of social law and a social function of the state.

These ideas are discussed worldwide. There exists already an arena, a "public." (*Publics* are a concept in the sociology of social movements: They are the groups that discuss certain ideas that specially concern them [Mauss, 1975:91].) Here are two examples: In 1890, the General Assembly of the International Criminalistic Association recommended in Christiania, Denmark, that in cases of simple assault, the accused should NOT be sentenced if he paid restitution to the victim. This was exactly in line with positivist thinking. The second example involved the International Prison Conference, in 1885, in Paris, which posited that because the state must effectively protect people from crime, the state must compensate crime victims. Compensation, as a public function of the state, should be financed by a fund from all fines collected.

At this time, scholars and legislators no longer assumed that the existing criminal procedure worked truly in the interest of the victims. The need for victim participation was already acknowledged, for example, by the German institution of *Nebenklage* (subsidiary or side prosecution, in which the victim, through a lawyer, can prosecute alongside the prosecutor). The *Partie Civile* in France was of a different character. Victim advocates argued in favor of a stronger position for the victim in criminal procedures, for example, by enlarging the array of offenses in which the victim can act as subsidiary prosecutor.

After World War I, involved states were forced to think about compensation for the countless wounded and killed soldiers and civilians. It is no surprise that Ferri's compensation doctrine was picked up. An example is the Draft Penal Law for the Czechoslovakian Republic, 1923: The state had to compensate injured parties from the fines collected, as a source of last resort. Moreover, the Italian Commission of Law Reform, 1921, saw three main areas to be protected in criminal proceedings, not just the public and the offender, but the victim as well. The commission was convinced that "If the Human Rights of the defendant are sacred, then the Human Rights of the victims of a crime are no less sacred" [English translation by the present author, Commentary to Article 99 of the Italian Code in *Relazione sul Progrettt Preliminare di Codice Penale Italiano*, Libro I; German translation by Harry Kahn, 1921, reprinted by Rutz, 1928]. In the fascist climate of the time, these ideas remained without visible reflection in American and European law but had greater impact in Latin America.

These late-nineteenth-century conferences were attended by many non-European scholars, who brought the ideas raised back to their home countries.

Elias Neuman, the Argentine lawyer and victimologist, discovered during his exile in Mexico a 1929 conference in Cuba, resulting in the publication *La Protección de la Víctima del Delito*. It informed the Spanish-speaking world, especially the members of the Cuban Lawyer's Association, about the results of the discussions in Europe and the impact already being felt in Argentina, Peru, Spain, and Mexico [Figueroa, Tejera, and Plá, 1930:99].

Edwin Sutherland, the father of American criminology, wrote in the first edition of his *Criminology* a chapter titled "The Victims of Crime" [Sutherland, 1924:62–72; rediscovered by Robert Jerin, 2003 in Stellenbosch]. This unique chapter did not survive later editions but is still of interest. At that time, the *Modern Criminal Science Series*, under the auspices of the American Institute of Criminal Law and Criminology, published the contributions of the Italian positivists Lombroso, Garofalo, and Ferri [Ferri, 1917]. Sutherland invoked Ferri and Lombroso; however, despite the fact that this chapter deals with losses caused by crime, the question of indemnification seemed apparently superfluous; Sutherland did not even mention the great positivist innovations of restitution and compensation. A critique of the backward methods of Lombroso as the incarnation of positivist thinking seemed more important to Sutherland, ruining a chance to include international victim-oriented discussions in the emerging American criminology.

4.2.6 Victim Issues in the Era of Interactionalism

The period after World War II was one of intense involvement with victims, the most salient cases of which were victims of the Holocaust and atomic bombs.

Victimologists are not completely correct in calling Hans von Hentig's *The Criminal and His Victim* [1948] the first text that deals with crime victims. However, this book became influential because it was theoretically new, sound, and practical. von Hentig picked up a new and epochal concept from sociology, that of interactionalism. Certainly a critical factor was that von Hentig—as later Schafer, Wolfgang, Amir, and others—published in English, reaching a great international audience. The European tradition of von Hentig and Schafer found a ready ear in an English-speaking world that increasingly became aware of its own relevance to the field.

Von Hentig interpreted crime, an interaction between offender and victim, as a social process. His use of this sociological viewpoint in criminology was new and revolutionary. It was not a "revived aspect of crime"—as Schafer expresses it in his rejection of victimology as a new science [Schafer, 1976:88]. Schafer was obviously not aware of the true importance of von Hentig. Never before had crime been seen as an interaction between two parties, and never before has the victim been seen as an active participant in it.

According to von Hentig, the concepts of "victims" and "offenders" are legal stamps imprinted on an essentially social process. This stamp creates the one who acts and the one who is acted on, subject and object, doer and sufferer, perpetrator and victim [von Hentig, 1948/1979:460]. His innovative formulation became a "classic": the victim molds and shapes the criminal. This inaugurated a new approach; hitherto, offenders were seen in their offending relationship to the state (social control through criminal procedure), whereas the victim played an accessory role as evidence. In paying increased attention to the crime-provocative function of the victim, whether an individual or community, von Hentig sets out to point the way to new techniques of control and prevention [von Hentig, 1948/1979:v]. The "crime provocative function of the victim" [von Hentig, 1948/78:460] was picked up by Stephan Schafer, in 1976, in his *Functional Responsibility of Victim and Criminal*; the victim has to omit all that could provoke the offender. The victim has to actively prevent his victimization. Schafer saw the central problems in victimology, namely, (1) the contribution of the victim to the genesis of crime; and (2) the necessity for a contribution by the criminal to reparation for the offense [Schafer, 1967:32]. Later, Saponaro interprets Schafer's approach as a "sociology of the victim"; victim blaming is now a means of social control [Saponaro, 2009].

In the interactionalist tradition, in 1948, the Dutchman W. H. Nagel (a World War II Dutch resistance figure) completed the second draft of his dissertation, *De Criminaliteit van Oss*, which posited a highly innovative applied approach (interviews with both victims and offenders). The first dissertation draft was confiscated by the Nazis. The second draft led to the 1949 publication of the dissertation in book form. Unlike the books of von Hentig and Schafer, Nagel's book, having been written in Dutch, reached a very limited audience outside the Netherlands. The *lingua franca* in social science was then, as now, English, and publication in other languages involved problems not yet properly considered.

4.3 Victim Issues: General Victimology

Outside the United States, Beniamin Mendelsohn presented his view on what he called "victimology" in March 1947 in a lecture to the Psychiatric Society of Romania at the Coltzea Hospital, Bucharest. Publication in French was in 1956, and 20 years later the text was published in English. Such language handicap did not prevent Mendelsohn's ideas from finding wide circulation: Mendelsohn was a passionate victimologist and a prolific letter writer. He sent his publications with personal letters to many people in medicine, psychiatry, psychology, law, sociology, and philosophy, an investment in time and energy that eventually paid off. Today every student of victimology is aware of his contributions [all references in Hoffmann, 1992].

Mendelsohn broadened his victimological interest, which had originally been stirred by his work as a defense lawyer, to include victims of all kind: of nature, technology, the environment, traffic accidents, and cosmic energy, as well as of crime. This came to be termed *universal* or *general* victimology. At the time of his writings, social scientists in the English-speaking world were generally unaware of his contributions. Moreover, the vast majority of them would have rejected his very broad notion of victimhood. Mendelsohn was not a scientist but rather a practicing lawyer. He did not hold an academic title or university chair. He published in French—all this might have contributed to difficulties in interacting with the English-speaking scientific world, in which criminology blossomed. However, he was eventually accorded the recognition he merited. The World Society of Victimology honored his lifework with the Hans von Hentig Award in 1992. In the same year, the Israeli Society of Criminology had a special award ceremony to honor him for his unparalleled value for victimology. Serious scientific analysis and discussion of his work started with Hanoch Hoffman's master thesis, *What Did Mendelsohn Really Say?* [Hoffman, 1992].

Among the developments Mendelsohn foresaw have been as follows:

1. Society of General Victimology. The World Society of Victimology (WSV) was founded in 1979 at the Third International Symposium on Victimology in Muenster, Germany. That founding was a courageous undertaking, and a very successful one.
2. The International Symposium. Such symposia have been held triennially since 1973 (the Jerusalem Symposium in 1973 and the Boston Symposium in 1976 were "adopted" by the WSV). The published proceedings of these symposia testify to the state of the science in that period.
3. The Journal of Victimology. Since 1976, Emilio Viano, well-known coeditor of the 1973 Jerusalem proceedings (with Israel Drapkin), has edited *Victimology—An International Journal*, the first professional journal in the field. Two other journals, *International Review of Victimology* (since 1991) and *International Perspectives on Victimology* (since 2003), enjoy excellent reputations. Numerous journals with special victimological focus also exist.
4. Institute of General Victimology. The first Institute of Victimology existed from 1968 to 1992, sponsored and directed by Koichi Miyazawa in Tokyo. The Tokiwa International Victimology Institute at Tokiwa University, Mito, Japan (founded in 2003), concentrates on problems of general victimology. The Intervict in Tilburg (the Netherlands) has a more special victimological focus, on legal, psychological, and social science issues. "Institute of Victimology" is not a reserved name for university-related academic institutes—it

may be the name of a private group of psychologists without further academic affiliation.

5. Victimological Clinics. The special clinics did not develop. However, a myriad of diverse victim assistance programs currently form a broad field of activities to counsel and to treat victims. There is no doubt that these grassroots organizations of victim assistance form "victim movements" in several countries, especially in the United States, the Netherlands, and the United Kingdom. Later the idea took root in Germany and generally in Europe, Australia, and Asia, especially Japan. The activist-driven social movements have placed the victim issue successfully on the agenda of national and international politics, in influencing the conditions of victims, especially as related to criminal justice systems.

Mendelsohn did not envision the entrance of victimology into university classrooms. Today, most criminology/criminal justice programs worldwide include some victimology courses in their curricula. Tokiwa University in Mito, Japan, is still the only university offering master's and doctoral programs with specialization in victimology [Kirchhoff-Morosawa, 2009] since 2003 (both degree programs can be pursued in English). Today, there is an abundance of victimological textbooks, readers, and monographs. The Tokiwa Institute of Victimology Library features dissertations concerned with victim in various contexts, including 128 from the United States.

4.3.1 Victim Issues in Research

The following paragraphs are based on the work of Hans Joachim Schneider [2007]. The classic and well-received empirical sociological investigation into victims of criminal homicide was conducted by M. E. Wolfgang (1924–1998), who analyzed homicide police files in Philadelphia [1958]. Drawing on von Hentig's idea that crime is an interaction, he identified "precipitated" cases in which the victim first used physical violence in the interaction that ended fatally for him. The notion of victim precipitation was later used by Amir [1967] in cases of forcible rape, in which he identified reciprocal interactions between perpetrator and victim. Later the concept became even more general and fluid to include all actions of the victim that could be interpreted as invitations to (further) sexual interaction.

In the 1960s and 1970s, the techniques of representative victim surveys were first developed in the United States [Bidermann et al., 1967; Ennis, 1967], leading to the National Crime Victim Surveys. Never before had so much scientific scrutiny (or money) been invested in an attempt to measure a social phenomenon. Victim surveys were soon being conducted in many countries. Under the guidance of van Dijk and his team, four sweeps of the International Victim Surveys in 1989, 1992, 1996, and 2000 have been conducted with a yield of about 220,000 cases in more than 60 countries [see the excellent summary in Schneider, 2007:401]. With these instruments, the burden of the population with victimizations can be measured, independently of police statistics, and various dimensions of victimization can be tested.

American emphasis on theoretically soundly based empirical social science research brought new insights. Influenced by the Philadelphia School of Criminology, a special theoretical approach developed with research into lifestyle, routine activity, and life opportunities [Hindelang, Garofalo, and Gottfredson, references in Miethe and Meier, 1990]. This research combined the neoclassical rational choice approach with Routine Activity Theory. Schneider [2007:400] summarizes:

> With social structural change in space and time, lifestyles are affected. Three elements of importance for victimization are identified: a motivated offender, an attractive target and an absent guardian. This has the potential to become an interaction theory. [Wikstroem in Schneider, 2007:348 FN 24]

In the meantime, excesses of sociopolitical activism, especially of a radical feminist orientation, tried to silence and criticize as "victim blaming" most attempts to see in the victim more than the sufferer from—usually male—terrorism.

In matters related to corporal punishment of children and domestic violence, Murray Straus and his team have uncovered social conditions that contradicted cherished beliefs (about the use of corporal punishment of children and about the harmonious way couples live together). The Conflict Tactic Scale and issues of victimization measurement were the center of lively discussions between different schools of thought and belief. One example is the "paradigm shift" [Winkel, 2007:36] in the field of domestic violence; while victim assistance groups and feminist research proliferated and an ideology of domestic violence emerged viewing predominantly female victimization, current research reconfirmed and re-established the role of victim characteristics in the partner dynamic. In the 1970s, it was already known that victims with aggressive personalities were often involved in conflicts [Stephan, 1976, for Germany; Ishii, 1979, in Japan]. For many years, research on the psychological characteristics of victims had little salience. Winkel states that the portrayal of female domestic violence victimization only in terms of terrorized victims suggests a social reality that overlooks important behavioral differences between victims [Winkel, 2007:44]. The prevalent ideological tone of the past decade permitted more balanced debate.

The program of the Thirteenth International Symposium on Victimology [Mito, 2009] reflects the context of the current victimology, thus:

1. Theory of victimology
2. The Draft United Nations (UN) Convention on Victims in the light of international instruments and national norms
3. The work of the UNHCR and victims of abuse of power, refugees, and displaced persons
4. Victims of human trafficking, sexual exploitation, and other transnational victimizations
5. Victim issues in national justice systems, restorative justice, and international crime victim surveys
6. Responses to disaster victimization
7. Psychotraumatological and psychological interventions, building of victim coordination and networks, and specialized interveners (professional and volunteer)
8. Victimization of indigenous peoples and other socially marginalized groups
9. Special victimizations, including family violence, torture, terrorist attacks, consumer fraud, and cybervictimization

4.4 The Structure of Victimology

Victimology does not have a theory of its own that explains all areas of victimological interest. But that does not mean that it is impossible to organize victimological ideas theoretically, something already done in the historical part of this text. This has been done to enable students to learn "the field." In the ensuing paragraphs, an attempt is made to organize the knowledge in our field. This will not be a new theory but rather a system of "drawers." These drawers make it possible to learn victimology, to place each scientific contribution, article, book, or research report into a somewhat suitable place on shelves, under suitable headings. We will not describe a theoretical canon that contributes to the knowledge in victimology [e.g., Saponaro, 2008].

Victimology is the social science of victims, of victimization, and of reactions toward both victimization and victims. This is a transfer of a classical definition of criminology to our field.

4.4.1 Definition of the Victim

Victimology must define the victim, a task for which three different directions exist. The first looks—following the ideas of von Hentig, Schafer, and

Wolfgang—at victims of crime, resulting in a special victimology of crime. Most contributions here deal with crime victims but that does not automatically mean that this would necessarily limit the victimological horizon to such victims. This limit is removed by the general victimology of the tradition of Mendelsohn, including all victims, ranging from natural disasters to traffic accidents. A third definition limits this wide view to victims of human rights violations, including crime. The *UN Declaration of Basic Principles of Justice for Victims of Crime and Abuse of Power* from 1985 follows this tradition, developed independently by Elias Neuman in Argentina, Robert Elias in the United States, and Zvonimir Paul Separovic in Croatia. It seems to be the most accepted definition of the victim in victimology.

A victim is an individual or a group forced to cope with important (at least) potentially uprooting events that can be actuated against him or her by other humans. Omissions are deemed equivalent to active deeds, provided there is a duty to be active. Living in miserable conditions is not enough. Victimization must be human-made—people cannot be victimized by alcohol or drugs [cf. Kosovski, 1993]—and against the will of the victim. The event must come from outside; therefore, suicide is usually not included in victimological theory [Separovic, 1985:20: Victims suffer "at the hands of other people"]. (This is different from the language of criminalistics, in which victimology is a method of investigating any crime; as such, criminalistics include suicide as an object of study [e.g., Patherick, 2008].) Finally, the victimization must be socially recognized. It is not enough that someone claims victim status without societal approval. Often activists fight for exactly this "social recognition" of their constituency. In this more static view, the victim suffers damage in three dimensions: emotional, physical, and financial. This is an important differentiation, even if after closer analysis, the limits between the categories are not so clear. Emotional damage can very well turn into physical damage.

4.4.2 Victim Measurement

Having defined the victim, victimology is interested in ways of measuring victimization. This is the entrance to the methods of empirical social science research. For many years, victimologists were rightly preoccupied with measurement problems. The methodological refinement of the Crime Victim Surveys (CVS) and the International Crime Victim Surveys (ICVS) is a prime example of careful application of methodological expertise. As a result, CVS have been conducted since 1972 in the United States, and the ICVS have been conducted in several sweeps, recently connected with the European Crime and Safety Survey (EU ICS). The data are collected by a standardized questionnaire, by telephone or personal interview, depending on the density of telephone penetration of a country. It is the most intensive analysis of crime, security, and safety ever conducted in the European Union (http://www.unicri.it/wwd/analysis/icvs/index.php) and focuses on the experiences of people in the European Union [Van Dijk et al., 2007]. These surveys divide victimization into the following categories: vehicle-related crimes (theft of cars, theft from or out of cars, and motorcycle and bicycle theft), burglary and theft (theft of personal property and pick-pocketing), contact crimes (robbery, sexual offenses, and assaults and threats), and unconventional crimes (consumer fraud, corruption, hate crimes, exposure to drug-related problems). These measurements are of necessity somewhat static because they rely on a static, nondynamic definition of victimization. In 20 years of comparative crime victim surveying, such research has become part of the international standard in victimology.

4.4.3 Correlates and Processes of Victimization

The next problem in the system of victimology involves the question: "What goes hand in hand with victimization?" Is victimization a randomly distributed chance event? Does it concentrate on certain groups? Is it dependent on gender, age, or social status? This is the question of the social correlates of victimization. Often the correlates of crime are similar: Victimization usually occurs within a group, not between groups.

In process of victimization, different kinds of damages are salient—some by their rapidity and unexpectedness, some by their incubation over a long period. Does it occur suddenly like a raid? Or is it likely to be adumbrated by special preconditions? Studies of victim precipitation [Wolfgang, 1958] in the early period of victimology belong here, as well as studies on victim-offender interactions during rape. The analysis of victimogenic situations and interactions aims to help understanding the event. Here we find Schneider's analysis of the genocide of the Jews by Nazi Germany, in which he describes the stepwise preparation of the victims, beginning with unequal protection and ending in mass victimization [Schneider, 1982:305–319]. Such stepwise victimizations in genocide correspond to similar gradual victimizations. In a different category are most traffic victimizations. These stepwise victimizations are intriguing because it might be possible to intervene early in the process. While we are used to imagining attacks as confrontational victimization (to borrow a term from Fattah), there are those that involve a probing of the parameters of the final confrontation. The victim is lured into a hopeless situation, and his or her ability to correctly diagnose the social situation is dulled. Human rights violations are often preceded by stepwise invasions of the victim's territory. Amnesty International's annual reports contain many examples of stepwise, escalating victimization. Some large-scale victimizations cannot be achieved without gradual preparation of both the victim population and the victimizers' social environment. Stepwise victimization becomes possible if the institutions of formal social control—police and courts—do not control the victimization of people regardless of group, but actively, one-sidedly, serve the powerful. Steps in this process can be seen when courts do not enforce existing laws against those with power and means. Discrimination to strengthen the position of power and privilege is crucial for many forms of victimization [generally Neuman, 1984:70–71; Fattah, 1989:31; Mueller, 1989].

All these categories involve a dynamic with feedback processes, loopings, and all the structures known from cybernetics. Nevertheless, for analytical purposes, it is indispensable that we keep the different factors apart for a while.

4.5 Reactions to Victimization

This does not mean that such factors are separate—they interact and impact each other. This becomes evident when we look into the dynamic definition of victimizations and into the department of victimology that deals with reactions. They are partly reactions toward victimizations, which become causes of further victimizations.

Victimology deals with reactions, which can be those of the victim and of the social environment. We describe the reactions of the victim in a dynamic model: Victimizations are invasions into the self of the victim.

This model permits differentiation of victimizations according to the depth of the penetration: like a cut into an onion, from the outer layers into deeper, softer areas, which never have seen the light of the sun. Victimizations may attack only the surface, without involving serious damage (theft of a cheap, mass-produced item). From that, escalation is possible to burglary (feeling of security is affected), street robbery, sexual invasion, and finally, murder.

4.5.1 Social Environment Reactions: Coping, Assistance, and Secondary Victimization

Many types of victim assistance groups claim to build their initiatives based on crisis theory and crisis intervention. These groups have immense importance in the national and international sphere. In the United States, under the leadership of the National Organization for Victim Assistance, tens of thousands of paid positions in victim assistance programs have been created in the past 30 years [Marlene Young, keynote address to the American Society of Victimology, Fresno, CA, 2007]. Victim assistance programs were originally the domain of enthusiastic grassroots volunteers. At the same time, the therapeutic professions have built on the enormous need for helpful interventions and therapies, responding to the need of helping volunteers and practitioners. Theories and practical implementations deal with grief and loss reactions, with stress and coping models, and with crisis intervention models. Special care is developed in the field of intimate partner and dating violence, sexual victimization of children and adults, victimization by school tyrants ("bullying"), victimization in the workplace (mobbing), homicide victims, traffic accident victims, abuse of the elderly population, mass victimization, and victims of terrorist attacks [e.g., in Green and Robertas, 2008]. The great variety of victim assistance programs in the United States are well reflected in the *Directory of Crime Victim Services* [U.S. Department of Justice, 2009].

These research contributions can be subsumed under the heading "Reactions toward Victimization." Concerning victim reactions, we typically look at emotional consequences. The negative reactions of the social environment can be subsumed under the heading "Secondary Victimization." As far as helping reactions are concerned, the heading "Coping Assistance and Therapeutic Interventions" contains all germane developments. Of course, the intersection with psychology, psychotherapy, and psychotraumatology is evident.

4.5.2 The Victim in the Criminal Justice System

Traditional formal reactions of society toward victimization have existed largely in the criminal justice system, criminal law being a means of formal social control *par excellence*. The importance of the criminal justice system for the fate of victims should not be underestimated; it is of overriding importance. However, it is deplorable that victims are often led to believe that these systems provide—or should provide—justice for them. The prime goal of criminal justice is and remains social control. Therefore, victims are necessarily disappointed and alienated when they experience this characteristic of the formal reaction toward crime, which often subjects them to secondary victimization. It cannot be overemphasized that avoidance of secondary victimization should be a prime goal of criminal justice systems—this is so important that it is repeated here yet again.

The messages "Victims must get their day in court" and "There will be criminal justice for victims" never cease to disappoint victims. These slogans belong to the repertoire of political activism. Victim-oriented politics mainly seeks a positive response in the departments of criminal law and procedure. It is often forgotten that criminal courts decide whether "this crime" must be "punished," not whether a person has been victimized.

Criminal procedure reform deals with the changing role of restitution, which is to become the central reaction, rather than fines and imprisonment, which are to lose their centrality. Restorative justice—instead of retaliative justice—is recommended. Victim participation in criminal procedure is advanced, enabling victims to participate in criminal proceedings, if they so wish.

There is also a strong movement promoting victim–offender mediation, instead of punishment. Here too, the various degrees in which the suggestions are implemented in national criminal justice systems must be taken in account. The successful attempts to achieve reparation of damages (emotional, physical, and financial) with a minimum of coercion (and the reasons for a possible failure) must be accounted for in the outcome of criminal procedures.

Victim-related political action can be observed worldwide, especially after the 1985 *UN Declaration of Basic Principles of Justice for Victims and Abuse of Power*, a decision preceded by developments in the United States and Australia. The Declaration has to be implemented at the national level. Schneider [2007:414] regards victim legislation in Australia and the United States as the most advanced in the world, clearly impacting legislation in the United Kingdom and Canada. In Europe, contributions from the United Kingdom and the Netherlands led to activities at the Council of Europe [1985, 2006], the European Parliament, and the Council of the European Union. In the meantime, the WSV, at its Twelfth Symposium, in Orlando, Florida, approved the work done by experts on a UN Convention for Justice and Support for Crime Victims.

Formal reactions toward victimization include state compensation systems in many countries, which have been discussed for about a century, but sadly, with little implementation around the world. The majority of countries do not have victim compensation schemes, although some (the United States, England, and Germany) do. The existing compensation schemes are often objects of justified criticism. However, critics often fail to take into account the general state of welfare and social security, above all the vastly different degrees and means of health insurance systems.

The area of "Formal Reactions of Social Systems to Victimization" includes victim support organizations, which exist in all developed countries. There concomitantly exists a growing body of laws and regulations for the financing, direction, and development of such organizations. Without formal reactions, their work to alleviate the burden of victims would be impossible. Without a caring response of such powerful groups, the social movement to pay better attention to the plight of victims could not be effectively channeled.

The Japanese approach is impressive by its systematic procedure: Fifty years ago, the field was introduced by Osamu Nakata [Richardson, 2006] and further developed by victimologists like Miyazawa [1970], Morosawa [1998], and Ohta [2006]. Their endeavors were backed by an active Japanese Society of Victimology and by a private victim support organization, Asunokai (since 1982). In the following years, the police introduced massive training of officers in victim-related services. In each of the provinces, victim assistance centers came into existence, often in close cooperation with the police, and there is a national network of such centers. The Japanese Association of Traumatic Stress (http://www.jstss.org/studies) supported the foundation of National Center for Traumatic Stress studies. The study of victimology became institutionalized in Tokiwa University's Graduate Schools of Victimology and Human Sciences. Based on all these developments, the Japanese central government enacted, as a first step, a basic law for crime victims, and promulgated the creation of a special council. This council in 1 year developed a Basic Plan for Victims, commencing in 2005, pointing to some 300 concrete areas in need of reform in the Japanese legal system. This plan is now being gradually implemented. Special laws, for example, for the elderly or victims of domestic violence, have been implemented. The legal order is stepwise reviewed to overcome the traditional negligence shown toward victims. All this has resulted in Japan receiving a central role in the developments in victim reform in Asia. This is underlined by regular study grants for Asian students and by special training courses for officials in public administration in underdeveloped countries, financed by public funds [Dussich et al., 2007; Kirchhoff & Morosawa, 2009].

4.6 Concluding Remarks

In recent decades, the victim movement has engendered political action that reach far beyond the traditional area of crime. Globalization does not exclude victimology, the attempts of scientists to understand, and the various steps societies undertake to cope with a new host of problems. Spurred on by the peace-preserving function of the Truth and Reconciliation Commission in South Africa, subsequent commissions have placed the victim's need for attention in an impressive salience on the political agenda (see the list and description of 20 such cases at http://www.usip.org/library/truth.htm). The audiences of victim-related discussions get broader and broader. Television and the Internet inform more and more people about the horrendous human neglect of victim care and prevention of victimization—especially after catastrophes like tsunamis, earthquakes, flooding, fires, and storms. The aftermaths of global warming are not even envisioned. This chapter did not cover these important emerging fields.

References

Agozino, B. 2006. Crime, criminology and post colonial theory: Criminological reflections on West Africa. In *Transnational and comparative criminology*, ed. J. Sheptycki and A. Wardak, 2nd ed., 117–34. Milton Park: Routledge-Cavendish.

Amir, M. 1971. *Patterns of forcible rape*. Chicago: University of Chicago Press.

Anonymous (ed.). 1788. *Des Herrn Marquis von Beccaria unsterbliches Werk von Verbrechen und Strafen*, Neueste Ausgabe von neuem vermehrt nebst dem

Commentar des Voltaire, Widerlegungen und anderen interessanten Werken verschiedener Verfasser, Erster Band, neu aus dem Italienischen uebersetzt. Breslau 1788 bey Johann Friedrich Korn dem Aelteren, Vol. I:1–194 (*Marquis de Beccaria's immortal book on Crimes and Punishments*, newest edition, anew enhanced, with the Commentary of Voltaire, Refutation and other interesting contributions of various authors, first volume, translated into German from the Italian by Johann Friedrich Korn).

_____. 1788. Antwort auf ein Schreiben welches den Titel fuehret: Anmerkungen und Betrachtungen ueber das Buch von Verbrechen und Strafen. In Zweyter Band: *Von Verbrechen und Strafen: Widerlegungen und anderes mehr.* Neueste Auflage, von neuem verbessert und vermehrt. Breslau bey Johann Friedrich Korn dem Aelteren, im Buchladen auf dem grossen Ring naechst dem Koenigl. Ober-Accis- und Zoll – Amt, Vol. II:1–63 (Reply to a document titled: Commentaries and reflections on the book of crime and punishments. In *Of Crime and Punishment: Refutation and different other items* Vol. II. Translated into German by Johann Friedrich Korn).

_____. 1788 (I) Eine ungedruckte Nachricht, betreffend die Veranlassung zu der Abhandlung von den Verbrechen und Strafen, 298–300. (Unprinted news concerning the occasion for the treatise on Crimes and Punishments).

_____. 1788 (II) Brief an einen Freund in welchem ein Gutachten gegeben wird ueber das Lehrgebaeude des Marchesa Beccaria von der Todestrafe, geschrieben von N. N. (Letter to a friend in which an expert statement is given on the dogmatics of Marchese Beccaria on the death penalty, written by N.N.). In Anonymous. 1788. (ed.) Zweiter Band: *Von Verbrechen und Strafen, Widerlegungen und anderes mehr* Vol. II:123–81.

Bassiouni, M. C. 1988. Preface to "International protection of victims." In *Nouvelles etudes penales*, vol. 7, ed. M. C. Bassiouni, 9. Paris: Eres.

Biderman, A. D., L. Johnson, J. McIntyre, and A. W. Weir. 1967. *Report on a pilot study in the District of Columbia on victimization and attitudes toward law enforcement.* Washington, DC: Government Printing Office.

Blumer, A. 1951. Collective behavior. In *New outline of the principles of sociology*, ed. A. M. Lee, 166–222. New York: Barnes and Noble.

_____. 1971. Social problems as collective behavior. *Social Problems* 18(3):298–306.

Botsman, D. V. 2005. *Punishment and power in the making of modern Japan.* Princeton, NJ: Princeton University Press.

Christie, N. 1977. Conflicts as property. *The British Journal of Criminology* 17(1):1–15.

Dussich, J. P. J., H. Morosawa, and N. Tomita (eds.). 2007. *Voices of crime victims change our society. Child abuse: International perspectives on causes and responses.* Proceedings of the 2nd symposium of the Tokiwa International Victimology Institute. January 20 and 21, 2005. Tokyo: Seibundo.

Elias, R. 1986. *The politics of victimization.* Oxford: Oxford University Press.

_____. 1993. *Victims still—The political manipulation of crime victims.* Newbury Park, CA: Sage.

_____. 1996. Paradoxes and paradigms. In *International victimology: Selected papers from the 8th International symposium on victimology*, ed. C. Sumner, D. Israeli, M. O'Conell, and R. Sarreeds, 9–34. Canberra: Australian Institute of Criminology.

Ennis, P. H. 1967. *Criminal victimization in the USA*. Washington, DC: Government Printing Office.

Fattah, E. A. 1992a. The need for a critical victimology. In *Towards a critical victimology*, ed. E. A. Fattah, 3–26. New York: St. Martin's.

_____. 1992b. Victims and victimology: The facts and the rhetoric. In *Towards a critical victimology*, ed. E. A. Fattah, 29–56. New York: St. Martin's.

_____. 2000. Victimology—Past, present, future. *Criminology* 33:17–46.

Ferri, E. 1917. *Sociologia criminale*. Trans. J. I. Kelly and J. Lisle, ed. W. S. Smithers. Boston: Little, Brown (Internet edition available as: Criminal Sociology. 1992. Trans. M. Zimmermann. http://emotional-literacy-education.com/classic-books-online-a/crsoc10.htm (accessed January 5, 2009).

_____. n.d. *Enrico Ferri Books*. Online Biography, Pictures and Portrait, trans. M. Zimmermann. http://emotional-literacy-education.com/classic-books-online-a/crsoc10.htm (accessed September 8, 2008).

Figueroa, J. R. H., D. V. Tejera, and F. F. Plà. 1929. *La Protección de la Víctima del Delito*. Biblioteca del Colegio de Abogados de la Havana Tomo II. Habana, Cuba: Imp. Julio Arroyo.

Guisepi, R. A. and F. R. Willis. 1980 and 2003. The history of ancient Sumeria (Sumer) including its cities, kings, religions and contributions or civilization. Laws: Ancient Sumerian/Mesopotamien Laws. http://history-world.org/sumerianlaws.htm (accessed January 5, 2009).

Hentig, H. von. 1948. *The criminal and his victim*. Reprint 1979, with a preface by Marvin E. Wolfgang, New York: Schocken Books.

Hitzig, F. 1874. *Das Buch Hiob*. Leipzig, trans. C. F. Winter. Digitized by Microsoft http://www.archive.org/details/dasbuchhiob00hitzuoft (accessed September 7, 2009).

Hoffman, H. 1992. What did Mendelsohn really say? In *International faces in victimology*, ed. S. Ben David and G. F. Kirchhoff, 89–104. Moenchengladbach: WWSV.

Hommel, K. F. 1784. *Philosophische Gedanken ueber das Criminalrecht*. Aus den Hommelischen Handschriften als ein Beytrag zu dem Hommelischen Beccaria, herausgegeben und mit einer Vorerinnerung und eigenen Anmerkungen begleitet von Karl Gottlob Roessig, ed. K. G. Roessig. (*Philosophical thoughts on criminal law* from the Hommelian manuscripts as a contribution to the Hommelian Beccaria, edited and accompanied by an introduction and own commentaries by the author). Breslau: Johann Friedrich Korn dem Aelteren. (In same series as Anonymous (ed.), 1788). In Roessig (ed.) 1784, 2–171.

Ishii, A. 1979. Die Opferbefragung in Tokyo. (The victim survey in Tokyo.) In *Das Verbrechensopfer. Ein Reader zur Viktimologie*, ed. G. F. Kirchhoff and K. Sessar, 133–58. Bochum: Studienverlag Dr. Brockmeyer.

King, L. W. 1997. Hammurabi's Code of Law. In *Exploring ancient world cultures. An introduction to ancient world cultures on the world-wide-web. The Near East.* Translated by King, L.W. http://eawc.evansville.edu/anthology/hammurabi.htm (accessed January 5, 2009).

Kirchhoff, G. F. 1991. The unholy alliance between victim representation and conservatism and the task of victimology. In *Victims and criminal justice*, vol. 2, ed. G. Kaiser, H. Kury, and H. J. Albrecht, 835–56. Freiburg: Max-Planck-Institut fuer auslaendisches und internationals Strafrecht.

_____. 1994. Victimology—History and basic concepts. In *International debates of victimology*, ed. G. F. Kirchhoff, E. Kosovski, and H. J. Schneider, 1–81. Moenchengladbach: WSVP.

_____. 2007a. Perspectives on victimology: The science, the historical content, the present. *Tokiwa Journal of Human Sciences* 10(3):37–62.

_____. 2007b. Prejudice against homeless as a victimological problem: Results from the Mito prejudice surveys. *Tokiwa Journal of Human Sciences* 15: 117–29.

Kirchhoff, G. F. and H. Morosawa. (2009). The study of victimology: Basic considerations for the study of the theoretical victimology. In *Victimization in a multidisciplinary key: Recent advances in victimology. Selections of papers selected at the 12th International Symposium on Victimology*, 2006, Orlando, FL, ed. F. W. Winkel, P. C. Friday, G. F. Kirchhoff, & R. M. Letschert, 271–312. WLP Nijmegen NL.

Kuhn, T. S. 1962/1970. *The structure of scientific revolutions*. Chicago: University of Chicago Press. (Trans. from German H. Vetter: *Die Struktur wuissenschaftlicher revolutionen*. Zweite revidierte und um das Postscriptum von 1969 ergaenzte Auflage. Frankfurt a. M.: Suhrkamp.

Luhmann, N. and P. Fuchs. 1998. *Reden und Schweigen*. Frankfurt: Suhrkamp.

Lyotard, J-F. 1988. *The différend: Phrases in dispute*. Trans. G. van den Abbeele. Manchester: Manchester University Press.

Mauss, A. 1975. *Social problems and social movements*. Philadelphia: Lippincott.

Miethe, T. D. and R. F. Meier. 1990. Opportunity, choice and criminal victimization. *Journal of Research in Crime and Delinquency* 27(3):243–66.

Miyazawa, K. 1970. *Hanzai to Higaisha*, vol. 1. Tokyo: Seibundo.

Modestin, G. 2001. Das Urfehdewesen im Deutschen Suedwesten im Spaetmittelalter und in der fruehen Neuzeit. *The Sixteenth Century Journal* 32(2):462–63.

Morosawa, H. 1998. *Higaishagaku nyomon*. Tokyo: Seibundo.

_____. 2001. *An interdisciplinary study of victim and victimization*, 2nd ed. Tokyo: Seibundo.

Nagel, W. H. 1949. De criminaliteit van Oss. Instituut voor Nederlandsche geschiedenis. http://www.inghist.nl/Onderzoek/Projecten/BWN/lemmata/bwn4/nagel (accessed September 8, 2008).

Neuman, E. 1994a. *Victimologia: El rol de la victim en los delitos convencionales y non convencionales*, 2nd ed. Buenos Aires: Editorial Universidad.

_____ 1994b. *Victimologia y control social: Las victimas del sistema penal*. Buenos Aires: Editorial Universidad.

_____ 1995. *Victimologia supranacional: El acoso a la soberania*. Buenos Aires: Editorial Universidad.

Ohta, T. 2007. Introduction: The development of victimology and victim support in Asia. In *Victim and criminal justice: Asian perspective*, ed. T. Ohta, 1–7. Tokyo: Seibundo.

Patherick, W. 2008. Victimology: The study of victims in criminal investigations. At http://www.trutv.com/library/crime/criminal_mind/profiling/victimology/1.html (accessed September 9, 2008).

Richardson, S. 2006. Osamu Nakata and the beginnings of victimology in Japan. *The Victimologist* 9(4): online publication, http://www.worldsocietyofvictimology.org/publications/wsc94.pdf (accessed January 5, 2009).

Rock, P. 2007. Theoretical perspectives on victimization. In *Handbook of victims and victimology*, ed. S. Walklate, 37–61. Uffculm: Willan.

Roessig, K. G. 1784. (ed.): *D. Karl Ferdinand Hommels Philosophische Gedanken ueber das Criminalrecht aus den Hommelischen Handschriften als ein Beytrag zu dem Hommelischen Beccaria* herausgegebenen und mit einer Vorerinnerung und eigenen Anmerkungen begleitet von Karl Gottlieb Roessig. Breslau, bey Johann Friedrich Korn, dem aelteren, im Buchladen neben dem koenigl. Ober-Zollamt am Markte.

Rutz, W. 1928. *Die Genugtuung des Verletzten in der staatlichen Reformbewegung und in den Entwuerfen* (Satisfaction for the injured in governmental reform movements and in the drafts). Stolp, Pommern: Delmanzosche Buchdruckerei.

Saponaro, A. 2004. *Vittimologia: Origini-concetti-tematiche*. Milano: Guiffre Editore.

_____. 2009. Victimology: A sociology of victim as well? In *Victimization in a multidisciplinary key: Recent advances in victimology. Selections of papers selected at the 12th International Symposium on Victimology*, 2006, Orlando, FL, ed. F. W. Winkel, P. C. Friday, G. F. Kirchhoff, & R. M. Letschert, 247–69. WLP Nijmegen NL.

Schafer, S. 1968. *The victim and his criminal: A study in functional responsibility*. New York: Random House.

Schneider, H. J. 2007. Viktimologie. In *Internationales Handbuch der Kriminologie. Band 1: Grundlagen der Kriminologie*, ed. H. J Schneider, 396–433. Berlin: de Gruyter.

Separovic, Z. P. 1985. *Victimology: Studies of victims*. Zagreb: Samobor.

_____ (ed.). 1988. *Victimology: International action and study of victims*. Paper presented at the 5th international symposium on victimology 1985. Zagreb, Yugoslavia.

Sessar, K. 1986. Literaturbericht Viktimologie. Teil I. *Zeitschrift fuer die Gesamte Strafrechtswissenschaft* 98:919–46.

_____. 1987. Literaturbericht Viktimologie Teil II: *Zeitschrift fuer die Gesamte Strafrechtswissenschaft* 99:82–108.

Sonnenfels, H. von. 1788. Bittschrift und Verteidigung des Herrn von Sonnenfels. In: Anonymous. 1788. Vol. II:183–202.

Stefan, E. 1976. *Die Stuttgarter Opferbefragung: Eine kriminologisch–viktimologische Analyse zur Erforschung des Dunkelfeldes unter besonderer Beruecksichtigung der Einstellung der Bevoelkerung zur Kriminalitaet. (The Stuttgart Victim Survey: A criminological–victimological analysis to investigate the dark field with special reference to the attitudes of the population towards criminality)*. Wiesbaden: BKA.

Voltaire [Pen name of Francois Marie Arouet]. 1788. Anmerkungen des Herrn Voltaire ueber das Buch von Verbrechen und Strafen. (Commentary of Mr. Voltaire on the book on Crimes and Punishments. In Anonymous (ed.). 1788. Vol. I:207–73.

Walklate, S. 1998. *Understanding criminology: Current theoretical debates*. Buckingham, PA: Open University Press.

Weitekamp, E. G. 1999. The history of restorative justice. In *Restorative juvenile justice: Repairing the harm of youth crime*, ed. G. Bazemore and L. Walgrave, 75–102. Monsey, NY: Criminal Justice Press.

Wertham, F. 1949. *The show of violence*. Garden City, NY: Doubleday.

Wikstroem, P. O. 2007. The social ecology of crime. In *Internationales Handbuch der Kriminologie. Band 1: Grundlagen der Kriminologie*, ed. H. J. Schneider, 333–58. Berlin: De Gruyter.

Winkel, F. W. 2007. *Post traumatic anger. Missing link in the wheel of misfortune.* Nimegen: Wlp.

Wolfgang, M. E. 1958. *Patterns of criminal homicide*. Philadelphia: Patterson Smith.

Zacchiroli, F. 1788. Brief an den Herrn Franz Albergati Capacelli. Nachricht an das Publicum ueber die dem Calas and Sirven zugerechneten Mordtaten. Eine ungedruckte Nachricht, betreffende die Veranlassung zu der Anhandlung von den Verbrechen und Strafen. (Letter to Mr. Franz Albergati Cappacelli. Message to the public on the homicides that are attributed to Calas and to Sirven. Until today not published message concerning the reason for the treatise on Crime and Punishment. In Anonymous. 1788. Vol. I:273–81.

_____. Der andere Brief des Herrn Zacchiroli an den Herrn Franz Albergati Capacelli. (The other letter of Mr. Zacchiroli to Mr. Franz Albergati Capacelli). In Anonymous. 1788. (ed.) Vol. I:281–98.

Research Methods in Victimology

II

Property Crimes and Repeat Victimization
A Fresh Look

5

ANDROMACHI TSELONI AND KEN PEASE

Contents

5.1 Repeat Victimization in Context

It has long been recognized that people and organizations vary in their experience of victimization by crime. Pioneers in the field like Nelson [1980] and Sparks [1981] drew out the central facts of uneven victimization. Polvi et al. [1990] drew attention to the time course of repeated victimization whereby victimizations tended to follow each other swiftly. More sophisticated analyses have subsequently confirmed this [e.g., Robinson, 1998]. Overviews of the research literature have been provided by Farrell [1995, 2006] and Eck, Clarke, and Guerette [2007]. Additional useful information may be gleaned from the Problem-Oriented Policing Web site.[*]

Despite substantial research literature on the topic, there are two key reasons to think that the central importance of the concentration of victimization has yet to be recognized in crime theorizing and policing practice. The first is that counting conventions in victimization surveys massively understate that concentration, and that policing attention does not reflect that concentration. The

[*] http://www.popcenter.org/Tools/tool-repeatVictimization.htm; accessed May 2, 2007.

second is that crime decreases may involve a dynamic in which concentration is centrally involved. These points will be briefly developed.

There is ample reason to believe that concentration of victimization is understated in official statistics and in particular national victimization surveys. Planty and Strom [2007] contend that the excision from crime counts of repeated offenses against the same victim by the same perpetrator (so-called series crimes) results in the absence of some 60% of all violence from the U.S. National Crime Victimization Survey (NCVS). Farrell and Pease [2007] report huge undercounting of victimization resulting from similar British Crime Survey (BCS) counting conventions. Ross and Pease [2008] show how variation in police resourcing from the force to the beat level fails to mirror variation in crime concentration, with the result that the most crime-challenged beats in the most crime-challenged areas in the most crime-challenged forces are the most under-resourced in relation to the presenting crime problem. Repeat victimization is evidenced across the world for all crime types [Farrell and Bouloukos, 2001]. Burglaries are arguably best suited for cross-national comparisons, especially in the industrialized world [Mayhew, 1987]. Similar patterns of burglary events have been evidenced across eight European countries [Tseloni and Farrell, 2002] or the United States, the United Kingdom, and the Netherlands [Tseloni et al., 2004] based on the International Crime Victims Survey (ICVS) and corresponding national crime surveys, respectively. The only contrast of note is that affluent households in the United States experience substantially fewer burglaries than average income ones in contrast with findings from the United Kingdom and elsewhere [Tseloni et al., 2004].

Burglary overdispersion is much higher in the United States than in the United Kingdom or the Netherlands [Tseloni et al., 2004] but strikingly similar to overdispersion estimates from a common pan-European model [Tseloni and Farrell, 2002]. In plain English it seems that the extent of unexplained differences in burglary frequency across U.S. and European Union (EU) households is similar, once one controls for household characteristics. By contrast "the distribution of burglaries between U.S. households is over three times more idiosyncratic, namely unpredicted by what is known about them, than in the U.K. or the Netherlands ... [a]ssuming this is not a sampling design effect" [Tseloni et al., 2004:86]. The following chapter of this volume is devoted to comparative studies in victimology, and cross-national comparisons will not be further discussed here.

The mechanism by which crime decreases (or increases) is not fully understood. It may do so by a reduction in the number of people, households, or organizations suffering crime and/or a reduction in the number of crime events each suffers, or (of course) both. That crime rate decreases mostly reflect reduction of repeats is suggested by recent Home Office work [Jansson et al., 2007]. It is difficult to overstate the importance of this analysis. If more generally true, it means that overall crime rates are generally responsive to rates of repeats. This sets the search for precisely how a decrease happens on a distinct course.

Perhaps most fundamental is the issue of distributive justice. Liberal democracies set out to allocate resources according to need. Without understating the concentration of victimization makes resource allocation impossible in relation to crime.

In this chapter, we will set out approaches to statistical modeling of crime rates that reflect the known facts of repeat victimization. We will use one such approach (negative binomial modeling) to clarify risk and protective factors in repeat victimization. We will not however, artificially exclude consideration of first-time victimization risks. This is because we believe that the approach taken enables good measurement of what may be thought of as risk and protective factors in relation to victimization generally.

5.2 The Distribution of Crime

Crime is in most places a rare event, and people vary widely in their encounters with it. Some may be victimized regularly, some frequently, others occasionally, and many never. This is manifest in what statisticians term the *overdispersion* of the observed crime distribution, whereby the variance exceeds the mean. This attests to the wide range in extent of victimization suffered, as alluded to above. Overdispersion is evident in respect of all crime categories. Visually the crime distribution for the general population is positively (right-hand) skewed with zero its most frequent value and a persistent tail, that is, a nonnegligible number of values greater than 2, each relatively infrequent.

The fact that victimization is concentrated on particular people and households makes it crucial to explain the conventional measures of crime, and how these reflect, or fail to reflect, that concentration. Conventional crime rates measure the number of events or the number of victims in the population. These are crime *incidence* and crime *prevalence* rates, respectively, and they are separately reported in national or international crime reports [e.g., Van Dijk et al., 2007]. Crime incidence is usually greater than prevalence, meaning that the number of crimes exceeds the number of victims, with some victims experiencing repeat crimes. In the very rare case that crime incidence and prevalence rates coincide, each event happened to a different victim (e.g., see Japanese car theft rates in 2000, in Van Dijk et al. [2007:238, Table 1; 250, Table 3]).

All Western victimization statistics have incidence higher than prevalence for virtually all crime types. The exception is murder and manslaughter because the same person cannot die twice, whatever the title of Bond movies may imply.* The contrast between the measures is particularly great for threats and assaults and particularly small for thefts of vehicles [Chenery et al., 1996; Tseloni and Pease, 2005]. Repeat victimization is most predictive for many of the crime categories of current concern. Nor should we think in terms of victim "careers," which are homogeneous, with burglary following burglary and assault following assault as the case described here attests.

> Mark Dyche Murdered Tanya Moore: The pair had met at a Young Farmers' ball and were soon engaged. But in February 2003 Miss Moore, fed-up over Dyche's jealous and threatening behaviour, ended the relationship. For a year he waged a hate campaign against her, which included repeated threats to kill her. In June 2003 he even paid three men armed with baseball bats … to rob and beat her at her family's farmhouse home in Alkmonton, near Ashbourne, Derbys. Nottingham Crown Court heard that Dyche, who has a history of terrorising women, "wanted her hurting, wanted her legs breaking, wanted her eyes gouging out, wanted to be in control." He offered criminal associates £50,000 to kill her but, when no one came forward, did it himself, lying in wait on a country road in March 2004 and blasting her in the face with a shotgun. A few days before she was murdered, Miss Moore presented officers with a bundle of threatening text messages from Dyche. [*Daily Telegraph*, November 2, 2006:12]

Because victim careers may incorporate a wide variety of experiences, the wider the category of victimization, the higher the concentration of incidents, insofar as the tendency to be victimized in different ways is positively associated.

Lorenz curves† traditionally demonstrate the extent of income inequality and how government's fiscal policy (taxes and subsidies) redistributes wealth for the benefit of the economically vulnerable. The same approach can be deployed to measure other forms of inequality, such as crime distribution, especially over victims based on national victimization survey data. Figure 5.1 plots the cumulative frequency of crimes over the cumulative frequency of victims, both totaling 100. Therefore, Lorenz curves are confined within a square. Lack of repeats would yield a right-hand diagonal line whereby the cumulative frequencies of victims and incidents coincide. The further away the Lorenz curve is from this diagonal, the higher the disagreement of the proportions of crimes and victims or the number of crimes per victim. The curve in Figure 5.1 shows that some 30% of crime is suffered by the 10% most victimized households. At the other end of the scale, the least victimized 60% accounts for only 40% of total crime suffered. Analysis of major crime categories using the 2000 BCS showed that within

---

* For example, *You Only Live Twice* and *Die Another Day*.
† http://demonstrations.wolfram.com/LorenzCurvesAndTheGiniCoefficient/; accessed September 29, 2008.

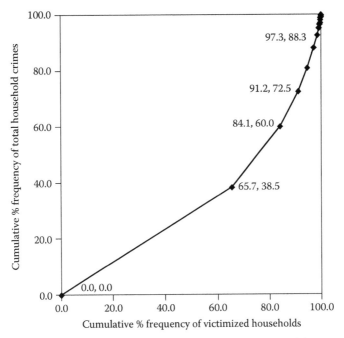

Figure 5.1 Lorenz curve of total household crimes. (Adapted from Tseloni, A. and K. Pease, *International Review of Victimology*, 12, 82, 2005.)

an annual reference period, threat and assault proved the most recurring single crime type, with fewer than 20% of victims experiencing more than 40% of incidents [Tseloni and Pease, 2005]. The contrasts presented in Figure 5.1 are even more marked because, as mentioned, aggregate crime types such as property, which comprises burglary, theft, criminal damage, and vehicle theft, are more likely to be repeated simply because of the longer list of events that count.

The *percentages of repeat crimes* and/or *repeat victims* are directly deducible from Lorenz curve graphs. Crime *concentration*, that is, the ratio of incidents over victims or incidence over prevalence, is an alternative statistic, important but was not hitherto routinely included in statistical reports. In 1999, each victimized household had on average 1.71 property crime incidents, 61.5% of household crime comprised repeats, and 34.3% of victimized households experienced two or more property crimes [Tseloni and Pease, 2005:79]. The success of (repeat) crime prevention will be reflected in changes over time in the above statistics and by displaying Lorenz curves in a use equivalent to that common in the economic policy literature in a more economic way than current practice.* Lorenz curves with constituent

---

* For example, Jansson et al. [2007] demonstrate that the crime reduction of the past 12 years in England and Wales closely follows reduction of repeat incidents via pairs of graphs of total number of incidents and single and repeat victim proportions, respectively.

percentages of crimes and victims display at a glance the extent of crime repetition. We think this a worthwhile form of representation, although it does not clarify the entire distribution of recurrence for each successive event. The distribution of repeat crime was originally used to draw attention to the problem [Farrell, 1992] and is now routinely given in Home Office BCS reports [see, for example, Nicholas et al., 2007:21–24].

5.2.1 Statistical Approximation and Interpretation

In this section, approaches to statistical modeling that are defensible or promising are described. There are two reasons for doing this. First, conceptual clarity is aided by thinking through the possible ways in which people, households, and circumstances interact. Second, some models yield results that do not fit the data about victimization, that is, they cannot be true as they stand. Thus, for both heuristic and policy development reasons, the reader is invited to persist with this section.

The number of crime events per victim is a count, that is, it comprises successive natural (whole nonnegative) numbers including zero. If crimes were random events their distribution would approximate the Poisson theoretical distribution [Nelson, 1980]. This specification is based on the assumption of equal mean and variance. Crime distributions are overdispersed and thus violate that assumption. Higher rates of victimization are far greater than could be attributed to chance recurrence [Osborn and Tseloni, 1998:325]. As a result, the simple Poisson specification fits observed crime counts only poorly. From a policy perspective, this reinforces the notion that random patrolling is not optimal, and that concentrating on the prevention of repeats takes people to where the action is. This is important given the evidence that high crime areas are systematically underpoliced [Ross and Pease, 2008]. Its importance is elevated when one considers the communication of risk in "near repeats" discussed later.

What are the promising theoretical distributions that one could apply to crime counts? These include the hurdle model and Poisson-based models [Cameron and Trivedi, 1998; McCullagh and Nelder, 1989]. The most parsimonious for approximating and predicting observed crime distributions is the *negative binomial* theoretical distribution, a compound Poisson [Irwin, 1968; Xekalaki, 1983]. This specification is the most frequently used to model crimes, partly because of the increasing availability of relevant software over the past 20 years.

Three substantive explanations for the nonrandomness of event repetition have been suggested in the statistical literature [Xekalaki, 1983], which can be applied to victimization as follows: event or state dependence, whereby current victimization increases the likelihood of near future events; unobserved heterogeneity of potential victims that is unknown and/or unmeasured characteristics and behaviors, which are lumped together as erratic deviations from the mean number of events; and spates of victimization events preceded and followed by the absence of victimization [Tseloni, 1995]. The first two explanations have been largely discussed and investigated in the criminological literature [Pease, 1998; Tseloni and Pease, 2004], whereas, to our knowledge, only a study of burglaries, which is mentioned later, points to spates.

The BCS, as for most national and international crime surveys, offers a snapshot of the distribution of crime typically within 1 year preceding the respondent interview [Hales et al., 2000; Van Dijk et al., 2007].[*] This is a problem for differentiating the explanations set out above because event dependence and unobserved heterogeneity are confounded in the (precision parameter of the) negative binomial empirical distribution when it is estimated via cross-sectional data [Heckman, 1981]. Thus, despite much attention in the literature, event dependence and (household) unobserved heterogeneity have not been adequately disentangled in empirical negative binomial models of (property) crime events. That said, such models represent an improvement over the more widely used binary models of victimization risk, that is, logit, which confound repeats altogether [Tseloni et al., 2002].

The NCVS of the United States is, to our knowledge, the only exception to the snapshot approach to national victimization surveys. It uses a rotating sample of 3.5 years with interviews taking place every 6 months. Thus, each respondent reports on successive 6-month victimization recall periods. Analysis of personal crimes based on the NCVS yielded the conclusion that "Event dependence is contingent on what is elusive about the individual" [Tseloni and Pease, 2003:209], especially over successive periods for which the direct event dependence effect varies according to lifestyle and area of residence [Tseloni and Pease, 2005]. This finding has yet to be replicated for property crimes.

The closest research has come to measuring event dependence and unexplained heterogeneity of repeat property crimes simultaneously was when analyses of the 1992 BCS showed high associations between victimization by burglary, car crime, and assault in the 4 years before the reference period and the number of property crimes during the study period [Osborn and Tseloni, 1998]. Controlling for individual and area socioeconomic characteristics (see the "Household Clustering: Hierarchical Models" section) previous burglary was the best predictor of the previous year's burglaries. Those suffering burglaries before the 1-year recall period experienced 86% more burglaries during the recall period compared with households without previous burglary.

---

[*] Since 2001, when the BCS moved to continuous sampling, the snapshot refers to the previous fiscal year (April to March; Nicholas et al., 2007).

The effect of previous victimization of the same type is not event dependence in its proper sense. Previous victimization is about history, and event dependence is about change. Previous victimization is a history parameter and does not address transition probabilities between successive events. These latter are inherent in the negative binomial statistical model. They may be estimated via a recursive formula that is based on the model's estimated parameters but does not allow for effects within individual events [Tseloni et al., 2002]. The formula is identical whether one considers transition from the second to the third incident or from the tenth to the eleventh incident [Osborn and Tseloni, 1998:325; Tseloni et al., 2002]. Disentangling the two explanations of crime repetition would have been straightforward for a diary-type victimization survey covering a long enough period to register repeats, especially of rare individual crime categories, but short enough to minimize memory biases and respondent fatigue [Biderman and Cantor, 1984].

The transition from nonvictim to single victim, from the latter to repeat victim, and perhaps ideally with escalating levels of frequency can be thought of as a series of "hurdles" [Osborn et al., 1996]. One gets over the first hurdle (i.e., suffers a crime). Repeat victimization (jumping the second hurdle) is only an option when a first crime hurdle has been overcome. In its simplest form, the hurdle model is a bivariate binary choice, such as the Probit, model with censoring that identifies associated probabilities of two binary outcomes with the second being conditional on the first. Controlling for socioeconomic individual and area characteristics (see the "Household Clustering: Hierarchical Models" section), the "probabilities of repeat victimisation will tend to be more similar across households than are initial victimisation risks" [Osborn et al., 1996:241]. In other words, single victims have more similar repeat crime risks than initial victimization risk in the general population, which confirms the nonrandomness of the crime distribution. Put another way, there is something about the first victimization and/or the people who suffer it and/or the circumstances in which it is suffered that shapes the risks of subsequent victimization.

Mullahy [1986] developed the *hurdle count* data regression model that is generated by combining a binary outcome and a count model truncated at zero, whereby only values greater than zero enter the second part of the model. In our case, the binary outcome would determine the probability of being a victim versus nonvictim, whereas the count model would estimate the expected number of crimes experienced that are conditional on being a victim in the first place. To the best of our knowledge at the time of writing this model has not been applied in criminology. It is similar to the following statistical specification with a little twist.

Empirical modeling of victimization risk tests whether victims, regardless of event frequency, may be distinct from nonvictims. To take this further, it is arguable that there are two groups of households: potential victims and improbable victims. The former may well be victimized. The latter are not likely to be. In these circumstances, the distribution of victimizations follows the Poisson theoretical probability distribution for potential victims including zeros. Thus, there exist a disproportionate number of zero crimes in the general population, and this is called zero inflation. The *zero-inflated Poisson* (ZIP), which has been applied to study crime frequency at the area level, showed that an estimated 3% of English and Welsh areas, defined as quarter postcode sectors, suffer no (personal or property) crime [Tseloni et al., 2007].

Another conceptualization is that observed crime distributions are the consequence of a mixture of count processes. As people are very different regarding their crime rates, some may be victimized regularly, some frequently, others occasionally, and many never. As mentioned, this heterogeneity is statistically manifested in the overdispersion of the aggregate crime distribution. People may be crime-safe, occasional victims, frequent victims, and chronic victims. The groups' size may diminish from crime-safe to chronic victims, but the respective mean number of crimes they experience increases. This interpretation may be realized via the *finite mixture Poisson model* with multinomial logit mixing probabilities [Wang et al., 1998; McLachlan and Peel, 2000], which has not been applied to victimization yet, although it has featured in the study of delinquent behavior [Nagin and Land, 1993; Wikström et al., 2008]. The distribution of events within each group is Poisson with varying expected counts; therefore, crime repetition for repeat and chronic victims is taken to be random.

The ZIP and the negative binomial specifications are statistical alternatives (with the former having more parameters than the latter), but their interpretations differ substantially. In the ZIP model crime events are the result of chance for potential victims. Once households have been sorted into the two groups of putatively crime-safe and crime exposed, there is *no association between successive events*, including the transition from zero to single events, among those exposed. In fact, this statistical specification is the closest statistical approximation to the lifestyle theory, which places an important role on crime exposure. By contrast, the negative binomial specification implies *nonrandomness* of successive events.

The ZIP specification may look like but is not an extension of the hurdle model because there is no hurdle to get over before the first victimization, and the crime count for those exposed can be zero. The two models diverge formally in that the hurdle count model considers only crime counts per victim, that is, greater than one.

Having challenged the reader with the somewhat technical discussion above, let us conclude with what we think it all amounts to. In short, it suggests that there is a range of approaches available, reflecting a range of assumptions about how crime experience is shaped, which are available to develop risk tools that could optimize the deployment of crime reduction resources across the victimization landscape.

5.3 What Defines Observed Heterogeneity: Key Predictors

Households that experience repeat property crimes cannot be distinguished from once-victimized households via a unique set of characteristics [Osborn et al., 1996]. Repeat property crime victims just have more of the character- istics that one-off victims have some of! This is why the discussion below sometimes ventures into research about singly victimized homes. The nega- tive binomial regression model implies this quantitative rather than qualitative difference between single and repeat victims and, as already mentioned, is the most parsimonious model, namely, the one with the fewest parameters, from among plausible statistical approximations of crime. Therefore, it has been used to model individual or aggregate personal or property crime counts or, indeed, both hierarchically.

There follows an account of patterns that have become clearer during the past decade. The putative policing implications will be added. This overview is based on estimated negative binomial models of the entire distribution of property crimes. As discussed in an earlier section, this statistical specification estimates with parsimony the extent to which repetition of events is higher than chance would predict via its precision parameter and/or overdispersion, the reciprocal. Within cross-sectional data the model cannot establish whether overdispersion is caused by unexplained heterogeneity or event dependence (or spates). However, crime covariates or explanatory variables with significant parameters indicate *observed heterogeneity*: de facto predictors of (property) crime frequency.

Individual and area characteristics play separate and partly interacting roles in predicting property victimization events [Tseloni et al., 2002:318, 321; Tseloni, 2006:223]. They explain substantial proportions of the differences between households: about a quarter in respect of property crime generally, and half for burglary and theft [Osborn and Tseloni, 1998; Tseloni, 2006]. This means that individual risk attribution can be made sophisticated and tailored to individual homes. The practical factor limiting deploying such a sophisticated risk measure would be that neighbors would receive substantially different levels of recommended protection, which may lead to feelings of unfairness.

5.3.1 Household Predictors

Previous research showed that many cars in the household, household com- position, especially lone parents, social renting, less than 2 years' residence in an area, professional social class, household affluence, and young age of "head" of household are associated with more property crimes roughly in that order. The age effect is inverse U-shaped: Households experience more property crimes as the head of the household grows older into her/his 30s, but thereafter the association becomes negative [Tseloni, 2006:228]. Figure 5.2 displays the national average relationship between age of head of household and property crimes. Figure 5.4 will show that this is not uniform across England and Wales.

The effect of home type differs by property crime category: (semi-) detached house occupiers experience more burglaries but fewer thefts and less vandalism than other house structures; by contrast, terraced homes experience more thefts and vandalism but fewer burglaries. Affluent households are more prone to burglary, whereas the level of household affluence is not related to theft frequency [Tseloni et al., 2002:125]. Lone-parent households experience repeat thefts rather than burglaries [Osborn and Tseloni, 1998]. The repetition of such events decreases if they are of manual social class, earn more than £30,000 per year, or live in semidetached accommodation. By contrast, it is heightened if they live in flats [Tseloni 2006]. "Programmes directed at the elderly affluent should concentrate on first burglaries, and those directed at lone parents should focus upon the possibility of chronic theft" [Tseloni et al., 2002:126], considering the differential association of household characteristics across property crime types.

5.3.2 Area Predictors

Area of residence can predict repeat property crime independently and sometimes in the opposite direction from the effect at the household level. For example, it is well established that affluent households in deprived areas are most frequently burgled. Area deprivation and housing type interact. More

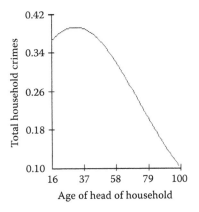

Figure 5.2 Total property crimes over age of "head of household."

households are repeatedly burgled and with higher frequency in deprived areas. Detached houses in deprived areas are most at risk of burglary and repeat burglary [Bowers et al., 2005]. As mentioned, "*household* affluence demonstrates a strong positive relationship with property crime and especially burglary" [Tseloni et al., 2002:120], whereas the opposite is true for *area* affluence. Inner-city and/or urban living, high population density or proportion of private rented accommodation, and general area deprivation increase the risk and repetition of property crimes in roughly the order stated.

It is interesting that area deprivation variables contributing to the empirical crime models based on BCS data are distinct from the Deprivation Index [e.g., DETR, 1999]. This is of huge practical importance because of the frequency with which local authorities and crime and disorder reduction partnerships use the latter as a proxy for area vulnerability to crime [see Bowers et al., 2005]. The more appropriate BCS-based model entails a number of correlated area characteristics, such as the percentage of lone-parent households, households without a car, the mean number of persons per room, the percentage of households renting from Local Authority and/or in housing association accommodation, households with a nonmanual head of household, owner-occupied households, crowded households (more than one person per room), households with three or more children, and male unemployment [Trickett et al., 1992; Tseloni, 2006].[*]

Table 5.1 [based on results from Osborn and Tseloni, 1998:319] lists the characteristics that are associated with crime frequency. Table 5.2 [drawn from Tables 3, 6, and 8 of Tseloni, 2006:214–215, 222, 224–225] repeats this with the additional insight of concordant or contrasting characteristics (interaction effects). It may be thought of in terms of risk ("+") and protective factors ("–") as is commonplace in delinquency research. For example, being a lone parent is a risk factor for repeat property victimization (see + in the sixth row and second column of Table 5.2), but a semidetached property is a protective factor for them (see – in the sixth column of Table 5.2).

5.4 Household Clustering: Hierarchical Models

It is of obvious interest to examine whether households within an area face similar numbers of property victimizations. If so, then risk of crime repetition is communicable to neighboring houses after initial victimization in an area. This defines near repeats. Risk of near repeats is more elevated in affluent areas [Bowers and Johnson, 2005] where burglaries happen during daylight in weekdays [Coupe and Blake, 2006; see also Townley et al., 2000].

---

[*] These enter victimization empirical models jointly via an aggregate factor with, depending on the study, equal or derived by principal components analysis weights (with appropriate signs) to avoid multicollinearity.

Table 5.1 List of Attributes That Are Systematically Related to High Number of Victimizations by Property Crime Type (England and Wales)

Crimes:	All Property Crime	Burglary	Theft	Criminal Damage
Household characteristics				
Younger "head" of household	+	+	+	
Household composition				
Fewer adults in the household	+	+		+
Children in the household	+			
Lone-parent household			+	
Ethnicity of "head" of household				
White			+	
Afro-Caribbean			−	
Indian subcontinent			−	
Chinese and "other"	−			
Increasing number of cars in the household	+	+	+	+
Nonmanual social class of "head" of household	+	+	+	+
Tenure				
Owner occupying	−		−	−
Private rented	−		−	−
Social rented	+		+	+
House structure				
Detached or semidetached		+	−	−
Terraced	+	−	+	+
Flat		− 2nd floor or above		
1–2 years length of residence in the area	+	+		
Area characteristics				
Higher mean number of cars per household in the area	−	−	−	−
More private rented housing	+		+	+
More single-parent households	+		+	
More population 5–15 years old	+	+	+	+
More Indian subcontinent	−			−
Inner city		+		
Victimization history				
Car theft	+	+	+	
Burglary	+	+	+	
Assault	+	+	+	+

+, Systematically more crimes; −, systematically fewer crimes or none.

Table 5.2   Combination of Attributes That Are Systematically Related to High Number of Property Crime Victimizations (England and Wales)

Household Characteristics	Manual	Household Income £30,000+	Household Income under £5,000	Semidetached	Flat	Urban
"Head" of household younger than 31 years old	+					
Household composition						
One or two adults	−					
Three or more adults	+					
Lone parent	+	−[a]	−[a]	−	+	
Tenure						
Owner occupying	−					
Private rented			+[a]			+
Social rented	+					
House structure						
Detached						
Semidetached	+					
Terraced	+					
Flat						
More than £30,000 annual household income	+					
Increasing number of cars	+					
Social class of "head" of household						
Manual	−					
Nonclassified	−					
Member of neighborhood watch	−					
Inner city	+					
Urban	+					

Table 5.2 (continued)

Household Characteristics		Manual	Household Income £30,000+	Household Income under £5,000	Semidetached	Flat	Urban
Area characteristics							
Poverty	+						
More private rented housing	+						
Higher population density	+						

+, Systematically more crimes; −, systematically fewer crimes or none.
[a] Refers to theft and burglary.

Analysis of local police-recorded data showed that burglary risks are com-municated to the neighboring (within 400 meters) houses, especially on the same street of a burgled house, for about 1 month, whereas for longer periods this elevated risk seems to move to other nearby neighborhoods [Bowers and Johnson 2004, 2005; Johnson and Bowers, 2004b]. Thus, neighborhoods go through spates of elevated burglary risks on initial burglary of some nearby house. The spates hypothesis is the least-considered explanation of repeat victimization (see earlier discussion), and in this (unique) evidence it seems entangled with event dependence in the production of near repeats.

The sample design of crime surveys is based on clusters of addresses within area segments, which in the case of the BCS are quarter postcode sectors [Lynn and Elliot, 2000]. Hierarchical or multilevel modeling [Goldstein, 1997] disentangles the within- and between-area variation of crime rates and overcomes the ecological fallacy, that is, confounding effects across different levels of aggregation of the data [Snijders and Bosker, 1999]. The terms *multi-level* and *hierarchical* are used interchangeably in this chapter.

5.4.1 Communicated Crime Incidence: Intraclass Correlation

Property crime experiences are to a large extent communicable across households within the same area. This *intraclass* correlation [ICC; Snijders and Bosker, 1999] is based on hierarchical crime count models yielding the proportion of (residual) crime variability attributable to area. The number of property crimes that are experienced by two randomly chosen households living in a randomly selected area (as defined in the BCS) are substantially correlated at .33.[*] This

---

[*] The above ICC was calculated via the estimated parameters of the baseline model by Tseloni [2006:225, Table 8] and the national average number of property crimes, .35, in 1999 recorded in the 2000 BCS, which coincides with the predicted property crimes from the same model [Tseloni, 2006:209 (Table 1), 225].

correlation coefficient is rather high considering that it comes from a nonlinear specification [Snijders and Bosker, 1999:226]. It is no surprise to find that there are areas that are consistently crime challenged.

With more insight on household profile via multilevel modeling across individual and area predictors and their interactions (as discussed earlier and displayed as Tables 5.1 and 5.2) the intraclass correlation can be calculated for any household type. For example, property crimes against two randomly selected "two adult household[s whose 'head' is 53 years old] of annual income between £10,000 and £29,999, owning two cars, manages well on its income, is of professional social class and lives in an owner-occupied detached house in a (randomly selected) rural South East area with sample mean characteristics but without Neighbourhood Watch" [Tseloni, 2006:218] are correlated by .23, that is, one-third less than any household.[*]

Event communicability within an area is higher when the crime category is narrowed down. Burglaries and thefts against two randomly chosen households living in a randomly selected area are highly correlated, .54.[†] ICC of burglaries and thefts, which refers to more tangible households, such as the above-described one "but without protection against intruders and regardless of car ownership" [Tseloni, 2006:218], is .46.[‡]

5.4.2 Area-Specific (Random) Effects

The association between crime and its predictors may vary across area. In statistical terms, the parameters of explanatory variables in multilevel models may be random. In this example the effect of a single predictor is given by a set of normally distributed values that are a random effect [Snijders and Bosker, 1999]. In multilevel negative binomial models of property crimes with area household clustering, a random effect is a set of normally distributed effect sizes across area. Thus, researchers can estimate the covariate's effect across area crime percentiles. For example, households in flats experienced between 0.21 and 6.17 total property crimes in the respective 2.5th and 97.5th percentiles of English and Welsh areas in 1999 [Tseloni, 2006:226]. Considering that the national (England and Wales) average for the same year was 0.35 property crimes per household [Hales et al., 1999], the above finding implies that flat dwellers experience from one-third less to nearly 18 times higher the national average property crimes, depending on area of residence for similar other characteristics.

---

[*] These calculations are based on Tseloni [2006:215, Table 3, Model 2] and the predicted number of property crimes for the reference household [ibid.:218].

[†] The calculation is based on Tseloni [2006:225, Table 8, baseline model] and the national average burglaries and thefts,. 15, in 1999 as recorded in the 2000 BCS [ibid.:209, Table 1], and also predicted from the same model.

[‡] The figure is calculated from Tseloni [2006:217, Table 4, Model 2], and .12 predicted events per calendar year [ibid.:218].

The highest between area variation was evidenced for lone parents (0.37, 7.03) [Tseloni, 2006:226]. Figure 5.3 the presents the number of property crimes for lone-parent households (x axis = 1) and others (x axis = 0) accounting for area clustering and this variable's parameter randomness (calculations based on Tseloni [2006:214–215, Model 3, Tables 3 and 8:214, 224]). The triangles in Figure 5.3 represent the estimated number of events across the 905 sampling points of England and Wales in the 2000 BCS [Hales et al., 1999]. In the 2.5th percentile of low-crime areas, lone parents experience effectively the national average number of events (0.37 versus 0.35). In average-crime areas, however, lone parents experience a high volume of property crimes. In the worst 97.5th and 100th percentiles they may experience roughly 20 and 28 times more events, respectively, than the national average.

From an earlier section it might be recalled that property crimes increase slightly with age of head of household until the early 30s and then decrease substantially each year as he or she grows older [Figure 5.2; Tseloni, 2006]. Figure 5.4 displays this nonlinear relationship between the age of head of household, ranging from 16 to 100 years old in the horizontal axis, and total household crimes (vertical axis) accounting for area clustering. Each curve represents the age–crime association for respective areas or sampling points. The lower curves refer to low-crime areas and the higher to high-crime areas. Most areas are clustered between 0.3 and 0.6 events in a year for a household whose head is 37 years old and well below 0.3 property crimes for the over-80s households. Household victimization is slightly associated (in terms of magnitude rather than proportionally) with age of head of household in low crime areas. The lowest curve in Figure 5.4 decreases from less than 0.3 to

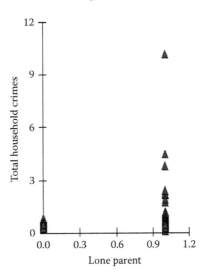

Figure 5.3 Total property crimes for lone parents (x axis = 1) and other household types (x axis = 0) with household clustering and random coefficient.

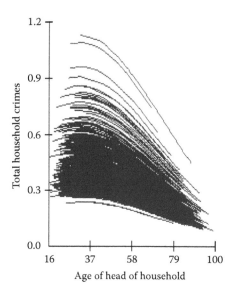

Figure 5.4 Total property crimes over age of "head of household" for households clustered within English and Welsh areas.

0.1 household crimes as age of head of household goes from 37 to 79 years. Property crimes reduce more in high crime areas as the head of household matures, but the lowest expected crimes for really elderly households are still higher than the national average. For example, crimes decrease from about 1.2 to less than 0.5 events as the head of household ages from 37 to 90 years (see the top curve of Figure 5.4) and from 0.9 to 0.5 crimes from the same starting age to 80 years (see fourth curve from top of Figure 5.4) depending on area of residence.

5.5 Parallels and Futures

The thrust of the work reported here is directed at understanding the drivers of victimization by deploying models that take into account the overdispersion of victimizations, which reflect the fact of risk concentration. We will outline specific pieces of research that seem urgently needed. Before addressing them, let us be more upbeat. The risk/protective factors identified by or inferable from the modeling reported above are already adequate to inform police deployment both before and after a first victimization. There will be practical barriers to implementing a thoroughgoing program based on these ideas, primarily because of the perceived injustice of treating close neighbors differently, even though they are properly categorized as having contrasting risks. Let us take an example that is likely to be particularly contentious. We know that detached houses in areas where terraced homes predominate experience higher burglary risk. Is it then appropriate to provide more police patrolling or security equipment subsidy to the people living in these more prestigious homes? It takes little imagination to predict the reaction were this to happen.

The work led by Shane Johnson and Kate Bowers has been cited already [Johnson and Bowers, 2004a, 2004b]. Their team has included Michael Townsley, Dan Birks, and Lindsey McLoughlin. Their approach contrasts with the statistical modeling approach reported here, but their software product, known as ProMap (short for Prospective Mapping), is capable of refinement when complemented by the insights gleaned from the modeling reported here. The work takes the phenomena of repeats and near repeats and puts them to work in prediction. Thus far, ProMap has been applied to domestic burglary in several countries and police force areas, to bicycle theft and to motor vehicle crime. It has imaginatively been used to predict the location of improvised explosive devices by Iraqi insurgents [Townsley et al., 2008]. Because the burglary research is furthest advanced, it will be used in illustration here.

Conventional crime mapping takes the past as a guide to the future. The work on near repeats makes it clear that the relationship of past and future is more subtle. Every burglary event confers an elevated level of risk on nearby homes. The closer the home to the one burgled, the greater the risk conferred. This risk is transient. In ProMap, every burglary event leads to the revision of risk for every nearby home, and every elapsed day leads to a diminution of that risk. Any new burglary event confers transient extra risk on homes nearby. ProMap substantially outperforms the most sophisticated alternatives in predictive accuracy and importantly the predictions of police officers serving the area. It has been trialed operationally with encouraging results [Johnson et al., 2007]. It will generally place police patrols where statistical modeling would also place them because places that suffer burglaries suffer burglaries! Supplemented by the results of statistical models, ProMap could make more precise risk distinctions within its existing tempospatial range. Modeling and ProMap should proceed in tandem.

As to more specific research questions that could usefully be addressed, the following provide illustrations where the policing and wider preventive implications are clear.

- Are there any crime types flagging escalation of repeat victimization, that is, from less to more serious and/or frequent incidents?
- Do disorders precede victimization?
- The evidence that repeat victims are only quantitatively different from one-time victims [Osborn et al., 1996] was based on the 1984 BCS and has not been replicated to date. Confirmation that the relationships still hold is needed.

It is worth (re-)testing whether single victims differ from repeat victims of escalating seriousness. This can be specified as a series of five "hurdles" of single victims versus nonvictims, single victims versus repeat victims of two to three crimes, these against four to five events repeat victims, and the last versus series victims. Partially different sets of covariates in the proposed specification will identify each probability and effectively distinguish across victimization risks of escalating frequency and seriousness. This can be extended via a finite mixture Poisson specification [McLachlan and Peel, 2000], where both the escalating risks for victim typology groups and the mean number of crimes per group can be estimated. This model addresses the twofold question: What are the characteristics that may sort households into the four (or five) groups of nonvictims (crime-safe), single (occasional) victims, low- and high-repeat (frequent) victims, and series (chronic) victims, and what predicts the mean number of crimes that repeat and series victims experience?

References

Biderman, A. D. and D. Cantor. 1984. *A Longitudinal analysis of bounding, respondent conditioning and mobility as a source of panel bias in the National Crime Survey*, 708–13. Proceedings of the Survey Research Methods Section, American Statistical Association. Washington, DC: American Statistical Association.

Bowers, K. J. and S. D. Johnson. 2004. A test of the boost explanation of near repeats. *Western Criminology Review* 5:12–24.

————. 2005. Domestic burglary repeats and space-time clusters: The dimensions of risk. *European Journal of Criminology* 2:67–92.

Bowers, K. J., S. D. Johnson, and K. Pease. 2004. Prospective hot-spotting: The future of crime mapping? *British Journal of Criminology* 44(5):641–58.

————. 2005. Victimisation and re-victimisation risk, housing type and area: A study of interactions. *Crime Prevention and Community Safety: An International Journal* 7:7–17.

Cameron, C. A. and P. K. Trivedi. 1998. *Regression analysis of count data*. Cambridge: Cambridge University Press.

Chenery, S., D. Ellingworth, A. Tseloni, and K. Pease. 1996. Crimes which repeat: Undigested evidence from the British Crime Survey 1992. *International Journal of Risk, Security and Crime Prevention* 1:207–16.

Coupe, T. and L. Blake. 2006. Daylight and darkness targeting strategies and the risks of being seen at residential burglaries. *Criminology* 44:431–64.

DETR. 1999. *Best value and audit commission performance indicators for 2000/2001*, vol. 1, The performance indicators including the publication of information direction 1999 (England). London: DETR.

Eck, J. E., R. V. Clarke, and R. T. Guerette. 2007. Risky facilities: Crime concentration in homogeneous sets of establishments and facilities. In *Imagination in crime prevention*, ed. G. Farrell, 1992. Multiple victimisation: Its extent and significance. *International Review of Victimology* 2:85–102.

Farrell, G. 1992. Multiple victimisation: Its extent and significance. *International Review of Victimology* 2:85–102.

———. 1995. Preventing repeat victimization. In *Building a safer society: Strategic approaches to crime prevention, crime and justice*, ed. M. Tonry and D. P. Farrington, 469–534. Chicago: University of Chicago Press.

———. 2006. Progress and prospects in the prevention of repeat victimisation. In *Handbook of crime prevention and community safety*, ed. N. Tilley, 143–70. Cullompton: Willan.

Farrell, G. and A. C. Bouloukos. 2001. A cross-national comparison of rates of repeat victimization. In *Repeat victimization*, vol. 12, ed. G. Farrell and K. Pease, 5–26. Monsey, NY: Criminal Justice Press.

Farrell, G. and K. Pease. 2007. The sting in the tail of the British Crime Survey: Multiple victimisations. In *Surveying crime in the 21st century*, ed. M. Hough and M. Maxfield, 33–54. Cullompton, UK: Willan.

Goldstein, H. 1995. *Multilevel statistical models*, 2nd ed. London: Arnold.

Hales, J., L. Henderson, D. Collins, and H. Becher. 2000. *2000 British Crime Survey (England and Wales): Technical report*. London: National Centre for Social Research.

Heckman, J. 1981. Statistical models for discrete panel data. In *Structural analysis of discrete data with econometric applications*, ed. C. F. Manski and D. McFadden. Cambridge, MA: MIT Press.

Irwin, J. O. 1968. The generalised Waring distribution applied to accident theory. *Journal of the Royal Statistical Society Series A-Statistics in Society* 131:205–25.

Jansson, K., S. Budd, J. Lovbakke, S. Moley, and K. Thorpe. 2007. *Attitudes, perceptions and risks of crime: Supplementary volume 1 to Crime in England and Wales 2006/07*. Home Office Statistical Bulletin 19/07. London: Home Office.

Johnson, S. D., D. J. Birks, L. McLaughlin, K. J. Bowers, and K. Pease. 2007. *Prospective crime mapping in operational context*. London: Home Office Online Report 19/07.

Johnson, S. D. and K. J. Bowers. 2004a. The burglary as clue to the future: The beginnings of prospective hot-spotting. *European Journal of Criminology* 1: 237–55.

———. 2004b. The stability of space-time clusters of burglary. *British Journal of Criminology* 44:55–65.

Johnson, S. D., K. J. Bowers, and K. Pease. 2005. Predicting the future or summarizing the past? Crime mapping as anticipation. In *Crime science: New approaches to preventing and detecting crime*, ed. M. Smith and N. Tilley, 145–63. Cullompton, UK: Willan.

Kershaw, C. and A. Tseloni. 2005. Predicting crime rates, fear and disorder based on area information: Evidence from the 2000 British Crime Survey. *International Review of Victimology* 12:295–313.

Lynn, P. and D. Elliot. 2000. *The British Crime Survey: A review of methodology*. London: National Centre for Social Research.

Mayhew, P. 1987. *Residential burglary: A comparison of the United States, Canada and England and Wales*. Washington DC: National Institute of Justice.

McCullagh, P. and J. A. Nelder. 1989. *Generalised Linear Models*, 2nd ed. London: Chapman and Hall.

McLachlan, G. J. and D. Peel. 2000. *Finite mixture models*. New York: Wiley.

Mullahy, J. 1986. Specification and testing of some modified count data models. *Journal of Econometrics* 33:341–65.

Nagin, D. S. and K. C. Land. 1993. Age, criminal careers and population heterogeneity: Specification and estimation of a non-parametric, mixed Poisson model. *Criminology* 31:327–61.

Nelson, J. F. 1980. Multiple victimisation in American cities: A statistical analysis of rare events. *American Journal of Sociology* 85:870–91.

Nicholas, S., C. Kershaw, and A. Walker, eds. 2007. *Crime in England and Wales 2006/07.* Home Office Statistical Bulletin 11/07. London: Home Office.

Osborn, D. R. and A. Tseloni. 1998. The distribution of household property crimes. *Journal of Quantitative Criminology* 14:307–30.

Pease, K. 1998. *Repeat victimisation: Taking stock.* Crime Detection and Prevention Series Paper No. 90. London: Home Office.

Planty, M. and K. Strom. 2007. Understanding the role of repeat victims in the production of annual US victimization rates. *Journal of Quantitative Criminology* 23:179–200.

Polvi, N., C. Humphreys, T. Looman and K. Pease. 1990. Repeat break-and-enter victimization: Time course and crime prevention opportunity. *Journal of Police Science and Administration* 17:8–11.

Robinson, M. 1998. Burglary revictimization: The time period of heightened risk. *British Journal of Criminology* 38:78–87.

Ross, N. and K. Pease. 2008. Community policing and prediction. In *Handbook of knowledge-based policing*, ed. T. Williamson, 305–20. Chichester: Wiley.

Snijders, T. A. B. and R. J. Bosker. 1999. *Multilevel analysis: An introduction to basic and advanced multilevel modeling.* London: SAGE.

Sparks, R. F. 1981. Multiple victimisation: Evidence, theory and future research. *Journal of Criminal Law and Criminology* 72:762–78.

Townsley, M., H. Ross, and J. Chaseling. 2000. Repeat burglary victimisation: Spatial and temporal patterns. *The Australian and New Zealand Journal of Criminology* 33:37–63.

Townsley, M., S. D. Johnson and J. Ratcliffe. 2008. Space time dynamics of insurgent activity in Iraq. *Security Journal* 21:139–46.

Trickett, A., D. Osborn, J. Seymour, and K. Pease. 1992. What is different about high crime areas? *British Journal of Criminology* 32:81–90.

Tseloni, A. 1995. The modelling of threat incidence: Evidence from the British Crime Survey. In *Crime and gender*, ed. R. E. Dobash, R. P. Dobash, and L. Noaks, 269–94. Cardiff: University of Wales Press.

——. 2000. Personal criminal victimisation in the U.S.: Fixed and random effects of individual and household characteristics. *Journal of Quantitative Criminology* 16:415–42.

——. 2006. Multilevel modeling of the number of property crimes: Household and area effects. *Journal of the Royal Statistical Society* Series A (Statistics in Society) 169(2):205–33.

——. 2007. Fear of crime, perceived disorders and property crime: A multivariate analysis at the area level. In *Imagination for crime prevention: Essays in honor of Ken Pease. Crime prevention studies*, vol. 21, ed. G. Farrell, K. Bowers, S. D. Johnson, and M. Townsley, 163–85. Monsey, NY: Criminal Justice Press.

Tseloni, A. and G. Farrell. 2002. Burglary victimisation across Europe: The roles of prior victimisation, micro and macro-level routine activities. In *Crime victimisation in comparative perspective: Results from the International Crime Victims Survey, 1989–2000*, ed. P. Nieuwbeerta, 141–61. The Hague: BOOM.

Tseloni, A., A. Nicolaou, and I. Ntzoufras. 2007. Bivariate zero-inflated Poisson modelling of personal and property crimes in England and Wales. Paper presented at the 7th Annual Conference of the European Society of Criminology, Bologna.

Tseloni, A., D. R. Osborn, A. Trickett, and K. Pease. 2002. Modelling property crime using the British Crime Survey: What have we learned? *British Journal of Criminology* 42:89–108.

Tseloni, A. and K. Pease. 2003. Repeat victimisation: 'Boosts' or 'Flags'? *British Journal of Criminology* 43:196–212.

———. 2004. Repeat personal victimisation: Random effects, event dependence and unexplained heterogeneity. *British Journal of Criminology* 44:931–45.

———. 2005. Population inequality: The case of repeat victimisation. *International Review of Victimology* 12:75–90.

Tseloni, A., K. Wittebrood, G. Farrell, and K. Pease. 2004. Burglary victimisation in the U.S., England and Wales, and the Netherlands: Cross-national comparison of routine activity patterns. *British Journal of Criminology* 44:66–91.

Van Dijk, J., J. Van Kesteren, and P. Smit. 2007. *Criminal victimisation in international perspective: Key findings from the 2004-2005 ICVS and EU ICS*. WODC Report 257. The Hague: BJU.

Wang, P., I. M. Cockburn, and M. L. Puterman. 1998. Analysis of patent data: A mixed Poisson regression model approach. *Journal of Business and Economic Statistics* 16:27–36.

Wikström, P. O., A. Tseloni, and D. Karlis. 2008. *Do people abide by the law because they fear getting caught?* Paper presented at the European Society of Criminology Meetings, Edinburgh.

Xekalaki, E. 1983. The univariate generalised Waring distribution in relation to accident theory: Proneness, spells or contagion? *Biometrics* 39:887–95.

Key Victimological Findings from the International Crime Victims Survey

6

JOHN VAN KESTEREN AND JAN VAN DIJK

Contents

6.1 Introduction

Victimization surveys have primarily been designed as a source of statistical information on the volume and trends of crime collected independently from police records. From this perspective, prevalence and incidence rates of victimization are the key findings. The surveys also yield estimates of the total numbers of crime reported to the police that can be compared with numbers of officially recorded offenses. Several developed countries conduct independent annual victimization surveys on a national scale, including Andalusia (Spain), Australia, England and Wales, France, Italy, the

Netherlands, Scotland, Sweden, Switzerland, and the United States. In the case of the International Crime Victims Survey (ICVS), data about crime at the macro level are collected in a comparative, international perspective. The ICVS dataset allows an analysis of the dynamics of actual and reported crime rates, fear of crime, and satisfaction with the police across countries [Van Dijk, Van Kesteren, and Smit, 2008]. Comparative victimization surveys are now generally recognized as an indispensable tool for the benchmarking of criminal policies in an international setting [*The Economist*, July 12, 2008]. In the meantime, Eurostat, the statistical arm of the European Commission, is preparing a similar, standardized victimization survey among its 27 Member States.

Victimization surveys typically collect data on the experiences or perceptions of individual persons (respondents interviewed) that are subsequently aggregated to calculate over all prevalence rates of populations. Unlike most police statistics of recorded offenses, victimization data can also be analyzed at the level of individuals. They can be used to analyze which types of individuals run the highest risks to be criminally victimized. Based on these findings, the relative vulnerability of various population groups can be determined in terms of age, gender, income level, or lifestyle. Surveys provide information on the central topic of early victimological writing: the proneness of persons to fall victim to crime [Von Hentig, 1948]. In addition, many surveys, including the ICVS, ask respondents who have been victimized about the consequences of the incident, their personal assessment of its seriousness, their treatment by the police, and whether they have received specialized help. The responses to these questions are of relevance to current victimological research agenda's centering around the impact of victimization on victims and on the provision of special victim services. Victimization surveys are not just useful tools to produce social indicators of crime, of obvious importance for criminological analyses, but they are also a rich source of victimologically relevant information. In this chapter results of the ICVS will be presented from a victimological perspective. We will mainly use data from the most recent round of the ICVS conducted in 2004–2005 in 30 industrialized countries and six main cities in developing countries. After a brief discussion of victimization rates of 30 different countries, we will present results on the differential victimization risks of main groups of the population. Next, comparative results will be presented on seriousness rating of offenses by victims, reporting rates, satisfaction with treatment by the police, and the reception of specialized help. Finally, we will compare the risk assessments of victims and nonvictims and the opinions of victims and nonvictims on the appropriate punishment for offenders across regions and countries. In the concluding paragraph, we will comment on the huge and largely untapped potential of victimization surveys to inform ongoing victimological debates.

6.2 Victimization Rates of Countries and Cities

The first round of ICVS was in 1989, followed by surveys in 1992, 1996, and 2000. The last round of surveys was done in 2004 and 2005. For complete information on the methodology of the ICVS and European Crime and Safety Survey (EU ICS), we refer to the reports with key findings [van Dijk, Manchin, van Kesteren, and Hideg, 2007; van Dijk, van Kesteren, and Smit, 2008] and to the web sites* of both projects. The results presented here are extracted from the integrated database of the ICVS [van Kesteren, 2007].

Almost 16% of the population of the 30 participating countries has been a victim of any crime in 2004. The overall victimization rates per country are shown in Figure 6.1. The four countries with the highest overall prevalence victimization rates in 2004 are Ireland, England and Wales, New Zealand, and Iceland. Other countries with comparatively high victimization rates are Northern Ireland, Estonia, the Netherlands, Denmark, Mexico, Switzerland, and Belgium. All these countries have overall victimization rates that are statistically significantly higher than the average of the 30 participating countries. The United States, Canada, Australia, and Sweden show rates near the average. Compared with past results, these countries have dropped several places in the ranking on overall victimization. The 10 countries with the highest rates comprise both very affluent countries, such as Switzerland, Ireland, and Iceland, and less affluent countries (Estonia and Mexico). This result puts into question conventional wisdom about poverty as the dominant root cause of common crime. Most of the high-crime countries are relatively highly urbanized, although this is not true for Ireland [Van Dijk et al., 2007]. For more comprehensive analyses of the social correlates of crime, see Van Wilsem [2004] and Van Dijk [2007].

Countries with victimization levels just under the mean include Norway, Poland, Bulgaria, Scotland, Germany, Luxembourg, and Finland. Lowest levels were found in Spain, Japan, Hungary, Portugal, Austria, France, Greece, and Italy. The latter eight countries all have victimization levels significantly below the average of participating countries. They can be regarded as low-crime countries in this context. This group is fairly heterogeneous, both geographically and in terms of affluence (gross domestic product per capita). Finland, Greece, and Poland are comparatively less urbanized than other European countries [Van Dijk et al., 2007].

6.2.1 Victimization in Capital and Main Cities

Figure 6.1 also shows the results of surveys conducted in 32 main cities concerning victimization by any crime. The results confirm that levels of

---

* http://rechten.uvt.nl/ICVS and http://www.europeansafetyobservatory.eu.

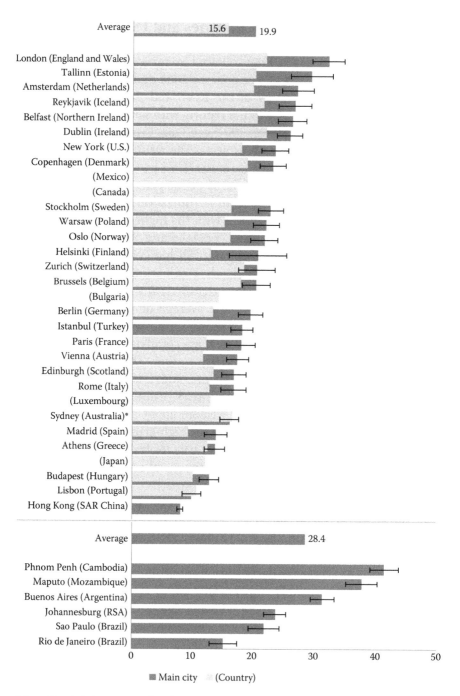

Figure 6.1 Overall victimization for 10 crimes; 1-year prevalence rates in 2003–2004 (percentages) of capital cities and national populations of 28 countries. (From 2002–2005 ICVS and 2005 EU ICS.)

* Australian victimization rate is based on nine crimes; sexual offenses were not asked, overall victimization about 1% lower here.

victimization by common crime are universally higher among city populations than among national populations. Lisbon forms the only exception to this criminological rule. The mean victimization rate of the participating cities in developed countries is 19.9%, whereas the mean national rate was 15.8%. In almost all countries, risks to be criminally victimized are one-quarter to one-third higher for main city inhabitants than for others.

On average, city rates are higher in developing countries (28.4%) than in developed countries (19.9%), but three of the six cities in developing countries are within the range of the main cities in developed countries. The ranking of cities in terms of victimization puts Phnom Penh and Maputo on top. Relatively high rates are also found in London and Buenos Aires. Tallinn, Amsterdam, Reykjavik, Belfast, Dublin, and Johannesburg have rates above the global mean. Victimization rates near the global city average of 21.7% are found in New York, Copenhagen, Stockholm, Sao Paulo, and Oslo. The five participating cities with the lowest victimization rates are Hong Kong, Lisbon, Budapest, Athens, and Madrid.

6.3 Trends in Crime

Trend data are available for 15 Western countries. Overall trends in victimization show a curved trend since 1988 with a peak in the early or mid-1990s. The survey also showed that levels of fear of property crime are decreasing, together with victimization rates, and that general levels of satisfaction with the police have increased.[*] The latest round of the ICVS confirms that most Western countries have emerged from a decades-long crime epidemic and that the public has started to become aware that this is the case.

The downward trend in car thefts in Europe cannot be explained by a decrease in car ownership because car ownership rates in Europe have increased [Van Dijk, et al., 2008]. The most plausible factor in the decrease of car theft rates across Europe is improved and more widely used antitheft measures, such as steering column locks, alarms, and electronic ignition systems. These measures are likely to have had the greatest impact on levels of joyriding and other forms of nonprofessional, opportunistic theft. The ICVS results confirm this hypothesis. The ratio between the number of stolen cars that have been returned to their owners and those that have not been returned has shifted. Now, most of the cars do not find their way back to their owners [Van Dijk et al., 2008]. If cars are stolen, it is now more often by professional gangs using sophisticated techniques or violence, breaking through protective devices installed.

ICVS trend data point to a universal growth in the possession and use of security measures over the past few decades. For example, the use of

[*] Victim satisfaction with the police will be discussed later in this chapter.

measures to prevent household burglaries has increased during the past 15 years across Western countries, especially among the middle classes [Van Dijk, 2007]. Potential victims of crime seem to have responded to higher crime rates with increased concerns about crime and additional investments in measures to avoid or reduce risks. It seems likely that "opportunities of crime" have shrunk as a result of improved self-protection of households and businesses in developed countries and that this has brought down levels of victimization. Property crimes have gone down more steeply than prevalent types of contact crimes. A possible explanation of the divergent trends in property and contact crimes is that improved security has reduced levels of many forms of property crime, such as burglary and nonprofessional car theft, but has had less impact on contact crimes.

6.3.1 Individual Risk Factors

The victimological literature shows that within countries some groups of the population are systematically more at risk to become victims of crime than others. Various theoretical models have been developed to explain how the differential vulnerability of individuals to criminal victimization is determined by their lifestyle or routine activities [Hindelang, Gottfredson, and Garofalo, 1978; van Dijk and Steinmetz, 1980; Felson, 2002]. Included in the ICVS questionnaire is a question on the frequency of outdoor activities in the evening, a variable known to impact on people's exposure to victimization. The ICVS also includes information on demographics such as age, gender, town size, marital status, income, and education of respondents. The ICVS dataset allows the execution of a victimological risk analysis using these variables. Because factors such as age and an outgoing lifestyle are interlinked, the independent effect of such factors on victimization must be determined with the help of a multivariate analysis. The results of a log-linear analysis given in Table 6.1 show which particular characteristics are most important in determining the risks of being criminally victimized, by different types of crime, independently of other factors. It shows the controlled risk factors for victimization expressed as odd ratios.

The results show that a young age and residence in a capital city are the most important independent risk factors for victimization by any of the 10 crimes included in the study. Not being married, and having a high income, a high educational level, and an outgoing lifestyle, all add to the risk to be victimized by any of these crimes. Therefore, most at risk are young affluent residents of major cities who are not married and who maintain an outgoing lifestyle (e.g., students). This finding could also be formulated inversely by stating that being a senior citizen, a resident of a village, poor, married, and not outgoing are important protective factors for criminal victimization by common crime.

Table 6.1 Controlled Effects of Risk Factors (Odd Ratios) on Victimization[a] in 2003 or 2004 for Overall Victimization of 10 Crimes,[b] Property Crime, and Contact Crimes

	Overall Victimization by 10 Crimes	Victimization by Seven Property Crimes	Victimization by Three Contact Crimes
Age			
Young (base)			
Middle	0.76*	0.78*	0.69*
Old	0.41*	0.45*	0.29*
Gender			
Male (base)			
Female	1.03	1.02	1.05*
Town size			
Rural (base)			
City	1.36*	1.42*	1.21*
Capital (or main) city	1.65*	1.72*	1.41*
Income			
Low (base)			
High	1.10*	1.12	0.97
Educational level			
Low (base)			
High	1.13*	1.10*	1.15*
Partner			
No (base)			
Yes	0.84*	0.90*	0.64*
Going out			
No (base)			
Yes	1.18*	1.16*	1.18

Source: 2004–2005 ICVS and 2005 EU ICS.

[a] Countries in the model are English-speaking/common law countries: Australia, Canada, England and Wales, Ireland, Northern Ireland, Scotland; Nordic countries: Denmark, Finland, Norway, Sweden; southern Europe: Greece, Italy, Portugal, Spain; western Europe: Austria, Belgium, France, Germany, the Netherlands; and eastern Europe: Hungary, Lithuania. The United States is kept separate from the English-speaking/common law countries in this analysis.

[b] Property crimes are theft of a vehicle, theft from a car, burglary, attempted burglary, and theft of personal property. Contact crimes are robbery, sexual offenses (women only), and assaults and threats.

* Statistically significant, $t > 1.96$, $p < .05$.

The risk analyses for property crimes and contact crimes are different from each other in some respects. The impact of risk factors such as being of young age, being single, entertaining an outgoing lifestyle, and being female are stronger for contact crimes than for property crimes. The risk factor urban residence is more salient for property crimes than for contact crimes. Finally, high income is a risk factor for property crimes but a protective factor for contact crimes. In terms of the lifestyle exposure models, high-income groups are more exposed to property crime because of their possessions but protected from contact crimes by their relative isolation from potential offenders.

The results raise the question whether differential risks of population groups are universal across the individual countries participating in the ICVS. Our results suggest that this is indeed largely the case, although the size of the odd ratios differs, and there seem to be some striking exceptions. Table 6.2A presents the results for five groups of countries/cities, and Table 6.2B presents the data from five main cities in developing countries and of the United States separately.

The degree of urbanization of places of residence appears to be a universal risk factor. There is a linear relationship between city size and risks of victimization in all countries included. There is also universally a linear, inverse relationship between age and risk. Risks to be criminally victimized tend to decrease with age universally. There is some evidence, however, that age is a stronger risk factor in more affluent countries, such as the United States, Canada, Australia, the United Kingdom, and the Scandinavian countries. This is probably because more young people in these countries can afford to entertain a distinct outgoing lifestyle, and the elderly population more often lives in secured places. In most countries females are slightly more at risk to be victimized by any crime. This positive link between gender and victimization is not found in southern and eastern Europe. Here the female gender acts as a weak protective factor. One possible explanation is that female labor participation is more limited in these countries (e.g., in Italy).

According to the results, high-income groups are more at risk in all regions, except in the United States. We have carried out log-linear analyses on risks for property crime and contact crimes separately.* High-income groups are universally more at risk for property crimes. Here the United States presents a striking exception, with risks being the highest among those with the lowest incomes. A focused trend analysis has shown that in the United States during

---

* In most developed countries, high-income groups are slightly less at risk to be victimized by contact crimes: The odd ratios are between 0.87 and 0.97 for high-income groups. In the Anglophone countries (except the United States) and in developing countries, the relationship is reversed: Those with higher incomes are more at risk (odd ratio 1.10). These findings suggest that the proximity of high-income groups to potential offenders of contact crimes is relatively great in developing countries and in Anglophone countries.

Table 6.2A   Controlled Effects of Risk Factors (Odd Ratios) on Victimization[a] in 2003 or 2004 for Overall Victimization of 10 Crimes in Six Regions

	All Countries	English Speaking / Common Law Countries	Nordic Countries	Southern Europe	Western Europe	Eastern Europe
Age						
Young (base)						
Middle	0.76*	0.59*	0.69*	0.82	0.77	1.05
Old	0.41*	0.24*	0.33*	0.58*	0.48*	0.84
Gender						
Male (base)						
Female	1.03	1.09	1.06	0.90*	1.26*	0.89
Town size						
Rural (base)	–					
City	1.38*	1.21*	1.49	1.30	1.62*	1.14
Capital	1.65*	1.70*	1.71*	1.49	2.34*	1.28
Income						
Low (base)						
High	1.10*	1.06	1.19*	1.12	1.04	1.03
Educational level						
Low (base)						
High	1.13*	1.09*	1.01	1.16	1.14	1.26
Partner						
No (base)						
Yes	0.84*	0.63*	0.82*	1.05	1.09	0.94*
Going out						
No (base)						
Yes	1.18*	1.09*	1.14*	1.14	1.37*	1.23

Source: 2004–2005 ICVS and 2005 EU ICS.

[a] Countries in the model are English-speaking/common law countries: Australia, Canada, England and Wales, Ireland, Northern Ireland, Scotland; Nordic countries: Denmark, Finland, Norway, Sweden; southern Europe: Greece, Italy, Portugal, Spain; western Europe: Austria, Belgium, France, Germany, the Netherlands; eastern Europe:Hungary, Lithuania. The United States is kept separately from the English-speaking/common law countries.

* Statistically significant, $t > 1.96$, $p < 0.05$.

Table 6.2B Controlled Effects of Risk Factors (Odd Ratios) on Victimization in 2003 or 2004 for Overall Victimization of 10 Crimes in Five Main Cities in Developing Countries and the United States

	Five Main Cities in Developing Countries[a]		United States[b]
Age		Age	
Young (base)		Young (base)	
Middle	0.68*	Middle	0.78*
Old	0.38*	Old	0.19*
Gender		Gender	
Male (base)		Male (base)	
Female	1.03	Female	1.01
		Town size	
		Rural (base)	
		City	1.30
Capital (or main) city	1	Capital (or main) city	1.58
Income		Income	
Low (base)		Low (base)	
High	1.25*	High	0.66*
Educational level		Educational level	
Low (base)		Low (base)	
High	1.23*	High	1.11
Partner		Partner	
No (base)		No (base)	
Yes	0.98*	Yes	0.84
Going out		Going out	
No (base)		No (base)	
Yes	1.03*	Yes	1.06

Source: 2004–2005 ICVS and 2005 EU ICS.

[a] The five main cities in developing countries are Buenos Aires (Argentina), Rio de Janeiro (Brazil), Sao Paulo (Brazil), Phnom Penh (Cambodia), and Lima (Peru).

[b] The United States is kept separately from the English-speaking/common law countries.

* Statistically significant, $t > 1.96$, $p < 0.05$.

the past 10 years, risks of victimization by property have decreased strongly among higher income groups and not among the poorest quartile [Van Dijk, 2007]. ICVS-based data on the use of security measures suggest that affluent people in developed countries have counteracted their higher exposure to crime with increased protection. Less affluent people are lagging behind in this respect, most likely because they can ill afford expensive measures of self-protection such as burglar alarms. Phenomena such as gated communities may have further reduced risks for well-to-do inhabitants in large cities. These trend data point at the emergence of a class-related security divide. A separate analysis of the 2005 ICVS data [Van Kesteren, 2006] has shown that in Europe migrant status is an independent risk factor of victimization by contact crimes. This finding suggests that immigrants are especially targeted for contact crimes (so-called hate crimes). Taken together, the latter findings suggest that the distribution of victimization risks across income groups is undergoing a structural change, with more affluent groups gradually become less and underprivileged groups more exposed to crime.

6.4 Reporting to the Police and Victim Satisfaction

The frequency with which victims (or relatives and friends on their behalf) report offenses to the police is strongly related to the type of offense involved. For ease of comparison, reporting levels were calculated for five offenses for which levels of reporting are variable across countries and/or experience of victimization is comparatively high.* The offenses are thefts from cars, bicycle theft, burglary with entry, attempted burglary, and thefts of personal property.

In the 30 countries and 12 capital cities, on average 41% of the five crimes were reported to the police. Among the 30 countries where national samples were drawn, roughly half of the five crimes were reported to the police (53%). The highest reporting rates were in Austria (70%), Belgium (68%), Sweden (64%), and Switzerland (63%). With the exception of Hungary, all counties with relatively high rates are among the most affluent of the world. As in previous rounds of the ICVS, reporting rates are very low in participating developing countries. Brazil (Sao Paulo), Cambodia (Phnom Penh), Peru (Lima), Mexico, and Mozambique (Maputo) stand out with reporting rate less than 20%. Reporting is also comparatively low in Hong Kong (24%). Countries with medium low reporting rates—between 35% and 45%—include South Africa (Johannesburg), Turkey (Istanbul), Bulgaria, Iceland, Estonia, and Poland.

The decision to report victimizations to the police is determined by costs–benefit assessments of the victims [Skogan, 1984]. An important factor behind the high reporting rates of property crimes in developed countries are high rates of insurance against theft and burglary. Another determining

---

* Omitted are car and motorcycle thefts (which are usually reported and are relatively uncommon), and robbery (for which numbers per country are small). Also omitted are sexual incidents and assaults/threats. Here, the proportion reported will be influenced by, respectively, the ratio of sexual assaults to offensive sexual behavior, and assaults to threats.

factor of reporting rates is public confidence in the police. Using data of the ICVS 2000, Goudriaan [2004] found that country-level variables, such as confidence in the police, account for a substantial amount of the cross-country variation in reporting property crimes.

Of special interest from a victimological perspective is whether reporting to the police shows any trend. Reporting rates overall have gone down since 1988 or 1992 in Belgium, Scotland, England and Wales, the Netherlands, France, New Zealand, the United States, and Canada, but this is largely caused by the changing composition of the crimes that are reported. In almost all countries reporting rates for bicycle theft have decreased significantly in recent years. More and more victims of bicycle theft tend to refrain from reporting the incident to the police. Few other significant trends can be discerned in the reporting rates for individual types of crimes. Reporting rates have gone up in Poland and Estonia, probably because of postcommunist reforms of national police forces that have increased trust among the community. Also, in Northern Ireland reporting has gone up since 1988 and 1992.

In the ICVS 2005, by far the most important reason for not involving the police was that the case was not serious enough. About one in three nonreporters nationally and one of five in capitals mentioned this. One-quarter of victims felt it was inappropriate to call the police or said they or the family solved it. The idea that the police could do nothing was mentioned fairly frequently (e.g., by one in five victims of thefts of cars who did not report). At the country level, 20% mentioned as reason that the police will not do anything. This percentage is higher at the level of capital cities. Within Europe nonreporting is more often mentioned in the capital (e.g., Rome and Amsterdam) than at the national level. Few victims mentioned fear or dislike of the police as a reason for not reporting a burglary. Fear of reprisals was also infrequently mentioned. Many victims mentioned other reasons for not reporting.

The 1996 ICVS introduced the open question why victims *did* report. The reasons why sexual incidents and assaults and threats were reported differed somewhat from those for other offenses. Victims here were especially concerned to stop what happened being repeated. Many victims also wanted help. For the two property offenses and robbery, more than one-third was reported because assistance was sought in recovering property. When a burglary or theft from a car was involved, about one-third reported for insurance reasons. About 4 in 10 victims overall referred to the obligation to notify the police, either because they felt a crime such as theirs should be reported or because what happened had been serious. Retributive motives— the hope that offenders would be caught and punished—weighed with nearly as many victims, although this was less evident when thefts from cars were involved.

6.4.1 Victim Satisfaction

If they had reported to the police, victims were asked whether they were satisfied with the police response.* To increase the number of cases, rates have been calculated on respondents who reported crimes over a 5-year period. On average, 53% of reporting victims were satisfied with the way the police had handled their complaint. Among the countries/cities, satisfaction levels did not differ between different types of crime.†

The respondents in Denmark (75%), Finland (72%), Switzerland (72%), Australia, Scotland, and Luxembourg (70%) were most satisfied after reporting any of the five crimes, although figures in several other countries were not far behind. The police response was considered least satisfactory in Estonia (17%), Peru (18%), Maputo (27%), Greece (28%), and Mexico (28%). Considerably lower than the average were also satisfaction levels in Japan (44%), Italy (43%), Hungary (41%), Bulgaria (40%), Johannesburg (36%), Istanbul (33%), and São Paulo (32%).

In many parts of the world, legislative and operational actions have been taken to improve the treatment of crime victims. In the European Union (EU), for example, legally binding minimum standards of victim reception went into force in 2003 (Council Framework Decision of 15 March 2001 on the Standing of Victims in Criminal Proceedings, SEC [2004]). Japan introduced victim-friendly legislation in 2002 as well. A cornerstone of these initiatives is a better treatment of victims by the police, including the right to be treated with consideration and respect and to be kept informed about follow-up and decisions. In view of these initiatives, it seems important to monitor trends in victim satisfaction with the police. Figure 6.2 shows results.

Although numbers are small, it is striking that in so many countries levels of satisfaction of the victims with the police have significantly gone down since 2000. This is most markedly the case in England and Wales and the United States (–10 percent points), the Netherlands (–9 percent points), Canada (–8 percent points), and Sweden (–7 percent points). This downward trend in satisfaction is more remarkable in view of the new victim-friendly legislation in force.

Nation-specific crime victim surveys in England and Wales and the Netherlands, using much larger samples, have also registered a decrease in satisfaction in recent years [Allan et al., 2006; CBS, 2006]. This intriguing result can be interpreted in different ways. One explanation is that victims are treated as professionally as before but that expectations among victims have

---

* This question was asked for the same five crimes as questions about reporting to the police: burglary with entry, thefts from cars, robbery, sexual incidents, and assault and threats.
† In developing countries, victims of property crimes tend to be more dissatisfied than victims of contact crimes because they would have liked more effective support in recovering stolen goods [Van Dijk, 1999].

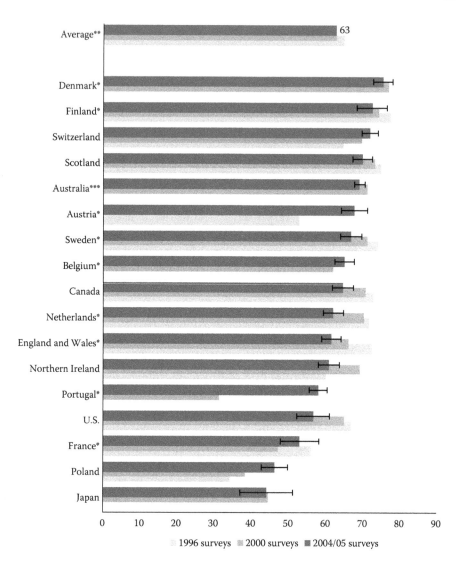

Figure 6.2 Satisfaction with report to the police for victims of five types of crimes (*) (percentages in a period of 5 years). (From 1996–2005 ICVS and 2005 EU ICS.)

(*) The five crimes are theft from a car, burglary, robbery, sexual offenses, and assault and threat.

** The average is based on countries taking part in each sweep. As countries included vary across sweeps, comparisons should be made cautiously.

*** The Australian rate for the 2004 survey is based on 4 crimes (sexual offenses were not asked in 2004).

been raised to the point that they can no longer be satisfied. For example, police forces may ask victims whether they would want to be informed about the investigation. If subsequently no information is given, victims might be more upset than when the issue had not been raised in the first place. Another possible interpretation is that police forces have become less service oriented,* especially in countries where special provisions for victims outside the police have been set up. In countries where victim support organizations are well established, police forces may feel that victim needs are duly met if a referral is made to such an agency. It seems striking in this respect that in Europe victims are more stably satisfied with the police in countries where victim support outside the police hardly exists, such as Denmark, France, Finland, and Luxembourg, than in countries such as the United States, Canada, United Kingdom, and the Netherlands, where police officers are instructed to refer victims to local victim support agencies.†

Those respondents who indicated that they were not satisfied with the way the police handled the matter were asked why not. Overall, the main reason for dissatisfaction was that the police "did not do enough." This held across all five crimes and was the complaint of two in three who answered. The second cause for dissatisfaction was that the "police were not interested"—mentioned by about half. The next most common complaint overall was that no offender had been caught. The exception was assaults and threats, where impoliteness on the part of the police was mentioned more often. An explanation for this might be that the police think that some assault incidents involve a degree of victim responsibility. For theft from cars and burglary with entry, around one-quarter were dissatisfied because the police did not recover any stolen goods.

One in five victims mentioned impoliteness as a source of dissatisfaction. One in three of those reporting sexual incidents did. Again, considering the European Commission 2001 instructions on the rights of crime victims to be treated with respect for their dignity, this result is disappointing.

To determine possible shifts in the relative importance of different types of complaints, a comparison was made of the relative frequency of response categories in the various sweeps. Of particular interest seemed the percentages of reasons given that fell into the category "did not give sufficient information." The complaint about lack of information made up 7% of all reasons given in 1996 and 2000 and 12% in 2005. This upward trend in victims complaining about lack of information is visible across the EU.

6.4.2 Victim Support

Victims who had reported to the police any of four types of crime with the most serious consequences for victims—burglary with entry, robbery, sexual incidents, and threats and assaults—were asked whether they had received

---

* A factor behind the decrease in satisfaction may be the gradual increase of victims reporting by telephone or via the Internet. There is some evidence that in England and Wales victims who have no face-to-face contacts with the police are somewhat less satisfied [Allan, 2005, 2006].

† The Dutch crime victim survey shows, for example, that the provision of crime prevention advice to reporting victims has gone down significantly since the 1990s.

support from a specialized agency. Such support was described as "information or practical or emotional support." Those who had not received any help
were asked whether they would have appreciated help in getting such information or practical or emotional support. Using this information, estimates
are made of the proportion of victims wanting specialized help that actually
receive it (the take-up rate of existing specialized victim support agencies).

For the victims of the four types of crimes together, 9% had received specialized support in 2005. Most likely to receive support are victims of sexual
offenses (30%). Fewer than 1 in 10 victims reporting robberies or threats and
assaults had received help (robbery, 8%; threat and assault, 8%). Victims of
burglaries with entry had much less often received help (4%).

In most countries support is mainly offered to victims of contact crimes
(robbery and crimes of violence) and only rarely to victims of burglary. Only
10% or more of burglary victims received support in the United Kingdom,
the Netherlands, and Belgium.

The coverage rates of specialized support agencies for crime victims are
the highest in New Zealand (24%), Scotland (22%), Northern Ireland (21%),
England and Wales (17%),* and the United States (16%). Comparatively high
rates were also found in South Africa/Johannesburg (15%), the Netherlands
(14%), Canada (13%), Hong Kong (13%), Austria (13%), Belgium (12%),
Denmark (10%), Norway (10%), and Sweden (9%). Within Europe victim
support is most developed in the northwest. The top position of New Zealand
is corroborated by statistics on the numbers of clients of victim support in
the country. In New Zealand, with a population of 4 million, some 100,000
victims are assisted annually. This is proportionally a higher number than in
England and Wales or the Netherlands.

The least support seems to be available in Hungary (0.4%), Lima (1%),
Bulgaria (1%), Finland (2%), Germany (2%), Greece (2%), Maputo (2%),
Turkey/Istanbul (2%), Italy (3%), and Spain (3%). No information is available
for Poland, but coverage was very low in 2000.

The proportion of victims contacted by victim support after they
have reported to the police seems to have grown since 1996/2000 in a
number of countries, although few differences are statistically robust.
Increases since 1988 can be observed in Austria (8–13%), Canada (9–14%),
Belgium (4–13%), Japan (0–8%), and the United States (11–16%), as well as
in Northern Ireland (11–21%) and Scotland (10–22%). In countries with
long-established nationwide infrastructures for victim support, such as
England and Wales, the Netherlands, and Sweden, the degree of coverage
has remained stable or decreased. Elsewhere the coverage of victim support has remained at the same comparatively low levels or even decreased

---

* Rates from England and Wales are extracted from the UK sample; the data from Scotland
and Northern Ireland are from independent samples.

further. Victim support figures for countries for which trend data are available are shown in Figure 6.3.

Victims who had *not* received support were asked whether it would have been useful. On average 42% of victims reporting any of the four types of crime felt such help would have been useful for them. Two of three victims of sexual offenses (68%) expressed a need of such help. Roughly four of ten of the victims of the three other types of crime would have appreciated such help. As reported above, victims of burglary are less likely to receive help in most countries. But the percentage of burglary victims who would have welcomed support is not much lower than among victims of robbery or threat and assault (burglary, 40%; robbery, 44%; threat and assault, 42%).

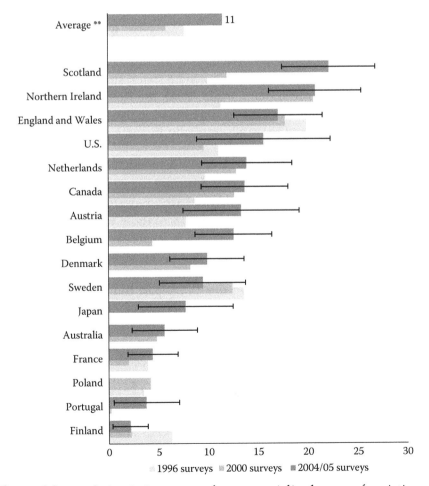

Figure 6.3 Trends in victim support from a specialized agency for victims of four crimes (percentage in a period of 5 years) in countries participating at least twice in the last three sweeps. (From 1996–2005 ICVS and 2005 EU ICS.)

The level of demand was highest in participating developing countries except Peru and in Portugal, Spain, Greece, and Turkey and, in 2000, Poland (no data on 2004 available). In all those countries such help is not readily available. Despite the relatively high level of support already given, unmet demand was also relatively high in the United Kingdom. The need of victim support seems relatively limited among victims in Bulgaria, Japan, Iceland, and Austria.

The results indicate that the need of help among victims of serious crime is widespread although not universal. Percentages of victims who would have appreciated help but did not receive it were 50 or higher in Asia, Africa, Latin America, and eastern Europe. In developed nations only 30% or 40% express such needs. The distribution of the need of help across regions is the reverse of that of its actual reception. In developing countries many more victims would have wanted such help. This is partly because in those countries such help is rarely offered and partly because fewer other general provisions of health care or social work are available. Among developed countries the percentages of victims who would have liked to receive victim support tend to be smaller in countries with extended welfare states, such as Iceland (23%), Austria (26%), Germany (27%), Canada (27%), the Netherlands (30%), and Denmark (30%). Higher percentages were found in the United States (38%), in England and Wales (45%), and especially in some southern European countries (Spain, 68%; Portugal, 70%).

6.4.2.1 Take-Up Rates of Victim Support

Globally, 8% of victims of serious crimes who reported the crime to the police received specialized help, whereas 43% of those who had not express a need of it. The proportion of victims whose expressed needs are met can be approached by dividing the number of victims who received support by the numbers of those who received it plus those who would have wanted it (times 100). Such calculation shows that in the past couple of years agencies of victim support provided services to roughly 21% of victims with manifest needs. Using the same formula, victim support organizations reach 38% of the victims of sexual offenses demanding specialized help, 20% of victims of robberies with such needs, 19% of victims of threats and assaults, and 10% of victims of burglaries. For all four groups the supply of specialized help falls short of the demand. The gap between supply and demand of victim support is by far the largest for the group of burglary victims.

Percentages of victims whose expressed needs are met by the agencies vary across countries. The proportions of victims of serious crimes with manifest support needs who were contacted by victim support are the highest in New Zealand (47%) and the United Kingdom, with percentages as high as 40 in Scotland, 37 in Northern Ireland, and 31 in England and Wales. Comparatively high satisfaction of expressed needs of victim support is also found in Austria (38%), Canada (37%), the Netherlands (35%), Japan (34%), the United States (33%), Belgium (28%), and Denmark (27%). Take-up rates in the range of 10–25% are achieved in Hong Kong, Norway, Iceland, Sweden, Ireland, Australia, France, and Luxembourg. In other countries less than 10% of the respondents who indicated that victim support would have been useful received it. This category of countries where victim support reaches only a tiny part of victims in need of help includes several affluent Western countries (Greece, Spain, Portugal, Finland, Italy, and Germany).

6.4.3 Attitudes toward Punishment

The ICVS asked respondents what sentence they considered most appropriate for a recidivist burglar—a man aged 21 who is found guilty of burglary for the second time, having stolen a color television. One of the most commonly raised arguments against the right of victims to be heard in court proceedings is that such participation would inevitably result in stiffer sentencing [Erez, 2000]. The ICVS data on the appropriate punishment for a burglar can shed some light on this issue. Table 6.3 shows sentencing preferences of victims and nonvictims of the five regions and for the main cities in developing countries.

The results show that, contrary to what is assumed by opponents of victims' rights, victims tend to be only marginally more punitive on average than the public at large in almost all countries. In Italy, Estonia, Australia, the Netherlands, Scotland, and Bulgaria, the victims are even a bit less punitive than the general public. The results also confirm the higher punitiveness of both victims and nonvictims in most of the English-speaking, common law countries. In 2005, England and Wales stood out with 51% of the public in favor of imprisonment compared with 19% in Germany and 12% in France. Most punitive, however, are the populations of Mexico (around 70% for both victims and nonvictims), Japan (around 53% for both victims and

Table 6.3 Percentage of the Public Opting for Imprisonment as Punishment for Recidivist Burglar in 2004–2005 in Five Regions in Developed Countries and Six Main Cities in Developing Countries, Broken Down by Victimization in the Year before the Survey

	No Victim	Victim
English-speaking/Common law countries	41.2	41.6
Nordic countries	23.4	25.2
Southern Europe	26.1	32.6
Western Europe	16.6	19.3
Eastern Europe	34.2	33.3
Six main cities in developing countries	57.1	57.2

Source: 2004–2005 ICVS and 2005 EU ICS.

Table 6.4   Log-Linear Analysis on Preference for a Prison Sentence

	21 Developed Countries
Age	
Young (base)	
Middle	.75*
Old	.67*
Gender	
Male (base)	
Female	.72*
Educational level	
Low (base)	
High	.65*
Region	
Other Western countries	

Source: 2004–2005 ICVS and 2005 EU ICS.
* Statistically significant, $t > 1.96$, $p < 0.05$.

nonvictims), Johannesburg (around 75% for both victims and nonvictims), and Phnom Penh (62% for nonvictims and 65% for victims).

Apart from the regional differences, the ICVS and EU ICS allow for an analysis of the correlates of punitivity at the individual level. Seven variables from the database were included in the initial analysis. The most important predictors of punitiveness were age, gender, and education (younger people, females, and those with less education being more punitive). These results are in line with the outcomes of previous analyses [Mayhew and van Dijk, 1997; Kuhnrich and Kania, 2005]. To determine the impact of national cultures controlling for these individual characteristics, a log-linear analysis was conducted. The results are given in Table 6.4.

The results of the log-linear analysis show that the factor most strongly associated with a preference for imprisonment is being Anglophone. The factors age, education, and gender are of secondary importance in predicting punitiveness.

6.5 Risk Assessments and Fear of Crime

In the ICVS a question is put to respondents to probe their perceptions of the likelihood of household burglary. The ICVS has previously found that perceptions of the likelihood of burglary at the national level are strongly related to national ICVS risks of burglary: that is, countries where the highest proportions feel vulnerable to burglary in the coming year are those where risks are highest. In the 2005 sweep, a relationship was again found between the proportions of those thinking burglary was very likely and national burglary rates. Among the 30 countries and 12 cities combined, perceived risks for burglary and actual risks were moderately strongly related ($r = .54$, $n = 35$, $p < .05$). The two Brazilian cities stand out because fear of burglary is out of proportion of actual victimization. This goes to a lesser extent for Japan and Istanbul as well. Maputo and Phnom Penh are so far off the regression line that we have considered them outliers.

In previous analyses, those who had recently been victimized by burglary were, not surprisingly, found to be more concerned than nonvictims [Van Kesteren, Mayhew, and Nieuwbeerta, 2000]. Figure 6.4 shows the percentages of those who deem a burglary likely among those victimized by burglary over the past 5 years, as well as among those who were not, per country. The results show at a glance that victims are universally more concerned than nonvictims. This is especially the case in countries where the public is generally less concerned about burglary risks. In many developing countries the differences between victims and nonvictims are less pronounced.

Since 1992, the ICVS has asked the below question, often used in other crime surveys, to measure vulnerability to street crime: "How safe do you feel walking alone in your area after dark? Do you feel very safe, fairly safe, a bit unsafe or very unsafe?" On average, a quarter of national populations felt very or a bit unsafe. The percentage is higher among inhabitants of main cities (37%), especially those in developing countries (>50%). Figure 6.5 gives details of the feelings of lack of safety of victims and nonvictims per country. Fear of street crime was lowest in the Scandinavian countries, Canada, the Netherlands, the United States, and Austria. At the country level, feelings of lack of safety were most widespread in Bulgaria, Poland, Greece, Luxembourg, Japan, and Italy.

As has been the case in previous sweeps of the ICVS, this measure of street safety is not consistently related to levels of contact crime (robbery, sexual incidents, and assaults and threats) ($r = -.07$; $n = 28$, not significant). In Portugal, for example, risks are low, but fear of street crime is much higher than, say, in Sweden, where actual national risks of contact crime are greater. One reason for this lack of a relationship between anxiety and risks is that fear of street crime may be influenced by nonconventional forms of crime such as drug dealing in public or other incivilities [Markowitz et al., 2001]. Previous analyses have found weak linkages between past victimizations by contact crimes and feelings of lack of safety [Van Kesteren, Mayhew, and Nieuwbeerta, 2000]. Figure 6.5 shows feelings of lack of safety of victims and nonvictims per country. The results confirm that those victimized by contact crime during the past 5 years exhibit somewhat higher levels of fear (35%) than those who have not (25%). In cities in developing countries the differences are smaller. The lack of a stronger relationship confirms that victimization by contact crimes is just one of the sources of anxiety about safety in the streets.

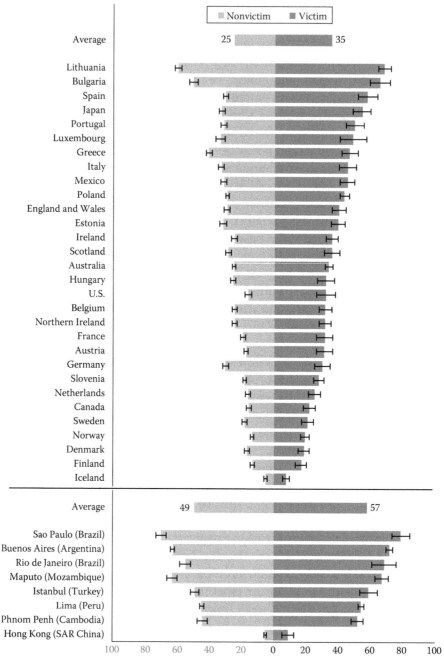

Figure 6.4 Percentage of the public feeling burglary is likely or very likely in the coming year data for countries and main cities, broken down by victimization by burglary and attempted burglary in a period of 5 years. (From 2004–2005 ICVS and 2005 EU ICS.)

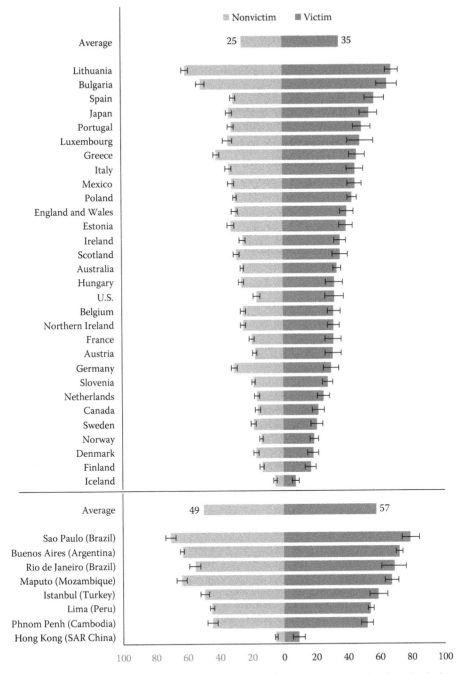

Figure 6.5 Percentage of the public feeling a bit or very unsafe after dark for countries and main cities, broken down by victimization by 10 common crimes in a period of 1 year. (From 2004–2005 ICVS and 2005 EU ICS.)

6.5.1 Analysis on the Individual Level

Apart from the experiences with victimization, there are a number of other individual characteristics that have an influence on the assessment of risk for burglary and feelings of lack of safety in the street. Results of a regression analysis show that a previous victimization by burglary or an attempt in the previous 5 years is the strongest predictor for assessing the risk for a burglary as high (regression coefficient of .174). Next strongest is town size; living in a larger city causes people to believe they run higher risks to see their houses burglarized. Less important but still significant predictors are gender (women feel themselves more at risk), educational level (higher income group considers themselves less at risk), living with a partner (lower perceived risks), and lifestyle (those going out often feel less at risk). The weakest predictor is age; older people feel they are less at risk. The results of the regression analysis are presented in Table 6.5. The multiple regression coefficient for this analysis is .20.

A similar analysis is carried out with feelings of lack of safety outdoors as the dependent variable. The results are given in Table 6.6. The multiple

Table 6.5   Regression Analysis on Assessment of Risk for Burglary

	Unstandardized Coefficients		Standardized Coefficients		
	B	Standard Error	Beta	t	Significance
(Constant)	2.720	0.017		158.171	<0.05
Going out	−0.012	0.003	0.023	−3.969	<0.05
Partner	−0.037	0.007	0.032	−5.708	<0.05
Educational level	0.006	0.001	−0.046	8.208	<0.05
Income	−0.022	0.007	0.019	−3.286	<0.05
Town size	−0.014	0.001	0.063	−11.766	<0.05
Gender	−0.056	0.006	0.049	−9.183	<0.05
Age	0.002	0.001	−0.010	1.789	<0.05
Victim	−0.288	0.009	0.174	−33.154	<0.05

Source: Data from 21 industrialized countries from the 2004–2005 ICVS and 2005 EU ICS.
Note: A 4-point scale was used except where noted below.
Multiple regression coefficient 0.20.
Going out is a variable on a 5-point scale from very often (1) to never (5).
Partner is a dichotomy: no partner (0), partner (1).
Educational level: number of years at school, from 0 to 40.
Income is a dichotomy: low income (0), high income (1).
Town size is a 6-point scale: small (1), capital city (7).
Gender is a dichotomy: male (0), female (1).
Age is in 12 categories of 5 years: 16–19 (1), 79+ (12).
Victim of a burglary or attempt in a period of 5 years is a dichotomy: no (0), yes (1).

Table 6.6 Regression Analysis on Fear after Dark

	Unstandardized Coefficients		Standardized Coefficients		
	B	Standard Error	Beta	t	Significance
(Constant)	1.489	0.027		54.64	<0.05
Going out	0.135	0.005	0.156	29.6	<0.05
Partner	−0.070	0.010	−0.034	−6.8	<0.05
Educational level	−0.026	0.001	−0.107	−20.7	<0.05
Income	−0.066	0.011	−0.033	−6.3	<0.05
Town size	0.062	0.002	0.164	33.2	<0.05
Gender	0.436	0.010	0.221	45.2	<0.05
Age	0.016	0.002	0.048	9.3	<0.05
Victim	0.179	0.013	0.067	13.8	<0.05

Source: Data from 21 industrialized countries from the 2004–2005 ICVS and 2005 EU ICS.
Note: A 4-point scale was used except where noted below.
Multiple regression coefficient 0.38.
Going out is a variable on a 5-point scale from very often (1) to never (5).
Partner is a dichotomy: no partner (0), partner (1).
Educational level: number of years at school, from 0 to 40.
Income is a dichotomy: low income (0), high income (1).
Town size is a 6-point scale: small (1), capital city (7).
Gender is a dichotomy: male (0), female (1).
Age is in 12 categories of 5 years: 16–19 (1), 79+ (12).
Victim of any of the 10 common crimes in a period of 1 year is a dichotomy: no (0), yes (1).

regression coefficient is .38. The three strongest predictors are gender (women are more afraid), lifestyle (people going out often are the least afraid), and town size (people living in large cities are more afraid). Educational level has a moderate effect in the sense that the higher educated are less afraid. All other variables in the model have very little predictive power. This is also the case with past victimization by any crime. The weak effect of victimization confirms that feelings of lack of safety are fueled by other factors besides actual experiences with crime.

6.6 Seriousness Rating of Types of Crimes by Victims

In the ICVS questionnaire, victims are asked to assess the seriousness of the incidents they reported to the interviewer on a simple 3-point scale, indicating serious (3), somewhat serious (2), and not very serious (1). For each of the 14 types and subtypes of crime, the mean scores were calculated for each region. On this basis, the scores of the regions were rank ordered. Crime types with the highest mean scores are considered the most serious and are given rank 1.

Table 6.7 presents the mean scores of the types of crimes and rank numbers. The results show that the 14 types of crime are rated very similarly by victims in the various regions. In the Nordic countries the mean scores of all crime types are consistently deemed less serious than in southern Europe. This finding confirms stereotypical images of Nordic coolness and Mediterranean emotionality, but it may also be simply the result of differences in connotation in the translations of the word *serious*. To control for such distortions, mean scores are translated into rank numbers per region. The ranking of the crime types in seriousness shows a striking similarity across regions, including the Nordic and southern European countries. The seriousness of victimizations by various types of crime is apparently perceived in much the same way across these world regions or language groups. This by itself is an important victimological finding because it refutes the notion of cultural relativism in the perception of victimizations by common crimes. However, there are some distinct divergences. Car theft and joyriding, as well as theft of a motorcycle, are considered to be the most serious in developing countries but less so in Western Europe, North America, and Australia. This difference is consistent over the various sweeps of the ICVS and seems to reflect a different appreciation of the economic value of motor cars and motorcycles [Van Dijk, 1999]. Armed robberies are rated as the most serious by victims everywhere. In the Nordic countries, where levels of violence are comparatively low, simple assaults and threats are considered as more serious than elsewhere.

6.6.1 Individual Factors Influencing Seriousness

Apart from the seriousness of the crime itself, there may be other factors influencing the opinions of the respondents. To explore this we have executed a regression analysis with the seriousness assessment as dependent variable and the 14 different types of crime and a number of individual characteristics, such as gender, age, marital status, educational level, income level, and town size, as independents. The analysis shows that the type of crime determines the serious rating by victims. Personal characteristics of the victims hardly play any role. After controlling for the type of crime, gender is the strongest predictor for the seriousness of the crime; women consider crimes somewhat more serious than men. The next strongest predictor is educational level; the higher educated consider crime less serious. The next strongest predictors are income and town size. Higher incomes consider crime less serious on average; people living in larger cities believe crime is more serious on average. Going out shows the least effect on the seriousness of the crimes. Living with a partner and age are not statistically significant. By and large the results confirm that seriousness ratings by victims of types of crime are little influenced by either national cultures or personal characteristics.

Table 6.7 Seriousness Scores* for 14 Crimes

	English-Speaking/ Common Law Countries		Nordic Countries		Southern Europe		Western Europe		Main Cities in Developing Countries	
1 Robbery with a weapon present	2.50	2	2.34	1	2.43	4	2.36	2	2.42	3
2 Sexual assault	2.52	1	2.30	3	2.43	3	2.37	1	2.29	4
3 Car theft	2.38	4	2.02	4	2.52	1	2.34	3	2.76	1
4 Assault and threat with a weapon	2.47	3	2.31	2	2.49	2	2.28	4	2.02	6
5 Joyriding	2.24	7	1.84	9	2.25	6	2.24	5	2.50	2
6 Burglary	2.29	5	1.90	8	2.31	5	2.06	6	1.98	7
7 Robbery without a weapon	2.24	6	1.93	6	2.13	7	2.01	8	1.96	8
8 Assault and threat without a weapon	2.11	8	1.94	5	2.12	9	2.04	7	1.90	9
9 Theft of motorcycle/moped	2.09	9	1.90	7	2.06	10	1.95	10	2.08	5
10 Pickpocketing	1.90	10	1.68	10	2.12	8	1.99	9	1.85	11
11 Theft of personal property	1.81	11	1.60	11	2.03	11	1.90	11	1.87	10
12 Attempted burglary	1.79	12	1.58	12	1.87	12	1.69	12	1.56	14
13 Bicycle theft	1.67	13	1.39	14	1.84	13	1.65	13	1.76	12
14 Theft from a car	1.62	14	1.44	13	1.82	14	1.60	14	1.58	13
Average for the region	2.12		1.87		2.17		2.03		2.04	

Source: 2004–2005 ICVS and 2005 EU ICS.

* Mean scores on a scale from 1 (not very serious) to 3 (very serious) and rank numbers.

6.7 Concluding Remarks and Policy Implications

The experiences with five rounds of the ICVS have demonstrated the viability of standardized crime surveying as a new avenue for comparative research on issues of crime and justice. Such surveys cannot only provide sound information on trends in victimization by common crimes at the aggregate level across countries, but also analyses at the individual level can provide insights in the distribution of victimization risks across population groups in a comparative perspective. Besides, follow-up questions to identified victims can yield comparative trend data on satisfaction with the police, pick-up rates of specialized services for victims, fear of crime of victims and nonvictims, seriousness ratings by victims, and attitudes toward punishment of offenders of victims and nonvictims.

Standardized surveys such as the ICVS provide basic facts about the state of crime victims across countries and their treatment by government agencies. They can help victimologists to identify what is universal and what is country specific in the world of victimization by common crimes and victim policies. Analyses of victimological risk factors show that risks to be victimized by common crime are everywhere closely linked to the factors of age and urbanization. In the provision of both crime prevention and victim services young urban residents should be given special attention. Traditionally high-income groups have been more at risk to be victimized by property crimes such as car theft, joyriding, and burglary. In the fifth sweep of the survey, high-income groups appeared no longer to be more at risk in Europe and the United States. In fact, low-income groups appeared to be more exposed to property crimes in the United States. The explanation for this recent shift in the distribution of risks is the differential increase of security measures across income groups. The growing divide between the poor and the rich in the use of security measures should be a wake-up call for policymakers across the Western world. Market forces in the field of crime prevention measures seem to produce an increasingly unequal distribution of victimization risks. In the United States, a veritable security divide between the rich and the poor is already in evidence.

In Austria, Germany, and Sweden, two of three victims are satisfied with how the police dealt with their case. In France and the United States, this is only one of two. In the corporate world such rates of satisfaction among clients would be regarded as a cause of great concern. Most notably, police forces in formerly socialist societies in Eastern Europe are still grossly under-performing in their handling of victim reports. Satisfaction is also comparatively low in Italy and Greece. The surprising decreases in satisfaction with police among reporting victims in many developed countries should also give cause for concern. The establishment of specialized victim support agencies seems to have caused the unintended negative side effect of diminished attention for victims by the police. This situation should be remedied by stricter instructions for the police and more recurrent on-the-job training and monitoring.

The supply of victim support itself does not yet fully meet demand even in those countries where such services are most firmly established, such as the United Kingdom, the United States, and the Netherlands. Fewer than one in three victims who would have appreciated such help received it. New Zealand is the only country that manages to reach out to at least half of all victims in need of help. Limited resources seem to have prevented a further growth of the pick-up rates of victim support organization during the past 10 years. The ICVS data on these issues can assist governments in policy setting by providing benchmarks based on the performance in other countries.

A recurrent issue in victimological research involves risk assessments and feelings of lack of safety. The ICVS data confirm that personal victim-izations by crime are an important source of anxiety but far from the only one. Feelings of lack of safety in the street seem to be fueled by many other cues besides personal victimization experiences. ICVS data on sentencing opinions refute the conventional wisdom that crime victims are intrinsi-cally punitive. Multivariate analyses have confirmed that opinions about punishment are influenced more by national cultures, notably Anglophones versus non-Anglophones, than by personal experiences with victimization. Comparative information on sentencing preferences can help to question conventional ideas about the punitiveness of the public at large. In many parts of the world, including the European continent, victims and nonvic-tims alike seem to prefer noncustodial sentences for run-of-the-mill offend-ers. Finally, the ICVS offers data on the serious rating of various types of crime by victims. The near universality of these ratings lends support to the conception of a standardized crime survey. This result also lends support to ongoing campaigns for universal standards for the treatment of victims such as a UN Convention on the Rights of Victims of Crime (for details, see www. Tilburg.edu/intervict). The notion that the moral suffering of victims is too culture bound to be usefully addressed in the framework of international standards seems unwarranted. Crime victims of the world seem to agree on the seriousness of the victimizations they have experienced and most likely also on their need to be better protected under national and international legislation.

References

Allen, J. (ed.). 2006. *Policing and the criminal justice system—Public confidence and per-ceptions: Findings from the 2004/2005 British Crime Survey*, Online report 07/06. http://www.homeoffice.gov.uk/rds/pdfs06/rdsolr0706.pdf (accessed January 3, 2009).

CBS. 2006. *Veiligheidsmonitor.* Voorburg: CBS.

Erez, E. and L. Rogers. 1999. Victim impact statements and sentencing outcomes and processes, the perspectives of legal professions. *British Journal of Criminology* 39:216–39.

Felson, M. 2002. *Crime and everyday life,* 3rd ed. Thousand Oaks, CA: Pine Forge/Sage.

Goudriaan, H. 2004. Reporting to the police in Western countries: A theoretical analysis of the effects of social context. *Justice Quarterly* 21(4):933–69.

Kuhnrich, B. and H. Kania. 2005. *Attitudes towards punishment in the European Union, results from the 2005 European Crime Survey (ECSS) with a focus on Germany.* Freiburg, Germany: Max Planck Institute for Foreign and International Criminal Law. http://www.europeansafetyobservatory.eu (accessed October 30, 2008).

Markowitz, F. E. 2001. Extending social disorganisation theory: Modeling the relationship between cohesion, disorder and fear. *Criminology* 39(2):293–320.

Mayhew, P. and J. J. M. van Dijk. 1997. Criminal victimization in eleven industrialized countries. *Key findings from the 1996 international crime victims survey.* The Hague: WODC.

Skogan, W. 1984. Reporting crimes to the police: The status of world research. *Journal of Research on Crime and Delinquency* 21(2):113–37.

Van Dijk, J. J. M. 1999. The experience of crime and justice, In *Global report on crime and justice,* ed. G. Newman, 25–43. New York: Oxford University Press.

———. 2007. *The world of crime. Breaking the silence on problems of security, justice and development across the world.* Thousand Oaks, CA: Sage.

Van Dijk, J. J. M., R. Manchin, J. N. van Kesteren, and G. Hideg. 2007. *The burden of crime in the EU, a comparative analysis of the European survey of crime and safety (EU ICS) 2005.* Brussels: Gallup Europe.

Van Dijk, J. J. M. and C. D. Steinmetz. 1980. *The RDC victim surveys, 1973–1979.* The Hague: WODC, Ministry of Justice.

Van Dijk, J. J. M., J. N. van Kesteren, and P. Smit. 2008. *Criminal victimization in international perspective, key findings from the 2004-2005 ICVS and EU ICS.* The Hague: Boom Legal.

Van Kesteren, J. N. 2006. Victimization of immigrants in Europe, results from the 2005 EU/ICS (ICVS). Paper presented at the 12th International Symposium of the World Society of Victimology, Orlando.

———. 2007. *Integrated database from the international crime victims survey (ICVS) 1989–2005, codebook and data.* Tilburg: INTERVICT, Tilburg University.

Van Wilsem, J. 2004. Criminal victimization in cross-national perspective: An analysis of rates of theft, violence and vandalism across 27 countries. *European Journal of Criminology* 1(1):89–109.

Wilcox Rountree, P. 1998. A reexamination of the crime-fear linkage. *Journal of Research in Crime and Delinquency* 35(3):341–72.

Patterns of Communal Violence Victimization in South India

A Geographic Information Systems (GIS) Analysis

7

K. JAISHANKAR

Contents

7.1 Introduction

In India, religion plays a very important role in governing people's clothing, food, marriage, and even occupations [Shah, 1998]. According to the 2001 census, the religious composition of India is Hindus, 80.5%; Muslims, 13.4%; Christians, 2.3%; Sikhs, 1.9%; Buddhists, 0.8%; Jains, 0.4%; and others, 0.7% [Census of India, 2001]. This diversity today reflects the fact that historically India has always been a meeting point for a large number of cultures and traditions. India is a secular country that believes in "Unity in Diversity." However, it is always difficult to keep unity among these diametrically different cultures. Many times religious intolerance has reached greater heights and caused significant disharmony and conflict among various religions in India. Of these conflicts, the relationship between Hindus and Muslims has been particularly salient, and it has a historical background [Hewstone and Voci, 2003].

A historical analysis of communal violence in India would emphasize that the roots of the communal disharmony and violence between the Hindus and Muslims could be dated several centuries back. However, contemporary historians like Sarkar [1983] would not agree with the view that the communal violence in India is a medieval phenomenon; rather, he argues that it is a modern one, as communal riots seem to have been significantly rare until the 1880s. Brass [2003] also agrees with this view and feels that there were no Hindu–Muslim conflicts before the nineteenth century. Despite historians' disagreement on the dates of communal violence, one can surely say that the victimization of one religious community by the other started as the suppression of rulers who invaded India [Ghosh, 1987]. Ghosh [1987:24] explores the invasion:

In 712 AD, Mohammad Bin al Q'asim overran Sind. The Arabs, the Turks, the Afghans and the Mughals invaded India in hordes from 1206 onwards, reducing temples to rubble, putting hundreds of thousands of Hindus to the sword, and forcibly converting the survivors to Islam. Later during the Mughal period relations between Hindus and Muslims were not cordial during the regimes of Babur, Jehangir, Shah Jehan, and Aurangazeb. Among the Mughal emperors, Aurangazeb reversed the enlightened policy of Akbar, the Great, and he was determined to make India a strictly Muslim empire. Under his orders, several Hindu temples were destroyed.

Mahajan [1993:45] further analyzes victimization of both these communities:

In 1669, a circular order was addressed to all appropriate officers in the Mughal Empire directing them to destroy all newly built temples and forbade the repair of old ones. Thousands of temples at Prayag, Kashi, Ayodhya, Hardwar, and other Holy places were destroyed. When these temples were destroyed, there were disturbances at many places on account or resistances of the Hindus against the demolition of temples. There was a prolonged fight between the Hindus and Muslims around the Mosque built on the ruins of the Veni, Madhava or Bindu Madhava temple at Banaras. The rioters destroyed some mosques in retaliation and when the Muslims got reinforcements, they destroyed all temples whether new or old.

From Mahajan's [1993] analysis it can be noted that communal rioting and victimization of both religious communities started during the Aurangazeb period. Later the British who invaded in India ignited animosity and conflict between the Hindu and Muslim communities. After the decline of Mughal power, the British often used "divide and rule" tactics to maintain governance over the vast area. In essence, the Hindu–Muslim conflict has existed in earnest since the British rule [Girdner, 1998]. As Eh Din [2002: paragraphs 35, 36] has put it:

The British organized communal violence because it provided them a pretext to further suppress the people and declare that it was not the colonial rule that was the cause of the problems of the Indian people, but that religion was the problem. They blamed the victims and their religions for the situation created by the colonial rule, and said that it is the policy of the British to be fair and pursue a Secular policy to "do justice to all religious communities".... Thus communal violence was institutionalised in the state structures, used to weaken the unity and resistance of the people and used as a pretext to further attack them and cause diversions. This communal nature of the institutions and state structure did not change with the transfer of power in 1947 and this transfer of power itself was done in the midst of a communal carnage.

The birth of Pakistan in 1947 did not settle Hindu–Muslim differences or end conflicts. To the contrary, all the old problems remained. However, the problem is more complex and involves more than simply a difference in values. Violence and communal strife have defined the relationship between Muslims and Hindus since partition [Shah, 1998]. India has regularly experienced communal rioting, particularly between Hindus and Muslims, but has occasionally involved other minority communities (Christians and Sikhs) since its independence in 1947. Even before independence, there were serious communal riots in Varanasi (1809), Bareilly (1871), Lahore and Delhi (1825), Kolkata (1851), Azamgarh (1893), Ayodhya (1912), Kolkata and Dhaka (1926), Ahmedabad and Mumbai (1941), and of course the horrendous countrywide riots of 1946 and 1947 [Dhar, 2002].

7.2 Communal Violence and Terrorism: Trends in Post–Babri Masjid Demolition Period

Even after 62 years of Indian independence, the seeds of hate between the two religious communities continue to sprout. If anything, it has been getting worse year after year. There has been not a single year in the postindependence period that has been free of communal violence, although the number of incidents may vary [Engineer, 2003]. The past decade and the start of the new millennium have been the worst era in this matter right from the beginning of the Babri Masjid demolition* (1992) to the Gujarat carnage (2002). After the Babri Masjid demolition in 1992, communal violence rose to a new dimension. Eight important trends are noticeable in the post-Babri period.

1. The first trend is the transition of communal violence to communal terrorism. The communal riots that occurred before the Babri Masjid issue were not planned. However, the post–Babri Masjid scenario has changed the facets of communal violence in India. Most of the riots are well planned, and spontaneous violence has been overtaken by planned terrorism. Earlier during the 1980s and before, a number of major communal riots had taken place, but no such bomb explosions occurred right up to the Babri Masjid period. However, now planned executions of bomb explosions have become a part of the communal terrorism scenario in various parts of India [Engineer, 2003].
2. The riots that occur in the post-Babri demolition period are not as horrendous as those in the 1980s. In the riots of the 1980s, the average number of deaths used to be more than 250–300; however, after the demolition of Babri Masjid, the average number of deaths has been around 25–30 [Engineer, 2002].
3. South India, which was relatively free of communalism and communal violence, began to experience outbursts of communal violence. Thus, the Coimbatore communal riots and subsequent bomb blast there in February 1998 is symptomatic of this [Engineer, 2001]. Kerala

---

* On December 6, 1992, a sixteenth-century mosque in Ayodhya, in the north Indian state of Uttar Pradesh, was demolished. During the preceding months, a movement of political parties, religious groups, and cultural organizations, including the BJP, Rashtriya Swayamsevak Sangh (RSS), Vishwa Hindu Parishad (VHP), and Shiva Sena, had called for the construction of a temple on the site of the mosque as an integral move in their struggle for Hindutva, or Hindu rule. More than 150,000 supporters known as *kar sevaks* (voluntary workers) converged on Ayodhya, where they attacked the three-domed mosque with hammers and pickaxes and reduced it to rubble [Human Rights Watch, 1996]. The destruction touched off Hindu–Muslim rioting across the country that has killed thousands in the past few years. Within 2 weeks of the destruction of the mosque, 227 were killed in communal violence in Gujarat, 250 in Bombay (Maharashtra), 55 in Karnataka, 14 in Kerala, 42 in Delhi, 185 in Uttar Pradesh, 100 in Assam, 43 in Bihar, 100 in Madhya Pradesh, and 23 in Andhra Pradesh.

also has become a safe haven for terrorists, and they have started operating from there. The recent Ahmedabad (2008) bomb blasts have witnessed the role of terrorists who had hideouts in Kerala.

4. There was an increase and a decrease of Muslim fundamentalist organizations like Jihad Committee, Al-Umma, and Islamic United Front seen in the post-Babri period. Also, there was a growth of new terrorist outfits like Indian Mujahideen (which played a great role in the bomb blasts of Ahmedabad in 2008) and Indian Islamic Security Force (which played a great role in the bomb blasts of Assam in 2008).

5. Blasts against Muslims in 1993 were a "business objective" for the Bombay underworld dons. However, the August 2003 blasts in Mumbai launched new intent from terrorists who commit crimes against Hindus. The Islamic militant Gujarat Revenge Group is growing active in Mumbai and works hand-in-hand with a banned militant students' organization, the Students Islamic Movement in India (SIMI) [Paul, 2003].

6. Infiltration of religious terrorists, such as Lashkar-i Tayyeba, was seen in the Mumbai (2003) and the Delhi bomb blasts (2005).

7. The data released by the Ministry of Home Affairs affirm that before the Babri demolition, the percentage of Muslim victims in these riots had been 80%. Post-Babri demolition the ratio might have become more adverse to Muslims [Puniyani, 2005].

8. The September 2008 bomb blasts in Malegeon, Maharashtra, showed a new trend. For the first time, Hindu right-wing terrorists were involved in the bombing.

9. Of these eight important trends, in this chapter, the first and third trends are analyzed from a victimological perspective.

7.3 Communal Violence and Terrorism in South India

All these years, the states in South India, particularly Tamil Nadu and Kerala, were free from communal violence. In fact, communalism and communal violence were considered a North Indian phenomenon. It is a well-known fact that people in South India, both the Hindus and Muslims, are generally more religious and orthodox and less fanatical than their counterparts in North India (Hussain, 1984). Hussain (1984:375) examines the differences between North Indians and South Indians:

The reasons for this glaring disparity between the attitudes of the people of the two regions may be traced to their different historical backgrounds. The North, having experienced the greater impact of invasion and rule by various foreign dynasties and powers from time to time, there are deeper traces of feudalism in the communities with strong feelings of the glory and grandeur of their pasts. This inhibits the normal process of national growth and integration. It is also to be remembered that only the states in the North had in fact borne the actual brunt of the partition of the country, when millions of people are uprooted and displaced on either side of the new political borders, leaving a trial of communal hatred and bitterness.

But of late, the virus of communalism has spread to the South too and has become more and more virulent. In Kerala, the Bharatiya Janata Party (BJP)[*] and the Rashtriya Suyam Sevak (RSS)[†] are trying to establish themselves, and in Tamil Nadu, the Hindu Munnani and Muslim fundamentalist organizations like the Al-Umma,[‡] for example, are spreading their tentacles. While Kerala has seen warfare between the Communist Party of India (Marxist) (CPM)[§] and RSS cadre, Tamil Nadu is witnessing warfare between Hindu Munnani and Al-Umma [Engineer, 1999]. At one time, Tamil Nadu was considered a haven of communal harmony, but now Tamil Nadu has also become one of the hotbeds of communal violence.

7.3.1 Communal Violence Victimization in Tamil Nadu

The long-considered belief of Tamil Nadu being a state of peace has been shattered during the past few years. A cursory survey of the map of Tamil Nadu (Figure 7.1) would show the growing incidents of communal tensions and violence.

The manifestation of communal terrorism varies in various parts of the state. It reflects sophistication in coastal areas like Chennai, Nagapattinam, Thanjavur, Tiruvarur, Ramanathapuram, and border districts of Coimbatore. Here, the fundamentalists use heavy doses of sophisticated explosives. In other districts like Dindigul, Theni, Madurai, Thoothukkudi, Tirunelveli, Neelagiri, and Coimbatore (rural), the communal terrorism is in preliminary stages. In these areas, the terrorists confine themselves to targeting killings. Vellore, Chengalpet, Namakkal, Karur, and Trichy serve as shelter points to acts of

---

[*] Bharatiya Janata Party is a political party in India. Propagating Hinduism is its main ideology, and this is the party presently in power in the central government of India.

[†] Rashtriya Suyam Sevak is a Hindu fundamentalist organization. The RSS is also a cultural organization, which seeks to promote a Hindu ethos within India and among Indians living abroad. Although an ostensibly cultural organization, RSS cells are involved in supporting political candidates for government, trade unions, and student organizations.

[‡] Al-Umma is a Muslim fundamentalist organization started by S.A. Basha, a Muslim fundamentalist in Coimbatore, India. After the arrest of S.A. Basha and other fundamentalists in connection with the Coimbatore bomb blasts in 1998, this organization was banned.

[§] The Communist Party of India is a political party in India that propagates Marxist ideology.

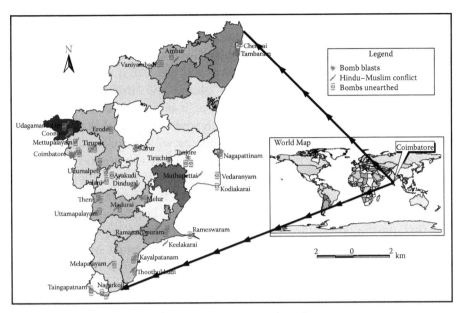

Figure 7.1 Communal violence scenario, Tamil Nadu.

communal terrorism. The situation in Tamil Nadu is a very complex one. There is a need to tackle the problem simultaneously at different stages, without any negligence or undermining of the gravity of the situation [ABVP, 1999].

7.3.2 Emergence of the Problem: Transition of Violence to Terrorism in Coimbatore City

The city witnessed brutal killings, arson, and riots in 1997, and bomb blasts in 1998 (Subramanian, 1998). The communal violence and bomb blasts that occurred at Coimbatore, which resulted in the loss of life of around 60 people and property worth millions of rupees, showed the proliferation of violent activities in Tamil Nadu. This incident put Tamil Nadu on the terror map.

In the history of Hindu–Muslim violence in Coimbatore during the past quarter century, there have been several turning points. The Hindu Munnani propaganda offensive in the early 1980s was followed by stray attacks on Hindu leaders. Simultaneously, Muslim gangs, thriving on extortion and petty crimes and seeking community acceptance, surfaced in the city. Around the same period, caste Hindu landlords pumped surplus funds into trade and merchandise that rivaled Muslim establishments. Slowly, the advantages of communalizing the situation became obvious. From isolated stabbings of known Hindu and Muslim activists to engineered riots to indiscriminate bomb blasts, it is a continuing story of communal elements finding a fertile ground for their dance of death in a *petit-bourgeois* environment. Shopkeepers and pavement vendors, divided not only communally but also geographically, found it necessary to obtain the protection of extremist elements. This was especially so in the case of Muslim traders who were repeatedly at the receiving end in riot situations [Gokulakrishnan, 1998, 2000].

The fact that the area prone to communal violence is contiguous to the region in neighboring Kerala, where the Islamic and Hindu fundamentalist outfits are known to have a strong presence, is of considerable significance. What compounds the problem, at least in some cases, is that the criminal and fundamentalist elements have joined forces, with the religious label serving as a cloak for the former's sinister activities. It is common knowledge that quite a few Islamic fundamentalist outfits, going by different names such as the Jihad Committee,* Al-Umma, and the Islamic United Front,† have become active in Tamil Nadu after the Babri Masjid demolition in 1992, and that, on the other side, the Sangh Parivar elements represented by the RSS, the Vishwa Hindu Parishad (VHP),‡ and the Hindu Munnani§ have been going all out to inject fanaticism and militancy into the ways of the majority community. Inevitably, this vicious and mutually destructive game of religious fundamentalism has manifested itself in retaliatory attacks and killings by the two sides, the like of which Tamil Nadu had not seen before [Gokulakrishnan, 1998, 2000].

On November 29, 1997, three youths belonging to Al-Umma, a Muslim fundamentalist organization, murdered a police constable, Mr. Selvaraj, which led to a virtual revolt by policemen. Police fired on "ferocious," "violent," and "belligerent" Muslim mobs and Al-Umma men, armed with petrol bombs, knives, sickles, stones, sticks, wooden logs, and swords. At the same time, large-scale arson and looting by Hindu fundamentalists of shops owned by Muslims happened. On the next day, many Muslims were killed [PUCL, 1997; Subramanian, 1997]. These events culminated in Al-Umma exploding a series of bombs in main places of the city on February 14, 1998, in which 58 people were killed [Subramanian, 1998]. These blasts were planned in revenge for the November 1997 riots in which Hindu Munnani played a key role. Rioting followed the bomb blasts, and a communal frenzy was generated [Engineer, 1998].

The past 10 years have witnessed an increase and a decrease in the terrorism graph of Coimbatore City. In tune with the general complexity of modern life, the Hindu–Muslim conflagration also has assumed complex dimensions. While a burgeoning population has aggravated several socioeconomic problems, old religious animosities have received fresh shots in the

---

* Jihad Committee is a Muslim fundamentalist organization.
† Islamic United Front is a Muslim fundamentalist organization.
‡ Vishwa Hindu Parishad is a Hindu fundamentalist organization. The VHP was established to unite Hinduism's regional and caste divisions under a single ecumenical umbrella. It is actively involved in Sanskrit education, the organization of Hindu rites and rituals, and converting Christians, Muslims, and animists to Hinduism.
§ Hindu Munnani is a Hindu fundamentalist organization.

arm and geared up the secular pitch of our society. As if this were not enough, power struggles between politicians are fueling these riots. Smugglers and other nefarious characters of the underworld too have found an avenue in communal violence to settle their personal scores. The diversity of the etiology and prognosis of this malady defies description and analysis. In brief, this particular manifestation of collective violence has become today a very complex and multilayered phenomenon, which creates issues for analysis [Saiyed, 1988]. A geographic information systems (GIS) approach may provide a comprehensive and systematic analysis of communal violence in Coimbatore City.

7.4 Purpose of the Study

Communal violence and terrorism in India had mostly been studied by political scientists and sociologists. Prominent among these is the efforts of Asghar Ali Engineer, who has conducted a large number of case studies of Hindu–Muslim riots and has deduced some explanations based on the empirical data [Saiyed, 1988]. However, the studies done have only analyzed the criminogenic factors underlying such violence. To understand the communal violence scenario, it is essential to study both the acts and victims in their wider contexts. Almost all the studies conducted on communal violence have reported the causes of such violence and measures to contain riots in the future, but no study has been done to analyze the victimization factors and victimization characteristics of communal violence.

The victimology of communal violence has become a neglected area of research. It is high time that victims are also given due consideration by studying such riots from both criminological and victimological perspectives. One could not forget the Coimbatore communal violence and the subsequent problems faced by the innocent victims (children, women, the aged) and indirect victims (victims of bomb blasts), which clearly revealed the untold misery and traumatic experience caused by the communal violence. In this context, the present investigation analyzes the Coimbatore communal terrorism from a victimological perspective.

In the present study, an innovative means for exploring the relationships among crimes of communal violence, victims, and sociodemographic characteristics of the city involves the use of GIS* or computer mapping

---

* A GIS is a computer system capable of capturing, storing, analyzing, and displaying geographically referenced information; that is, data identified according to location. Practitioners also define a GIS as including the procedures, operating personnel, and spatial data that go into the system. GIS allows us to view, understand, question, interpret, and visualize data in many ways that reveal relationships, patterns, and trends in the form of maps, reports, and charts.

software. GIS has been used for several years by researchers working in natural resources and environmental geography. Only recently, however, have social scientists begun to use this technology for their own purposes. GIS presents a powerful tool for the visualization and spatial analysis of practically any kind of phenomena that can be linked to geographical reference points [Herman, 1999]. Using such software has enabled the researcher to pinpoint the location of clusters of communal violence and victims in relation. More so, this software has enabled the creation of custom maps that overlay crimes of communal violence and victim data, thus allowing for visual assessment of the communal violence scenario in Coimbatore City. The application of GIS is a new venture in the field of victimology of communal violence and terrorism; therefore, it is believed that this may open up new areas of future research.

7.4.1 Review of the Literature

There is no dearth of spatial analysis and crime mapping studies in India. Srivastava [1963], Rao [1968], Sivamurthy [1980, 1988], Jos [1993], and Jaishankar, Shanmugapriya, and Balamurugan [2004] have done pioneering research in crime mapping and spatial analysis of crime in India. However, most of these studies focus on general crimes, and no spatial analysis had been done on crimes of communal violence in India. Existing literature on communal riots mostly deals with the causes of riots in contemporary structural terms in the political, economic, and socioculture perspective, tracking on occasion their origin to historical roots. The role of information technology in the prevention and control of riots has not been exclusively examined by any study in India. Whereas literature examining the geography of crime and GIS application in mapping crime is ample, only within the past few years have criminologists and GIS experts begun to research the dynamics of communal violence with GIS. As a result, research on analysis of communal riots using GIS is relatively limited.

European social scientists are the forerunners in the spatial analysis of crime. Guerry [1833] and Quetelet [1842] were the first scholars who noted that crime was not evenly distributed across geographic areas in France, and they pioneered the usage of maps to examine the spatial distribution of crime [Brantingham and Brantingham, 1981]. Guerry and Balbi first used crime maps in 1829, and Quetelet published ecological work shortly thereafter. Studies in England by Plint [1851] and Mayhew [1862] also noted the spatial variation in crime. However, scholars from the United States took over the spatial crime analysis and pioneered the art of making crime maps [e.g., Lottier, 1938a, 1939b; Shannon, 1954; Schmid, 1960a&b; Harries, 1971]. The transition of criminology from legal to sociological perspective was strongly grounded by Shaw and McKay [1969] and their Chicago School of criminological thought, which had significant components of spatial and temporal analysis of crime.

Since the 1920s, spatial analysis of crime became an integral part of American criminology [Harries, 1999; Canter, 2000], and later other countries emulated this model (e.g., the United Kingdom became the first country to start a master's of science program in crime science, which has a significant component of GIS and crime mapping). Many scholars have done research in this area. Examining various aspects of crime within a geographical context has contributed to a better understanding of geographical distribution of crimes. Some of the studies in this field are crimes of violence [McClintock, 1963], spatial patterns of victims [Curtis, 1972, 1974], offender travel patterns [Rengert, 1972; Pyle, 1974; Gabor and Gotthell, 1984; LeBeau, 1987; Rossmo, 1995], the building environment [Jeffery, 1971; Newman, 1972; Taylor, Shumaker, and Gottfredson, 1985], environmental criminology [Brantingham and Brantingham, 1981], social ecology [Shaw, 1929; Shaw and McKay, 1942, 1969; Harries, 1980; Schuerman and Kobrin, 1986; Sampson and Groves, 1989], patterns of crime [Brantingham and Brantingham, 1984], perception of crimes [Sivamurthy, 1984], and rates and trends of victimization [Laub, 1997].

The advent of GIS has made possible new types of spatial analysis of crime and created an explosion of interest in crime mapping [e.g., see Harries, 1990; Block and Dabdoud, 1993; Block, Dabdoud, and Fregly, 1995; Weisburd and McEwen, 1997]. The use of GIS to study patterns of riots/hate crimes [Herman, 1999; Umemoto and Mikami, 2000; Daihani and Purnomo, 2001] and terrorism [Molyneux, 1993; Elliott and Wagner, 2000; Harwood, 2002] is a modern trend. In this study, as we focus on the victims, the review further analyzes the use of crime mapping/GIS in the study of victims.

Curtis [1972, 1974] was the first researcher to develop victim maps using computer cartography. He used isopleth maps to study victims of robbery. Hirchfield [1995] also examined the victim location. Spelman [1989] estimated that 10% of victims are involved in approximately 40% of the victimization. Ratcliffe and McCullagh [1998] have also studied repeat victimization using GIS. McClung [2000] examined the study conducted by the Crime Victim's Institute, Texas: "The Impact of Crime on Victims: A Baseline Study on the Program Service Delivery." GIS played a key role in the planning, implementation, and evaluation of the study. The Institute used GIS to create a statewide thematic map to aid Texas Attorney General staff in determining the criteria for awarding the grants to local law enforcement agencies and prosecutor offices. The Crime Victims' Institute is one of the first agencies in the United States to apply GIS to victim services.

7.4.2 Resources and Data Used in the Study

The following software packages were used: ArcView GIS version 3.1, PC ArcInfo 3.5, ArcView Spatial Analyst, Crime Analysis Tools, ArcView Crime

Analyst extension, Demographics Analyst extension, and Count Points on polygons extension. Microsoft Excel 2000 was used as the relational database management system (RDBMS) to store the attribute data. Data were retrieved from RDBMS to be used in GIS by import and export functions within these packages. Internet sites about GIS, communal violence, and crime mapping were browsed to give a thorough understanding of the problem and its analysis.

Interviews and archival research were conducted to gather additional information on a number of identified "hot spots" to gain a better understanding of the nature of the phenomena in specific geographic areas. Interviews were conducted with police officers who tackle crimes of communal violence at Coimbatore City, Muslim fundamentalists, Muslim moderates, Hindu fundamentalists, and Hindu moderates. Archival materials included police reports, newspaper articles, charge sheets, correspondence, and flyers and announcements pertaining to Hindu–Muslim conflicts. Newspapers included *The Hindu*, *The Indian Express*, *Dinamani*, and *The Hindustan Times*, and magazines included *Frontline* and *India Today*. Articles from *The Frontline* were used extensively in the study. The charge sheet of bomb blasts in 1998 [SIT, 1999] and Justice Gokula Krishnan reports [1998, 2000] were intensively reviewed and used for this study, along with police preliminary investigation and follow-up reports for incidents that occurred in several areas.

The present study mainly relies on secondary data. Most of the spatial crime studies use secondary data instead of primary data [Harries, 1971; Sivamurthy, 1980, 1988]. The main reason is the mapping application, for which a large amount of data are needed for mapping, and it can only obtained from the secondary data. Moreover, there are time limitations for the collection of primary data. In the present study, because of the time limitation and the magnitude of the problem, primary data were not collected. Data for this study mainly come from three sources: the Police Department of the City of Coimbatore, Coimbatore Corporation, and the Land Planning Authority of the City of Coimbatore.

The data include crime statistics and land use, socioeconomic, and demographic characteristics. Crime statistics consist of the total number of crimes of communal violence by police boundaries. Land use characteristics encompass such categories as educational, industrial, public, residential, agriculture, water bodies, commercial, semipublic, and village boundaries. Socioeconomic and demographic characteristics include population, literacy, and urbanization. Data regarding the locations and characteristics of all crimes of communal violence that occurred during 1997 and 1998 in Coimbatore City were collected from the charge sheet of the communal violence [1998] and Justice Gokula Krishnan Commission reports [1998 and 2000]. The charge sheet was obtained from the religious organizations. The following characteristics were taken from the charge sheet: the street address where the crimes of communal violence occurred and the religion, sex, and age of the victim and the perpetrators; ward boundaries were obtained from Coimbatore municipal corporation, and population characteristics were linked to each one of the ward boundaries from the 1991 census. Police boundaries were obtained from the Commissioner of Police, Coimbatore City. The land use map was obtained from the Land Planning Authority of Coimbatore City.

7.5 GIS Methodology

A city map of Coimbatore of the year 1997 with a scale of 1:25,000 was scanned using a Deskan flatbed scanner. A base map* (Figure 7.2), consisting of the Coimbatore City boundary, main road networks, and ward boundaries was constructed by onscreen digitization† in ArcView 3.1 (a GIS software program), and topology‡ was constructed in PC ArcInfo 3.5 (a GIS software program). The base map is the one that is used for the present study. The base map was prepared with the help of three maps. The three maps are the police boundary map, ward map, and land use map.

As such, there was no police boundary map with the Coimbatore Police Commissioner. By the orders of the commissioner all the boundary maps were brought by the respective station in charge, and the researcher manually drew the boundaries on the ward map (Figure 7.3). Then, redrawing it on a tracing sheet segregated the police boundary. This map was scanned and digitized with ArcView GIS. A police station boundary map (Figure 7.4) evolved. Then it was overlaid on the land use map (Figure 7.5) to use the roads and streets. Finally, the base map consisting of police station boundaries, police stations, railway lines, and major roads evolved.

* A map showing planimetric, topographic, geological, political, and/or cadastral information that may appear in many different types of maps. The base map information is drawn with other types of changing thematic information. Base map information may include major political boundaries, major land use data, or major roads. The changing thematic information may be bus routes, population distribution, or migration routes.
† Digitization is the process of converting point and line data from source documents to a machine-readable format. A means of converting or encoding map data that are represented in analogue form into digital information of x and y coordinates.
‡ Topology is a mathematical procedure that defines the spatial relationships between connecting or adjacent coverage features (e.g., arc, nodes, polygons, and points). For example, the topology of an arc includes its from and to nodes and its left and right polygons. Topological relationships are built from simple elements into complex elements: points (simplest elements), arcs (sets of connected points), areas (sets of connected arcs), and routes (sets of sections that are arcs or portions of arcs). Primarily topology consists of three concepts: (1) contiguity (adjacency): features next to each other (usually polygons); (2) connectivity: features linked or connected (usually arcs); and (3) area (containment): arcs containing a polygon with given area.

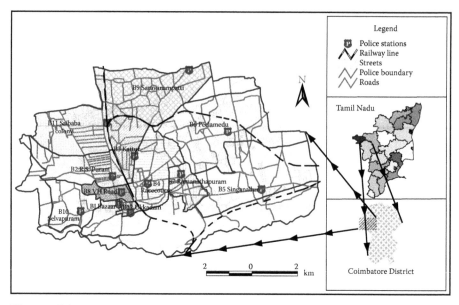

Figure 7.2 Base map. (From Coimbatore Corporation & Coimbatore Police Commissionerate.)

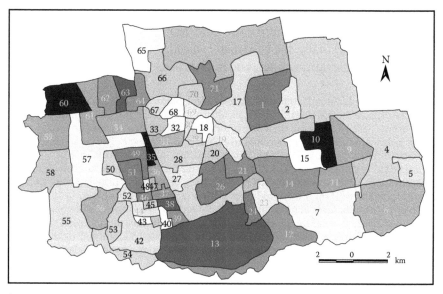

Figure 7.3 Ward map. (From Coimbatore Corporation & Coimbatore Land Planning Authority.)

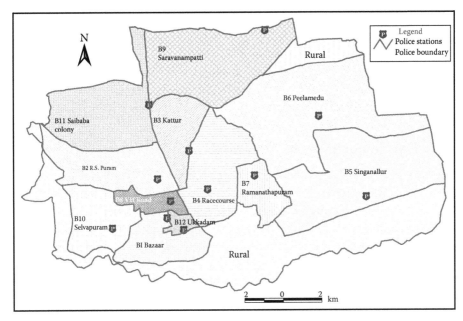

Figure 7.4 Police boundaries. (From Coimbatore Corporation & Coimbatore Police Commissionerate.)

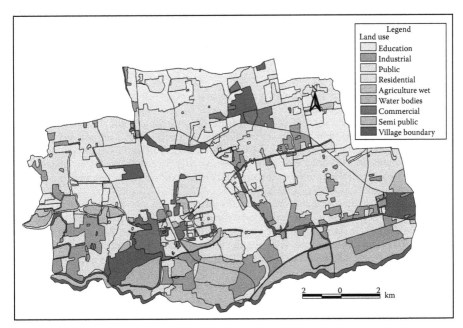

Figure 7.5 Land use. (From Coimbatore Corporation & Coimbatore Land Planning Authority.)

The GIS methodology of this study involves four steps:

1. Development of GIS database
2. Unification of sociodemographic data
3. Identification of spatial and temporal crime patterns
4. Visualization of the results

7.5.1 Development of GIS Database*

The first step in GIS methodology was to prepare the databases for import into ArcView. Census data were separated in an Excel spreadsheet because each type was to be added to ArcView as a separate theme and analyzed separately. The locations of crimes of communal violence were taken from the records, and the points were plotted as separate themes on the scanned raster† map in ArcView 3.1. Crimes of communal violence were added as a point theme. These shape files‡ were converted to arc files in PC ArcInfo 3.5 for constructing topology and for the projection§ and transformation of the coverages. These coverages¶ are brought again to ArcView 3.1. The crimes of communal violence for each year were compiled into separate coverages by matching the addresses where the crimes occurred with their geographic locations. The characteristics of each of the crimes were then added.

These coverages were superimposed on the ward boundary map to learn the number of crime incidents per ward and on the police boundary map to find out the number of crime incidents per police station boundary. Input of attribute** crime data was done in Microsoft Excel and imported into ArcView 3.1. Apart from the city and ward boundary maps, road maps, land use maps,

---

* Usually a computerized file or series of files or information, most diagrams, listings, location records, abstracts, or references on a particular subject or subjects organized by datasets and governed by a scheme of organization. "Hierarchical" and "relational" define two popular structural schemes in use in a GIS. For example, a GIS database includes data about the spatial location and shape of geographic entities, as well as their attributes.

† Machine-readable data that represent values usually stored for maps or images and organized sequentially by rows and columns. Each "cell" must be rectangular but not necessarily square, as with grid data.

‡ Shape files are the file format of ArcView GIS software.

§ Projection is the process of converting two-dimensional features into three-dimensional features; a mathematical model for converting locations on the Earth's surface from spherical to planar coordinates, allowing flat maps to depict three-dimensional features. Some map projections preserve the integrity of shape; others preserve accuracy of area, distance, or direction.

¶ Coverages are the file format of PC ArcInfo software.

** A numerical, text, or image field in a relational database table that describes a spatial feature such as a point, line, area, or cell. A characteristic of a geographic feature described by numbers or characters, typically stored in tabular format, and linked to the feature by an identifier. For example, attributes of a crime (represented by a point) might include time, crime type, location, and criminal address and victim address.

police station boundary maps, and the point location form the basis for this study. These maps could also be called *virtual pin maps* [Harries, 1999].

7.5.2 Unification of Sociodemographic Data

The data* are measured at three levels: wards, police boundaries, and land use. To incorporate the spatial factor in the analysis, the data were first unified from the three sources so that all data were in the same geographic unit. Overlaying functions were then used to combine these coverages with another coverage that contained the wards of the Coimbatore City and their corresponding demographic features that were obtained from the 1990 census. Because of the versatility of GIS, any combination of these coverages could be created to perform the needed analyses.

The sociodemographic data were in the ward map. These data were converted to the police station boundary map from the ward map. To do that, first a poly-on-poly overlay† (intersect) operation in ArcView GIS was conducted. The intersect process is used to integrate two spatial data sets while preserving only those features falling within the spatial extent common to both themes. After the overlaying operation is complete, the query builder in ArcView GIS is used to query the IDs (identification numbers) of police station boundaries. Then the following formula is used:

New population = Population / Total area of ward (sum of selected wards inside the police ID = 1 [Example: ward 10 + 11 + 20 + 30]). *Present area that is selected (or) police ID = 1 or ... (intersected area of each polygon that has been selected [Example: ward half of 10 + full 11 + half 20 + half 30])

Example: N_pop = population / w_area * p_area

Population is population field.
W_area is ward area field.
P_area is police area field.
N_pop is new population field.

In the same way, data were calculated for the other police boundaries, and data are calculated for all the remaining columns like male population, female population, male literacy, female literacy, and total literacy. In this map all data pertaining to police boundary are calculated from census data. Then the dissolve option in the geoprocessing in ArcView GIS is used. The

---

* A general term used to denote any or all facts, numbers, letters, and symbols that refer to or describe an object, idea, condition, situation, or other factors. These may be line graphics, imagery, and/or alphanumerics. It connotes basic elements of information that can be processed, stored, or produced by a computer.
† A set of data describing a single characteristic of each location within a bounded geographical area. Only one item of information is available for each location within a single layer. Major components of a layer are its resolution, orientation, and zone(s).

dissolve process is used to remove boundaries or nodes between adjacent polygons or lines that have the same values for a specified attribute. A new name is given to the theme, and the attribute field *police_id* is selected so that it merges with the map. The sum of each new field, which is created, is given to get the final data in the police station boundary map. Thus, census data of wards were incorporated to the police station boundary.

7.5.3 Identification of Spatial and Temporal Crime Patterns

To determine the spatial pattern of crimes of communal violence from 1997 and 1998, a combination of coverages and the ward coverage was used. The total number of crimes that occurred in each ward was calculated to determine where most crimes of communal violence took place in the Coimbatore urban area. The analysis was performed by assessing each one of the crime coverages separately in combination with the police station boundary coverage. A comparison of the number of crimes that occurred in each police station boundaries over the 2 years of interest determined the progression of crime over time for each area. The total number of crimes that occurred in each police station boundary was calculated to determine where most crimes of communal violence took place in the police boundary of Coimbatore City. Here the patterns of crimes of communal violence are calculated per police station boundary to give future directions to the police department for the prevention of such violence.

7.5.4 Visualization of the Results

A series of maps were generated to graphically display the location of the crimes and the demographic characteristics of the police station boundary limits in which the crimes were committed. In addition, statistics were compiled to show the findings of the analyses.

7.6 Results

The crimes of communal violence taken for this analysis in this study are clubbed together to get an annual picture of the crime scenario of the city for the years 1997 and 1998 (Figures 7.6 and 7.7). Maps in this section depict victimization in the following levels of severity: property damage (rioting, looting, arson), simple injuries (from which the victim recovers fully), grievous injury (from which the victim emerges maimed, disfigured, or disabled), killings. The distribution of crime incidents shows that only the southern part of the city is highly affected by these nefarious activities. The distribution is clustered in the south, and a rectangular pattern from north to down south is found.

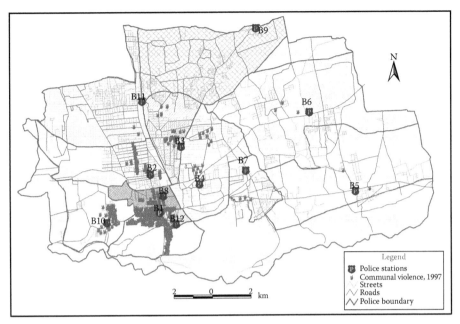

Figure 7.6 Crimes of communal violence (rioting, looting, arson, murder, and simple and grievous injuries), 1997.

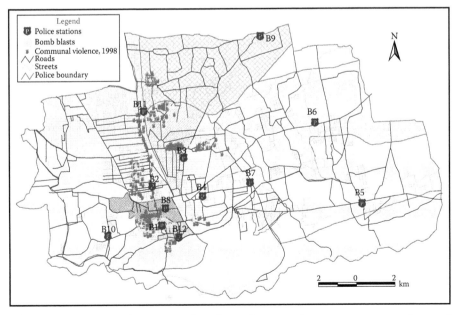

Figure 7.7 Crimes of communal violence (rioting, looting, arson, murder, and simple and grievous injuries), 1998.

The maps (Figures 7.8 and 7.9) examine the crimes of communal violence that occurred in the year 1997, with respect to specific police boundaries. It is found that the B1 police station B10 and B2 police station limits were heavily affected by these riots. Opannakkara Street and Bazaar Street in B1 police station limit and DB road in B2 RS Puram police limit are the most affected. The reason is that in these areas most of the shops and establishments belong to Muslims.

7.6.1 Victimization Patterns

The victimization pattern is analyzed based on the religion of the victim, age, sex, and compensation to the victims.

7.6.1.1 Religion

The map (Figure 7.10) shows the victims of communal murder in 1997 and police firing with relation to religion. As stated earlier, most of the victims of murder were Muslims. They were identified in places like hospitals where they went for treatment, and they were killed by the Hindu fundamentalists. During the police firing, also particularly Muslims were targeted. However, as those victims were a part of the rioting, they cannot be sympathized as victims because they were also the perpetrators who precipitated their victimization.

The map (Figure 7.11) shows the properties of victims damaged during communal violence in 1997. The most notable trend in this map is the

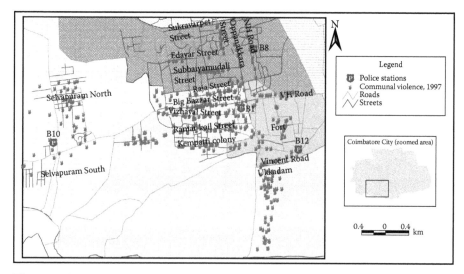

Figure 7.8 Crimes of communal violence (rioting, looting, arson, murder, and simple and grievous injuries), in police boundaries B1, B12, B10, and B8, 1997.

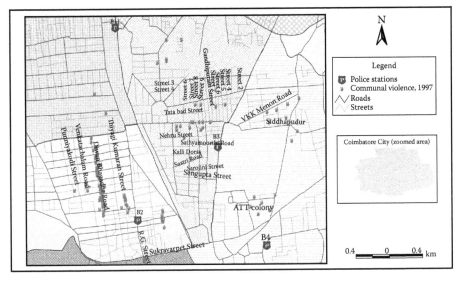

Figure 7.9 Crimes of communal violence (rioting, looting, arson, murder, and simple and grievous injuries), in police boundaries B2, B11, B4, and B3, 1997.

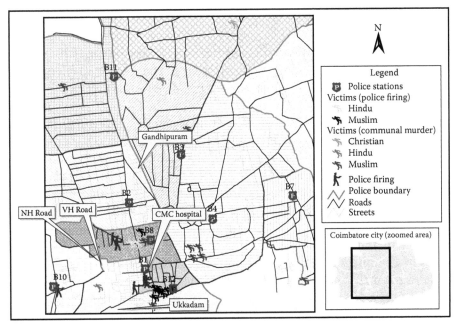

Figure 7.10 Victims of communal murder and police firing, categorized by religion, 1997.

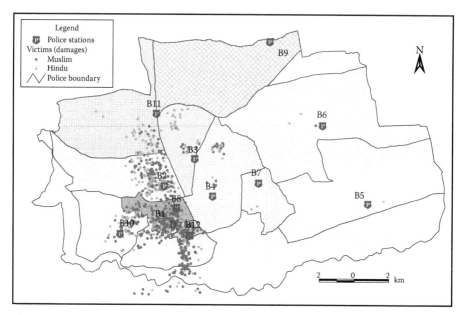

Figure 7.11 Property damage due to communal violence, categorized by religion, 1997.

disproportionate rate of increase in the victimization of Muslims than the crimes of communal violence committed against Hindus. The vandalism committed points to the fact that Muslim shops were identified, attacked, and their properties were looted by the antisocial elements.

The maps (Figures 7.12, 7.13, and 7.14) show the victims of the bomb blasts in relation to the religion. As these bomb blasts were masterminded by the Muslim fundamentalists, the majority of the victims were from the Hindu community. However, some of the victims who died in the bomb blasts also were from the Muslim community. This gives the impression that only in certain areas the Muslim fundamentalists have taken care to ensure that Muslims are not victimized in the bomb blasts. Moreover, the fundamentalists and terrorists are persons who are not bothered about the victimization of innocent lives. The bomb blasts, which occurred in B2 RS Puram police limits, have a great role in the victimization. Eight to 12 of the victims died from these bomb blasts, and this shows the gravity of the bomb blasts, which was blasted in B2 police station limits. The majority of the victims who died in the bomb blasts came from other parts of Coimbatore City apart from the places of bomb blasts, which is evident from the map. Because the bomb blasts were planned to disrupt the political and commercial activity in Coimbatore City, most of the victims who died were either a party of political or commercial activity that took place on February 14, 1998. This corroborates with routine activities theory.

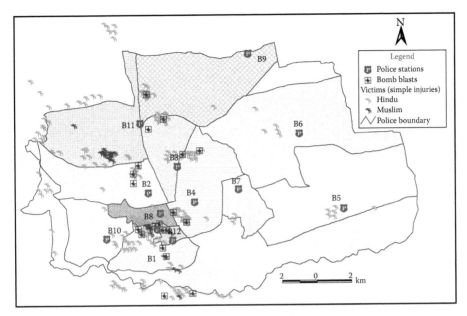

Figure 7.12 Bombing fatalities, categorized by religion, 1998.

The map (Figure 7.15) shows the victims of communal violence in 1998 (damages) in relation with the religion of the victims. Even though these bomb blasts and violence were targeted toward the Hindus, the majority of the victims were from the Muslim community. However, the bomb blasts have seriously affected the Hindu community and their establishments.

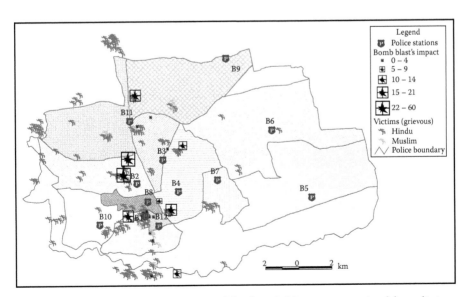

Figure 7.13 Grievous injuries caused by bomb blasts, categorized by religion, 1998.

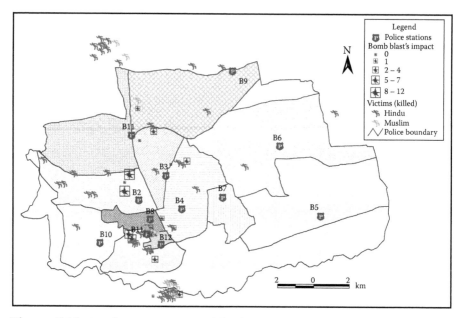

Figure 7.14 Simple injuries caused by bomb blasts, categorized by religion, 1998.

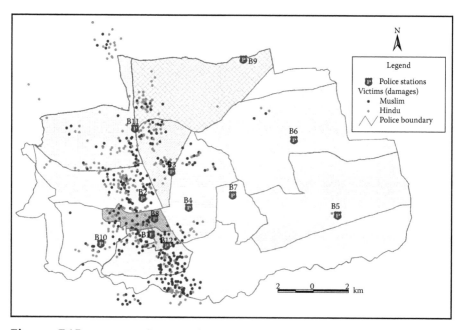

Figure 7.15 Property damage due to communal violence, categorized by religion, 1998.

7.6.1.2 Age

The maps (Figures 7.16, 7.17, and 7.18) show the victims of bomb blasts in relation with the age of the victims. It is found that majority of the victims were youth. This shows the vulnerability of young people toward these heinous crimes. As a bomb blast is vulnerable to hurt anyone irrespective of age, then why most of the victims happened to be in the younger age group needs to be assessed. The reason could be that most of the bomb blasts have occurred in places where people congregate. The political activity that was going on that day (Mr. Advani, the president of the BJP, was participating in a rally on February 14, 1998) is one of the key factors in victimization. Throngs of young people were pulled by the centrifugal force of the political activity, and they mostly came from the peripheral regions of Coimbatore City. Apart from this, Muslim fundamentalist youths were involved in communal rioting after the bomb blasts. These rioters used pipe bombs on the Hindu rioters. The bombs affected the Hindu rioters, who were significantly composed of a group of youths.

7.6.1.3 Sex

The maps (Figures 7.19, 7.20, and 7.21) show the victims of bomb blasts in relation with the sex of the victims. It is found that the majority of the victims were males. Only males participate in outdoor activity in larger groups. Except in certain places, like the hospital where a female nurse may be killed and several other female nurses severely injured, the majority of other victims

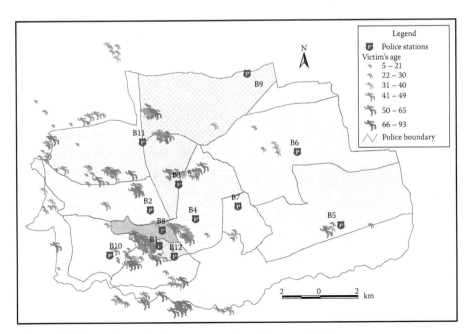

Figure 7.16 Bombing fatalities, categorized by age, 1998.

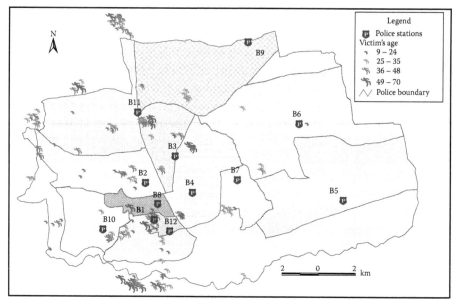

Figure 7.17 Grievous injuries caused by bomb blasts, categorized by age, 1998.

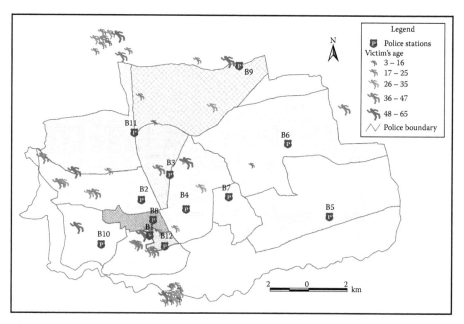

Figure 7.18 Simple injuries caused by bomb blasts, categorized by age, 1998.

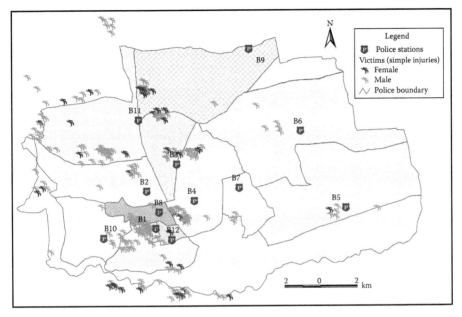

Figure 7.19 Bombing fatalities, categorized by sex, 1998.

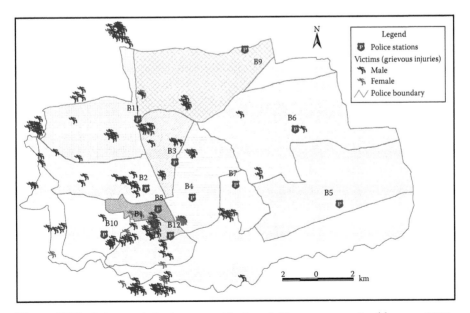

Figure 7.20 Grievous injuries caused by bomb blasts, categorized by sex, 1998.

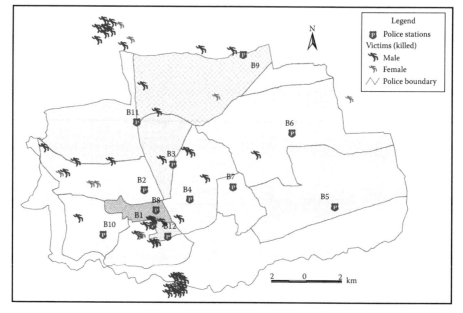

Figure 7.21 Simple injuries caused by bomb blasts, categorized by sex, 1998.

are males. Therefore, the relationship of sex of the victim with victimization cannot be generalized in bomb blast victimization.

7.6.2 Victim Compensation

Figure 7.22 shows the victim compensation given to the victims of communal violence in 1997. Most of the victims were platform vendors, who are poor and downtrodden. The Tamil Nadu government swiftly provided compensation to those poor people. Even though the loss was estimated to several crores (crore = 10 million) of rupees, a ceiling was fixed, and the government has awarded a total amount of Rs. 4,92,35,995/- as compensation [Gokulakrishnan, 1999, 2000].

The map (Figure 7.23) shows the victim compensation given to the victims of communal violence and bomb blasts in 1998. The total amount of compensation awarded was Rs. 3,15,35,091/-. After careful consideration the government decided to restrict the maximum compensation as Rs. 1,000,00 lakh (1 million) to an individual [Gokulakrishnan, 1999, 2000].

7.7 Discussion and Conclusion

The results of the analysis of victimization patterns indicate that individuals with varying sociodemographic characteristics experience distinctive

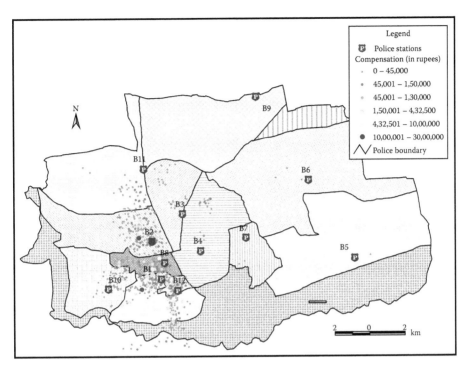

Figure 7.22 Victim compensation for crimes of communal violence (rioting, looting, arson, murder, and simple and grievous injuries), 1997.

patterns of communal violence victimization. The probable location of crimes of communal violence is significantly related to the sex, age, and religion of the victim, and the likely relationship between the victim and the offender is appreciably associated with religion. All the significant associations observed in the data are compatible with the routine activities perspective. The consistent pattern of the findings is striking. Although not every sociodemographic characteristic has a substantial effect on each dimension of crimes of communal violence, none exhibits a significant association with either dimension in a way opposite to the predictions of routine activity.

Several criminologists have argued that risk of criminal victimization is linked to lifestyle, routine activities, and opportunities [Hindelang, Gottfredson, and Garofalo, 1978; Cohen and Felson, 1979; Cohen, Klugel, and Land, 1981]. What people do, where they go, and whom they associate with all affect their likelihood of victimization. Variations in lifestyle are important because they are associated with differences in exposure to "high risk times, places and people" [Hindelang et al., 1978]. In a large part, lifestyle and routine activities are adaptations to various role expectations and structural constraints. There is considerable evidence that victimization follows the patterns suggested by the idea of lifestyle and routine activity theorists [Laub, 1997].

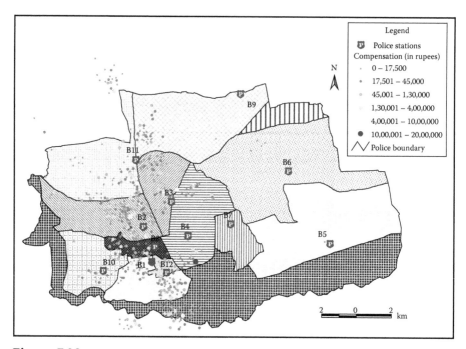

Figure 7.23 Victim compensation for crimes of communal violence (rioting, looting, arson, murder, and simple and grievous injuries), 1998.

The routine activity approach [Cohen and Felson, 1979] to crime rate analysis specifies three elements of crime: a likely offender, a suitable target, and the absence of a capable guardian. The theory suggests when all three elements are available, crime will occur. For all three elements to be present, a large population is needed for the chances of a victim and an offender to "converge in one place at the same time." Routine activities that bring together potential offenders and criminal opportunities are especially effective in explaining the role of place in encouraging or inhibiting crime. The resulting crime locales often take the form of facilities—places that people frequent for a specific purpose—that are attractive to offenders or conducive to offending. Victimization occurs when a target is "exposed" to crime, i.e., if a person spends large amounts of time in public places at night, there is a better chance of that individual becoming a victim of a crime than someone at home. The activity areas tend to be on major highways, near schools, shopping areas, and recreational centers. The results of the victimization pattern of bomb blast correlate with the lifestyle and routine activities theory.

Apart from corroborating theories of crime with the victimization a simple reasoning is also made in the ensuing paragraphs. Another reason for the victimization of communal violence is the bias of the police force in Coimbatore City. Lower-ranking police officials colluded with the Hindu fundamentalists, and either they abetted the crimes of communal violence or were mere spectators of those crimes. There was bias in police firing also. Rai [1997] conducted a study into the behavior of police in the communal riots. The study is based on the interviews with the community leaders, feedback from serving and retired police personnel, records of the police academy, and study of the reports of different communal riots. While we know that 65% of the victims of communal riots have been Muslims, the arrest and casualty Figures are very revealing. In the Bhiwandi riots in 1970, of those arrested in cognizable offenses, 21 were Hindus, whereas 901 were Muslims; casualty-wise, 17 were Hindus and 59 were Muslims. In the Meerut riots of 1982, the pattern is no different: 124 Hindus were arrested versus 231 Muslims, and 2 Hindus and 8 Muslims were the victims of casualty. As in Mumbai, here also police bullets selectively hit the body of Muslims and the soul of secular values. In Bhiwandi (1970), Firozabad (1972), Aligarh (1978), and Meerut (1982), there was not a single Hindu victim of police bullets, where the number of Muslims dying of police bullets was 9, 6, 7, and 6, respectively. The results of the present study also corroborate with the above study.

Because of the heavy communalization of the police force, police personnel believe that communal riots are caused by Muslims, and this is what guides their conduct. Their communalized consciousness is supplemented by brutal savagery, which gets further compounded by their nonprofessional approach in dealing with these situations. Many Muslim-predominant areas are termed as *mini-Pakistan* (e.g., Kottaimedu in Coimbatore city), and police enter these areas with the preparation and spirit as if they are entering enemy territory. This also makes them investigate the riot in an apathetic manner, and for years they sit on available evidence, which goes against their deep-set biases [Punyani, 2000].

This spatial exploration of crimes of communal violence and victimization in Coimbatore City reveals a number of insights that are relevant to crimes of communal violence generally and to our understanding of the phenomenon in Coimbatore more specifically. This study also helps to identify directions for future research. Crimes of communal violence in Coimbatore City tend to be more brutal and socially divisive than those conventional crimes perpetrated by individuals acting alone. Victimization is found to be higher in crimes of communal violence than in conventional crimes. The present study of communal violence and victimization by GIS analysis will be helpful in charting the framework for police patrol planning, measures for controlling and preventing communal violence in future. The quantification of mass victimization by the present study will be helpful for policymaking for victim compensation and victim assistance for the victims of communal violence, such as anticipating and predicting number of victims, types of victims, gravity of victimization, award of compensation to different levels of victimization, etc.

7.8 Limitations of the Study

The description and analysis of communal violence and victimization in the present study are confined to the metropolitan areas of Coimbatore City. The study mainly concentrates on spatial analysis done in GIS. The period chosen for the study is 2 years (1997–1998). Police crime reports reflecting criminal acts of communal violence in Coimbatore City for the years of 1997 and 1998 were chosen as the case subjects. Only crimes of communal violence and victims of communal violence were studied, and general crimes and victims did not come under the scope of the present study.

Because of the time limitation/constraints, data on victims and perpetrators of communal violence in 1997 were not obtained in a detailed manner (the charge sheet of 1997 communal violence was not prepared by the police during the data collection). The limitations regarding the police boundaries are that two new police stations (B8 Police Station at VH Road and B12 Police Station at Ukkadam) were created after the communal violence incidents. These data are incorporated in the study, and data pertaining to crimes of communal violence were also distributed in those particular police boundaries to give a clear distribution trend even though those stations did not exist before occurrence of the communal violence incidents (1997, 1998).

Care has been taken to ensure the accuracy in locating the crimes, perpetrators, victims, and police stations. The use of global positioning systems (GPS) will provide greater accuracy level. In future studies, this issue will be taken into account, and GPS will be used to locate the exact locations. Because of the inaccessibility of aerial photographs to the researcher, the crime incidents were approximately plotted around the main locations. If aerial photographs had been available, it would have enhanced the accuracy of the results. These are certain limitations that require immediate attention for a proper utilization of GIS in crime/victim analysis.

Acknowledgments

The author thanks Professor K. Chockalingam, currently Professor of Victimology at Tokiwa International Victimology Institute, Mito, Japan, for supervising this research work, which is part of the author's PhD thesis. The author also thanks Professor Keith D. Harries, Professor Emeritus, Department of Geography and Environmental Systems, University of Maryland, Baltimore, Maryland, for his constant guidance and comments that improved this study.

References

Akila Bharatiya Vidya Parishad (ABVP). 1999. *Islamic terrorism in Tamilnadu*. Tamil Nadu: ABVP.

Block, C. R. and M. Dabdoud. 1993. *Proceedings of workshop on crime analysis through computer mapping*. Chicago: Illinois Criminal Justice Information Authority.

Block, C. R., M. Dabdoud, and S. Fregly (eds.). 1995. *Crime analysis through computer mapping*. Washington, DC: Police Executive Research Forum.

Brantingham, P. J. and P. L. Brantingham. 1981. *Environmental criminology*. Prospect Heights, IL: Waveland.

_____. 1984. *Patterns of crime*. New York: Macmillan.

Brass, P. 2003. *The production of Hindu-Muslim violence in contemporary India*. Seattle: University of Washington Press.

Canter, P. 2000. Using a geographic information system for tactical crime analysis. In *Analyzing crime patterns: Frontiers of practice*, ed. V. Goldsmith, P. G. McGuire, J. H. Mollenkopf, and T. A. Ross, 3–10. London: Sage.

Census of India. 2001. *Percentage of population of major religions, 2001*. New Delhi: Office of the Registrar General, India. http://www.censusindia.gov.in/Census_Data_2001/India_at_glance/religion.aspx (accessed October 28, 2008).

Cohen, L. and M. Felson. 1979. Social change and crime rate trends: A routine activities approach. *American Sociological Review* 46:588–608.

Cohen, L., J. R. Klugel, and K. Land. 1981. Social inequality and predatory criminal victimization: An exposition and test of a formal theory. *American Sociological Review* 46:505–24.

Curtis, L. A. 1974. *Criminal violence: National patterns and behavior*. Lexington, MA: Lexington Books.

Daihani, D. U. and A. B. Purnomo. 2001. The May 1998 riot in Jakarta, Indonesia, analyzed with GIS. *Arc News*, Fall 2001. http://www.esri.com/news/arcnews/arcnews.html (accessed July 13, 2001).

Dhar, T. N. 2002. Politics, governance and conflict management. *The Indian Journal of Public Administration* 47(3):284–94.

Eh Din. 2002. *Genesis of communal violence in India*. Eh Din. http://www.panjab.org.uk/english/genesis.html (accessed June 5, 2004).

Engineer, A. A. (ed.). 1984. *Communal riots in post-independence*. Hyderabad: Sangam Books.

_____. 1998. Communal violence in 1998. *The Hindu*, December 12.

_____. 1999. *Communal violence in Coimbatore 1997*. Progressive Dawoodi Bohras. http://www.dawoodi-bohras.com/perspective.htm (accessed February 20, 2000).

Gabor, T. and E. Gotthell. 1984. Offender characteristics and spatial mobility: An empirical study and some policy applications. *Canadian Journal of Criminology* 26:267–81.

Ghosh, S. K. 1987. *Communal riots in India (Meet the challenge unitedly)*. New Delhi: Ashish Publish House.

Girdner, E. J. 1998. *Muslims in India*. College of behavioral and social sciences, University of Maryland. http://www.bsos.umd.edu/cidcm/mar/indmus.htm (accessed June 5, 2004).

Gokulakrishnan, P. R. 1998. *Report of justice Thiru P. R. Gokulakrishnan Commission of Inquiry constituted to inquire into the murder of Thiru Selvaraj, Traffic Constable (Grade-I) on 29th November 1997, Police Demonstration on 30th November 1997 and subsequent law and order disturbances, etc., in Coimbatore City.* Dated November 27, 1998.

_____. 1999. *Report of justice Thiru P. R. Gokulakrishnan Commission of Inquiry regarding compensation for property damages during the violent incidents in Coimbatore City on 29.22.1997 and 30.11.1997.* Dated May 6, 1999.

_____. 2000. *Report of justice Thiru P. R. Gokulakrishnan Commission of Inquiry constituted to inquire into the causes and circumstances leading to the bomb blasts that occurred in Coimbatore city and its suburbs on 14th February 1998 and other law and order disturbances including damages to the public and private properties, etc.- Vide G.O. Ms. No. 254, Public (Law and order-F) Department, dated 22nd February 1998.* Dated May 18, 2000.

_____. 2000. *Report of justice Thiru P. R. Gokulakrishnan Commission of Inquiry regarding compensation for property damages during the violent incidents in Coimbatore city on 29th and 30th November 1997.* Dated January 31, 2000.

Guerry, A. M. 1833. *Essai sur la statisque morale de la France.* Paris: Crochard.

Harries, K. 1971. The geography of American crime, 1968. *Journal of Geography* 70:204–13.

_____. 1980. *Crime and the environment.* Springfield, IL: Charles C. Thomas.

_____. 1990. *Geographic factors in policing.* New York: McGraw-Hill.

_____. 1999. *Mapping crime: Principle and practice.* Washington, DC: U.S. Dept. of Justice, Office of Justice Programs, National Institute of Justice.

Harwood, S. 2002. Managing chaos relies on fast, accurate information New York City—Creating a disaster management GIS on the fly. *Arc User Magazine* July-September 2001. http://www.esri.com/news/arcuser/0701/julsep2001.html (accessed January 2, 2002).

Herbert, D. 1982. *The geography of urban crime.* London: Longman.

Herman, M. A. 1999. *Fighting in the streets: Ethnic succession, competition, and riot violence in four American cities.* PhD diss., University of Arizona.

Hewstone, N. T. M. and A. Voci. 2003. *Intergroup contact between Hindus and Muslims in India, Its role in reducing perceived threats, intergroup anxiety and intergroup bias.* Paper presented in the Social Inclusion/Exclusion Meeting, University of Kent.

Human Rights Watch. 1996. INDIA: Communal violence and the denial of justice. *Human Rights Watch Short Report* 8(2):1–27.

_____. 2002. WE HAVE NO ORDERS TO SAVE YOU: State participation and complicity in communal violence in Gujarat. *Human Rights Watch Short Report* 14(3):1–68.

Hussain, S. 1984. Communal riots in the post-partition period in India: A study of some causes and remedial measures. In *Communal violence in post independence India,* ed. A. A. Engineer, 374–90. New Delhi: Ajanta.

Hutchins, B. 2000. Counter-terrorism exercises a success using GIS. *Arc User Magazine* Summer:1–3. http://www.esri.com/news/arcuser/0701/julsep2001.html (accessed January 2, 2002).

Jeffery, C. R. 1971. *Crime prevention through environmental design.* Beverly Hills, CA: Sage.

Jaishankar, K., S. Shanmugapriya, and V. Balamurugan. 2004. Crime mapping in India: A GIS implementation in Chennai city policing. *Geographic Information Sciences* 10(1):20–34.

Jos, M. 1993. The structure of crime and determinants in Delhi: A socio-spatio analysis. PhD diss., Jawaharlal Nehru University.

Laub, J. H. 1993. Patterns of criminal victimization in the United States. In *Victims of crime*, ed. R. C. Davis, A. J. Lurigo, W. G. Shogan, 9–25. London: Sage.

LeBeau, J. L. 1987. The journey to rape: Geographic distance and the rapist's methods of approaching the victim. *Journal of Police Science and Administration* 15:129–36.

Mahajan, V. D. 1993. *India since 1526*. New Delhi: S. Chand.

McClintock, F. H. 1963. *Crimes of violence*. London: MacMillan.

Molyneux, J. I. 1995. Experiments in terrorism: The geography of sectarian violence in Central Belfast 1972–1992 (Northern Ireland). PhD diss., University of New Orleans.

Newman, O. 1972. *Defensible space: Crime prevention through urban design*. New York: Macmillan.

People Union for Civil Liberties. 1998. 1997 An Anti-Muslim pogrom. Report on Coimbatore Communal violence in late. *Frontline* 15(5):115–99.

Puniyani, R. 2005. *Is riot free India possible?* Binu Mathew, Countercurrents.org. http://www.countercurrents.org/comm-puniyani150905.htm (accessed September 15, 2008).

Pyle, G. F. 1974. *The spatial dynamics of crime*. Research paper no. 159. Chicago: University of Chicago, Department of Geography.

Quetelet, M. A. 1973. A treatise on man and the development of his faculties. Farnborough, UK: Gregg International. (Original work published, 1842).

Rai, V. N. 1997. A study into the behavior of police in the communal riots record of police neutrality in communal riots. *Indian Journal of Secularism* 2:25–36.

Rao, V. S. 1968. *Murder: A pilot study of urban pattern with particular reference to the city of Delhi*. New Delhi: Research Division, Central Bureau of Investigation, Ministry of Home Affairs, Government of India.

Ratcliffe, J. H. and M. J. McCullagh. 1998. Identifying repeat victimization with GIS. *British Journal of Criminology* 38(4):651–62.

Rengert, G. F. 1972. *Spatial aspects of criminal behavior: A suggested approach*. Paper presented at East Lake division, Association of American Geographers annual meeting, Philadelphia.

Rossmo, D. K. 1995. Overview: Multivariate spatial profiles as a tool in crime investigation. In *Crime analysis through computer mapping*, ed. C. R. Block, M. Dabdoub, and S. Fregly, 65–97. Washington, DC: Police Executive Research Forum.

Saiyed, A. R. 1988. Changing urban ethos: Some reflections in Hindu-Muslim Riots. In *Collective violence-genesis and response*, ed. K. S. Shukla, 97–119. New Delhi: Indian Institute of Public Administration.

Sampson, R. J. and W. B. Groves. 1989. Community structure and crime: Testing social disorganization theory. *American Journal of Sociology* 4:774–802.

Sarkar, S. 1983. *Modern India 1885–1947*. Delhi: Macmillan India.

Schmid, C. 1960a. Urban crime areas, Part I. *American Sociological Review* 25:526–43.

____. 1960b. Urban crime areas, Part II. *American Sociological Review* 25:655–78.

Schuerman, L. and S. Kobrin. 1986. Community careers in crime. In *Crime and justice: A review of research, communities and crime*, ed. A. J. Reiss, Jr. and M. Tonry, 67–100. Chicago: University of Chicago Press.

Shah, A. 1998. Epic enemies: A discussion of Hindu-Muslim relations in India. *Online edition of Perspectives: The Davies County High School Journal of Social Sciences.* http://members.aol.com/megxyz/ankur.html (accessed October 29, 2004).

Shannon, L. W. 1954. The spatial distribution of criminal offenses by states. *Journal of Criminal Law and Criminology, and Police Science* 45:264–73.

Shaw, C. R. 1942. *Delinquency areas: A study of geographic distribution of school truants, juvenile delinquents, and adult offenders in Chicago.* Chicago: University of Chicago Press.

Shaw, C. R. and H. D. McKay. 1942. *Juvenile delinquency and urban areas.* Chicago: University of Chicago Press.

Sivamurthy, A. 1980. The spatial pattern of crimes and criminal behaviour in Madras City: A crimino-geographic study. PhD diss., University of Madras.

____. 1988. *The public perception of crimes in Madras City.* Project submitted to Indian Council for Social Sciences Research, New Delhi.

Special Investigation Team, Tamil Nadu Police (SIT). 1999. *Charge sheet of Coimbatore bomb blasts.* Tamil Nadu: Tamil Nadu State Police.

Srivastava, S. S. 1963. *Juvenile delinquency: A socio-ecological study of juvenile vagrants in the cities of Kanpur and Lucknow.* Bombay: Ashish Publishing House.

Subramanian, T. S. 1997. Confrontation in Coimbatore. *Frontline,* December 26, 112–15.

____. 1998. Fundamentalism and a flare-up. *Frontline* December 18, 113–45.

Taylor, R. B., S. A. Shumaker, and S. D. Gottfredson. 1985. Neighborhood-level links between physical features and local sentiments: Deterioration, fear of crime, and confidence. *Journal of Architectural Planning and Research* 2:261–75.

Umemoto, K. and M. C. Kimi. 2000. A profile of race-bias hate crime in Los Angeles County. *Western Criminology Review* 2(2):21–56. http://wcr.sonoma.edu/v2n2/umemoto.html (accessed September 26, 2000).

Weisburd, D. and T. McEwen (eds.). 1997. *Crime mapping and crime prevention.* Monsey, NY: Criminal Justice Press.

Patterns of
Victimization

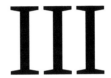

Secondary Victims and Secondary Victimization

8

RACHEL CONDRY

Contents

8.1 Introduction

When instances of victimization are surveyed and quantified they can appear to be contained events, suspended in time, in a fixed location, and involving only the primary actors. The experience of victimization is in reality much more complex. Victims can continue to experience the effects of victimization long after the event, and those effects can reach into the lives of many more people than just the primary victims; the ripple effect of crime travels across time, across place, and through kin and friendship ties.

This chapter explores the meaning of "secondary victimization" and examines three distinct ways in which the concept has been defined. First, secondary victimization is said to result from victimization or the consequences of victimization extending to another party, so distinguishing the status of *primary victim, secondary victim, tertiary victim,* or *indirect victim.* Second, victims of crime are said to experience secondary victimization when they are subject to processes and responses that cause further victimization or compound their feelings of victimization, a notion which is said to have particular salience for victims of rape or sexual assault. A third understanding of secondary victimization is that it can be created by a social reaction to a primary victim's status that leads to that status becoming entrenched and central to that person's identity, a conception which parallels other concerns with the negative consequences of adopting and internalizing a victim identity.

8.2 Secondary Victims

"Victims" means persons who, individually or collectively, have suffered harm, including physical or mental injury, emotional suffering, economic loss, or substantial impairment of their fundamental rights. The term *victim* also includes, where appropriate, the immediate family or dependants of the direct victim and persons who have suffered harm in intervening to assist victims in distress or to prevent victimization [United Nations Declaration of Basic Principles of Justice for Victims of Crime and Abuse of Power, Annex, 1985].

What does it mean to lay claim to the status of victim? Why is it a status that some want but others are keen to reject? What are the processes through which we come to assign victim status and come to understand individuals and groups as victims? Claims to the status of primary victim are often contested, provisional, and evolve through complex processes, processes that are perhaps even more complex, provisional, and contested when claims to secondary victim status are mobilized. We live in a climate that is sympathetic to claims to victimhood, and those claims are ever increasing[*] [Best, 1999]. Although secondary victims tend to be less visible than primary victims, there has been some official recognition of the extension of victim status to other parties for more than 20 years, as we can see in the quotation above.

How are we to understand and interpret claims to secondary victimhood? Holstein and Miller advocate an interactional approach to analyzing victimization that focuses on the social processes through which people come to be known and understood as victims and the descriptive processes through which victim status is assigned to individuals or groups [Holstein and Miller, 1990:103], an approach that is of particular benefit when analyzing claims to different degrees and different types of victimization. By focusing on these social processes it is possible to bracket the rather simplistic question of who "is" and who "is not" a victim, and to try to understand instead the meaning of victimhood to those who claim (and reject) it, the processes through

---

[*] Although there has been a backlash to increasing claims to victim status, see for example Sykes [1992] and Lamb [1999].

which claims and counterclaims are (and are not) honored, the processes through which people become victims, and the consequences of those processes for people's lives.

Claims to the status of victim can be made by individuals and groups experiencing a wide range of predicaments. We can be victims of illness, of addictions, of psychological problems, or of a plethora of other circumstances. Each condition can generate further claims to secondary victim status from those connected to primary victims, and some of these claims give rise to various support groups, campaigning groups, and entire social movements—the codependency movement, Al-Anon for families of alcoholics, Adfam for families of drug addicts, and numerous caregiver support groups are such examples. Through these groups claims to the status of secondary victim of alcoholism, heroin addiction, or Alzheimer's disease are mobilized. Although these claims have interesting parallels, our focus here will be mainly restricted to the secondary victims of crime.

I intend to consider three groups for whom the claim of "secondary victim" is made: kin of primary victims; kin of offenders; and a broader group who are seen to be affected by their association with events rather than their direct tie to the primary actors, such as witnesses to crimes or emergency workers who are sometimes said to experience vicarious trauma. Although it is analytically useful to distinguish between kin of victims and kin of offenders, it is important to note that in reality much crime is intrafamilial, and many people will be both; similarly, perpetrators of crimes can also be relatives of victims, a point missed in much of the existing research on secondary victims [see Hendricks et al., 1993; Morrison et al., 2007:7], so my focus here is on what might be described as nonperpetrator relatives.

The act of naming someone a victim or making claim to the status for oneself has a resonance that is widely understood: "Calling someone a victim encourages others to see how the labelled person has been harmed by forces beyond his or her control, simultaneously establishing the 'fact' of injury and locating responsibility for damage outside the 'victim'" [Holstein and Miller, 1990:106]. The label provides "interpretive instructions," advising others "how they should understand persons, circumstances, and behaviors under consideration" [ibid.:107]. As Holstein and Miller explain, describing someone as a victim serves a number of purposes: It can deflect or remove responsibility from that person; it can assign causes or identify the source of harm by designating its opposite, the victimizer; it can specify responses or remedies—that a person is deserving of help or compensation, or that another should be sanctioned or provide restitution (and failure of these expectations can be another form of secondary victimization, as we will consider later in the chapter); and it can account for personal failings or not living up to expectations that, it is claimed, might have been otherwise were it not for this victim status, so preserving the personal integrity of the claimant [ibid.].

So it appears that a single label, "victim" (or for our purposes "secondary victim"), has immense interpretive power. The *Cambridge English Dictionary* defines a victim as "someone who has suffered the effects of violence, illness, or bad luck" to which we might add a definition of a secondary victim as someone who has suffered the effects of violence (or indeed any crime), illness, or bad luck, indirectly or through their relationship with another. The interpretive instructions of the term *secondary victim* may be even more important than they are to a primary victim as the harm a secondary victim endures is indirect, less clear-cut, and open to a wider range of different interpretations.

8.2.1 Relatives of Victims

How do crimes affect the relatives of victims? The answer to this question depends on a number of factors, not least the type and seriousness of the crime and the degree of harm caused, as well as the kin relationship in question. A wide range of crimes have the potential to affect a victim's relative, trigger an emotional reaction, or present practical consequences. A relative might feel frustration, annoyance, or anger if the crime is a minor theft, for example, or might need to come to the aid of a family member who is burgled. However, it is violent or sexual crimes that will have the most significant consequences and cause harm to the most people.

If asked about secondary victims, the group that would first come to mind for most people would be the relatives of homicide victims. As a group their status as victims would be the least contested, offering the least challenge to the notion of secondary victimhood because the harm the crime has inflicted on them, the impact on their lives, and their suffering is immediately apparent from their traumatic bereavement. Although not experienced by all in the same way, the grief of people bereaved by homicide has particular characteristics and differs from the bereavement that follows a death by natural causes, leaving relatives with a distinct range of practical and emotional needs [Rock, 1998; Paterson et al., 2006].

Rock [1998] plots the phenomenology of this grief, providing an ideal type of the bereavement of homicide "survivors." For these relatives, their experience is more terrible than anything they can imagine; one woman whose husband was murdered said, "There is no worse crime. There is no worse thing that anyone can do to hurt you"* [Rock, 1998:31]. Rock describes how these relatives feel a group apart, different in a number of significant ways from those bereaved by "natural" causes.

---

* Other groups of victims may make similar claims—suffering is ineffable and defies quantification, and there is often an element of competitive grief between groups and individuals.

First, murder and manslaughter tend to be sudden and unexpected, events for which one can never be prepared. There may be unfinished emotional or practical business and often no opportunity to say goodbye. The shocking revelation of a homicide can be impossible to assimilate, and life is thrown into disarray. Second, a death from homicide is not natural or inevitable but rather "intended and purposive or reckless and negligent—someone actually wanted the victim to die or was indifferent to the consequences of his actions" [1998:43]. Survivors see the murder as a moral assault and the murderer as the manifestation of evil. They can be left with feelings of vulnerability, fearful of what else might happen and what else fate might have in store, and isolated and alienated from the rest of the world and the mundane problems of everyday life. Different family members deal with their grief in different ways, and this can lead to conflict and rifts within the family, particularly as many survivors are struggling with feelings of anger and rage.

The third distinctive characteristic of bereavement by homicide is "the sheer ugliness of violent death. Stabbing, strangulation, and hitting and kicking, the most common methods of killing, can maim the victim and leave behind hideous visual images" [1998:51]. Survivors are prone to dreams and fantasies about what might have happened and how their relative might have suffered; homicide is a violation of the natural order and cannot possibly be constructed as a "good death." Fourth, homicide is inextricably linked to images of powerlessness—of the victim to resist, the bereaved to intervene, and loss of control of events afterward. Survivors are preoccupied with how and why the homicide happened and whether it could have been prevented, which can amplify feelings of survivor guilt and self-blame.

Finally, bereavement acquires a "clear, career-like organization" from without as relatives are pulled through the various, prolonged stages of the criminal justice process dealing with the police, the inquest, and a trial, often under the watchful eye of the mass media [Rock, 1998]. This can lead to very particular needs, as a recent Victim Support report details. Contact with criminal justice agencies can exacerbate trauma and interfere with grief processes, and relatives frequently describe dissatisfaction with how they are treated by criminal justice agencies, citing problems with poor communication, insensitivity, and lack of information. Key points for relatives in these processes included being notified of the death, being called on to identify the victim, the post mortem, the police investigation, and the trial and sentencing [Paterson et al., 2006]. Furthermore, families are often, legitimately, objects of police and more general suspicion during an inquiry. One mother whose son was murdered said she received little information from the police:

I felt very alone and angry at being ignored by the police. They left me by myself, they didn't come to see me, they didn't come to ask how I was, they didn't even phone. I felt as if I was rejected. [My son] is dead and I count as nothing. It makes me feel as if I am a bad mother. It leaves a very bitter taste in my mouth till this day. [Mother, 58, in Paterson et al., 2006:36]

The difficulties these families face do not end with the trial and sentencing, as expressed in a statement from the self-help national charity Support after Murder and Manslaughter (SAMM): "Most people need emotional support more after the trial than before. The trial is very traumatic and most people are unhappy with the outcome. The anger comes in more then" [Paterson et al., 2006:20]. Time for the relatives in Rock's study was not linear but rather cyclical, with events playing over again and again and anniversaries being particularly significant times [Rock, 1998]; this was an experience that relatives claimed not to recover from. Many families continue to endure financial problems and difficulties with employers and schools, and need to manage practical domestic problems and take on new responsibilities—four of the families in the Victim Support research had to take on new childcare responsibilities overnight when caring for children whose mothers were murdered by their fathers [Paterson et al., 2006:27].

Therefore, the act of homicide changes the lives of the relatives of victims forever. Homicide survivors who are members of support organizations are very vocal in their claims to victim status (although different groups vary in the degree to which they are activist or campaigning) [Rock, 1998]. Government policy in England and Wales has begun to recognize their status as secondary victims. The needs of survivors of homicide have been specifically acknowledged in the recent *Victims' Code of Practice*, which has been in force since April 2006, and states that relatives of victims who have died as a result of relevant criminal conduct should have access to a range of support services in their area and that they should be assigned a dedicated family liaison officer [Home Office, 2005a]. There has also been a growing right to make impact statements in court, to receive information about such matters as the impending release of an offender, and to sit in the well of the court and thereby to receive a special, spatially defined status [Home Office, 2005c; Attorney General's Office, 2007].

What of crimes that do not result in death and bereavement? How do the relatives of victims of other serious crimes fare, and can they be described as secondary victims? The range of crimes that could be considered here is potentially limitless; therefore, the discussion will be restricted to one type of crime, rape and sexual assault, which can have very significant and prolonged effects on relatives of victims. The experiences of the relatives of adult victims of sexual offenses can be distinguished from those of the relatives of child victims. There has been comparatively little research on the impact of rape and sexual assault on the relatives of adult victims, and when these relatives are considered, the focus is usually on how they respond to the victim or help or hinder the victim's recovery, rather than their own needs or difficulties [Smith, 2005; Morrison et al., 2007]. One study categorized the reactions of male partners of rape victims as either "modern," viewing the rape as an act of violence causing injury to the woman, or "traditional," focusing on the rape as sexual and causing harm and stigma to themselves. Those who took the traditional view focused on their own hurt and tended to blame their partner [Holstrom and Burgess, 1979, in Morrison et al., 2007:9]. Morrison et al. compare this study with more recent work [e.g., Nelson and Wampler, 2000, 2002] and suggest that there has been a shift over time in the way that the effects on the male partner of victims is represented in the research, from conceptualizing the male partner's responses as being unsupportive and traditional in earlier work to viewing these reactions as symptoms of the male partner's trauma in more recent studies. They suggest that this might be the result of the development of clinical concepts of trauma in the sexual assault field, but they warn that although the shift might represent a more compassionate understanding of male partners as secondarily victimized, there is the danger that harmful reactions might be justified or reinforced if such stereotypical or pejorative views are not challenged [Morrison et al., 2007a:9–10].

Smith [2005] conducted an in-depth study with five male partners of female sexual assault victims, asking the men about their feelings, thoughts, and behavior. She found that the men described many of the same psychological and interpersonal difficulties that female victims of sexual assault experience, including depression, guilt, self-blame, loss of trust, withdrawal from others, sleep disturbances, and symptoms of post-traumatic stress disorder [Smith, 2005:163]. For the male partner "it is an experience that has left him feeling angry, helpless, and guilty, prompted him to self-inspection, and thus changed him forever" [Smith, 2005:149]. Robert, one of the partners in Smith's study, described his feelings when his partner was raped:

> ... it felt like he raped me as well ... I felt traumatized by it. I went into a horrible depression.... They took her in for a rape examination and basically they left me out in the waiting room to deal with it on my own.... I felt abandoned. I was concerned about her, I wanted to be with her ... nobody told me how the hell she was doing.... I spent most of my time out in the parking lot chain smoking and crying. [Smith, 2005:156–65]

There was little social support for these male partners, and they often felt they could not share their experiences with anyone.

The little research that does exist on the relatives of adult victims of sexual assault focuses overwhelmingly on male partners of female victims. We know very little of the experiences of the parents, children, or siblings, or of partners in gay or lesbian couples.* A male partner may be the most important person to the primary victim in terms of initial reaction to a sexual assault and the support they provide afterward [Cwick, 1996], but as Morrison et al. [2007] suggest, this one-sided focus might also reflect traditional gendered assumptions about heterosexual relationships. The assumption that the "wounds" are greatest for the male sexual partner might reflect traditional notions of sexual ownership and entitlement. It is important to recognize that the effects on other relatives and also on friends [e.g., see Ahrens and Campbell, 2000] may also be profound [Morrison et al., 2007:10]. The small body of research on families of sexual assault victims shows that they experience considerable emotional, physical, and psychological symptoms [Silverman, 1978; Cwick, 1996] and that the crisis of rape has a very significant impact on family and marital relationships [Morrison et al., 2007].

Most of the research on relatives of child victims of sexual assault focuses on their parents and particularly on mothers. Finding out about the sexual abuse of their child is extremely distressing for parents, and research shows that they experience "secondary traumatization" [e.g., Newberger et al., 1993; Manion et al., 1996] with serious and long-lasting consequences: "The message from … studies is clear. The sexual abuse of their children represents a fundamental crisis for women that threatens to be overwhelming and which has seriously disruptive long-term effects of their lives" [Hill, 2001:386]. Hill conducted detailed interviews with 11 women from a UK support group for mothers of children who had been sexually abused and found that these mothers struggled with an overwhelming feeling of guilt at their own sense of failure as mothers and their feeling that they ought to have been able to protect their children (which might be seen as part of a larger syndrome of survivor guilt). They described the impact of finding out about their children's abuse as serious, distressing, and intense; they found it difficult to accept help from their families and friends; and most felt misunderstood by professionals and thought their interventions had made things worse [Hill, 2001].

The sense of guilt and failure experienced by the mothers in Hill's study is not without foundation, having roots in strong discourses of parental—and particularly maternal—responsibility that permeate all aspects of social life. Mothers are often constructed as idealized nurturers [Davies and Krane, 1996], and they are blamed for problems within the family. Research within families that experience father–daughter incest has shown that the father is often not held totally accountable, and the mother is centrally implicated and blamed as collusive or even thought to be orchestrating the abuse through her inadequacies or emotional absence [Davies and Krane, 1996]. These kinds of

---

* It would also be interesting to know something about the management of information by those involved—how disclosing abuse is managed within the family, and who is allowed to know what and when, that is, different types of "awareness contexts" [Glaser and Strauss, 1965] and their consequences.

assumptions have been found in the accounts of some child protection professionals [Kelley, 1990] and in the child sexual abuse literature, which "carries a legacy of at least twenty-five years of blaming non-offending mothers either partially or fully for the sexual abuse of their children" [Humphreys, 1994:50]. Although the mothers in Hill's study did not use the term *secondary victim*, we might surmise that this would be a reasonable claim: They themselves were not responsible for the abuse; the perpetrator was responsible for his actions; and those actions had caused serious, distressing consequences for the mothers. Mothers in these circumstances might want to lay claim to the status of victim to deflect the blame and responsibility inherent in discourses of family responsibility and mother-blame—as we saw earlier in this chapter, one of the important interpretive instructions of the victim label is locating responsibility for the damage outside that person—but as Hill's study shows, many of those mothers are themselves struggling with their own sense of culpability or failure and whether there was anything they might have done to better protect their children.

Studies of the partners of adults who experienced childhood sexual abuse (often referred to as *sexual abuse survivors*)* show how the secondary effects on relatives can be very long-lasting, with the abuse still having a significant impact many years later. Chauncey studied 20 male partners of female sexual abuse survivors and found they were struggling with conflict between their own needs and the needs of their partner, and had difficulties with achieving emotional and physical closeness, difficulties with spontaneity or unpredictability, sexual problems, and feelings of guilt, anger, and shame. She argues that it is important that these male partners' experiences are understood so that they can begin to feel less ashamed, less isolated, and less helpless, and calls for more research on the long-term course of surviving childhood sexual abuse [Chauncey, 1994].

Ten female partners of male survivors of child sexual abuse were studied by Jacob and Veach [2005]. They asked the female partners to describe their perceptions of the intrapersonal and familial effects of their male partner's abuse, and their findings correspond to a model of "trauma contagion" [Maltas and Shay, 1995] based on threatened beliefs and shattered assumptions as a result of their partner's disclosure of sexual abuse; chronic stress, including feelings of increased irritability, anger, depression, and anxiety; and repetition and re-enactment of emotional and traumatic aspects of the child sexual abuse, including lack of trust, emotional disconnection, and power and control struggles. They conclude that female partners, male partners, and their children experience significant distress as a result of male partner childhood sexual abuse [Jacob and Veach, 2005]. We need to be cautious about generalizing from studies with relatively small sample sizes and participants sourced from a support group [Hill, 2001], a therapy group

---

* The etymology of *survivor* is said to date back to the Holocaust.

[Chauncey, 1994], therapist referral [Jacob and Veatch, 2005], or self-referral from flyers or advertisements [Jacob and Veatch, 2005; Smith, 2005]. These participants may not be representative of all relatives of abuse survivors, but taken together these studies do suggest that the effects of victimization can travel through kin ties and that harm from sexual offenses has a broad reach.

8.2.2 Relatives of Offenders

More controversially, and not necessarily successfully, relatives of offenders are sometimes claimed to be secondary victims. In this context, the claim has its root in the literature on prisoners' families who have been variously described as the "hidden victims of crime" [Bakker et al., 1978], the "inno-cent victims of our penal system" [Matthews, 1983], and "the innocent, and often 'forgotten' victims within the criminal justice system" [Howard League, 1994]. As Light explains, "the victims of crime include not only those who have had offences committed against them, but also families and dependents of those convicted of offences, particularly if the offender is sentenced to a period in prison" [Light, 1993:324–25].

The claim here is usually that some of the punishment meted out to the offender is experienced vicariously by the offender's family, and a consider-able body of research evidence shows this to be so. Studies going back some 40 years have found the families of prisoners to experience numerous diffi-culties, including severe stresses on family relationships, financial problems stemming from the loss of wages or benefits and the additional expenses of supporting a prisoner, social stigma, and an array of problems faced by children suddenly separated from imprisoned parents [for a detailed review of this literature, see Codd, 2008; Comfort, 2008:Appendix 2]. Research from the United States has looked at the impact of imprisonment on families of prisoners and on communities (and how this impact is unevenly distributed, particularly hitting African American communities) and draws our attention to a range of "collateral consequences" [e.g., see Hagan and Dinovitzer, 1999; Mauer and Chesney-Lind, 2002; Harris and Miller, 2003].

Do these consequences merit describing prisoners' families as second-ary victims? The idea of collateral consequences is taken from the military euphemism of collateral damage, referring to the deaths of civilians or other indirect, secondary, or unintended consequences of warfare; it could be argued that the consequences of imprisonment are similarly to be seen as somehow unavoidable in the pursuit of the higher aim of the punishment of offenders, or even that they form part of that punishment, necessary pains of imprisonment if imprisonment is to have any force and a deterrent effect. From this perspective, responsibility for the consequences experienced by family members would lie with the prisoner, not with the State, as expressed by one Conservative Member of the Scottish Parliament:

I recognise the soul-destroying effect that a parent's imprisonment must have on a youngster, but there should be no off-loading of responsibilities for who caused this anguish. The responsibility lies firmly with the individual who landed in prison as a result of their decision to break the law. The offender must take full responsibility. [Gallie, 2002, quoted in Codd, 2008:41]

As Codd argues, there is a question about how this responsibility could be borne and exercised by prisoners because while they are in prison there is little they can do to help their family—prison wages are not "real" wages for the work prisoners do; family contact is limited, and visiting conditions are difficult; and there are aspects of prison life and the prison establishment that make the difficulties families face even worse [Codd, 2008:42].

Prisoners' families might also be seen as somehow culpable themselves, as "criminal families" or as having colluded with or protected the offender or profited from crime, and therefore not blameless and not entitled to claim victim status. Children of prisoners may be more easily designated as innocent victims because they are not deemed responsible for their parents' imprisonment, and their plight might garner more sympathy or funding. One study estimates that around 1% of children in England and Wales experience the imprisonment of a parent in each year and argues that prisoners and their children experience multiple types of social exclusion and poor future prospects [Murray, 2007]; the figures for the United States are much higher [Martone, 2005]. However, the status of children of prisoners as secondary victims and the difficulties they face are not generally acknowledged: They remain under-researched, unmonitored, and unsupported by the statutory sector [Murray, 2007].

Describing prisoners' families as secondary victims and encouraging prisons to develop "family-friendly" policies have been criticized for obscuring the question of why families face such difficulties in the first place. Writing in the newsletter of the abolitionist organization *No More Prison*, for example, one partner of a serving prisoner describes feeling disillusioned with some of the more established organizations for prisoners and their families who "tend to see families as 'forgotten victims' who the Prison Service should be nicer to" [*No More Prison*, 2006:4]. She argues that these organizations should be expressing outrage at the suffering of these families:

There is a general silence that surrounds so much of that pain and humiliation. Prisons cannot possibly be family-friendly. They are designed to break up families, to separate people from those they love, and to observe and threaten them constantly when they are together, with no respite. We know that family ties are the single biggest factor in preventing re-offending but there is no consideration given to the maintenance of those ties, with some rare exceptions. The prisons run courses like "Family Man" to encourage better parenting without any questioning of the manner in which prisons themselves undermine and, in many cases, destroy family life. [*No More Prison*, 2006:4]

From this perspective, a claim to victim status for prisoners' families masks the real problem and suggests that their difficulties can be remedied by policy changes, rather than seeing their suffering as at the very core of imprisonment. However, others have argued that viewing families as victims of penal policy is not incompatible with a critical perspective on imprisonment and its expansion in contemporary society:

> Prisoners' families could be argued to be the innocent victims of current penological policies; they are the casualties of the move towards mass imprisonment and the dominance of imprisonment as the paradigmatic criminal sanction. A critique of penology and the use of imprisonment, therefore, entails a recognition and understanding that families are suffering along with inmates. [Codd, 2008:41]

One study of the partners of prisoners from the United States warns against taking an oversimplified and one-sided view of the impact of prison on the lives of prisoners' families. Comfort's [2008] study of women visiting male partners at San Quentin prison in California found the women to be themselves fundamentally changed by their interaction with the prison, assuming the status of quasi-inmates as they came under its rules and discipline, and as the boundary between home and prison became blurred. However, the roles that the prison played in their lives were "convoluted and counterintuitive." With severely declining welfare and other sources of assistance for poor women, the prison provided a "peculiar refuge," becoming a resource for the women who were able to reframe and manage their relationships through the prison, "transforming incarceration into a readily accessible tool provided to them by the state" [Comfort, 2008:17].

Paradoxically, collateral consequences coexisted with positive functions that enabled the women to sustain and shape relationships in ways that would not have been possible on the "outside." Comfort is critical of previous studies on prisoners' families that construct families' experience of prison as entirely damaging and fail to address the conditions of these families' lives before imprisonment and to question whether imprisonment mitigated or altered those conditions—as Comfort says, the "collateral damage" experienced by these families might have a source other than the prison [Comfort, 2008:11]. Comfort's study shows the need for a more nuanced approach to the impact of imprisonment on families' lives, capturing the complexities and contradictions of their experience. They may be victimized in particular ways by penal policy, but this conceptualization alone is not enough to understand what families *do* with the situation in which they find themselves; furthermore, it is difficult to disentangle the impact of penal policy from the impact of poverty, social disadvantage, and the innumerable problems these bring.

Some relatives of serious offenders have claimed to be the "other victims" of crime, suffering from the fact of the serious offense itself and from the consequences that follow [Howarth and Rock, 2000; Condry, 2007]. In a book based on several years of research with these relatives in England, I describe how the impact of the offense reached into every corner of their lives [Condry, 2007]. Finding out that a relative has committed an offense such as murder, manslaughter, rape, or child sex offenses can be shocking and devastating. The time they found out about the offense was etched with clarity in the minds of these relatives as the point at which their lives were forever changed. It was a moment that precipitated feelings of distress and grief that would continue for many months and even years. Gill described how she felt when she discovered her husband had committed child sex offenses:

> I can actually remember physically what I felt like that day, half dead. It's like when you've got the worst dose of the flu but double-fold, it's like you just, your limbs have got no weight but they feel dead heavy, you know, I can feel how I felt but you couldn't describe how you felt. You weren't floating, they were heavy but there was nothing in them, you were just nothing, you were just hollow. [Gill, in Condry 2007:25]

Their distress was centered on loss: of their relationship with the offender or of free contact with him or her following imprisonment, of their hopes and dreams for the offender and what his or her life might hold, of other family members and friends, and of other practical losses of money and time that would now be devoted to the offender and his or her needs. There was also a less tangible but nevertheless devastating loss of what the relatives had thought they had known and of how they understood their lives to be. As Gill said, "my world as I knew it: gone" [Condry, 2007:40]. Many relatives said they were traumatized and compared the devastating impact to bereavement. One mother of a man given a life sentence for murder said: "It's grief, a form of grieving, but you haven't got the respectability of them being dead" [Condry, 2007:27]. This respectability was important as their distress was also rooted in a deep-seated sense of personal shame.

Bringing shame on the family is a notion that has been more commonly associated with "other" distant cultures and close-knit extended families, but the shame associated with such serious offenses flows freely through kin ties. Relatives felt that their grief was not legitimized because they themselves were causally implicated and perceived to be somehow contaminated. They would be blamed because it was imagined that they knew, or should have known, about the offending and failed to stop it, or that their own deeds in the immediate or distant past might have caused or contributed to the offender's actions. Frances, another wife of a sex offender, was shocked when a doctor who had been called to visit her at home implied she had known about her husband's offending:

... his first words to me were, "Did you know it was going on and did you condone it?" And I thought if somebody of a professional nature has said that, how many other people were saying that? And whether some people thought that I knew it was going on I don't know, but I have lost a hell of a lot of friends. [Frances in Condry, 2007:74]

Relatives wrestled privately with self-blame, wondering if their past actions might have contributed in some way to what had happened. As Beryl, whose son was convicted of murder, said, "You wonder where you've gone wrong. You think, 'Why did it happen? Is it something I've done?'" [Condry, 2007:136].

The relatives felt they were perceived to be the same as the offender because of their close association—"tarred with the same brush"—or because of a genetic connection that could provoke very primitive ideas of bad blood. Mothers, for example, often spoke of their horror that someone born of their body had committed a heinous offense, and sons worried whether they might inherit some of their offending father's traits. The consequences of being blamed and stigmatized could be severe. Friendships were lost; a mother was spat at in the street; another had eggs thrown at her windows and abuse from neighbors; and another received abusive phone calls. One wife had all the windows of her house broken, and another was taunted in the street: "You murderer's wife."

The stories of the relatives I spoke to are often echoed in very high-profile cases where relatives of serious offenders are simultaneously the subject of intense public curiosity and outright vilification. Witness, for example, the criticism directed at Primrose Shipman, the wife of the UK serial killer Harold Shipman, and the fury that erupted over the decision to award her a widow's pension, or the world's media camped outside the house of Virginia Tech Campus killer Cho Seung-Hui in 2007, chewing over every detail of his family's life—from their dry cleaning business to the vegetable patches in their back garden and their Princeton graduate daughter—and the Cho family's devastation expressed in their statement released to the press: "We could never have believed that he was capable of so much violence. He has made the world weep. We are living a nightmare."

Explanations that locate the source of deviant behavior within the family have a long history and are woven through political, media, and lay discourse, as well as expert and therapeutic analyses. The families I met felt they were constantly faced with the belief that serious offenders were "made" by their families. Does this devastating, life-changing impact make relatives of serious offenders the "other victims" of crime? Much of the fieldwork for the study was conducted with Aftermath, a self-help organization specifically for families of serious offenders that has now closed. Aftermath existed for 17 years and in that time supported hundreds of families through self-help meetings, newsletters, and telephone support. Aftermath maintained that there were many victims of an offense, and that families of offenders were indeed the unrecognized victims of crime. One of Aftermath's leaflets, *The Forgotten Victims*, stated:

> Whilst we support the offender and his family, we never condone the offence. We do, however, sympathise with the unique and difficult circumstances in which these families find themselves. These are the Forgotten Victims. Our aim is to offer them support, love and understanding. [Aftermath leaflet, no date]

As we saw at the start of this chapter, the victim label has powerful interpretive instructions. Aftermath's narrative about the experiences of its members was constructed around resisting relatives' own feelings of shame and worthlessness and notions of kin contamination and culpability. Constructing relatives as the other victims encompassed both blamelessness and suffering: They were not to blame for the circumstances in which they found themselves; the crime was not their fault; and they were not to be blamed if they chose to support the offender.

However, interviewees had different interpretations of what it meant to claim the status of victim, whether relatives of serious offenders were victims, and varied in the degree to which they incorporated the status into their own personal narratives. Some accepted outright that they were victims, whereas others were less categorical. Like most relatives, Lisa accepted that relatives of serious offenders were victims and explained why:

> It must be so difficult for … a wife whose husband's gone inside and she has to explain to the children, she has to try and stop them being bullied and tormented in the school playground, she's confronted with media pressure, she's confronted with conversations in shops that suddenly stop as she goes in, I mean all those must be dreadful pressures and I think this is something that people don't understand…. We'll read *The Sun* and we'll take on board all these ridiculous stories about yes they're living on lobster and caviar and Whitemoor [prison] is a hotel, what they won't take on board is how a little girl goes back to wetting the bed and cries herself asleep at night because she's lost her daddy and she doesn't understand why, and because of what people are saying to her about it. [Lisa, partner convicted of homicide, in Condry, 2007:174]

However, Lisa said she did not see herself as a victim. Frances, on the other hand, did so define herself and said that this was what had attracted her to Aftermath in the first place: "Um, well it was you know, what it said, you know 'for the other victims', um, because there was no help for me, everybody else seemed to get help but me, you know I did take it quite badly"

[Condry, 2007:174]. Harriet, whose son was accused of sex offenses, was less sure about the claim because she felt the term *victim* did not differentiate between different types of harm:

> H: I've always taken issue with Aftermath that we are victims. I think that must be dreadfully annoying to the people who have had someone murdered or raped. You know, how dare they say they are victims? You know. We've suffered greatly as a result, but I think the word victim is the wrong word. And I think it must lose us a lot of public sympathy. I can't think of another word other than victim, but it is the wrong word.

> R: And you don't feel like a victim yourself?

> H: Possibly, but I think it's worse for the actual people whose brother has been murdered ... we're a victim once removed, aren't we? There are many different types of victim—the immediate victim, the relatives of that victim, and then another tier on the other side, the relatives of those that have done it. [Harriet, son accused of sex offense, in Condry, 2007:175–76]

Harriet was unusual in "taking issue," as she describes it, with Aftermath over its claims to the status of victim; there appeared to be, on the surface at least, a general acceptance that this term captured the experience of relatives of serious offenders. However, by probing the use of this term in interviews, it emerged that *victim* was a flexible category and part of a narrative that was used contingently as a *resource* by relatives. Different aspects of victimization were emphasized, and the degree to which relatives were prepared to incorporate this status into their own personal narratives varied and was dependent on their circumstances and the other resources they used to understand those circumstances [Condry, 2007]. This illustrates what Holstein and Miller [1990] describe as the descriptive processes through which victim status is assigned to individuals or groups and the importance of trying to unpack the interpretive instructions of such a claim.

Aftermath members attempted to resist culpability through their claim to victim status, but this was a claim that was often not honored as they experienced stigma, blame, and exclusion. Although on the "other side" of a serious crime, their claim had parallels with the claims made by survivors of homicide: "Both have lost control. Both point to catastrophically invasive knowledge that is impossible to absorb, accept or integrate. Both point to a disintegration of meaning; to feelings of oppression, vulnerability, guilt, stigma, and isolation; and to a profound sense of bereavement and loss" [Howarth and Rock, 2000:70]. Their intimate connection to the offender meant their claim to victim status was not usually publicly accepted; they made their claims much more quietly and privately and had "little of the righteous anger, vociferous campaigning and denunciation of outsiders that so beset the politics of other survivors' groups" [Howarth and Rock, 2000:73].

Aftermath found it difficult to generate support and funding, and as a result closed in 2005; in the United Kingdom there is now no national organization of the same kind specifically supporting families of serious offenders.[*]

8.2.3 Vicarious Trauma and Victimization

The notion of vicarious trauma has been further extended beyond the family and friends of a primary victim to professionals working with victims, witnesses to crime, and even as far as the level of the community. Numerous studies have found professionals such as counselors or therapists, lawyers, and the police working directly with victims of rape, sexual assault, and other forms of interpersonal violence experience high levels of vicarious trauma [see Dunkley and Whelan, 2006, for a review of this literature; Morrison, 2007]. Vicarious trauma can also be experienced by researchers listening to the stories of victims of crime. Jordan describes in detail how she experienced "vicarious victimization" while undertaking research on rape, suffering a range of emotional effects, feeling increased fear, and sleeping poorly. However, the emotional dimensions of researching sexual violence are rarely addressed [Jordan, 2004:238–39].

Therefore, we can see a broader category of tertiary or indirect victims that could potentially be infinitely expanded. If we take crimes of great enormity, such as a terrorist attack, we can see how one event can have many levels of victims. In July 2005, suicide bombers killed 52 people on the transport system in London. The 52 primary victims who were killed had many relatives and friends; around 700 further victims were injured, and they also would have had kin and friends; there were a significant number of witnesses to the attacks; there were the emergency services and others who worked with the victims on the day and for some time after; or consider even the people in London who were not directly involved but were unable to leave the city as public transport shut down and were fearful of what was happening, and possibly even those who witnessed events unfolding on television and felt that their own sense of security and safety was threatened. Literature on the fear of crime attests to people experiencing indirect victimization when hearing about the victimization of others produces anxiety and increased perception of risk [see Jackson et al., 2007, for discussion].

Expanding the category of vicarious trauma or victimization in this way can be useful to illuminate who is affected by crime, but it is important to acknowledge that as the category is expanded further and further the degree of harm may be very much diluted, with increasing numbers of people identifying as victims and increasing claims competing for degrees of harm.

---

[*] There is a smaller organization, AFFECT, based in the south of England and run by some former Aftermath members, but it too exists on a very low income and risks closure if funds cannot be found: http://www.affect.org.uk.

One example can be seen in the anger that erupted when a police officer was awarded more than £300,000 compensation in 2001 for the trauma he had suffered attending the 1989 Hillsborough football stadium disaster when 96 Liverpool fans died. The Hillsborough Family Support Group condemned the award, saying people who had lost sons, daughters, and loved ones had received nothing or payouts of only a few thousand pounds [BBC, 2001]. Relatives of victims had also had to contend with significant victim blaming [Taylor et al., 1995]. These relatives deemed their secondary victimization to be worse than that experienced by a police officer doing his job [BBC News Online, 2001].

8.3 Secondary Victimization: Processes That Inflict Further Harm on Victims

Our second way of conceptualizing secondary victimization is as something that happens to primary victims after the offense as their victimization is prolonged, compounded, and made worse by the reactions of others and their treatment in the criminal justice process. There has been a growing awareness in recent years of the needs of victims and the difficulties they face within the criminal justice system, and victims have become an increasing focus of academic research, policymaking, government legislation, and activist and voluntary sector groups. There are a number of factors that can compound or worsen victimization: a lack of involvement in the criminal justice process; no opportunity to express views and be listened to; a lack of information about the process and decisions made; a lack of coordination between criminal justice agencies or support services; and a feeling that justice has not been achieved, whether because a case fails or if there is no compensation or reparation.

I intend to very briefly sketch only a few of the key developments in policies for victims in England and Wales [for a more detailed review of these developments, see Rock, 2004; Dignan, 2005; Spalek, 2006; Hoyle and Zedner, 2007]. Governments internationally have introduced a range of measures that aim to tackle the problems victims face and their experiences within the criminal justice process. The needs of victims were placed firmly on the agenda by the United Nations Declaration of Basic Principles of Justice for Victims of Crime and Abuse of Power in 1985. It sought to set standards for how victims should be treated and what they should be entitled to, including compassion and respect for their dignity, access to justice and prompt redress, information about their rights and the timing and progress of their case, consideration of their views, and restitution and compensation [United Nations, 1985], all aspirational rather than justiciable rights. Some of these entitlements are echoed in declarations on victims made by the Council of

Europe. However, these rights are highly generalized and give wide scope for how they should be implemented by member states [Dignan, 2005:66].

The Home Office in Britain introduced two Victims' Charters [Home Office, 1990 and 1996] setting out the standards of service victims should expect. These have since been replaced with The Code of Practice for Victims of Crime, which was introduced in the Domestic Violence, Crime, and Victims Act 2004 (section 32), which has been in force since April 2006, setting out to represent a minimum level of service for victims in England and Wales and the obligations of service providers to victims at different stages of the criminal justice process: the police, the Crown Prosecution Service, Witness Care Units, the Crown Court, the Magistrates Court, the Court of Appeal, Youth Offending Teams, the National Probation Service, the Prison Service, the Parole Board, the Criminal Injuries Compensation Authority and Appeals Board, and the Criminal Cases Review Commission, all of whom must ensure that victims and their families receive information, protection, and support. More specifically, victims have a right to information about their crime within specified time scales, including the right to be notified of any arrests and court cases; clear information from the Criminal Injuries Compensation Authority (CICA) on eligibility for compensation under the Scheme; being told about Victim Support and either referred to them or offered their service; provision of an enhanced service to vulnerable or intimidated victims; and flexibility for victims with regard to opting in or out of receiving services to ensure that they receive the level of service they want [Home Office, 2005a]. The Government has also established 165 Witness Care Units across England and Wales acting as a single point of contact to provide information and coordinate support, and proposed the appointment of a Commissioner for Victims and Witnesses, although no appointment has yet been made.

Vulnerable victims (defined as those under the age of 17 or with mental or physical disabilities) and intimidated victims need further protection through the criminal justice process. The Youth Justice and Criminal Evidence Act 1999 put in place special measures to protect child and other vulnerable witnesses, including screening the witness from the accused, the opportunity to give evidence by means of a live link or to give evidence in private, the removal of wigs or gowns, the use of video recordings in the questioning of witnesses as evidence, and the opportunities for witnesses to be examined through an intermediary and for aids to communication to be used in court. However, as Goodey has said, the judiciary retains a considerable degree of discretion in deciding who is a vulnerable or intimidated witness, and there is still inconsistency in service provision [Goodey, 2005].

Victim Support, the national organization for victims in Britain, has received core funding from the Government since 1986 and currently receives more than £30 million. In its 2007 annual report, Victim Support reports having supported more than 1.4 million people through its services in the community, and its Witness Service helped around 380,000 people in Crown and Magistrates courts in the preceding year [Victim Support, 2007].

There have, then, been numerous efforts made to improve the experience of victims and witnesses, to place their needs on the criminal justice agenda, and to provide some protection from secondary victimization, but as Dignan says, these safeguards are both partial and limited in scope: "Many victims continue to experience secondary victimisation, both with regard to the 'regular' and, for some also, ironically, as a result of the victim-focused reforms themselves" [Dignan, 2005:85]. Raising expectations that cannot be delivered—when the information victims receive is incomplete or late arriving, when their input into the criminal justice process is one-directional and very limited—can in itself increase secondary victimization [Dignan, 2005:85].

Some proponents of restorative justice argue that it places the victim center stage and better meets victims' needs, therefore reducing secondary victimization, but this has been the subject of much debate, and research evidence on whether it serves the interests of victims is mixed [for a more detailed discussion see Strang, 2002; Dignan, 2005; Hoyle and Zedner, 2007]. Although victim surveys show an appetite for restorative justice [Hoyle and Zedner, 2007] and some studies have found high levels of victim satisfaction [e.g., McCold and Wachtel, 1998; McGarrell et al., 2000; Hoyle et al., 2002], many schemes have low rates of victim participation, and development of restorative justice in Britain has been somewhat patchy. Miers conducted an international review of restorative justice programs and found that only one jurisdiction, Denmark, claimed to be primarily victim oriented—the rest were either offender oriented or of mixed orientation [Miers, 2001]. Although there may be positive signs from some of the recent research evidence on restorative justice [e.g., see Sherman and Strang, 2007], it would be a step too far to suggest that it provides the solution to secondary victimization. The place of restorative justice in the criminal justice system is far from clear, and as Hoyle and Zedner point out, low participation of victims in many restorative justice schemes leaves open the question of the degree to which restorative practice (rather than theory) is victim centered [Hoyle and Zedner, 2007:486].

8.3.1 Secondary Victimization of Rape and Sexual Assault Victims

The subject of secondary victimization has received the most attention in studies of victims of rape and sexual assault, and analyses of how criminal justice processes can inflict further harm on victims have been particularly powerful in this context. These victims recount feeling retraumatized as they report the crime, undergo invasive medical examinations and intensive questioning, and—if their case ever reaches court—find that they are under scrutiny and their own credibility brought into question: "Women who are raped continue to be embarrassed, doubted, and abused by the legal organizations that process them" [Martin and Powell, 1994:856]. This prolonged experience of harm has been characterized as a "second assault" [Martin and Powell, 1994], "the second rape" [Madigan and Gamble, 1991; Campbell et al., 2001], or "secondary victimization" [Campbell and Raja, 1999, 2005].

Rape victims experience secondary victimization when they are failed by the justice system and when they are treated insensitively by professionals in the health and justice systems when they report rape. In a newspaper article, a young woman subjected to a sexual attack said: "The experience of the investigation and court process is not terribly dissimilar to the attack itself: there is the lack of control, the humiliation and the enforced submission. I needed far more counselling after I had gone through the police investigation and court case than I had after the attack itself" [Hill, 2005].

Victims can also experience secondary victimization from informal sources in their everyday lives: from kin, friends, or others in their local communities. Whether to report rape is a difficult decision, and we know that many choose not to do so, but many rape victims are also fearful of disclosing their status to friends or kin because of fear of the reaction it might elicit; in a UK survey of women who had experienced rape or sexual assault, for example, 40% said they chose not to tell anyone about their worst experience [Walby and Allen, 2004]. Why do rape victims choose not to tell? Lievore [2003] makes a distinction between personal barriers to disclosure and barriers at the level of the criminal justice system. Personal barriers include a victim's perception of the crime and whether it is a "real" crime or inappropriate to report to the police; regarding it as a private matter and not wanting family or others to know; shame, embarrassment; fear of reprisals; self-blame or fearing blame from others; and a desire to protect the perpetrator, a relationship, or children [Lievore, 2003:28]. It is clear from this list of factors that the act of disclosure has the potential to trigger consequences that exacerbate, prolong, or compound the experience of victimization. Barriers to disclosure at the level of the justice system include concerns that the police would not or could not do anything or would not think it serious enough; fear of not being believed by the police; fear of being treated hostilely by the police or others in the justice system; fear or dislike of the police; fear of the legal process; lack of proof that the incident happened; or not knowing how to report the incident [Lievore, 2003:28].

Feelings of shame, stigma, and fearing blame from others will be stronger in patriarchal cultures with strong moral codes and prohibitions around female sexuality and proprietary attitudes toward women. Furthermore, in armed conflicts sexual violence is often used as a weapon of war on a vast scale; Amnesty International reports that tens of thousands of women and girls are currently subjected to sexual violence in Darfur, for example, and one-third of the women in Sierra Leone faced sexual violence during the conflict [Amnesty International, 2007]. It is impossible to do justice to the complexities of this topic in this chapter, but it is important to note that when strong cultural stigmas are attached to rape, women can experience incredibly severe secondary victimization, including rejection by their communities and families.

Human Rights Watch, in a web page entitled "the stigma of rape," describes how in Somalia rape victims face being ostracized by their families. It describes the case of Hibaq, a woman aged 40, who was raped by three unknown assailants. When her husband discovered what had happened, he sent her away from the compound in which they were living, took her belongings, and denied her access to her children. Staff members from the UN High Commissioner for Refugees were eventually able to negotiate access to her children, but her husband refused to have anything to do with her, and she now lives alone. Perhaps not surprisingly, women in Somalia often refuse to acknowledge publicly that they have been raped for fear of stigmatization [Human Rights Watch, 2008], which is secondary victimization on a devastating scale.

Research on victims of rape in the justice system in Britain and in many other jurisdictions tells us that they do not fare well. When rape is reported to the police, it is unlikely to result in a conviction. The "problem of attrition" in rape cases is severe and growing; in the United Kingdom in 2004–2005, only 5.3% of reported rapes resulted in conviction [Home Office, 2005b, in Temkin and Krahe, 2008:9], whereas in 1977, the conviction rate was 32% [Regan and Kelly, 2003:13]. Therefore, despite increasing rates of reporting, a victim of rape who reports only has a slim chance of seeing the perpetrator brought to justice. Considerably less than 5.3% of rapes actually result in conviction because of the stark fact that most victims never report rape, and many of those who do find their report rejected by the police and therefore do not enter the recorded crime figures [Temkin and Krahe, 2008:10]. The problem of attrition has been the subject of a considerable body of research that seeks to understand why the problem occurs and what might be done to remedy it. Lees and Gregory clearly identified four major points in the judicial process where attrition might take place: when the police reject a report of rape; when the police fail to refer a case to the Crown Prosecution Service (CPS); when the CPS decides not to proceed or to reduce a charge through plea bargaining; and when a jury finds a defendant "not guilty" [Lees and Gregory, 1993], each decision a source of distress to a victim seeking justice.

The police rejection of reports of rape is often referred to as "no-criming," and "numerous studies over the past few decades testify to the overzealous and inappropriate no-criming practices of the police" [Temkin and Krahe, 2008:17; see Clark and Lewis, 1977, Women's National Commission 1985,

Harris and Grace, 1999, cited in Temkin and Krahe]. It is at the stage of police investigation that the highest rate of attrition takes place, with complaints either being withdrawn by victims or discontinued by the police [Kelly et al., 2005]. Recent UK research examining 3,527 cases of alleged rape found that 20% were no-crimed and that "the vast majority of cases did not progress beyond the investigative stage" [Kelly et al., 2005:xi].

In England and Wales the proportion of recorded rapes that are prosecuted each year is low; some rape cases stall at the stage of the CPS, whereas others do not progress from the Magistrates Court to a Crown Court trial [see Temkin and Krahe, 2008: Chapter 1 for a review of the evidence at each stage]. Home Office figures from 1998 to 2002 show that only a quarter of cases of rape and attempted rape that were prosecuted resulted in conviction [Kelly et al., 2005]. Therefore, the figures tell us that around 95% of those who report rape and three-quarters of those whose cases proceed to the prosecution stage are failed by the justice system.

The experience of prosecution itself has been found to cause harm to victims. One study found that rape victims whose cases were prosecuted were psychologically worse off with lower self-esteem 6 months after the rape than those whose cases were not prosecuted [Cluss et al., 1983], and other studies have similarly documented harm caused to victims by criminal justice processes [Matoesian, 1993; Sloan, 1995, in Campbell et al., 2001]. If a rape case reaches court, the experience for the victim can be an ordeal, and in an adversarial system rape victims can find that it is they who are under scrutiny as defense counsel attempt to introduce doubt and call into question their version of events. Despite legislation intended to place limits on invasive and unnecessary questioning about a rape victim's personal life and sexual history, judges still use their discretion and allow this kind of questioning to happen [Temkin and Krahe, 2008]. In a study of rape cases in U.S. courts, Taslitz similarly found progress through rape law reform to be modest because police, prosecutors, judges, and defense counsel use their discretion to circumvent reforms [Taslitz, 1999:7]. Reliving the events of a rape in a public arena can be traumatic in itself. One rape victim who was 16 when she was attacked said:

> The court experience had been so disturbing and brought the experience back in such clarity that, although I thought a successful judgement would give me closure, instead it triggered an even deeper despair. I could not imagine an end to the way I was feeling, and that left me suicidal. [in Hill, 2005]

In recent decades there have been numerous reforms intended to improve the experience of rape victims, decrease attrition, and minimize further harm to victims, with varying levels of success. In Britain, the feminist movement of the 1970s and the Rape Crisis Movement brought the treatment of rape victims to the fore. The subject was then placed firmly in the public consciousness by Roger Graef's 1982 television documentary *A Complaint of Rape*, showing police officers interrogating and bullying a woman who had reported being raped, provoking public outcry and leading to changes in how rape was investigated. During the decades since, the police have introduced a raft of guidance and reforms in how cases are investigated and have made this a central concern. A conference on improving police responses to rape held in July 2008 was attended by senior police officers from all 47 police forces in England and Wales [Westmarland, 2008]. Legislation has been introduced to try to offer rape victims further protection—yet still the attrition rate remains, and other than Ireland, the United Kingdom has the lowest conviction rate in Europe [Kelly et al., 2005:34].

What lies beneath the failure to bring perpetrators to justice? There is the problem of uncorroborated testimony, with rape trials often turning on one person's word against another. But there may be more complex reasons why complainants are disbelieved. Temkin and Krahe say that rape stereotypes and myths that involve derogatory beliefs about rape victims are deeply embedded in our culture. These myths include a restrictive definition of what constitutes "real rape" (an attack out of doors on a stranger using force, with the victim actively resisting), normative expectations about how rape victims behave (e.g., reporting an offense immediately), and other misconceptions about the offense and the victim's role. Victim-blaming myths are prevalent—an Amnesty International study found that 26% of respondents believed that a woman was totally or partially responsible if she was wearing sexy or revealing clothes, and 22% thought she was totally or partially to blame if she had had many sexual partners [Amnesty International UK, 2005, in Temkin and Krahe, 2008].

There is a substantial body of research that shows wide acceptance of rape myths. These myths cast doubt on complainants' allegations, and Temkin and Krahe argue that this affects women's self-definition of rape and each stage of the criminal justice process: "not only are rape myths widely shared in many countries across the world, they are also endorsed by members of professional groups involved in different stages of the prosecution of rape complaints" [Temkin and Krahe, 2008:209]. This affects every stage, from a decision to report rape through to the decision of a jury, and complainants are secondarily victimized as they experience victim blaming, disbelief, and a failure to achieve justice. Police initiatives and legislation do not change these deeply embedded beliefs, although perhaps acknowledging their existence in the first place is an important step—the Metropolitan Police's specialist rape investigation unit Project Sapphire lists 10 of these myths, explaining why they are false, on its web site (http://www.met.police.uk/sapphire/myths.htm). Temkin and Krahe stress that "designing effective strategies for changing these misconceptions is an urgent task, not only to improve the fate of rape victims in the criminal justice system and avoid 'secondary victimisation', but to reduce the prevalence of sexual assault in the first place" [Temkin and Krahe, 2008:199].

8.4 Secondary Victimization and Identity

Our final interpretation of secondary victimization is as something that can be created by a social reaction to a primary victim's status that leads to that status becoming entrenched and central to that person's identity, a notion that owes much to labeling theory and particularly Lemert's [1951] conception of "secondary deviance." The concern here is with secondary victimization as a new status—a secondary status—created by the reaction to the primary victim whose original victimization may well otherwise have been short-lived. In his book about the rise of Victim Support in England and Wales, Rock [1990:135–36] describes how a key actor in the working group of an early 1970s influential local scheme for victims was drawn to the then-fashionable tenets of labeling theory. Ideas about secondary deviation were straightforward to transpose to a description of victimization, and victimization was said therefore to have the potential to become frozen into secondary victimization, a form of learned helplessness or disablement [Rock, 1990].

This understanding of secondary victimization with its opposition to the reification and stabilization of victim status is significant because it was one of a number of founding ideas fused together in the early development of services for victims and was important to how those services developed and evolved in England and Wales [Rock, 1990:409]. This was not a rejection of claims to victimhood—these groups were very much concerned with the recognition of the plight of victims, and the emergent victims' movement of the time was working to place victims on the criminal justice agenda—but it was instead a concern with the shape that helping victims might take and the consequences of adopting a victim status. Similarly, some other groups have rejected outright claims to victim status because of concerns that taking on a victim identity would engender powerlessness and passivity, preferring instead the term *survivor*. This was particularly a concern of the feminist movement, although debate over the appropriate terminology continues today.

8.4.1 Claims about Victims and Victimization

To conclude, claims to secondary victim status and to secondary victimization can be seen as part of an era of ever-increasing claims to victim status and "new victims" [Best, 1999]. During the past three decades or so the climate has been increasingly receptive to such claims as more and more groups have come forward. As Best [1999] says, victims' crusaders, like equal rights movements, have argued that society has neglected millions of victims and that victims' problems need to be recognized and addressed. Victims have become far more visible and an increasingly common focus in contemporary society. Therapeutic professions have expanded; the self-help movement has grown; and different types of trauma and harm have been brought to the fore. Claims to secondary victimhood are being made in a sympathetic climate along with untold other claims to direct and indirect harm. These claims are not identical but are constructed around similar ideology and are mutually reinforcing, borrowing language, orientations, explanations, tactics, and solutions from each other as elements of claims become "cultural resources" that can be adapted to different kinds of victimization [Best, 1999:103]. Hence how people talk about being secondary victims or experiencing secondary victimization is shaped by how people talk about a variety of kinds of victimization—as Best says, these narratives cross-fertilize, creating a powerful set of ideas about victims and victimization [Best, 1999].

Simultaneously, something in our culture tends to distrust the victim. Victims are taken to be somehow unsavory, having a "pariah identity" [Rock, 1998:167]. Their status reflects victim blaming and our need to believe that victims of misfortune deserve what happens to them—what Lerner [1980] called our "belief in a just world."* We are left asking whether something a victim did could have contributed to his or her misfortune, not wanting to believe that the same could happen to us. Secondary victims are even more bedeviled with the problem of culpability, which taints the claims of relatives of victims and relatives of offenders. The stigma for relatives of offenders can be particularly powerful—they can be seen as culpable for particular acts or stigmatized for being the same as the offender, from the same stock, or contaminated by their kin tie [Condry, 2007]. Claims to victim status can be an attempt to counter this culpability and contamination, although as we have seen, they often have rather limited success.

Victims provoke complex and contradictory responses. Even in a sympathetic climate, some claims are more likely to be honored than others, and some claims receive greater prominence. Although the secondary victimization of rape victims has received academic attention and been the focus of legislation and policymaking, the attrition rate remains. Secondary victims have tended to fall outside the conventional criminological and policymaking gaze, with the exception of the more recent recognition of homicide "survivors."

---

* Although it has been suggested that notions such as this might be culturally specific, underpinned by Western values and assumptions [see Spalek, 2006:90].

We should note that there are many types of crime and many types of victim—just as the experience and impact of victimization are mediated by factors such as age, gender, socioeconomic status, and ethnicity, so the experience and impact of secondary victimization will vary, too. The impact of crime is contingent, and people vary in the extent to which they are willing to identify as victims (or secondary victims). Furthermore, the meanings of crime and victimhood change over time. They have their own histories and important cultural and spatial differences: (secondary) victimization will not necessarily mean the same in the United Kingdom, Rwanda, or Australia. However, this does not detract from the importance of recognizing that many more people are affected by crime than a cursory look at crime figures might suggest. Criminology will be richer for including in its focus those who are swept up in the aftermath of crime. By thinking about the various ways in which the experience of victimization can potentially extend and expand, a more nuanced picture begins to emerge of who is affected by crime and how they are affected, and the consequences and structures that crime generates can be better understood.

Acknowledgments

I thank Paul Rock for comments on an earlier version of this chapter.

References

Ahrens, C. E. and R. Campbell. 2000. Assisting rape victims as they recover from rape: the impact on friends. *Journal of Interpersonal Violence* 15(9):959–86.

Amnesty International. 2007. Violence in conflict and post conflict. http://www.amnesty.org/en/campaigns/stop-violence-against-women/issues/implementation-existing-laws/violence-in-conflict (accessed June 14, 2008).

Amnesty International UK. 2005. *Sexual assault research summary report*. London: Amnesty International.

Attorney General's Office. 2007. Prosecutors to support victims' families across England and Wales—national scheme is announced by Baroness Scotland, 1st October 2007. News Release, Attorney General's Office. http://www.attorneygeneral.gov.uk/attachments/prosecutors%20to%20support%20victims%20families.01.10.2007.pdf (accessed August 3, 2008).

Bakker, L. J., B. A. Morris, and L. M. Janus. 1978. Hidden victims of crime. *Social Work* 23:143–48.

BBC News Online. 2001. Hillsborough Police Payout Condemned. BBC News. http://news.bbc.co.uk/1/hi/uk/1197720.stm (accessed July 22, 2008).

Best, J. 1999. *Random violence: How we talk about new crimes and new victims*. Berkeley and Los Angeles: University of California Press.

Campbell, R. and S. Raja. 1999. Secondary victimisation of rape victims: Insights from mental health professionals who treat survivors of violence. *Violence and Victims* 14: 261–75.

_____. 2005. The sexual assault and secondary victimisation of female veterans: Help-seeking experiences with military and civilian social systems. *Psychology of Women Quarterly* 29:97–106.

Campbell, R., S. M. Wasco, C. E. Ahrens, T. Sefl, and H. E. Barnes. 2001. Preventing the "second rape": Rape survivors' experiences with community service providers. *Journal of Interpersonal Violence* 16(12):1239–59.

Chauncey, S. 1994. Emotional concerns and treatment of male partners of female sexual abuse survivors. *Social Work* 39(6):669–76.

Clark, L., and D. Lewis. 1977. *Rape: The price of coercive sexuality.* Toronto: The Women's Press.

Cluss, P.A., J. Boughton, E. Frank, B. Duffy Steward, and D. West. 1983. The rape victim: Psychological correlates of participation in the legal process. *Criminal Justice and Behavior* 10:342.

Codd, H. 2008. *In the shadow of the prison: Families, imprisonment and criminal justice.* Cullompton, UK: Willan.

Comfort, M. 2008. *Doing time together: Love and family in the shadow of the prison.* Chicago: University of Chicago Press.

Condry, R. 2007. *Families shamed: The consequences of crime for relatives of serious offenders.* Cullompton, UK: Willan.

Cwick, M. S. 1996. The many effects of rape: The victim, her family, and suggestions for family therapy. *Family Therapy* 23:95–116.

Davies, L. and J. Krane. 1996. Shaking the legacy of mother-blaming: No easy task for child welfare. *Journal of Progressive Human Services* 7(2):3–22.

Dignan, J. 2005. *Understanding victims and restorative justice.* Maidenhead, UK: Open University Press.

Dunkley, J. and T. A. Whelan. 2006. Vicarious traumatisation: Current status and future directions. *British Journal of Guidance and Counseling* 34(1): 107–16.

Gallie, P. L. 2002. Prisoners responsible for family anguish—not prison system. Press Release, July 8.

Goodey, J. 2005. *Victims and victimology: Research, policy and practice.* Harlow, UK: Longman.

Hagan, J. and R. Dinovitzer. 1999. Collateral consequences of imprisonment for children, communities, and prisoners. In *Prisons*, ed. M. Tonry and J. Petersilia, 121–62. Chicago: University of Chicago Press.

Harris, J. and S. Grace. 1999. *A question of evidence? Investigating and prosecuting rape in the 1990s.* Home Office Research Study 196. London: Home Office.

Harris, O. and R. Miller. 2003. *Impacts of incarceration on the African-American family.* New Brunswick, NJ: Transaction.

Hendricks, J. H., D. Black, and T. Kaplan.1993. *When father kills mother: Guiding children through the trauma and grief.* London: Routledge in association with the Royal College of Psychiatrists.

Hill, Amelia. 2005. Scandal of justice revolution that betrayed rape victims. *The Observer*, May 1. http://www.guardian.co.uk/uk/2005/may/01/ukcrime.prison sandprobation (accessed July 22, 2008).

Hill, Andrew. 2001. "No-one else could understand": Women's experience of a support group run by and for mothers of sexually abused children. *British Journal of Social Work* 31:385–97.

Holstein, J. A. and G. Miller. 1990. Rethinking victimisation: An interactional approach to victimology. *Symbolic Interaction* 13(1):103–22.

Holstrom, L. L. and A. W. Burgess. 1979. Rape: The husband's and boyfriend's initial reactions. *The Family Coordinator* 28(3):321–30.

Home Office. 1990. *Victim's charter: A statement of the rights of victims.* London: HMSO.

_____. 1996. *Victim's charter.* London: HMSO.

_____. 2005a. *The code of practice for victims of crime.* London: HMSO.

_____. 2005b. *Crime in England and Wales 2004/5.* Home Office Statistical Bulletin 11/05. London: Home Office.

_____. 2005c. Hearing the relatives of murder and manslaughter victims: The government's plans to give the bereaved relatives of murder and manslaughter victims a say in criminal proceedings—Consultation. London: Home Office. http://www.restorativejustice.org.uk/Resources/pdf/murder_mansl.Consultation.pdf (accessed August 3, 2008).

Howard League. 1994. *Families matter.* London: Howard League for Penal Reform.

Howarth, G. and P. Rock. 2000. Aftermath and the construction of victimisation: "The other victims of crime." *The Howard Journal* 39(1):58–78.

Hoyle, C., R. Young, and R. Hill. 2002. *Proceed with caution: An evaluation of the Thames Valley police initiative in restorative cautioning.* York: York Publishing Services.

Hoyle, C. and L. Zedner. 2007. Victims, victimisation, and criminal justice. In *The Oxford handbook of criminology*, ed. M. Maguire, R. Morgan, and R. Reiner, 461–95. Oxford: Oxford University Press.

Human Rights Watch. 2008. The stigma of rape. http://www.hrw.org/about/projects/womrep/General-78.htm#P1447_354428 (accessed June 14, 2008).

Humphreys, C. 1994. Counteracting mother-blaming among child sexual abuse service providers: an experimental workshop. *Journal of Feminist Family Therapy* 6(1):49–65.

Jackson, J., S. Farrall, and E. Gray. 2007. *Experience and expression in the fear of crime* (working paper 7). http://ssrn.com/abstract=1012397 (accessed January 9, 2009).

Jacob, C. M. A. and P. M. Veach. 2005. Intrapersonal and familial effects of child sexual abuse on female partners of male survivors. *Journal of Counseling Psychology* 52(3):284–97.

Jordan, J. 2004. *The word of a woman: Police, rape and belief.* Basingstoke, UK: Palgrave Macmillan.

Kelley, S. J. 1990. Responsibility and management strategies in child sexual abuse: A comparison of child protective workers, nurses, and police officers. *Child Welfare* 69(1):43–51.

Kelly, L., J. Lovett, and L. Regan. 2005. A gap or chasm? Attrition in reported rape cases. Home Office Research Study 293. London: Home Office. http://www.crimereduction.homeoffice.gov.uk/sexual/sexual13.htm (accessed June 13, 2008).

Lamb, S. 1999. *The trouble with blame: Victims, perpetrators and responsibility.* Cambridge, MA: Harvard University Press.

Lees, S. and J. Gregory. 1993. *Rape and sexual assault: A study of attrition—multi-agency investigation into the problem of rape and sexual assault in the borough of Islington.* London: Islington Council.

Lemert, E. 1951. *Social pathology*. New York: McGraw Hill.

Lerner, M. J. 1980. *The belief in a just world: A fundamental delusion*. New York: Plenum.

Lievore, D. 2003. *Non-reporting and hidden recording of sexual assault: An international literature review*. Canberra: Australian Institute of Criminology. http://www.aic.gov.au/publications/reports/2003-06-review.pdf (accessed July 22, 2008).

Light, R. 1993. Why support prisoners' family-tie groups? *The Howard Journal* 32(4):322–29.

Madigan, L. and N. Gamble. 1991. *The second rape: Society's continued betrayal of the victim*. New York: Lexington Books.

Maltas, C. and J. Shay. 1995. Trauma contagion in partners of survivors of childhood sexual abuse. *American Journal of Orthopsychiatry* 65:529–39.

Manion, I. G., J. McIntyre, P. Firestone, M. Ligezinska, R. Ensom, and G. Wells. 1996. Secondary traumatization in parents following the disclosure of extrafamilial child sexual abuse: Initial effects. *Child Abuse and Neglect* 20(11):1095–109.

Martin, P. Y. and R. M. Powell. 1994. Accounting for the second assault: Legal organizations' framing of rape victims. *Law and Social Inquiry* 19:853–90.

Martone, C. 2005. *Loving through bars: Children with parents in prison*. Santa Monica, CA: Santa Monica Press.

Matoesian, G. M. 1993. *Reproducing rape: Domination through talk in the courtroom*. Chicago: University of Chicago Press.

Matthews, J. 1983. *Forgotten victims: How prison affects the family*. London: NACRO.

Mauer, M. and M. Chesney-Lind (eds.). 2002. *Invisible punishment: The collateral consequences of mass imprisonment*. New York: New Press.

McCold, P. and B. Wachtel. 1998. *Restorative policing experiment: The Bethlehem, Pennsylvania police family group conferencing project*. Pipersville, PA: Pipers.

McGarrel, E., K. Olivares, K. Crawford, and N. Kroovand. 2000. *Returning justice to the community: The Indianapolis restorative justice experiment*. Indianapolis, IN: Hudson Institute.

Miers, D. 2001. *An international review of restorative justice*. London: Home Office.

Morrison, Z. 2007. "Feeling heavy": Vicarious trauma and other issues facing those who work in the sexual assault field. Melbourne: Australian Centre for the Study of Sexual Assault. http://www.aifs.gov.au/acssa/pubs/wrap/acssa_wrap4.pdf (accessed July 22, 2008).

Morrison, Z., A. Quadara, and C. Boyd. 2007. "Ripple effects" of sexual assault. Melbourne: Australian Centre for the Study of Sexual Assault. http://www.aifs.gov.au/acssa/pubs/issue/acssa_issues7.pdf (accessed July 22, 2008).

Murray, J. 2007. The cycle of punishment: Social exclusion of prisoners and their children. *Criminology and Criminal Justice* 7(1):55–81.

Newberger, C. M., I. M. Gremy, C. M. Waternaux, and E. H. Newberger. 1993. Mothers of sexually abused children: Trauma and repair in longitudinal perspective. *American Journal of Orthopsychiatry* 63(1):92–102.

No More Prison. 2006. Family unfriendly. http://www.alternatives2prison.ik.com/p_Family_Unfriendly.ikml (accessed July 22, 2008).

Paterson, A., P. Dunn, K. Chaston, and L. Malone. 2007. In the aftermath: The support needs of people bereaved by homicide: A research report. London: Victim Support. http://www.victimsup port.org.uk/vs_england_wales/about_us/publications/homicide/in_the_after math.pdf (accessed July 22, 2008).

Regan, L. and L. Kelly. 2003. Rape: Still a forgotten issue. London: Child and Women Abuse Studies Unit. http://www.rcne.com/downloads/RepsPubs/Attritn.pdf (accessed June 19, 2008).

Rock, P. 1990. *Helping victims of crime: The home office and the rise of victim support in England and Wales.* Oxford: Oxford University Press.

____. 1998. *After homicide: Practical and political responses to bereavement.* Oxford: Oxford University Press.

____. 2004. *Constructing victims' rights: The home office, new labor, and victims.* Oxford: Oxford University Press.

Sherman, L. W. and H. Strang. 2007. *Restorative justice: The evidence.* London: The Smith Institute.

Silverman, D. C. 1978. Sharing the crisis of rape: Counseling the mates and families of victims. *American Journal of Orthopsychiatry* 48(1):166–73.

Sloan, L. M. 1995. Revictimisation by polygraph: The practice of polygraphing survivors of sexual assault. *Medicine and Law* 14:255–67.

Smith, M. 2005. Female sexual assault: The impact on the male significant other. *Issues in Mental Health Nursing* 26(2):149–67.

Spalek, B. 2006. *Crime victims: Theory, policy and practice.* Basingstoke, UK: Palgrave Macmillan.

Strang, H. 2002. *Repair or revenge: Victims and restorative justice.* Oxford: Oxford University Press.

Sykes, C. J. 2002. *A nation of victims: The decay of the American character.* New York: St. Martin's.

Taslitz, A. E. 1999. *Rape and the culture of the courtroom.* New York and London: New York University Press.

Taylor, R., A. Ward, and T. Newburn. 1995. *The day of the Hillsborough disaster: A narrative account.* Liverpool: Liverpool University Press.

United Nations. 1985. Declaration of basic principles of justice for victims of crime and abuse of power. United Nations Office of the High Commissioner for Human Rights. http://www.unhchr.ch/html/menu3/b/h_comp49.htm (accessed June 15, 2008).

Victim Support. 2007. Annual report & accounts 2007. London: Victim Support. http://www.victimsupport.org.uk/About%20us/Publications%20section/~/media/Files/Publications/AboutOurCharity/report-accounts-2007 (accessed January 13, 2009).

Walby, S. and J. Allen. 2004. *Domestic violence, sexual assault and stalking: Findings from the British Crime Survey.* Home Office Research Study 276. London: Home Office.

Westmarland, N. 2008. Rape's a real crime. *New Statesman,* July 10. http://www.newstatesman.com/law-and-reform/2008/07/rape-conference-police-women (accessed August 4, 2008).

Women's National Commission. 1985. *Violence against women: Report of an ad hoc working group.* London: Women's National Commission.

Drugs and Alcohol in Relation to Crime and Victimization

9

MARILYN CLARK

Contents

9.1 Introduction

The study of the links between substance abuse and offending and substance abuse and victimization has been underway for some years. Various research questions relating to this agenda have been explored, evidence brought forward, and recommendations for interventions, policy, and further research made. Still, many questions remain unanswered, and the complexity of the issues continues to be highlighted. Simplistic causal explanations are refuted, and more dynamic process-based accounts of the phenomenon have been proposed. Both topics are well researched, and reviews have been written on both issues. Thus far, however, they have been treated separately, with authors tackling either substance abuse in the offender or substance abuse in the victim. This chapter is novel in that it attempts to explain both phenomena using the same conceptual frameworks and adopting a multidisciplinary, cross-cultural perspective.* The question as to the association between drugs, alcohol, crime, and victimization is of more than mere academic relevance. Different conceptualizations of the links influence society's response to substance users and inform debates about drug legislation, crime prevention, drug and alcohol treatment, and law enforcement.

9.2 Trends in Drug and Alcohol Use

The incidence of drug and alcohol use for experimental, recreational, and social reasons is widespread [e.g., see Miller and Plant, 1996; Ramsay and Percy, 1996; Balding, 1998]. A recent survey conducted by the World Health Organization (WHO) research consortium in 2008 examined patterns of licit and illicit drug use in 17 countries representing the six WHO regions. The survey examined the lifetime use of alcohol, tobacco, cannabis, and cocaine and found that in the Americas, Europe, Japan, and New Zealand alcohol had been used by a vast majority of the population, whereas smaller lifetime prevalence rates were found in the Middle East, Africa, and China. There was an uneven distribution in the global distribution of drug use. The United States had the highest levels of both legal and illegal drug use. Males and younger adults had the highest prevalence rates, and there were also differences in terms of socioeconomic groups. Drug policies do not seem to have an effect on prevalence rates as countries with strict policies like the United States did not have lower rates than countries with liberal policies like the Netherlands. In its 2007 annual report, the European Monitoring Centre for Drugs and Drug Addiction (EMCCDA) claims that after a decade of increasing use, Europe may be reaching a stable phase in illicit drug use. Heroin and cannabis use are stable, but cocaine use continues to increase. Alcohol remains the most common drug used by young and old alike [Parker et al., 1998]. The results of the 2003 European School Survey Project on Alcohol and Other Drugs (ESPAD) survey show that among 16 year olds in Europe frequent drinking is most prevalent in Western Europe, as is drunkenness. Among young people, illicit drug use is dominated by the use of marijuana. An increasing proportion of ESPAD students perceive cannabis to be easy to obtain.

Illegal drugs are widely used, and the average age of initiation to substance use is becoming lower [NACRO, 2000]. Recent studies demonstrate

---

* This chapter will refer to drug and alcohol use in Europe, the United States, and Australia.

that the use of illegal drugs—particularly cannabis—is becoming an increasingly "normal" aspect of young people's leisure, transcending class and gender boundaries [Anderson and Frischer, 1997; Parker et al., 1998]. Most people who use both illegal and legal drugs such as alcohol become neither problematic users nor involved in further crime. In the careers of most illegal drug users, "escalation" to "harder" drugs and long-term continuation of use remains confined to a minority [NACRO, 2001]. In other words, most young drug users are not at a significant risk of becoming casualties—their experimentation is too fleeting, and their involvement too occasional [South, 1999:73]. However, there is no doubt that some young people are at "high risk of addiction and social exclusion" [Gilman, 1998:17]. Such risk is particularly associated with certain background factors in their lives.

9.3 Theorizing the Nexus

Research provides ample evidence that offender populations contain large numbers of substance abusers and that substance abusers commit a substantial number of undetected crimes [Innes, 1988; Fagan, 1990; Bennett, 1991; Lipton, 1995]. Research also indicates that the victims of crime are more likely to be involved with both licit and illicit substances [NVAA, 2000].

Several central concerns are of relevance to theorizing the substance use/ crime/victimization connection: Does substance use cause crime and victimization, or is substance use a consequence thereof? Is there some intrinsic property associated with certain substances that leads the user to engage in criminal behavior or that makes the victim more vulnerable? Does substance use cause violence and destroy communities? Does crime or criminal behavior or being a victim of a crime, perhaps, lead people into substance use? What types of substance use and what types of crime are we talking about? What is the temporal sequence of the substance use/crime/victimization nexus? This debate is constantly confounded by media-generated myths and consequent simplistic interpretations of the issues. According to Newburn [2007], as far as alcohol is concerned it is the possibility of its association with violent crime and victimizations that is paramount in people's minds. In relation to drugs, fears that usage may be linked to acquisitive crime dominate public concerns. However, the drug/alcohol/crime nexus is far more complex than this.

That substance use, criminality, and victimization are correlated cannot be debated [Goode, 1996]. It is almost axiomatic to state that substance abuse is considered to be a major contributing factor to both crime and victimization [Chaiken and Chaiken, 1990; Collins and Lapsley, 2002]. Although this correlation is well documented, the precise nature of the relationship between these phenomena is not. Thus, it is not sufficient to simply examine the correlation between substance use, crime, and victimization. This chapter will also examine the nature of the relationship and the way in which a range of factors impact on the nature of that relationship.

9.3.1 Substance Abuse by the Offender: A Note on Methodology

The most common research designs to examine the relationship between the commission of crime and substance abuse involve examining the extent of substance use in offending populations and the extent of offending in substance-using populations. A large part of early research on the links between drugs and crime comprised an attempt to establish the proportion of drug users among samples of criminals, usually using prison populations or the proportion of criminals among drug users, usually using in-patient or out-patient treatment groups [Bennett, 1991]. However, these populations tend to include only the most chronic cases of criminals or drug users, and information about drugs and crime tends to be collected a long time after the event. Besides this, although such research shows that many arrestees test positive for one or more drugs, to show a link between drug use and crime it would have to be shown that the prevalence rates among arrestees are higher than a comparable noncriminal or less criminal sample, a control sample that is very difficult to find. In fact, there exists no sample of noncriminal nonarrestees that is comparable with arrestee populations, and hence comparisons can only suggest and not prove a link between drug use and the commission of criminal behavior.

9.4 Substance Use in Offending Populations

In Britain, Maden et al. [1992] found that 43% of 1,751 male prisoners had misused drugs in the 6-month period before being imprisoned. About one-third of these (34%) said that they had used cannabis, and about 5% said that they had used cocaine. In 1998, Bennett, in a Home Office research study, found that the proportion of arrestees who used at least one drug in the past 12 months and who thought that their drug use and criminal behavior were connected ranged from one-third (36%) to more than one-half (57%) in different English cities. The majority of these arrestees believed that their drug use caused crime. The two most frequent reasons given were that drug use affected their judgment and that they broke the law to support a habit. In relation to alcohol use and crime, the proportion of arrestees who thought that their alcohol use and criminal behavior were connected ranged from 33% to 46% in different cities. The majority believe that alcohol use causes crime mainly by affecting judgment. In the 1998 study, Bennett concluded that three of four arrestees tested positive for at least one substance (including alcohol), and one in three arrestees tested positive for multiple substances (including alcohol). One in 2 arrestees tested positive for cannabis, 1 in 5 for opiates, and 1 in 12 for methadone. One in 10 tested positive for amphetamines, cocaine, and benzodiazepines, and 1 in 5 arrestees tested positive for alcohol [Bennett, 1998].

In 2000, Bennett again found that drug use among arrestees is prolific. Two-thirds of arrestees tested positive for one or more drugs; one-quarter tested positive for opiates; and one-fifth tested positive for cocaine (including crack). Younger arrestees were more likely to test positive for cannabis, whereas older arrestees were more likely to test positive for opiates and cocaine. Arrestees testing positive for polydrug use reported three times as many offenses as those who had negative tests. They also reported twice as many arrests in the previous year.

McKeganey et al. [2000] report very high levels of illegal drug use and criminality in Scotland. Seventy-one percent of urine samples among arrestees tested positive: 52% tested positive for cannabis, 33% for benzodiazepines, 31% for opiates, 12% for methadone, and 3% for cocaine. Twenty-five percent of arrestees said they had generated illegal income in the past month, and 25% of arrestees either owned or had access to a gun. Of arrestees, 65% also believed there was a connection between illegal drugs and violence, and 93% believed there was a connection between alcohol and violence.

Research on drug use by criminal justice populations in Australia provides similar evidence. Studies show that the majority of offenders have used illicit drugs at some point in their careers [Makkai, 1999a; Loxley, 2001] and that intravenous use is common [Loxely, 2001]. Smaller numbers have used drugs in the period before their offense [Putnins, 2001]. Australian studies also find that illicit drug use is much higher in criminal justice populations than in the general population, and multiple drug use is common [Makkai et al., 2000]. The use of alcohol is the most prominent [Kevin, 1999].

Raskin, White, and Gorman [2000] report high levels of drug use among criminals in the United States. The results published in the 1998 Annual Report of the Arrestee Drug Abuse Monitoring program, covering findings from 35 survey sites, show that about two-thirds of adult arrestees test positive for one or more drugs [National Institute of Justice, 1999, cited in Raskin et al., 2000]. In 1998, the median rate of positive tests for cocaine was 37% and 40% for male and female arrestees, respectively. The rates for opiates were lower. In 2002, 29% of convicted inmates reported they had used illegal drugs before crime. Cannabis and cocaine were the most common drugs convicted inmates said they had used at the time of the offense. In 2002, 56% of jail inmates convicted of robbery, 56% of those convicted for weapons violations, 55% of those convicted of burglary, and 55% of those convicted of motor vehicle theft reported using drugs at the time of the crime [Karlberg and James, 2002]. In 2004, 17% of state prisoners and 18% of federal inmates said they committed their current offense to obtain money for drugs

[Mumola and Karberg, 2006]. Among state prisoners in 2004, property (30%) and drug offenders (26%) were more likely to commit their crimes for drug money than violent (10%) and public-order offenders (7%) [cited in Raskin et al., 2000].

In the Mediterranean context, the Malta Probation Services report that from all their registered clients ($n = 440$) in 2005, 48% (211 persons) had a drug problem, predominately heroin. Of clients with a drug problem, 86% were male. The average age of all clients was 25 years (median, 24 years). On entry into prison, 39% (154 persons) of all inmates tested positive for opiates, cocaine, or cannabis. Of all 391 admitted inmates, 26% tested positive for heroin [EMCCDA, 2006].

9.4.1 Offending among Problem Drug Users

According to Parker et al. [1998] illicit drug use has become "normalized," especially among the younger generation, and many young people will have tried an illicit substance at some point in their lives. Much of this use is recreational, a "time out" from the stresses and strains of postmodern life. Studies on drug-using careers show how users may continue to use even addictive substances in a controlled manner and that those who get seriously committed to drug-using careers constitute a small proportion of the drug-using population [Zinberg, 1984; Faupel, 1991; Carnwath and Smith, 2002]. Consequently, the proportion of all illicit drug users who are involved in criminal activity is likely to be small. However, these users commit a disproportionately large amount of crime.

Australian research indicates that there are high rates of crime among problem drug users. Maher et al.'s [2002] study of Sydney heroin users found that 70% were active property offenders. Darke et al. [2000] report that nearly half of users from all jurisdictions in Australia in both 1999 and 2000 reported that they had been arrested in that period, most often for property and drug possession/use offenses. This trend has not changed since 2000 [Breen et al., 2003]. Valuri et al. [2002] studied a large sample of people in Western Australia arrested for at least one drug offense and found that 49.3% had previous convictions for other offenses. In a study by Larson [1996] of 77 injecting drug users living in the Brisbane area, 89.6% had undertaken some type of illegal activity to earn money to buy drugs. The most commonly reported activities were dealing drugs, buying drugs for somebody else against payment, committing burglary, and receiving stolen goods. Around 40% reported doing these activities more than once. Other activities frequently mentioned were shoplifting, stealing cars, and stealing from cars.

A study of the criminal histories of drug offenders in Scotland shows that 70% had previous convictions, and 41% of those with previous convictions had at least 10. Of those addicts with previous convictions, 61% had previous convictions for theft, 41% for housebreaking, 26% for theft of a motor vehicle, 38% for the possession of drugs, and 15% for supplying or attempting to supply drugs [McGallagly and Dunn, 2001].

Maher et al. [1998] cite a range of research from Europe, North America, and Australia that indicates that many dependent heroin users are involved in theft and sale of stolen goods [e.g., Dobinson and Ward, 1985; Johnston et al., 1985; Parker, Baks, and Newcombe, 1988; Hammersley et al., 1989; Dorn, Murji, and South, 1994; Grapendaal, Leuw, and Nelen, 1995]. Hall, Bell, and Carless [1993], in an Australian study, found that 90% of patients applying for methadone treatment had one or more convictions. Similarly, Maher et al. [1998] found that 70% of a sample of heroin users from Western Sydney were active property offenders. Dobinson and Ward [1985] found that among heroin users, as their heroin careers escalated, their involvement in crime also increased. This is not necessarily interpreted as increased drug consumption causing addicts to increase criminal behavior. It is also likely that heroin use will escalate once users come into a fair amount of money. Faupel [1991] in his ethnographic study of drug-using careers writes how controlled users may develop from stable addicts into "free-wheeling" addicts once they have access to larger amounts of heroin.

In a qualitative study on the development of criminal careers among young male prisoners in the Mediterranean island of Malta, Clark [1999, 2006] found that more than half of her sample reported being active heroin users when on the outside, and many spoke about how they financed their addictions via crime. However, most of these users reported having started deviant behaviors long before they developed an addiction, but that when they did so they escalated their involvement in crime and became considerably more committed to their criminal career. The criminal addicts in the sample reported feeling more constrained than the nonaddicts in the sample to continue with their criminal career. Thus, addiction is seen to constitute an important contingency for the continuation, escalation, and development of the career. Irrespective of whether crime or drug use appears first, continued drug use increases the rate at which crimes are committed and maintains criminal careers [Dobinson and Ward, 1985; Clark, 1999]. Heroin addicts are estimated to commit up to six times as many crimes while using as when abstaining [Nurco et al., 1988]. However, it is also unreasonable to assume that someone with little criminal experience will suddenly develop the criminal skills to be able to illegally sustain a costly habit daily. Conversely, it is also unreasonable to expect a criminally entrenched lifestyle to be terminated simply because of a cessation of addictive behavior [Hammersly, 2008]. Hammersly writes:

> Crime provides funds that can facilitate a growing and eventually very large drug habit. Many drug users would be unable to develop a full blown dependence without being competent criminals because this can easily cost

upwards of 80 sterling a day. When more funds are available from crime, then heroin injectors tend to take more heroin; when little cash is to be had they may not be able to get any heroin at all.

Chaiken and Chaiken's [1990] summary of U.S. research indicates that a progression from casual misuse to dependence and then to property crime occurs for some drug users, but that for others, possibly most, a history of acquisitive crime may predate and facilitate drug use escalation.

If illicit drug use is linked to crime, then a reduction in use should also bring about a reduction in offending behavior. In a review of the literature, Hall [1996] concludes that in randomized controlled trials, methadone maintenance therapy has been shown to reduce both heroin use and crime. Effective treatment has been shown to reduce the level of shoplifting and other drug-related crimes [NTORS, 1999].

Thus, problem drug misuse is a crucial factor in a large number of acquisitive crimes, and both dependent and other very heavy users report financing at least part of their habit through theft and other crimes. Typically drug-related crime is nonviolent and acquisitive, involving theft, shoplifting, forgery, or burglary [Chaiken and Chaiken, 1990] or prostitution [Plant, 1990; McKeganey et al., 2000].

9.4.2 Violent Crimes

Violence as part of the process of acquiring drugs does occur but is less common than nonviolent acquisitive crime. High levels of violence are associated with crack dealing [Bean and Pearson, 1992; Dorn et al., 1992], and substance-related violence, murder, large-scale trafficking, and money laundering are on the increase [South, 1997]. The intoxicating effect of drugs may provoke violence or may facilitate the victimization of a person but varies by type of drug. Cannabis and opiates do not predispose users to violence. The use of "dance drugs" at raves is said to promote "benign collectivist hedonism" [Saunders, 1993]. They may, however, predispose users toward victimization by making them more trusting. Regular use of stimulants can foster anxiety, psychotic symptoms, and paranoid behavior [Fagan, 1990; Ghodse, 1995]. It is alcohol that is probably most closely associated with violence [Russell, 1993]. D'Orban [1991] suggests that "criminality and alcohol abuse tend to run in parallel, as both have their peak incidence in young adults and tend to diminish with age. Those who continue with heavy drinking and petty crime into mid-life tend to become habitual drunkenness offenders" [D'Orban, 1991:298]. D'Orban also observes that "studies of offences of violence show that the majority of the offenders, the victims or both, had consumed alcohol prior to their offence" [1991:296]. Excessive intake of alcohol is much more closely linked with violence than most illegal drugs [Russell, 1993]. Taking various drugs to excess in combination substantially increases the chances of violent behavior [Hough, 1996]. Young men who have been drinking heavily are more likely than moderate drinkers to become both perpetrators and victims of violence [Cookson, 1992]. Disorderly conduct and violent offenses have repeatedly been found to be strongly related to recent alcohol consumption.

9.5 Substance Use and Victimization

Victimization is associated with a number of economic and health consequences. According to Miller, Cohen, and Wiersema [1996] in the United States a rape incident is likely to cost nearly $90,000 and an assault costs nearly $10,000. Physical and mental health consequences include chronic pain, miscarriage, sexually transmitted diseases, irritable bowel syndrome, post-traumatic stress disorder (PTSD), and substance abuse. Although there is a clear link between substance abuse and victimization, research on this relationship has been limited with the focus traditionally remaining on drug use by offenders. According to Stevens et al. [2007:402], this is a politicized agenda; they write

> In Anglo American political discourse at least, the idea that drug use causes crime has come to be one of the main drivers of drug and penal policy … the identification of dependent drug users as belonging to the class of predatory offenders has been used to reinforce the bifurcatory separation of drug users from the "law abiding citizens who need protection from their crimes."

However, since the 1990s, the emphasis has shifted somewhat onto substance abuse among victims [NVAA, 2000]. Still, because the war on drugs seems to have developed into a war on drug users, it seems unlikely that research on drug users as victims will reverse the focus on them as offenders. Seeing substance users as at increased risk of victimization may help to challenge stereotypical views of substance abusers.

Victimization has been associated with substance use and abuse in a fair number of recent research studies [Dunn, Ryan, and Dunn, 1994; Covington, 1997; Kilpatrick et al., 1997; Brewer et al., 1998]. High rates of substance abuse are often found among crime victims. Logan et al. [2002] partition contributing factors to this link into four main categories. These are trauma and coping factors, lifestyle factors, sociological factors, and contextual factors. These form the basis of their conceptual model on the link between substance abuse and victimization. By trauma and coping factors, Logan et al. [2002] are referring to postvictimization efforts at restoring adjustment by the victim. These authors cite how substance abuse is more likely among people victimized in childhood and adolescence. Substance abuse may be used as a coping strategy but may also bring about biological changes and hence contribute to further vulnerability. Substance abuse may be compounded by mental health problems. Stevens et al. [2007] found that the strongest links with victimization were with indicators of mental health problems. In their sample of drug-dependent individuals, people who report histories of serious depression and anxiety were significantly more likely to suffer from various types of victimization. In terms of lifestyle factors, the environment the substance abuser finds him- or herself in is likely to increase the risks of victimization. The impairment caused by substance abuse is also a risk factor, as is revictimization. Sociological factors are also seen by these authors as contributing to both victimization and substance abuse and include poverty, cultural norms, family environment, and mating patterns [Logan et al., 2002]. Stevens et al. [2007] in their study of victimization of drug-dependent users found that dependent drug users who face several aspects of social exclusion are extremely vulnerable to victimization. Finally, contextual factors refer to structural and psychological barriers and relationship dynamics. Although these authors' model was developed with female victimization in mind, it can also readily apply to male victims.

Substance use or abuse or addiction leads the user to place him- or herself at greater risk of assault. Offenders and victims are also often the same people. Stevens et al. [2007] found that in a sample of dependent drug users, those who reported recent offending were more likely to report being victims of crime. This may be the consequence of participation in the "violent subculture" [Wofgang and Ferracuti, 1967]. Thus, substance abuse places a potential victim at greater risk of being victimized and is an issue in relation to domestic violence, sexual assault, and homicide and affects adults, adolescents, and children. According to Christie [1986], criminally involved dependent drug users are increasingly portrayed as the ideal offender. However, the separation between offender and victim is not as clear as suggested by popular discourse on crime [Farrall and Matby, 2003]. The risk factors for offending are also the same risk factors for victimization. These include lifestyle factors, situational circumstances, and individual responses to structural difficulties and exposure to social exclusion. According to Stevens et al. [2007], because dependent users contain a higher proportion of socially excluded people than the general population, one can hypothesize that it will also contain higher proportions of victims of crime. In the United States this has been shown to be the case in various research studies [McClenna et al., 1997; Inciardi and Surratt, 2001; DeKeseredy et al., 2003]. European studies are less common, but one by Stevens et al. [2007] found similar results. The realization that problem illicit drug users are often victims of crime as well as being perpetrators of crime provides a further insight into the dynamics involved in the relationship between substance abuse and crime. There is evidence that illicit drug users are victimized at a much greater rate than the rest of the community. McElrath, Chitwood, and Comerford [1997] found that 15.3% of their sample of 308 heroin, cocaine, and crack cocaine users from Miami, Florida, had been victims of violent crime in the preceding 6 months. A further 23.4% had been victims of property crime in the 6 months before interview. The use of crack cocaine increased the likelihood of property crime victimization in the study. In comparing the illicit drug user group with crime statistics for the population as a whole, they found that the illicit drug users were approximately 23 times more likely to be victims of personal larceny, 8 times more likely to be victims of robbery, twice as likely to be victims of rape, 1.4 times more likely to be victims of burglary, and 1.3 times more likely to be victims of motor vehicle theft [cited in Stevens et al., 2007]. In a 2005 Scottish study by Neale et al. [2005], 560 dependent drug users entering treatment were researched. High levels of offending and victimization were found. Fattah [1992] highlights how a goal of critical victimology is to use such research to challenge and resist the political use of the victim in justifying repressive crime policies. In Vienna, a qualitative study by Waidner [1999, cited in Stevens, 2007] undertook interviews with 24 dependent heroin users. Most of the interviewees had been victimized but refused assistance from the police. The users reported seeing themselves as rejected from society and were unlikely to cooperate with criminal justice officials who they felt would treat them unfairly. Rather, they expressed solidarity with the perpetrators of the crimes and were generally uncooperative with the police. In a European study of dependent drug users [Stevens et al., 2007] where data on 545 dependent drug users entering treatment in four European countries were analyzed, members of the sample were found to have been exposed to high levels of criminal victimization. Subgroups found to be particularly vulnerable were women, women sex workers, the homeless, recent offenders, and the mentally ill. The data from this study "suggest that dependent drug users are highly vulnerable to criminal victimization, whether it threatens their property or their person, compared with people who respond to general surveys" [Stevens et al., 2007:392]. Repeat victimization was also very common. In terms of the types of property crime, dependent drug users are vulnerable to petty thefts of small items and cash. The females in the sample were more likely to be subject to criminal victimization and violence.

Research has shown that alcohol misuse and intimate partner violence are significantly related [Kantor and Straus, 1989; Miller, Downs, and Gondoli, 1989; Leonard and Senchak, 1996; O'Farrell, Van Hutton, and Murphy, 1999; Caetano, Schafer, and Cunradi, 2001]. Studies with incident-specific measures show that alcohol use by the perpetrator and the victim increases the risk for violence. Among prisoners and jail inmates convicted of committing a violent crime against an intimate partner, almost half were drinking alcohol at the time of the assault [Greenfeld et al., 1998]. Alcohol was detected in

70% of the suspects and 45% of the victims in interpersonal violence–related homicides [Slade, Daniel, and Heisler, 1991].

9.5.1 Alcohol and Sexual Violence

Alcohol is perhaps the most implicated of all substances in terms of sexual violence. Both men and women suffer sexual violence that can have long-lasting physical and mental health consequences. A report by the Home Office [Finney, 2004] puts together key findings from published UK and international research on the relationship between alcohol, crime, and victimization. Alcohol use is common in the event of sexual violence in both the perpetrator and the victim. Alcohol use is more common in sexual violence incidents among people who do not know each other very well. Finney [2004] concludes that alcohol problems are common among victims and that in many cases the problems followed victimization.

9.6 A Causal Link?

Although, as shown above, the link has been established by international research, identifying the precise causative connection between substance abuse, criminal offending, and victimization remains a primary preoccupation of many writers in this area. The link actually refers to a wide range of behaviors that may be connected in many different ways. Consequently, explanations have drawn on widely disparate theories [Brochu, 1995].

9.6.1 Hypothesis 1: Drug Use Comes First

Because its simplicity is appealing, the hypothesis that drug use leads to criminal offending and/or victimization is perhaps the most popular explanation proposed by both laypersons and academics alike. Within this hypothesis three models may be identified that incorporate the dynamics that may be in play. The psychopharmacological model argues that acute or chronic intoxication or withdrawal causes criminal behavior and/or victimization. Typical effects of intoxication like disinhibition, cognitive and perceptual changes, attention deficits, poor judgment, faulty decision making, and neurochemical changes cause criminal, especially violent, behavior and increase the potential for victimization [Collins, 1981; Fagan, 1990]. Sleep deprivation, nutritional deficits, and impaired neuropsychological functioning aid deviant behavior. The use of certain substances may cause predisposed individuals to become excitable and irrational [Virkkunen, 1974]. Research studies attempting to attribute violent behavior to the use of opiates and marijuana have been mainly discredited [Finestone, 1967; Inciardi and Chamber, 1972]. Although the consumption of opiates is unlikely to directly lead to violence, the irritability associated with withdrawals may do so. For example, Goldstein [1979] found that heroin-using prostitutes often linked robbing and/or assaulting clients with the withdrawal experience. Studies have, on the other hand, consistently established links between intoxication by alcohol and aggression [Bushman, 1997]. Parker and Auerhahn [1998:307], in a review of the literature on the link between alcohol, drugs, and violence, conclude: "study after study indicates that…violent events are overwhelmingly more likely to be associated with the consumption of alcohol than with any other substance." The pharmacological effects of some substances make users more vulnerable to victimization. This has been termed the *victim precipitation theory*. It has been suggested that the victim-to-be may trigger a violent situation because of his or her own intoxication. In other words, drug use may alter a person's behavior in such a manner as to bring about that person's violent victimization.

A route whereby drug use may lead to victimization is through impaired decision making, risk assessment, and consequent risky behavior. Drugs or alcohol may reduce the user's ability to perceive, integrate, and process information, increasing the risk for violence. Substance use causes cognitive and emotional changes that reduce self-awareness and accurate assessment of risks [Bushman, 1997]. For example, an intoxicated young person on ecstasy might accept a lift home from an undesirable individual when under the influence. Gustafson [1994] found that drinking constricts an intoxicated person's attention span. Pernanen [1991] documents how both men and women report consuming more alcohol than they normally would before their recent victimization incident. Kevin [1999] provides evidence that a notable percentage of victims are intoxicated at the time of the offense. Alcohol has been found to be a significant factor in a large number of violent homicides and suicides [Roizen, 1993].

Pernanen et al. [2002] also suggests another explanation to understand how drug use places one at greater risk of victimization. Drinking and violence occur in "time-out" or leisure situations where deviant behavior is more acceptable. The diminished sense of responsibility may cause the user to engage in exceptional behaviors. According to Parker and colleagues [Parker, 1993; Parker and Rebhun, 1995; Parker and Auerhahn, 1998], alcohol's effect on behavior is strongly influenced by the social and cultural context in which it is consumed. Zinberg [1984] discussed this in his classic text *Drug, Set and Setting*. Parker and Auehahn [1998] argue that in potentially violent situations, a conscious effort is needed to resolve disputes nonviolently, but people may be less likely to make this effort in contexts where violence is more accepted, such as bars.

Research indicates relatively high frequencies of alcohol consumption in rape [Amir, 1971; Rada, 1975] and homicide victims [Shupe, 1954; Wolfgang, 1958]. Public intoxication may invite a robbery or mugging. Alcohol affects decision making at blood alcohol levels as low as 0.5 and has negative effects on judgment and the ability to resist aggression, making for an easily entrapped victim [Finney, 2004]. Borrill, Rosen, and Summerfild [1987, cited in Finney, 2004] showed how just two drinks in a 1-hour period impaired the user's ability to recognize angry faces. Expectancies associated with substance abuse also impact on decision-making abilities. Substance abuse is associated with expectancies of pleasure and fun and is likely to attend to the environmental cues involving socializing and pleasure, consistent with their expectancies, rather than the incongruent cognitions involving danger and assault, reducing their ability to recognize danger cues. One study found that in rapes where only the victim was intoxicated, she was significantly more likely to be physically injured [Johnson et al., 1976].

This is not in any way to insinuate that victims are responsible for the actions perpetrated against them. The victim precipitation approach is not without problems because it risks stereotyping problematic drug users and blaming the victim. The National Victim Assistance Academy (NVAA) [2000] warns:

> Both victimization and substance abuse carry weighty societal stigmas, and when the stigma of victimization is combined with the stigma of substance abuse, victims can fall prey to a "double-edged sword." Moreover, substance use or abuse by victims may be viewed as a "reason" for their victimization.

Many instances of psychopharmacological violence go unreported and unrecorded. Intoxicated victims may be reluctant to report their victimization, not wishing to talk to the police while drunk or "stoned." They feel that reporting the event would be futile because they may be confused about the event and perhaps unable to remember what their assailant looked like. Assuming that the psychopharmacological violence is not precipitated by the victim, the victim can then be just about anybody and can occur in any context.

The economic or drug enslavement model [Bean, 1994] is applicable only to offending behavior and not to victimization. According to this model, drug users generate income through crime to support their drug habit. Heroin and cocaine, both expensive and addictive substances, are mostly implicated in this model. This model proposes that addicts are motivated not by violent tendencies but by economic need. Although heroin users avoid violent crime if nonviolent alternatives are available [Swezey, 1973; Cushman, 1974; Gould, 1974; Goldstein and Duchaine, 1980; Goldstein, 1981; Johnson et al., 1985], violence may be present in the context. In 1937, Dai wrote:

> The small percentage of addicts committing such crimes as robbery, assault and battery, homicide and others that involve the use of force seems to discredit the view shared by many that the use of drugs has the effect of causing an

individual to be a heartless criminal. On the contrary, our figures suggest that most of the crimes committed by addicts were of a peaceful nature that involves more the use of wit than that of force. [1937:69]

The economic motivation to commit crime to purchase drugs manifests itself in an increase in such crimes following addiction and the reduction of crimes following successful participation in treatment. Addiction appears to be an important contingency for the escalation of the criminal career, whereas cessation of addictive behavior may facilitate desistance from crime. However, this model is overly simplistic, fueled by public opinion on the enslaving potential of addictive substances, especially heroin. Not all drug users are addicts. There are many regular heroin users who are not addicted, and for addicts, the drive to maintain a particular level of consumption is much weaker than popularly believed [Zinberg, 1984]. Zinberg [1984] investigated and found ample evidence for controlled use of the opiates. Kaplan [1983:38] examined how heroin addicts or "problem" users voluntarily abstain from use for substantial periods for many reasons. Addicts' use patterns have been shown to vary considerably. If research indicates that an addict's demand for the drug of choice may be flexible and if the withdrawal pains for addicts are much milder than popularly portrayed [Kaplan, 1983], then the economic compulsive mode becomes less tenable.

The systemic model maintains that drug distribution and use are inherently connected with violent crime and violent victimization [Goldstein, 1985]. Typical crimes surrounding the distribution of illicit substances include territorial arguments, enforcement of distribution rules, and punishments targeted against rule breakers. Transaction-related crimes, such as robberies of dealers or buyers, collecting debts, and resolving disputes over quality or amount, are also common [Miczek et al., 1994]. Drug markets create community disorganization, which, in turn, affects the norms and behaviors of individuals who contribute to the development of the violent subculture. Such community disorganization may be associated with increases in crime not directly related to drug selling [Fagan and Chin, 1990; Skogan, 1990; Blumstein, 1995]. In the systemic model, violence is intrinsic to involvement with any illicit substance and hence places the user at risk of being both a perpetrator and a victim. Studying the area of systemic violence may be more important than the study of the relationship of drug use to crime on the level of the individual user.

Routine activities theory may be drawn on to explain how drug use contributes to crime and victimization. Illicit drug users are exposed to a large pool of motivated offenders; they are viewed as attractive targets; and few, if any, capable guardians are present [McElrath et al., 1997]. Substance abuse and victimization may be associated because the environment in which substances are used makes it more likely that individuals come into contact with criminally motivated others who are perpetrating multiple criminal offenses. This is particularly applicable to illicit drug use, which, by virtue of its illegality, may place the previously law-abiding individual in contact with criminal others. Violence may occur during the process of obtaining and using substances. Procuring drugs increases the opportunity for exposure to criminals, weapons, and violent subcultures. Routine activity theory argues that criminal events are the product of the intersection in time and space of three variables: motivated offenders, suitable targets, and absence of capable guardians—all three needing to be present for a crime to occur. Within the context of drug-using subcultures, the three variables are likely to come together. Hence a dependent drug user is likely to come into contact with motivated offenders because the context of purchasing and consuming illicit substances is likely to be characterized by the presence of criminals. Even if the substance is legal, such as alcohol, hanging around in bars is more likely to place one in contact with motivated offenders than if one were at home. Frequenting bars has been associated with increased substance use and victimization [McElrath et al., 1997]. As discussed previously, dependent drug users also make suitable targets because their use might impair their functioning and make them more likely to be victimized and less likely or willing to call the police if they have engaged in risk behavior. The role of the double stigma of victimization and substance abuse cannot be discounted. The fact that substance-abusing victims are likely to be blamed for their victimization makes it less likely that they will report crimes. Capable guardians are likely to be absent in places where both legal and illegal substances are consumed.

Hence routine activities theory suggests that when one associates with or comes into contact with individuals engaged in activities such as illegal behavior one may be more likely to experience victimization. Inciardi [1990] found a relationship between proximity to the crack market and victimization. According to Sampson and Lauritsen [1994], associating with individuals in the drug culture will increase an individual's vulnerability to being victimized. For example, ethnographic studies such as those by Amaro [1995] document the common practice of victimization and degradation of women in the crack-using subculture. Reig [1996, cited in Logan et al., 2002] found that 78% of female crack users interviewed had been victims of a violent crime at least once during their adulthood. Falck et al. [2001, cited in Logan et al., 2002] found that 62% of women reported a physical attack since initiation of their crack use, and 325 reported having been raped since initiation of use. Of those who have been raped, 83% were high when that happened.

9.6.2 Hypothesis 2: Crime and Victimization Cause Drug Use

The second hypothesis is that crime and victimization cause drug use. In terms of offending behavior, one way this may happen is when offenders use drugs to facilitate the commission of a criminal act. Sex workers often cite that they use substances to minimize the stressors they encounter in their illicit work. Burglars may drink alcohol before breaking and entering a property. Criminal individuals use drugs to self-medicate anxiety or give themselves an excuse to commit deviant activities [Raskin, White, and Gorman, 2000]. This model argues that it is not addicts who turn to crime but criminals who turn to drugs. Long before they become dependent on heroin and cocaine, those who eventually do so were already engaging in a variety of criminal activities. Persons who eventually become drug addicts and abusers were delinquents and criminals first; only later do they turn to drug use. Addiction has nothing to do with their criminal behavior; they are not enslaved to a drug so much as participants in a criminal lifestyle. Their drug use is a reflection or an indicator of that lifestyle; it is a later phase of the deviant career. In this model, cessation of addictive behavior will not result in cessation of criminal behavior. It might contribute to a reduction in criminal behavior but not a complete termination of the criminal career [Inciardi, 1992]. The intensification model argues that criminal careers are already well established long before someone abuses, becomes dependent on, or even uses illegal drugs [Inciardi, 1992]. If they stop using substances they may reduce their criminal involvement, but these same persons would still commit crimes vastly in excess of the general population. Many drug-dependent persons are deeply entrenched in a criminal lifestyle [Anglin and Speckart, 1988; Nurco et al., 1988]. Ethnographic studies of addiction careers show how drug use is intensified in times of superfluous cash, such as after a successful robbery. In these times the addict may move from a period of stable and controlled use to a stage of free-wheeling addiction where availability and lack of structure facilitate unrestrained use [Faupel, 1991]. Criminal individuals are also more likely to choose to be or find themselves in social situations and subcultures in which drug use is condoned or encouraged. Aspects of the criminal subculture such as being only periodically employed and being geographically mobile may encourage heavy drug use. According to this explanation, involvement in a criminal subculture provides the context, the reference group, and the definitions of a situation that are conducive to subsequent involvement with drugs [White, 1990]. For example, rather than the need for a drug compelling an individual to commit robbery, the income generated from a robbery might provide the individual with extra money to secure drugs and therefore place the individual in an environment that supports drug use [Collins, Hubbard, and Rachal, 1985]. In addition to subcultural and lifestyle explanations, it has been proposed that deviant individuals may use drugs to self-medicate [Khantzian, 1985] or to give themselves an excuse to act in a deviant manner [Collins, 1993]. Drugs may be used to facilitate the commission of crime. Stimulants and alcohol are often used for this purpose. Drugs may be then used to celebrate successful crime or to handle the day-to-day stress associated with the criminal lifestyle, for example, in prostitution, which in turn supports use. There is some support for this theory in that the drugs/crime career research indicates that offending usually precedes drug use. However, this does not necessarily demonstrate that the two are causally related, that is, offending causes drug use.

In relation to victimization, much research has addressed the hypothesis that victimization brings about the use of drugs and alcohol. If victimization causes feelings of powerlessness and humiliation, people may attempt to self-medicate these negative emotions through the use of substances. The clinical observation that addictively involved individuals tend to be more anxious, depressed, and angry than the norm served as a catalyst for development of the self-medication hypothesis. This hypothesis, with roots in psychoanalytic theory, holds that substances are used and other addictive activities engaged in for the express purpose of alleviating psychiatric symptoms and painful emotional states. Individuals who abuse substances characteristically exhibit higher level of anxiety and depression [Clark et al., 2001] than those who do not abuse substances. Likewise, people diagnosed with anxiety disorder [Helzer, Burnam, and McEvoy, 1991, cited in Logan et al., 2002] and major depressions are at elevated risk for drinking and other substance misuse problems [Davidon and Ritson, 1993, cited in Logan et al., 2002]. Khantzian [1985], writing from a psychodynamic perspective, highlighted how substance abuse might be an attempt at medicating emotional distress. In this regard, the research often deals with victims of domestic violence, sexual assault, child and adolescent abuse, and homicide. Research indicates that there is a relationship between victimization, trauma, and subsequent substance use and abuse [Arellano, 1996; Kilpatrick et al., 1997; Kilpatrick et al., 2000, cited in Logan et al., 2002]. Miller et al. [1990, cited in Logan et al., 2002] found that women undergoing treatment for alcohol dependency were more likely than a household sample of women to report verbal abuse (69% vs. 22%), sexual abuse (66% vs. 35%), and severe childhood physical violence (46% vs. 22%). According to Miller [1990, cited in Logan et al., 2002], being a victim of domestic violence is associated with an increased incidence of substance abuse. Miller and Downs [1993, cited in Logan et al., 2002] calculate that approximately 50% of all female alcoholics have been victims of domestic violence. Kantor and Strauss [1989] found that victimized wives were more likely than nonvictimized wives to have been high on drugs or drunk during the year of the survey. Substance abuse may be used as a coping mechanism for the physical and emotional pain consequent of being abused [Collins et al., 1997]. Substance abuse may be viewed as a reason for the abuse, but this would often constitute an inaccurate assessment.

The link between childhood victimization and an increased risk of substance abuse in adults and adolescents [Clark et al., 2001] is particularly strong. In a study of therapeutic community treatment for adolescents, approximately one-third of the sample reported a history of sexual abuse [Hawke et al., 2000]. One of the more striking findings of recent literature on adolescent substance abusers is the high prevalence rates of childhood physical and sexual abuse [Blood and Cornwall, 1994, 1996]. Substance abuse clients who report histories of childhood abuse also typically exhibit more severe drug abuse problems and greater psychopathology [Blood and Cornwall, 1996] and are more likely to drop out [Roman, 1988; Root, 1989] and relapse [Gil-Rivas, Fiorentine, and Anglin, 1996]. Similarly, adult victims of sexual abuse who address abuse issues during treatment tend to make better progress in recovery than those who do not [Chiavaroli, 1992]. Those substance abusers who experienced early victimization are likely to have early age of onset [Cavaiola and Schiff, 2000], higher drug use frequency, multiple drug use, and increased severity of use [Brown and Anderson, 1991; Harrison et al., 1997].

Sexual assault is also correlated with substance abuse. According to the NVAA [2000], victims of sexual assault and rape are much more likely to use alcohol and other drugs to cope with the trauma of victimization than nonvictims. In a review of studies on rape victims, Resnick [1993] concludes that individuals who experience rape and other sexual victimization report high levels of fear and anxiety, PTSD, depression, suicidal ideation, and alcohol and substance abuse. Kilparick, Edmunds, and Seymour [1992] found that rape victims were 5.3 times more likely than nonvictims to use prescription drugs nonmedically and to have used cocaine and marijuana.

A strong relationship exists between victimization, PTSD, and substance abuse [Kilpatrick et al., 1998]. Because victimization can bring about PTSD, research has addressed the issue of whether PTSD and substance abuse are related. The NVAA [2000] reports that women with PTSD were 2.48 times more likely to suffer alcohol abuse or dependence and 4.46 times as likely to suffer drug abuse or dependence. However, the issue of chronology is difficult to establish. Rather than substance abuse being a function of self-medicating from emotional and physical trauma, substance abuse could be putting individuals at risk of victimization that could lead to PTSD. Using data from the National Women's Study, Kilpatrick et al. [2000] tested and found support for three major hypotheses. A history of violent assault increases the risk of alcohol dependence even after controlling for family history of substance abuse and sensation seeking. PTSD also increased the risk of alcohol dependence after controlling for family history, sensation seeking, and violent assault. The hypothesis that a history of substance use or abuse increases the risk of violent assault was partially supported, and the hypothesis that risk of alcohol dependence at follow-up is predicted by a history of violent assault, substance abuse, past-year violent assault, and PTSD was also partially supported. This study provided some evidence that assault tended to precede alcohol use or dependence rather than vice versa. Assault victims with PTSD are much more likely to have alcohol dependence than victims without PTSD. The NVAA [2002] concludes regarding the substance abuse, victimization, and PTSD issue that:

> Because of their exposure to trauma, crime victims are at high risk of developing PTSD (20% or one in every five victims) and at additional risk of abusing drugs and alcohol (three or four times the normal prevalence) if the PTSD persists—as it will for over one third of the cases. Extrapolating from these frequencies brings the stark realisation that many thousands of crime victims are at high risk for suffering the co-morbid disorders of PTSD and alcohol abuse. If they remain untreated, these absolute numbers would be accumulative.

9.6.3 Hypothesis 3: Drugs, Crime, and Victimization Have a Reciprocal Relationship

It is likely that both of the above models are correct and that the relationship between substance use, crime, and victimization is in fact reciprocal. Substance use, crime, and victimization may be causally linked and mutually reinforcing; thus, drinking and drug use may lead to more criminal behavior or victimization, and criminal behavior and victimization may lead to more drinking and drug use [Collins, 1986; Fagan and Chin, 1990]. The research evidence for both models is impressive, but common sense tells us that the pathways into drugs and crime are complex and various. Contingencies operate at various stages of the lifespan that facilitate or impede involvement in the addictive or criminal career. Contingencies are also present that make it more or less likely that victimization will occur. For example, when an addict has an easy opportunity to commit robbery, he or she will commit it and then buy drugs with the money gained, not out of a compulsion but rather as a consumer expenditure. Conversely, when the need for drugs is great, users will commit crimes to get money to buy drugs [Goldstein, 1981; Chaiken and Chaiken, 1990]. If an addict starts to sell drugs, his or her consumption is likely to increase as a result of the available cash. Involvement in the drug trade will also place the user at greater risk of systemic violence. Similarly, a battered woman may find solace at the bottom of a bottle, but her substance abuse makes her more vulnerable to further attacks from a partner who also abuses substances.

The relationship between substance abuse and victimization by partners appears to be bidirectional. Substance use may increase their risk of victimization through numerous paths, such as impairing both their judgment and the perpetrator's judgment alike, increasing financial dependency, and exposing women to violent men who also abuse substances [El-Bassel et al., 2000]. Women's risk for alcohol and drug abuse is also increased by their victimization [Stark and Flitcraft, 1996; Harris and Fallot, 2001].

Substance abuse and domestic violence toward women appear to have a reciprocal relationship.

9.7 Final Note

This chapter has presented evidence in support of the idea that substance abuse, crime, and victimization are correlated. The chapter has also discussed the main models that attempt to explore that relationship. It differs from other reviews in two ways. First and foremost, it attempts to explain the relationship between substance abuse and offending behavior and substance abuse and victimization using the same conceptual frameworks. Thus far, these two issues have been treated separately. Second, it adopts a cross-cultural perspective, reviewing data mainly from the United States, the United Kingdom, and Australia.

The models of the drugs/violence nexus discussed above should be viewed as ideal types, and overlap does occur between them. For example, a heroin user preparing to commit an act of economic compulsive violence, for example, a robbery, might ingest some alcohol or stimulants to give him- or herself the courage to do the crime. This event now contains elements of both economic compulsive and psychopharmacological violence. If the target of his or her robbery attempt was a drug dealer, the event would contain elements of all three types of drug-related violence. The user would then celebrate his or her successful criminal endeavor with drug use and might find him- or herself victimized when attempting to purchase drugs in the midst of the criminal subculture. The complexities of the connections between substance abuse, crime, and victimization and their embeddedness in social structure have far-reaching implications for penal policy and for criminal justice interventions.

Drugs, crime, and victimization may also owe their existence to some other variable. They are seen to have common causes and similar risk factors. Hammersly writes in relation to drugs and crime that the links are often heavily overdetermined: "This overdetermination means that while it is correct that drugs and crime are strongly associated, it is false that one causes the other" [2008:73]. Perhaps drugs, crime, and victimization are more likely to occur among individuals who form part of deviant social networks or because they possess particular personality traits. Other common factors that have been explored include disturbed or disrupted childhoods, social exclusion, and mental health problems [Stevens et al., 2007]. Drug use, crime, and victimization may be linked to other underlying socioeconomic and subcultural factors.

Substance use and crime and victimization are mutually reinforcing—they can precede and reinforce the others and are influenced by any contingencies encountered in the course of the development of the lifespan. In a process-based career account of the phenomenon, there is no search for inevitable causal links between substance use, crime, and victimization. Motivation for addictive and criminal behavior changes in the course of the career, which is individually negotiated although influenced by structural variables.

References

Amaro, H. 1995. Love, sex and power: Considering women's realities in HIV preven-tion. *American Psychologist* 50:437–47.

Amir, M. 1971. *Patterns in forcible rape*. Chicago: University of Chicago Press.

Anderson, S. and M. Frischer. 1997. *Crime and criminal justice research findings 17: Drug misuse in Scotland*. Findings from the 1993 and 1996 Scottish crime sur-veys. Edinburgh: SO.

Anglin, M. and G. Speckart. 1988. Narcotics use and crime: A multisample, multim-ethod analysis. *Criminology* 26:197–233.

Asnis, S. and R. Smith. 1978. Amphetamine abuse and violence. *Journal of Psychedelic Drugs* 10:317–77.

Balding, J. 1998. *Young people and illegal drugs in 1998*. Exeter: University of Exeter Press.

Bean, P. 1994. Drugs and crime in Britain: An overview. *Drugs: Education, Prevention and Policy* 1(2):93–99.

Bean, P. and Y. Pearson. 1992. Crack and cocaine use in Nottingham in 1989/90 and in 1991/92. In *Cocaine and crack in England and Wales*. Research and Planning Unit Paper No. 70, ed. J. Mott, 27–31. London: Home Office.

Bennett, T. 1991. The effectiveness of a police-initiated fear-reducing strategy. *British Journal of Criminology* 31(1):1–14.

_____. 1998. *Drugs and crime: The results of research on drug testing and interviewing arrestee*. Home Office Research Study 183. Great Britain: Home Office Research Development and Statistics Directorate.

_____. 2000. *Drugs and crime: The results of second developmental stage of the NEW-ADAM programme*. Home Office Research Study 205. London: Home Office.

Bensley, L., J. Van Eenwyk, and K. W. Simmons. 2000. Self-reported childhood sexual and physical abuse and adult HIV-risk behaviors and heavy drinking. *American Journal of Preventive Medicine* 18(2):151–58.

Blood, L. and A. Cornwall. 1994. Pretreatment characteristics that predict comple-tion of an adolescent substance abuse treatment program. *Journal of Nervous Mental Disorders* 182:14–19.

_____. 1996. Childhood sexual victimization as a factor in the treatment of substance misusing adolescents. *Substance Use and Misuse* 31(8):1015–39.

Blumstein, A. 1995. Youth violence, guns and the illicit-drug industry. In *Trends, risks, and interventions in lethal violence: Proceedings of the third annual spring symposium of the Homicide Research Working Group*, ed. C. Block and R. Block, 265–78. Research Report, NCJ 154254. Washington, DC: U.S. Department of Justice, National Institute of Justice.

Blumstein, A., J. Cohen, J. A. Roth, and C. A. Visher. 1986. *Criminal careers and "career criminals."* Washington, DC: National Academy Press.

Boles, S. and K. Miotto. 2003. Substance abuse and violence: A review of the literature. *Aggression and Violent Behavior* 8:155–74.

Borrill, J., B. Rosen, and A. Summerfield. 1987. The influence of alcohol on judgments of facial expressions of emotion. *British Journal of Medical Psychology* 60:71–77.

Breen, C., L. Degenhardt, A. Roxburgh, et al. 2003. *Australian drug trends, 2002.* Findings of the Illicit Drug Reporting System (IDRS), NDARC Monograph No. 50. http://ndarc.med.unsw.edu.au/ndarc.nsf/website/Publications.monographs (accessed August 15, 2008).

Brewer, D., R. Catalano, K. Haggerty, R. Gainey, and C. Fleming. 1998. A meta-analysis of redictors of continued drug use during and after treatment for opiate addiction. *Addiction* 93:73–92.

Brochu, S. 1995. *Drogue et criminalité: Une relation complexe.* Montréal and Brussels: Presses de l'Université de Montréal and De Boeck Université.

Bushman, B. J. 1997. Effects of alcohol on human aggression: Validity of proposed explanations. In *Recent developments in alcoholism,* ed. M. Galanter, 227–43. New York: Plenum.

Caetano, R., J. Schafer, and C. Cunradi. 2001. Alcohol-related intimate partner violence among White, Black, and Hispanic couples in the United States. *Alcohol Research and Health* 25:58–65.

Carnwath, T. and I. Smith. 2002. *Heroin century.* New York: Routledge.

Cavaiola, A. and M. Schiff. 2000. Psychological distress in abused, chemically dependent adolescents. *Journal of Child and Adolescent Substance Abuse* 10(2):81–92.

Chaiken, J. and M. Chaiken. 1990. Drugs and predatory crime. In *Drugs and crime: Crime and justice,* vol. 13, ed. M. Tonry and J. Q. Wilson, 241–320. Chicago: University of Chicago Press.

Chermack, S. and P. Giancola. 1997. The relation between alcohol and aggression: An integrated biopsychosocial conceptualization. *Clinical Psychology Review* 17:621–49.

Chiavaroli, T. 1992. Rehabilitation from substance abuse in individuals with a history of sexual abuse. *Journal of Substance Abuse Treatment* 9:349–54.

Christie, N. 1986. Suitable enemies. In *Abolitionism: towards a non-repressive approach to crime,* ed. H. Bianchi and R. Van Swaaningen, 46–54. Amsterdam: Free University Press.

Clark, H., C. Masson, K. Delucchi, S. Hall, and K. Sees. 2001. Violent traumatic events and drug abuse severity. *Journal of Substance Abuse Treatment* 20(2):121–27.

Clark, M. 1999. The pursuit of a criminal career. PhD diss., University of Sheffield.

———. 2006. Commitment to crime: The role of the criminal justice system. *European Journal of Criminology* 3(2):201–20.

Cohen, M., M. Lipsey, D. Wilson, and J. Derzon. 1994. *The role of alcohol consumption in violent behavior: Preliminary findings.* Nashville, TN: Vanderbilt University Press.

Collins, D. and H. Lapsley. 2002. *Counting the cost: Estimates of the social costs of drug abuse in Australia in 1998–9.* Monograph series no. 49. Canberra: Department of Health and Ageing.

Collins, J. 1986. The relationship of problem drinking to individual offending sequences. In *Criminal careers and career criminals,* vol. 2, ed. A. Blumstein et al., 89–120. Washington, DC: National Academy Press.

_____. 1993. Drinking and violence: An individual offender focus. In *Alcohol and interpersonal violence: Fostering multidisciplinary perspective*, ed. S. Martin, 221–35. Rockville, MD: U.S. Department of Health and Human Services, National Institutes of Health.

Collins, J., R. Hubbard, and J. Rachal. 1985. Expensive drug use and illegal income: A test of explanatory hypotheses. *Criminology* 23:743–64.

Collins, J. and P. Messerschmidt. 1993. Epidemiology of alcohol-related violence. *Alcohol Health and Research World* 17:93–100.

Collins, J. and W. Schlenger. 1988. Acute and chronic effects of alcohol use on violence. *Journal of Studies on Alcohol* 49:516–21.

Cookson, H. 1992. Alcohol use and offence type in young offenders. *British Journal of Criminology* 34:189–93.

Cushman, P. 1974. Relationship between narcotic addiction and crime. *Federal Probation* 38:38–43.

Dai, B. 1937. *Opium addiction in Chicago*. Montclair, NJ: Patterson Smith.

Darke, S., L. Topp., and S. Kay. 2000. *The illicit drug reporting system (IDRS) 1996–2000*. NDARC Technical Report No. 117, http://ndarc.med.unsw.edu.au/ndarcweb.nsf/resources/TR_18/$file/TR.117.PDF.

Degenhardt, L., W. T. Chiu, N. Sampson, et al. 2008. *Toward a global view of alcohol, tobacco, cannabis, and cocaine use*. Findings from the WHO World Mental Health Surveys. PLoS Med 5(7):e141. http://medicine.plosjournals.org/perlserv/?request=get-document&doi=10.1371%2Fjournal.pmed.0050141&ct=1 (accessed August 13, 2008).

DeKeseredy, W., M. Schwartz, S. Alvi, and E. Tomaszewski. 2003. Crime victimization, alcohol consumption, and drug use in Canadian public housing. *Journal of Criminal Justice* 31:383–96.

Dembo, R., L. Williams, E. Berry, et al. 1988. The relationship between physical and sexual abuse and illicit drug use: A replication among a new sample of youths entering a juvenile detention center. *International Journal of the Addictions* 23:1101–23.

Dembo, R., L. Williams, A. Getreu, et al. 1991. A longitudinal study of the relationship among marijuana/hashish use, cocaine use and delinquency in a cohort of high risk youths. *Journal of Drug Issues* 21:271–312.

Dembo, R., L. Williams, L. LaVoie, and E. Berry. 1989. Physical abuse, sexual victimization and illicit drug use. *Violence Victims* 4(2):1212–38.

Derzon, J. and M. Lipsey. 1999. A synthesis of the relationship of marijuana use with delinquent and problem behaviors. *School Psychology International* 20:57–68.

Dobinson, I. and P. Ward. 1985. *Drugs and crime*. Sydney: NSW Bureau of Crime Statistics and Research.

D'Orban, P. 1976. Barbiturate abuse. *Journal of Medical Ethics* 2:63–67.

_____. 1991. The crimes connection: Alcohol. In *The international handbook of addiction behavior*, ed. I. Glass, 295–301. London: Routledge.

Dorn, N., K. Murji, and N. South. 1992. *Traffickers: Drug markets and law enforcement*. London: Routledge.

Duncan, R., B. Saunders, D. Kilpatrick, R. Hanson, and H. Resnick. 1996. Childhood physical assault as a risk factor for PTSD, depression, and substance abuse: Findings. *American Journal of Orthopsychiatry* 66(3):437–48.

Dunn, G., J. Ryan, and C. Dunn. 1994. Trauma symptoms in substance abusers with and without histories of childhood abuse. *Journal of Psychoactive Drugs* 26(4):357–60.

Dunnegun, S. 1997. Violence, trauma and substance abuse. *Journal of Psychoactive Drugs* 29:345–51.

El-Bassel, N., L. Gilbert, R. Schilling, and T. Wada. 2000. Drug abuse and partner violence among women in methadone treatment. *Journal of Family Violence* 15(3):209–28.

Ellinswood, E. 1971. Assault and homicide associated with amphetamine abuse. *American Journal of Psychiatry* 127:1170–75.

EMCCDA. 2006. *Malta National focal point: Valletta*. National Report 2006: http:// www.emcdda.europa.eu/html.cfm/index45007EN.html (accessed August 12, 2008).

_____. 2007. *Annual report: The state of the drugs problem in Europe*. EMCDDA: Lisbon. http://www.emcdda.europa.eu/html.cfm/index44682EN.html (accessed August 14, 2008).

Fagan, J. 1990. Intoxication and aggression. In *Drugs and crime: Crime and justice*, vol. 13, ed. M. Tonry and J. Q. Wilson, 241–320. Chicago: University of Chicago Press.

Fagan, J. and K. Chin, 1990. Violence as regulation and social control in the distribution of crack. In *Drugs and violence: Causes, correlates and consequences*, ed. M. De La Rosa, E.Y. Lambert, and B. Gropper. Research Monograph 103. Rockville, MD: U.S. Department of Health and Human Services, National Institute on Drug Abuse.

Farrall, S. and S. Maltby. 2003. The victimisation of probationers. *Howard Journal* 42:113–23.

Fattah, E. 1992. *Towards a critical victimology*. London: Macmillan.

Faupel, C. E. 1991. *Shooting dope: Career patterns of hard-core heroin users*. Gainesville: University of Florida Press.

Feldman, H., M. Agar, and G. Beschner. 1979. *Angel dust: An ethnographic study of PCP users*. Lexington, MA: Lexington Books.

Finestone, H. 1967. Narcotics and criminality. *Law and Contemporary Problems* 22:60–85.

Finney, A. 2004. Alcohol and intimate partner violence: Key findings from the research. Home Office Findings no. 216. London: Home Office. http://www.homeoffice. gov.uk/rds/pdfs04/r216.pdf (accessed August 24, 2008).

Friedman, A. 1998. Substance use/abuse as a predictor to illegal and violent behavior: A review of the relevant literature. *Aggression and Violent Behavior* 3:339–55.

Gerson, L. and D. Preston. 1979. Alcohol consumption and the incidence of violent crime. *Journal of Studies on Alcohol* 40:307–12.

Gilbert, L., N. El-Bassel, R. F. Schilling, and E. Friedman. 1997. Childhood abuse as a risk for partner abuse among women in methadone maintenance. *American Journal of Drug and Alcohol Abuse* 23(4):581–95.

Gillmore, M., S. Butler, M. Lohr, and L. Gilchrist. 1992. Substance use and other factors associated with risky sexual behavior among pregnant adolescents. *Family Planning Perspectives* 24:255–68.

Gilman, M. 1998. Onion rings to go: Social exclusion and addiction. *Druglink*, May/ June 1998:14–18.

Gil-Rivas, V., R. Fiorentine, and M. Anglin. 1996. Sexual abuse, physical abuse, and posttraumatic stress disorder among women participating in outpatient drug abuse treatment. *Journal of Psychoactive Drugs* 28:95–102.

Glaser, D. 1974. Interlocking dualities in drug use, drug control and crime. In *Drugs and the criminal justice system*, ed. J. A. Inciardi and C. D. Chambers, 39–56. Beverly Hills, CA: Sage.

Goldstein, P. 1979. *Prostitution and drugs*. Lexington, MA: Lexington Books.

Goldstein, P. and N. Duchaine, 1980. *Daily criminal activities of street drug users*. Paper presented at annual meetings of the American Society of Criminology, Chicago.

Goode, E. 1996. *Drugs in American society*. New York: McGraw-Hill.

Gould, L. 1974. Crime and the addict: Beyond common sense. In *Drugs and the criminal justice system*, ed. J. Inciardi and C. Chambers, 57–75. Beverly Hills, CA: Sage.

Graham, K. and P. West. 2001. Alcohol and crime: Examining the link. In *International handbook of alcohol dependence and problems*, ed. N. Heather, T. Peters, and T. Stockwell, 439–70. Chichester, UK: John Wiley.

Grapendaal, M., E. Leuw, and H. Nelen. 1995. *A world or opportunities: Life-style and economic behaviour or heroin addicts in Amsterdam*. Albany: State University of New York Press.

Greenberg, S. and F. Adler. 1974. Crime and addiction: An empirical analysis of the literature, 1920–1973. *Contemporary Drug Problems* 3:221–70.

Grella, C. and V. Joshi. 2003. Treatment processes and outcomes among adolescents with a history of abuse who are in drug treatment. *Child Maltreatment* 8:7–18.

Gustafson, R. 1993. What do experimental paradigms tell us about alcohol-related aggressive responding? *Journal of Studies on Alcohol* September:20–29.

Hall, W. 1996. *Methadone maintenance treatment as a crime control measure*. Contemporary Issues in Crime and Justice, no. 29. Sydney: NSW Bureau of Crime Research and Statistics.

Hall, W., J. Bell, and J. Carless. 1993. Crime and drug use among applicants for methadone maintenance. *Drug and Alcohol Dependence* 31:123–29.

Haller, D. and D. Miles. 2003. Victimization and perpetration among perinatal substance abusers. *Journal of Interpersonal Violence* 18:760–89. http://jiv.sagepub.com/cgi/content/abstract/18/7/760 (accessed August 12, 2008).

Hammersley, R. 2008. *Drugs and crime*. Glasgow: Polity Press.

Hammersley, R., A. Forsyth, V. Morrison, and J. Davies. 1989. The relation between crime and opioid use. *British Journal of Addiction* 84:1033–34.

Harris, M. and R. Fallot. 2001. Envisioning a trauma-informed service system: A vital paradigm shift. *New Directions for Mental Health Services* 89:3–22.

Harrison, P., J. Fulkerson, and T. Beebe. 1997. Multiple substance use among adolescent physical and sexual abuse victims. *Child Abuse and Neglect* 21:529–39.

Harrison, P., N. Hoffmann, and G. Edwall. 1989. Differential drug use patterns among sexually abused adolescent girls in treatment for chemical dependency. *International Journal of the Addictions* 24:499–514.

Hawke, J., N. Jainchill, and G. DeLeon. 2000. The prevalence of sexual abuse and its impact on the onset of drug use among adolescents in therapeutic community drug treatment. *Journal of Child and Adolescent Substance Abuse* 9:35–49.

Inciardi, J. 1992. *The war on drugs II*. Mountain View, CA: Mayfield.

Inciardi, J. A. and C. Chamber. 1974. *Drugs and the criminal justice system*. Beverly Hills, CA: Sage.

Inciardi, J. A. and H. L. Surratt. 2001. Drug use, street crime, and sex-trading among cocaine-dependent women: Implications for public health and criminal justice policy. *Journal of Psychoactive Drugs* 33:379–89.

Innes, C. A. 1988. *Drug use and crime*. Bureau of justice statistics special report. Washington, DC: Justice Statistics Special Clearinghouse/NCJRS. U.S. Department of Justice

Ito, T., N. Miller, and V. Pollock. 1996. Alcohol and aggression: A meta-analysis on the moderating effects of inhibitory cues, triggering events, and self-focused attention. *Psychological Bulletin* 120:60–82.

Jarvis, T., J. Copeland, and L. Walton. 1998. Exploring the nature of the relationship between child sexual abuse and substance use among women. *Addiction* 93(6):865–75.

Johnson, B., P. Goldstein, E. Preble, J. Schmeidler, S. Lipton, and T. Miller. 1985. *Taking care of business: The economics of crime by heroin abusers*. Lexington, MA: Lexington Books.

Johnson, S., L. Gibson, and R. Linden. 1976. Alcohol and rape in Winnipeg: 1966–1975. *Journal of Studies on Alcohol* 39:1887–94.

Kantor, G. and M. Straus. 1989. Substance abuse as a precipitant of wife abuse victimization. *The American Journal of Drug and Alcohol Abuse* 15(2):173–89.

Kaplan, J. 1983. *The hardest drug: Heroin and public policy*. Chicago: University of Chicago Press.

Karberg, J. and D. James. 2002. *Substance dependence, abuse and treatment of jail inmates, 2002*. Washington, DC: U.S. Department of Justice Office of Justice Programs. http://www.ojp.usdoj.gov/bjs/pub/pdf/sdatji02.pdf (accessed August 23, 2008).

Kevin, M. 1999. *Violent crime, alcohol and other drugs: A survey of inmates imprisoned for assault in New South Wales*. Sydney: NSW Department of Corrective Services.

Khantzian, E. 1985. The self-medication hypothesis of addictive disorders: Focus on heroin and cocaine dependence. *American Journal of Psychiatry* 142:1259–64.

Kilpatrick, D., R. Acierno, H. Resnick, B. Saunders, and C. Best. 1997. A two-year longitudinal analysis of the relationships between violent assault and substance abuse in women. *Journal of Consulting and Clinical Psychology* 65:834–47.

Kilpatrick, D., C. Edmunds, and A. Seymour. 1992. *Rape in America: A report to the nation. Arlington, VA: National centre for victims of crime*. Charleston: Medical University of South Carolina.

Kozel, N., R. Dupont, and B. Brown. 1972. A study of narcotic involvement in an offender population. *International Journal of the Addictions* 7:443–50.

Kramer, J. 1976. From Demon to Ally-How mythology has and may yet alter national drug policy. *Journal of Drug Issues* 6:390–406.

Larson, A. 1996. *What injectors say about drug use: Preliminary findings from a survey of indigenous injecting drug users*. IDU Project Working Paper. Brisbane: Australian Centre for International and Tropical Health and Nutrition.

Leonard, K. and M. Senchak. 1996. Prospective prediction of husband marital aggression within newlywed couples. *Journal of Abnormal Psychology* 105:369–80.

Lipton, D. S. 1995. *The effectiveness of treatment for drug abusers under criminal justice supervision*. Washington, DC: National Institute of Justice.

Logan, T., R. Walker, J. Cole, and C. Lekefld. 2002. Victimization and substance abuse among women: Contributing factors, interventions and implications. *Review of General Psychology* 6(4):325–97.

Loxley, W. 2001. Drug use, intoxication and offence type in two groups of alleged offenders in Perth: A pilot study. *The Australian and New Zealand Journal of Criminology* 34(1):91–104.

Macandrew, C. and R. Edgerton. 1969. *Drunken comportment: A social explanation*. Chicago: Aldine.

Maden, A., M. Swinton, and J. Gunn. 1992. A survey of pre-arrest drug use in sentenced prisoners. *British Journal of Addiction* 87:27–33.

Maher, L., D. Dixon, W. Hall, and M. Lynskey. 2002. Property crime and income generation by heroin users. *The Australian and New Zealand Journal of Criminology* 35(2):187–202.

Makkai, T. 1999. Harm reduction in Australia: Politics, policy and public opinion. In *Harm reduction and drug control: Concepts and policies*, ed. J. Inciardi and L. Harrison, 171–92. Thousand Oaks, CA: Sage.

Makkai, T., J. Fitzgerald, and P. Doak. 2000. *Drug use amongst police detainees*. Crime and Justice Bulletin, no. 49. Sydney: NSW Bureau of Crime Statistics and Research.

Martin, S., B. Kilgallen, D. L. Dee, S. Dawson, and J. Campbell. 1998. Women in a prenatal care/substance abuse treatment program: Links between domestic violence and mental health. *Maternal and Child Health Journal* 2(2):85–94.

McCauley, J., D. E. Kern, K. Kolodner, et al. 1997. Clinical characteristics of women with a history of childhood abuse: Unhealed wounds. *Journal of the American Medical Association* 277(17):1362–68.

McElrath, K., D. Chitwood, and M. Comerford. 1997. Crime victimization among injecting drug users. *Journal of Drug Issues* Fall:771–83.

McGallagly, J. and B. Dunn. 2001. *The criminal histories of 372 suspected drug offenders*. Scottish executive central research unit, crime and criminal justice research findings, no. 52. Edinburgh: Scottish Executive.

McKeganey, N., C. Connelly, J. Knepil, J. Norrie, and L. Reid. 2000. *Interviewing and drug testing of arrestees in Scotland: A pilot of the arrestee drug abuse monitoring (ADAM) methodology*. Edinburgh: Scottish Executive Central Research Unit.

Medrano, M. A., W. Zule, J. Hatch, and D. P. Desmond. 1999. Prevalence of childhood trauma in a community sample of substance-abusing women. *American Journal of Drug and Alcohol Abuse* 25(3):449–62.

Miczek, K., J. DeBold, M. Haney, J. Tidey, J. Vivian, and E. Weerts. 1994. Alcohol, drugs of abuse, aggression, and violence. In *Understanding and preventing violence*, vol. 3, ed. A. J. Reiss and J. A. Roth, 186–98. Washington, DC: National Academy Press.

Miller, B., W. Downs, and D. Gondoli. 1989. Spousal violence among alcoholic women as compared to a random household sample of women. *Journal of Studies on Alcohol* 50(8):533–40.

Miller, P. and M. Plant. 1996. Drinking, smoking, and illicit drug use among 15- and 16-year-olds in the United Kingdom. *BMJ* 313:394–97.

Miller, T. R., M. A. Cohen, and B. Wiersema. 1996. *Victim costs and consequences: A new look*. Washington, DC: National Institute of Justice.

Mumola, C. and J. Karberg. 2006. *Drug use and dependence, state and federal prisoners, 2004.* U.S. Department of Justice, Office of Justice Programs, NCJ 213530. http://www.ojp.usdoj.gov/bjs/abstract/dudsfp04.htm (accessed August 23, 2008).

NACRO. 2001. *Drink and disorder.* London: NACRO.

NACRO Briefing. 2000. *Young people, drug use and offending.* London: NACRO.

Naranjo, C. and K. Bremmer. 1993. Behavioral correlates of alcohol intoxication. *Addiction* 88:25–35.

Neale, J., M. Bloor, and C. Weir. 2005. Problem drug users and assault. *International Journal of Drug Policy* 16:393–402.

Newburn, T. 2007. *Criminology.* Devon, UK: Willan.

NTORS. 1999. *NTORS at one year: The national treatment outcome research study,* 3rd bulletin. London: Department of Health.

Nurco, D., T. Hanlon, T. Kinlock, and K. Duszynski. 1988. Differential criminal patterns of narcotic addicts over an addiction career. *Criminology* 26:407–23.

O'Farrell, T., V. Van Hutton, and C. Murphy. 1999. Domestic violence before and after alcoholism treatment: A two-year longitudinal study. *Journal of Studies on Alcohol* 60:317–21.

Palacios, W., C. Urmann, R. Newel, and N. Hamilton. 1999. Developing a sociological framework for dually diagnosed women. *Journal of Substance Abuse Treatment* 17(1/2):91–102.

Parker, H. 1996. Alcohol, young adult offenders and criminological cul-de-sacs. *British Journal of Criminology* 36:282–98.

Parker, H., J. Aldridge, and F. Measham. 1998. *Illegal leisure: The normalization of adolescent recreational drug use.* London: Routledge.

Parker, H., K. Baks, and R. Newcombe. 1988. *Living with heroin: The impact of a drugs 'epidemic' on an English community.* Milton Keynes, UK: Open University Press.

Parker, R. 1993. The effects of context on alcohol and violence. *Alcohol Health & Research World* 17:117–22.

Parker, R. and K. Auerhahn. 1998. Alcohol, drugs and violence. *Annual Review of Sociology* 24:291–311.

Parker, R. and L. Rebhun. 1995. *Alcohol and homicide: A deadly combination of two American traditions.* Albany: State University of New York Press.

Pernanen, K. 1991. *Alcohol in human violence.* New York: Guilford.

Pernanen, K., M. Cousineau, S. Brochu, and F. Sun. 2002. *Proportions of crimes associated with alcohol and other drugs in Canada.* Toronto: Canadian Centre in Substance Abuse.

Plant, M. 1990. *AIDS, drugs and prostitution.* London: Routledge.

Preble, E. and J. Casey. 1969. Taking care of business: The heroin users life on the street. *International Journal of the Addictions* 4:1–24.

Putnins, A. 2001. *Substance use by South Australian young offenders.* Adelaide: Office of Crime Statistics.

Rada, R. 1975. Alcoholism and forcible rape. *American Journal of Psychiatry* 132:444–46.

Ramsay, M. and A. Percy. 1996. *Drug misuse declared: Results from the 1994 British crime survey.* Research Findings, 33. London: Home Office.

Raskin-White, H. 1990. The drug use-delinquency connection in adolescence. In *Drugs, crime, and criminal justice,* ed. R. Weisheit, 215–56. Cincinnati, OH: Anderson.

_____. 1997. Alcohol, illicit drugs, and violence. In *Handbook of antisocial behavior*, ed. D. Stoff, J. Brieling, and J. D. Maser, 511–523. New York: John Wiley.

Raskin-White, H. and D. Gorman. 2000. *Dynamics of the drug-crime relationship.* Washington, DC: U.S. Department of Justice. http://www.ojp.usdoj.gov/nij/criminal_justice2000/vol1_2000.html (accessed July 18, 2008).

Raskin-White, H. and S. Hansell. 1998. Acute and long-term effects of drug use on aggression from adolescence into adulthood. *Journal of Drug Issues* 28:837–58.

Raskin-White, H., P. Tice, R. Loeber, and M. Stouthamer-Loeber. 2002. Illegal acts committed by adolescents under the influence of alcohol and drugs. *Journal of Research in Crime and Delinquency* 39:131–52.

Reiss, A. and J. Roth. 1993. *Understanding and preventing violence.* Washington, DC: National Academy Press.

Resnick, P. 1993. The psychological impact of rape. *Journal of Interpersonal Violence* 8(2):223–55.

Robert, N. 1993. The effects of context on alcohol and violence. *Alcohol Health & Research World* 17:117–22.

Rohsenow, D., R. Corbett, and D. Devine. 1988. Molested as children: Hidden contribution to substance abuse? *Journal of Substance Abuse Treatment* 5:13–18.

Roizen, J. 1993. Issues in the epidemiology of alcohol and violence. In *Alcohol and interpersonal violence: Fostering multidisciplinary perspectives*, ed. S. E. Martin, 3–36. NIAAA Research Monograph no. 24. Rockville, MD: U.S. Department of Health and Human Services and National Institutes of Health.

Roman, P. 1988. *Women and alcohol use.* Rockville, MD: National Institute on Alcohol Abuse and Alcoholism.

Rounds-Bryant, J., P. Kristiansen, J. Fairbank, and R. Hubbard. 1998. Substance use, mental disorders, abuse, and crime: Gender comparisons among a national sample of adolescent drug treatment clients. *Journal of Child and Adolescent Substance Abuse* 7(4):19–34.

Russell, J. 1993. *Alcohol and crime.* London: Mental Health Foundation.

Sampson, R. and J. Lauritsen. 1997. Racial and ethnic disparities in crime and criminal justice in the United States. In *Crime and justice: An annual review of research*, vol. 22, ed. M. Torry, 311–74. Chicago: University of Chicago Press.

Saunders, N. 1993. *E for ecstasy.* London: 14 Neal's Yard.

Schatzman, M. 1975. Cocaine and the drug problem. *Journal of Psychedelic Drugs* 56:7–18.

Seymour, A., M. Murray, J. Sigmon, et al. 2000. *NVAA text.* National Victim Assistance Academy, 2000. http://www.ojp.usdoj.gov/ovc/assist/nvaa2000/academy/welcome.html (accessed August 25, 2008).

Shupe, L. M. 1954. Alcohol and crime: A study of the urine alcohol concentration found in 882 persons arrested during or immediately after the commission of a felony. *Journal of Criminal Law, Criminology and Police Science* 44:661–64.

Singer, M., M. Petchers, and D. Hussey. 1989. The relationship between sexual abuse and substance abuse among psychiatrically hospitalized adolescents. *Child Abuse and Neglect* 13:319–25.

Skogan, W. 1990. *Disorder and decline: Crime and the spiral of decay in American neighborhoods.* Berkeley: University of California Press.

Slade, M., L. Daniel, and C. Heisler. 1991. Application of forensic toxicology to the problem of domestic violence. *Journal of Forensic Science* 36:708–13.

Smart, R. and A. C. Ogborne, 1994. Street youth in substance abuse treatment: Characteristics and treatment compliance. *Adolescents* 29(115):733–45.

Smith, R. 1972. Speed and violence: Compulsive methamphetamine abuse and criminality in the Haight-Ashbury district. In *Drug abuse: Proceedings of the international conference*, ed. C. Zarsfonetis, 120–33. Philadelphia: Lea and Febiger.

South, N. 1997. Drugs, crime, and control. In *The Oxford handbook of criminology*, ed. M. Maguire, R. Morgan, and R. Reiner, 393–440. Oxford: Clarendon.

_____. 1999. Debating drugs and everyday life. In *Drugs: Cultures, controls and everyday life*, ed. N. South, 123–28. London: Sage.

Stark, E. and A. Flitcraft. 1996. *Women at risk: Domestic violence and women's health.* Thousand Oaks, CA: Sage.

Stevens, A., D. Berto, U. Frick, et al. 2007. The victimization of dependent drug user findings from a European study. *European Journal of Criminology* 4(4):385–408.

Swett, C., C. Cohen, J. Surrey, A. Compaine, and R. Chaves. 1991. High rates of alcohol use and history of physical and sexual abuse among women outpatients. *American Journal of Drug and Alcohol Abuse* 17(1):49–60.

Swezey, R. 1973. Estimating drug-crime relationships. *International Journal of the Addictions* 8:701–21.

Teets, J. 1997. *Childhood sexual trauma of chemically dependent women.* 27(3):231–38.

Testa, M. and K. A. Parks. 1996. The role of women's alcohol consumption in sexual victimization. *Aggression and Violent Behavior* 1:217–34.

Tinklenberg, J. 1973. Drugs and crime. In *National commission on marijuana and drug abuse, drug use in America: Problems in perspective*. Appendix, vol. 1: Patterns and consequences of drug use, ed. R. P. Shafer, 107–15. Washington, DC: U.S. Government Printing Office.

Valuri, G., D. Indermaur, and A. Ferrante, 2002. *The criminal careers of drug offenders in Western Australia*. University of WA, Perth: Crime Research Centre.

Virkunnen, M. 1974. Alcohol as a factor precipitating aggression and conflict behavior leading to homicide. *British Journal of the Addictions* 69:149–54.

Virkkunen, M. and L. Markku. 1993. Brain serotonin, type II alcoholism, and impulsive violence. *Journal of Studies on Alcohol* September:163–69.

Waidner, G. 1999. Die Viktimisierungserfahrungen drogenabhängiger Personen. MA thesis, University of Vienna.

Watts, W. and A. Ellis. 1993. Sexual abuse and drinking and drug use: Implications for prevention. *Journal of Drug Education* 22(3):183–200.

Wilsnack, S., N. Vogeltanz, A. Klassen, and T. Harris. 1997. Childhood sexual abuse and women's substance abuse: National survey findings. *Journal of Studies on Alcohol* 58(3):264–71.

Windle, M., R. C. Windle, D. M. Scheidt, and G. B. Miller. 1995. Physical and sexual abuse and associated mental disorders among alcoholic inpatients. *American Journal of Psychiatry* 152(9):1322–28.

Wolfgang, M. 1958. *Patterns in criminal homicide.* Philadelphia: University of Pennsylvania Press.

Wolfgang, M. and F. Ferracuti. 1967. *The subculture of violence: Toward an integrated theory in criminology.* London: Tavistock.

Zinberg, N. 1984. *Drug, set, and setting.* New Haven, CT: Yale University Press.

Victims of Sex Trafficking

10

Gender, Myths, and Consequences

SANJA MILIVOJEVIC AND SANJA ĆOPIĆ

Contents

10.1 Introduction

Trafficking in people, and particularly trafficking in women for the purpose of sexual exploitation ("sex trafficking"), has been widely referred to as "modern-day slavery" [Bales, 1999; Bertone, 2000; Hughes, 2001; Jeffreys, 2002; Boyd, 2003; King, 2004; van den Anker, 2004; Roby, 2005] and "the dark side of globalization" [Sanghera, 2005:6], and described within the rhetoric of "evil" [U.S. Department of State, 2004; Abrams, 2005; Kwon, 2005]. This phenomenon re-emerged on the international agenda in the early 1990s, coinciding with the fall of the Berlin Wall and a period of increased mobility from the global south to the global north [Rijken, 2003:91; Saunders and Soderlund, 2003:16; Tyldum et al., 2005:9]. A range of actors across the developed and developing world, from international organizations, state and nonstate institutions, politicians, and the media, to academics, feminists, civil rights activists, and the clergy, warned of the "dramatic increase" in trafficking [Rijken, 2003:101; O'Connell Davidson, 2006], particularly women and children, portraying "sex slavery" as a peril that threatens basic values of modern civilization. This "21st century abolitionist movement" [U.S. Ambassador John Miller, U.S.

House of Representatives' Subcommittee on Africa, Global Human Rights and International Operation Hearing, June 14, 2006:27] called for the "abolition of slavery" by firmly locating antitrafficking responses within a "law and order" framework.

At the same time, critics suggested that although the process of acknowledgment of the "trafficking problem" had occurred particularly in the past 2 decades, trafficking itself has existed throughout history [Petersen, 2001; Truong, 2001; Zhao, 2003; Bennett, 2004; Coontz and Griebel, 2004; Long, 2004; Kelly et al., 2005:141; Kempadoo, 2005]. They questioned whether such promotion of sex trafficking was motivated by its actual magnitude or by its appeal [Kleimenov and Shamkov, 2005:39] and the fact that "sex sells." Finally, they called for a critical approach to the "trafficking hype" [Murray, 1998], and a more pragmatic gaze into the causes of trafficking and consequences of countertrafficking policies [Doezema, 2000; Ditmore, 2002; Miller, 2004; O'Connell Davidson, 2006].

Trafficking in people came to the attention of Serbian nongovernmental organizations (NGOs) in the late 1990s. The Serbian government, however, largely ignored the issue until the fall of Milosevic's regime in October 2000, when numerous antitrafficking initiatives and campaigns were launched, with support and pressure from international organizations engaged in combating trafficking in the Balkans [Lindstrom, 2004; Simeunovic-Patic, 2005; U.S. Department of State, 2005]. In 2000 Serbia signed the United Nations (UN) Protocol to Prevent, Suppress, and Punish Trafficking in Persons, Especially Women and Children, Supplementing the UN Convention against Transnational Organized Crime (The Palermo Protocol),* and after its ratification in 2001 and following intensive lobbying by local NGOs and the international community, trafficking in people was defined as a criminal offense.† In relation to trafficking in women, it has been suggested that Serbia represents a country of origin, destination, and transit [Nikolic-Ristanovic et al., 2004; Bjerkan, 2005; Surtees, 2005; U.S. Department of State, 2008]. In the 2008 U.S. Department of State Annual Trafficking in Persons (TIP) report, Serbia has been ranked in Tier 2, as a country that makes "significant efforts to meet the minimum standards" for the elimination of trafficking, as defined by the U.S. Trafficking Victims Protection Act of 2000 [U.S. Department of State, 2008:12]. Although engagement around trafficking intensified in the past decade, there is still a lack of research, and there are many dilemmas in relation to trafficking in women in Serbia [Nikolic-Ristanovic, 2005b].

---

* As the Federal Republic of Yugoslavia, a federal union of Serbia and Montenegro.
† Article 111b of the Criminal Code of the Republic of Serbia was passed in April 2003. In January 2006, the Criminal Code was revised, and trafficking in people is now regulated in Article 388 [Ćopić and Nikolic-Ristanovic, 2006].

Based on a survey on trafficking in people conducted in Serbia[*] and research by one of the authors[†] on sex trafficking in Serbia and Australia, this chapter aims to identify predominant discourses around women victims of trafficking in Serbia, as seen by practitioners (judges, prosecutors, lawyers, NGO/victim support activists, scholars, and policymakers) who engage with this issue through various governmental and nongovernmental agencies. It will highlight the ways in which women's victimhood is tied to their gender and desired performances of femininity and explore the consequences of these discourses to women's victim status. The authors conclude that although in Serbia some women are unconditionally perceived as victims, others might slip through the net, and call for deconstruction of these contrasting discourses and understanding trafficking within all its complexities.

10.2 Women Trafficked for Sex: A Global Framework

Women victims of crime—especially rape, sexual assault, and domestic violence—have been commonly represented through the contrasting processes of blaming the victim and creating the "ideal victim" [Christie, 1986]. Women's "contribution" to their own victimization, or lack of it, has historically been considered an important element in achieving victim status [Stanko, 1982; Hawkesworth, 1990; Ward, 1995; Korn and Efrat, 2004]. Trafficked women have often been scrutinized through the same lens [Doezema, 1998, 2000; Demleitner, 2001; Petersen, 2001; Long, 2004; Kantola and Squires, 2004; Wijers, 2004]. The female victim of sex trafficking was historically constructed through the "white slave" narrative that implied their virginity and pureness [Doezema, 2000; O'Connell Davidson, 2006]. This powerful "sex slavery" discourse still resonates in the contemporary trafficking debate [Wijers and van Doorninck, 2002; Goodey, 2004; O'Connell Davidson, 2006] as the official discourses reinforce the notion of a naïve, young, impoverished, and disadvantaged woman from developing countries as the typical victim of trafficking. She is kidnapped, lured, and/or forced into sex work [Bertone, 2000; Clark, 2003; Lehti and Aromaa, 2003; Oberloher, 2003; Rijken, 2003; King, 2004; Roby, 2005; Stoecker, 2005; U.S. Department of State, 2006], and once trafficked, her resistance is broken by violence. Similar to discourses around rape, the female body is perceived as weak and vulnerable [Stanko, 1985; Clark, 2003; Agustin, 2005]. Trafficked

---

[*] Research on trafficking in Serbia was conducted by the Victimology Society of Serbia in 2004. The book *Trafficking in People in Serbia* is available in Serbian and English at www.vds.org.yu.

[†] Selected chapters of Sanja Milivojevic's doctoral thesis, "Sex Trafficking in Serbia and Australia," are published in *Sex trafficking: International context and response*, with Marie Segrave and Sharon Pickering, by Willan.

women are portrayed as "completely disposable tools," "under the total control" of traffickers [Bales, cited in O'Connell Davidson, 2006:7]:

> Forced abortions, beatings and threats were all part of their new life in
> America.... They worked six days a week, having sex in 15-minute sessions
> with men who paid their bosses $20 or $25. Thirty men a day was not unusual,
> and after the brothels closed for the night, the men who guarded the girls took
> their turn.

This sex slavery discourse, although undoubtedly one possible (and perhaps not uncommon) scenario of trafficking, has been criticized by feminist scholars and criminologists because it creates the ideal victim [Christie,
1986] of trafficking, thus possibly delegitimizing women who do not fit into
this narrow category. They are "frequently labelled by much of society and
officialdom as 'common prostitutes'" [Roby, 2005:140] and are either dismissed as victims of crime [Doezema, 2000; Goodey, 2003:68] or forced
to validate their legitimacy in the criminal justice system [Renzetti, 1999;
Doezema, 2000]. Indeed, practitioners who work with/assist women trafficked for sex in Serbia identified the resilience of these discourses in the
Serbian context.

10.2.1 Trafficked Women in Serbia: Discourses and Impact

> The premise is that (women) are poor victims with the history of violence,
> stupid and naïve ... or the moral one: they are all whores.
>
> **Sandra Ljubinkovic**
> *NGO Anti-Trafficking Centre, Belgrade*

10.2.1.1 Acknowledging the Female Victim

The task of identifying victims of trafficking in Serbia has been given to the
Service for Coordination of Protection of Victims of Trafficking (commonly
referred to as "the Service"), a governmental body established in March
2004, and the "Mobile Team," a group that combines representatives of
both governmental and nongovernmental agencies engaged in combating
trafficking [Simeunovic-Patic, 2005]. However, the first "filter" women go
through in the process of identification is the police: the "'gate-keepers' who
decide *who* will enter the system and *how* they will enter" [Cunneen, 2001:132,
emphasis in the original]. Interviews with practitioners in Serbia indicate
that whether a woman—a potential victim of trafficking—will be identified
as such does not depend exclusively on the crime through which she has been
victimized. Rather, her position is determined by "traits"—her perceived
"contribution" to victimization, and whether she fits a desired victim role.

These traits, or identities, group all potential victims of trafficking into two contrasting narratives: "otherness" and "innocents."

The first predominant narrative identified around trafficked women in Serbia has been constructed within the discourse of otherness. From this discourse three critical identities have emerged: the prostitute, the foreigner, and the "unworthy" woman. The more these identities intersect, the less likely a trafficked woman will be granted victim status. Practitioners in Serbia generally agreed that women victims of trafficking are still commonly and primarily identified as prostitutes:

> The first thing that comes across someone's mind when you say "sex trafficking" is a prostitute who came here voluntarily, and the conclusion is: "She's got what she's been looking for."
>
> **Respondent**
> *Ministry of Labour, Belgrade*

> The majority of people (in Serbia) do not believe in sex trafficking. I often find myself arguing with people who say, "Don't tell me that she didn't know, that she was forced to do it—she is doing it because she wants to and she loves it." They are not seen as victims but as prostitutes. And that is the end of the story.
>
> **Vesna Stanojevic**
> *Shelter for Women Victims of Trafficking, Belgrade*

The question of whether a woman willingly opted for or was forced into sex work is one of the crucial arguments in achieving victim status. The connection between women's victimization and expected and desired performances of femininity results in the notion that women's "appropriate" behavior—"keeping the 'Lady' safe" [Campbell, 2005]—is considered to be an essential tool in preventing their victimization. Here we find the starting point of the "blaming the victim" process that generates the construction of trafficked women as sex workers.

> It is believed that women have to be careful with whom they talk to or go out, and that's unacceptable. It is still believed that a woman must not do certain things and (if she does) that she somehow indirectly...contributed to her own victimisation.
>
> **Judge**
> *District Court, Belgrade*

> People often say: "She's got what she wanted—if she *wasn't doing what she was doing* it would never (have) happened to her."
>
> **Police officer**
> *Department for Combating Illegal Migrations and Trafficking in Human Beings, Belgrade (emphasis added)*

The interviews also revealed that the construction of trafficked women as sex workers is strongly linked to an additional aspect of otherness: They are predominantly considered to be foreigners, that is, migrant women:

> (Victims) are seen as foreign women who came here to "ruin" our youth, make money and go back.

Respondent
Service for Coordination of Protection of Victims of Trafficking, Belgrade

In Serbia, the stereotype of trafficked women as foreigners—as eastern Europeans (especially Russians and Ukrainians)—gained currency in the early 1990s with an increase in women's migration flows from the former Eastern bloc.

> There is the stereotype that women victims of trafficking are "whores" and this is the continuum of the stereotype we have had since the beginning of the 1990s that portrayed victims as "easy" women from Eastern Europe.

Vesna Nikolic Ristanovic
Belgrade University, NGO Victimology Society of Serbia, Belgrade

The notion of "women from the East" as typical victims of trafficking in Serbia has been reinforced by some international organizations and agencies engaged in combating trafficking in the Balkans [European Commission, 2001; IOM Counter-Trafficking Service, 2004; Mendelson, 2005; UN Office on Drugs and Crime, 2006]:

> International organisations love to create patterns, how the victim from one country looks like.

Police officer
Belgrade Police

> Every book about trafficking starts with the same intro, like the Bible: "With the fall of Berlin's Wall"….(Stereotypes are) put on the agenda by the international organisations and donors.

Tamara Vukasovic
NGO ASTRA, Belgrade

Although it could be argued that media coverage, lack of debate, and the standpoint set by international organizations and local NGOs have been instrumental in constructing such images of women trafficked for sex [Nikolic-Ristanovic, 2005b:12–13], there are additional factors in Serbian culture that need to be acknowledged, such as xenophobia and patriarchy. As sex trafficking is perceived as a problem that comes from outside, acting on the nation, the "trafficked woman" is "the other" to women of the nation. Therefore, the problem is in an alien, racialized "other" that represents a threat to the security and identity of the nation-state [Kapur, 2005:25; Guiraudon, 2006].

As practitioners in Serbia indicate, the intersection of the two identities within the discourse of otherness—a racialized, "oriental" or "Eastern" woman and a prostitute—creates a third: the "unworthy" woman:

> A trafficked woman in Serbia is an absolute loser: because she is a woman, because she is from Ukraine or Moldova, and because she is, according to the people here, a prostitute…. They are women from "inferior" countries, former or future prostitutes, regardless of whether it was willingly or not, and that is the end of the story.
>
> **Olivera Simonov**
> *Attorney and victims' representative, Belgrade*

Once perceived as such, trafficked women have been portrayed as *lawbreakers* [Demleitner, 2001:262]—somewhere between being a victim and an offender, manipulative and opportunistic, ready to take advantage of everyone: their clients, support services, law enforcement agencies, and the State.

> She is very skilful, both with criminals and law enforcement, to get what she wants. She is not an angel or Mother Theresa. That is the problem: It is always a question whether you can rely on her. If someone offers her more money one day she might decide she is not [a] victim anymore.
>
> **Public Prosecutor**
> *Department for Public Prosecution, Belgrade*

> I think that they develop a mechanism of manipulation in order to survive, and when they come out of the situation of trafficking they continue to employ it. They manipulate in order to get some privileges and survive, and continue to behave like that in the Shelter.
>
> **Respondent**
> *Service for Coordination of Protection of Victims of Trafficking, Belgrade*

Here, agency is entirely attributed to women: They are represented as manipulating the authorities for financial, immigration, or other purposes. Therefore, not women, but the State and state agencies, are identified as victims [Cyrus and Vogel, 2006]. This shift in allocating victimization completes the process of denying victim status to women who fall within this discourse.

The second narrative identified through interviews with practitioners in Serbia depicts women trafficked for sex as "innocent" and "deserving" victims and encloses three key identities: an "abused" woman (kidnapped and/or raped, beaten up, locked in), an unfortunate (poor and/or uneducated, with previous history of abuse), and blameless (not "responsible" for what happened). The more these identities intersect, the closer women get to "ideal victim" status:

> They would go out … and the traffickers would stop their cars next to them and pull them into their cars. Just like in crime films.
>
> **Vesna Stanojevic**
> *Shelter for Women Victims of Trafficking, Belgrade*
> *[Nikolic-Ristanovic et al., 2004:75]*

> (S)he went to a taxi…. After a while the taxi slowed down and two guys got violently inside … and grabbed her bag with documents and money. From that moment (on) she became nobody, a person without identity.
>
> **Respondent**
> *[Nikolic-Ristanovic et al., 2004:77–78]*

Practitioners in Serbia confirmed the notion that women are often "broken in" and physically forced into the sex industry:

> (When) she refuses to engage in (sex) work, because she doesn't want to do it at all, or did not agree to such (job) conditions, she is deprived of liberty, abused and tortured until she does.
>
> **Judge**
> *District Court, Belgrade*

> (T)he owner of the café had kept them locked-up, raped them and forced them into prostitution.
>
> **District Public Prosecutor**
> *Department for Public Prosecution, Sabac*
> *[Nikolic-Ristanovic et al., 2004:62]*

This "initiation" is more than rape—it sends a message to women that there is no alternative [Nikolic-Ristanovic, 2005a:90–91], and they become the traffickers' "property" [Fergus, 2005:23].

> The initial rape, especially if a girl is a virgin, is like ceremonial initiation. He breaks her resistance, and lets her know what will happen to her in the future.
>
> **Tamara Vukasovic**
> *NGO ASTRA, Belgrade*

> A girl … was raped in front of other girls immediately after she came to the house, to show her who is the boss.
>
> **Olivera Simonov**
> *Attorney and victims' representative, Belgrade*

Within the predominant trafficking discourse, after the initial rape, or after women who willingly entered into sex work are coerced to work under conditions they did not agree to, traffickers execute unconditional power over their helpless victims in a gruesome scenario of sex slavery that entirely removes women's agency. Migrant women, as argued in the literature [Feher, 2002; Gulcur and Ilkkaracan, 2002; Kelly, 2002; Konrad, 2002; Goodey, 2003; Sullivan, 2003; Aghatise, 2004; Sanghera, 2005], are particularly vulnerable to control and manipulation by traffickers, especially if the process of migration is situated outside legitimate migration flows. Practitioners in Serbia confirmed that traffickers often use relentless and disempowering control, particularly over their foreign victims:

> He takes her documents, takes her money. They are illegally here, often isolated, their mobility limited.... They're stripped of basic human rights and turned (in)to objects, real slaves.
>
> **Judge**
> *District Court, Belgrade*

> Victim is stripped of her documents; they change her name, and she loses her identity.... She loses one personal freedom after another, and becomes a thing.... (The trafficker) is her unlimited owner, with the unlimited power.... She will never walk freely, never be able to choose a customer; if a customer has a special request, for example to beat her up, she won't be able to stop it.
>
> **Olivera Simonov**
> *Attorney and victims' representative, Belgrade*

> She was enslaved.... She had a room with two guards in front of it. She had no freedom of movement.... In the evening they would take her to the bar.
>
> **Respondent**
> *[Nikolic-Ristanovic et al., 2004:84]*

The second element within the discourse of innocents is "unfortunate" victim. This identity is linked to women's age, class, education, and family history: Trafficked women are perceived as young, poverty stricken, helpless, uneducated women from the global south, with a previous history of victimization [Clark, 2003]. Thus, women who end up in trafficking are victims of their culture, inexperience, ignorance, illiteracy, and tradition [Lyons, 1999; Kapur, 2002] and therefore cannot be blamed if they try to find a better life.

> The typical victim is from Eastern Europe, 17–20 years old, completed primary or high school. She is completely uninformed; she idealises the West, and lacks basic knowledge of geography and culture. Many think they are in Italy, and are in fact in Serbia. A complete ignorance – that is the (victim)

profile.... They are mostly uninformed, uneducated, below the poverty line ... and from dysfunctional families with divorced parents.

Police officer
National Bureau of INTERPOL, Belgrade

Unfortunately, all of them have had the same characteristic: every single one experienced or witnessed horrible violence in (their) family, whether it was murder or suicide, alcohol, incest, or rape.... We had girls who were from horrid rural areas in Moldova; they didn't know to use the bathroom, and saw an electric stove for the first time.

Vesna Stanojevic
Shelter for Women Victims of Trafficking, Belgrade

However, there are limits women should not cross, as the third identity within this discourse requires women's blamelessness: They cannot "contribute" to their victimization, whether it is the illegality (illegal migrations) or immorality (previous engagement in the sex industry or knowledge about their future job) of their actions. In addition, women's "guilt" can also be generated through a lack of agency in obtaining information about their job and/or journey, trusting information without corroboration, and failing to acknowledge the warning signs before victimization:

A girl's mother told her not to trust her boyfriend, and that she might become a victim of trafficking. She didn't believe and indeed became a victim.... She was not only uninformed, but also reckless and trusted people who betrayed her. Majority of women is like that, even if they are from good families and educated.

Respondent
Ministry of Labour, Belgrade

Women (victims of trafficking) are uninformed, naïve and reckless.... Traffickers buy their trust, and that is very much related to naiveté and recklessness. What is the difference between (trafficking) and a school kid who has been offered a candy? If you don't want to buy a vacuum cleaner, you're not going to buy it. But if you're reckless and you think that the salesperson is telling the truth, you will buy it even though it's untrustworthy and has no warranty.

Police officer
National Bureau of INTERPOL, Belgrade

While women are held responsible for their own victimization, a reverse process of "purification" [Lamb, 1996] of victims of trafficking could also be identified, as practitioners stressed that women's "choice" of sex work or "recklessness" in the migration processes is sometimes the direct consequence of the conditions women live in. In other words, women's resistance to complex social/personal circumstances pushes them to engage in sex work and ignore or reject information that might prevent their victimization:

> If you sit in a dump, of course you want to try to change something....Even if you know what is going to happen, you want to run away and try something different. A woman has no way out; she wants to make something of her life.... Why would you live in a dump? You want to try. That is not naiveté.
>
> **Representative**
> *International organization working on trafficking, Belgrade*

> They run away because of rigid, patriarchal control, or violence (in their families)....The mixture of a family situation, rigid patriarchal socialisation ... and economic problems pushes them to trafficking.... I think there is a difference in not having information and refusing to know because they are in trouble. Even when they hear stories (about trafficking) they ignore it, as that would stop them (in the decision-making process).... They are trying to find the way out.
>
> **Vesna Nikolic-Ristanovic**
> *Belgrade University, NGO Victimology Society of Serbia, Belgrade*

> (A)lmost all victims replied to an advert in their country, eager to escape the poverty and hoping to provide themselves a better future.
>
> **Respondent**
> *[Nikolic-Ristanovic et al., 2004:75]*

Here, the (re)construction of the "ideal victim" [Christie, 1986] of sex trafficking is almost complete: Victims are seen as weak—young and poor women who are not capable of protecting themselves, severely victimized and innocent/purified, and thus women who should readily be given victim status, rescued, and protected. Agency is explicitly attributed to the State—the protector of the female victim [Coomaraswamy, 2003]—whereas women are voiceless and helpless.

The most important consequence of this narrative is that women who have not been "abused enough" or those who are considered to be "guilty" might not be perceived as victims of trafficking. In addition, an absence of unlimited control by traffickers alongside a lack of active resistance strategies by women trafficked for sex, similar to discourses around rape and sexual assault [Benedict, 1992; Ullman and Knight, 1993; Ward, 1995; Korn and Efrat, 2004], might result in the delegitimizing of women trafficked for sex as victims of crime.

However, women's identification as a victim of trafficking in Serbia depends not only on how much they fit into the ideal victim framework, but also on whether they will uphold such status in the criminal justice system.

10.2.1.2 *Maintaining Victim Status*

Practitioners in Serbia warn that once the construct of "sex slaves" fails before the court, women are promptly stripped of their victim status:

> The judge said: "They are not 'real' victims. I've seen them walking around in the park; ... they were free and could run away if they wanted to".... Then the lawyers tear (women) apart, they get confused and scared, don't know the language well enough, and that's it. They are all prostitutes.

Vesna Stanojevic
Shelter for Women Victims of Trafficking, Belgrade

Because women's experiences rarely mirror such extreme narratives, they need to prove that they are "genuine" victims. Usually that requires cooperation with law enforcement to establish that they did not contribute to victimization by engaging in illegal/immoral ventures such as illegal migration and sex work:

> It is a big burden to prove they are innocent. They can do it only if they accept to testify, and by exceptional efforts during the criminal procedure.

Respondent
Ministry of Labour, Belgrade

In this process of "cleansing," trafficked women have routinely been exposed to questions about their personal history and involvement in the sex industry. Practitioners in Serbia identified this reinforcement of the discourse of otherness before the court: Trafficked women are simply viewed as prostitutes who testify for money, visas, or permanent residence.

> The judge allowed a question (about the) victim's engagement in the sex industry three years ago. Legally speaking, that was irrelevant question.... In some cases those questions have an effect (to women's status and the outcome of the case), in some they don't.

Olivera Simonov
Attorney and victims' representative, Belgrade

Women who have voluntarily engaged in sex work prior to being trafficked are in an especially difficult position and that fact might disqualify them as both victims and/or witnesses:

> An attitude from public prosecutors and judges ... is that, if a woman has been involved in prostitution that is something that disqualifies her.

Olivera Simonov
Attorney, Belgrade, Serbia

The defence lawyers asked, "What were you doing in 2002?" and she said: "I was a prostitute." And they said: "This is the third time that you're a prostitute." Some judges don't allow such questions, some do, and then we engage in discussion about prostitution and morality—she got what was she looking for, she was playing with the devil.... That is the point where we might change our mind and start to think that maybe she really is somehow guilty?

Marija Andjelkovic
NGO ASTRA, Belgrade

However, some practitioners conclude that women's innocence in terms of their contribution to victimization sometimes plays no role in the criminal procedure: The bare fact that women have engaged in sex work, even against their will, is enough to disqualify them as victims. No matter how hard they try, victims of sex trafficking could never really be treated as such:

A victim's husband was a police officer. She was tricked to come to Serbia. Finally she managed to escape—she jumped (over the balcony) and injured her back. It was all irrelevant to the judge, didn't move him at all.

Tamara Vukasovic
NGO ASTRA, Belgrade

Women are treated as prostitutes, regardless of whether they entered prostitution voluntarily or not. An entirely different approach is used toward ... victims of family violence, compared to women who were ... prostitutes, even if it was forced prostitution.

Respondent
Ministry of Labour, Belgrade

10.3 Conclusion

Sex trafficking raises many issues in relation to women's sexuality, mobility, human rights, and representation [Kapur, 2005; Sanghera, 2005; Segrave and Milivojevic, 2005; Milivojevic and Pickering, 2008]. As Sanghera [2005:5] notes, "The dominant discourse of trafficking is based upon a set of assumptions. These, in a large measure, merely flow from unexamined hypotheses, shoddy research, anecdotal information, or strong moralistic positions."

This chapter highlights that women—potential victims of trafficking in Serbia—are constructed through contrasting processes of blaming the victim and the ideal victim [Christie, 1986]. They are located, according to their "traits" in relation to gender and performances of femininity, into two sharply divided discourses—the innocents and otherness. This dichotomy is believed to be facilitated by media representations of women trafficked for sex, predominant narratives set by international organizations and local NGOs engaged in combating trafficking, and xenophobia and patriarchy.

The discourse of innocents encloses three key identities—the abused, unfortunate, and blameless victim. The more these three identities intersect, the more likely it is for women who are victims of trafficking to be recognized as such by governmental agencies (police and the Service) and to maintain the victim status before the court. Those who fit the narrowly defined discourse of sex slaves and who have been severely abused, constructed as unfortunate, and perceived as blameless, both in terms of legality and morality of their actions, are certain candidates to be acknowledged as victims of crime in Serbia. Innocent and violated women's bodies are perceived as helpless, and the ideal victim narrative is a perfect tool for reinforcing a law and order agenda [Spalek, 2006:27] that aims to restore injured identities. Defining women as vulnerable, weak, abused, and under traffickers' unconditional control sets the response to trafficking firmly within this discourse, in which the prosecution of traffickers and the "rescuing" of victims are the main tasks of the nation-state.* However, criminalization, as Vernier [2006:38] argues:

> ... does not clearly provide for the prohibition of exploitation ... (but) tends to deny the very existence of such exploitation, and consequently, that of its victims, both symbolically (they are not recognized as victims) as well as practically (they are not protected as victims).

What antitrafficking initiatives based on a law and order response do succeed in, as indicated in this chapter, is to generate a range of categories of victims, with various degrees of legitimacy, and expose them to secondary victimization. The construction of the ideal victim of sex trafficking leaves those who do not fit into such a narrow category outside the system. The discourse of otherness incorporates three identities—the prostitute, the foreigner, and the unworthy. The more these identities intersect, the more women fall into the category of *lawbreakers*. Women's contribution to victimization through the choices they make—willing participation in sex work or illegal migration—makes them guilty and disqualifies them as victims of crime. To claim such status, women who fall into this category need to go through the process of "purification" by justifying wrong choices (engaging in sex work or illegal migrations) or recklessness in the migration processes, and/or are required to assist the authorities in the criminal proceedings.

Once before the court, trafficked women are compelled to prove they are genuine victims: This process of cleansing consists of exposing their personal and sexual history, and eliminating any illegal, immoral, or manipulative

---

* This "rescue," however, often implies objectification and silencing of victims of trafficking. For further discussion on this topic, see Segrave et al. [2009] *Sex trafficking: International context and response* (Willan).

elements that might jeopardize their perceived innocence. Mistreatment, insults, and threats are common incidents, and yet trafficked women in criminal proceedings often remain viewed simply as prostitutes.

This chapter argues that it is time to acknowledge sex trafficking "not as the enslavement of women, but as *the trade and exploitation of labor under conditions of coercion and force*, analyzed from the lives, agency, and rights of women and men who are involved in a variety of activities in a trans-nationalised world" [Kempadoo, 2005:viii–ix, original emphasis). It calls for deconstruction of contrasting and exclusive narratives that define women trafficked for sex and for understanding trafficking in its all complexities. Sex trafficking needs to be debated within the context of the reality of women's lives, particularly women from the global south, as they negotiate the challenges and changes of contemporary global developments [Wonders and Michalowski, 2001]. It is essential that the multiple identities of women trafficked for sex are acknowledged, and that women's victimization in the context of various forms of subordination and oppression is given a voice. In addition, it is necessary to give recognition to *all* strategies women use to survive, particularly those that are difficult to locate. The universal victim subject needs to be deconstructed, as narrowing women's experiences to mutually exclusive identities further violates women's rights.

In doing so, voices of women are the first necessary step, as they can provide us with firsthand testimonies and brave encounters of the complex matrix of victimization, criminalization, agency, and survival that characterizes trafficking in women for the purpose of sexual exploitation. We need women's voices in this debate, as such an approach will assist us in developing strategies that will truly respect and strengthen the human rights of women—victims and survivors of trafficking.

References

Abrams, C. 2005. Sex trafficking duo jailed, *The Sun Online*, November 2, http://www.thesun.co.uk/article/02-2005500738,00.html (accessed July 2, 2008).

Aghatise, E. 2004. Trafficking for prostitution in Italy: Possible effects of government proposal for legalization of brothels. *Violence against Women* 10(10):1126–55.

Agustin, L. 2005. Migrants in the mistress's house: Other voices in the trafficking debate. *Social Politics* 12(1):96–117.

Bales, K. 1999. *Disposable people: New slavery in the global economy.* Berkeley, Los Angeles, London: University of California Press.

Benedict, H. 1992. *Virgin or vamp: How the press covers sex crimes.* Oxford: Oxford University Press.

Bennett, T. 2004. Preventing trafficking in women and children in Asia: Issues and options. *Impact on HIV*, vol. 1, no. 2:9–13.

Bertone, A. M. 2000. Sexual trafficking in women: International political economy and the politics of sex. *Gender Issues* 18(1):4–22.

Bjerkan, L. (ed). 2005. *A life on one's own: Rehabilitation of victims of trafficking for sexual exploitation.* Oslo: Fafo.

Boyd, R. 2003. Implementation of the trafficking victims protection act. In Troubnikoff, A. (ed) *Trafficking in women and children: Current issues and development.* New York: Nova Science Publishers.

Campbell, A. 2005. Keeping the "lady" safe: The regulation of femininity through crime prevention literature. *Critical Criminology* 13(2):119–40.

Christie, N. 1986. The ideal victim. In *From crime policy to victim policy*, ed. E. Fattah. New York: St Martin's.

Clark, M. 2003. Trafficking in persons: An issue of human security. *Journal of Human Development* 4(2):247–63.

Coomaraswamy, R. (ed.). 2003. Fishing in the stream of migration: Modern forms of trafficking and women's freedom of movement. In *Stemming the tide or keeping the balance—The role of judges.* Fifth Conference of International Association of Refugee Law Judges, Wellington, New Zealand.

Coontz, P. and C. Griebel. 2004. International approaches to human trafficking: The call for a gender-sensitive perspective in international law. *Women's Health Journal* April:47–48.

Ćopić S. and V. Ristanovic-Nikolic. 2006. Mechanism for the monitoring of trafficking in human beings in Serbia. In *Mechanism for the monitoring of the trafficking in human beings phenomenon*, ed. J. Škrnjug. Belgrade: IOM.

Cunneen, C. 2001. *Conflict, politics and crime: Aboriginal communities and the police.* Crows Nest, Australia: Allen and Unwin.

Cyrus, N. and D. Vogel. 2006. Social working of criminal law on trafficking and smuggling in human beings in Germany. In *Immigration and criminal law in the European Union: The legal measures and social consequences of criminal law in member states on trafficking and smuggling in human beings*, ed. E. Guild and P. Minderhound. Leiden, Boston: Martinus Nijhoff.

Demleitner, N. 2001. The law at a crossroads: The construction of migrant women trafficked into prostitution. In *Global human smuggling: Comparative perspective*, ed. D. Kyle and R. Koslowskis. Baltimore, London: The Johns Hopkins University Press.

Ditmore, M. 2002. Trafficking and sex work: A problematic conflation, PhD thesis, City University New York, New York.

Doezema, J. 1998. Forced to choose: Beyond the voluntary v. forced prostitution dichotomy. In *Global sex workers: Rights, resistance, and redefinition*, ed. K. Kempadoo and J. Doezema. New York and London: Routledge.

_____. 2000. Loose women or lost women? The re-emergence of the myth of "white slavery" in contemporary discourses of trafficking in women. *Gender Issues* 18(1):23–50.

_____. 2002. Who gets to choose? Coercion, consent and the UN trafficking protocol. *Gender and Development* 10(1):20–27.

European Commission. 2001. Trafficking in women—The misery behind the fantasy: From poverty to sex slavery. European Commission, Justice and Home Affairs, http://ec.europa.eu/justice_home/news/8mars_en.htm (accessed July 2, 2007).

Feher, L. 2002. Trafficking in human beings in candidate countries. Paper presented to the EU/IOM STOP European Conference on Preventing and Combating Trafficking in Human Beings: A Global Challenge for the 21st Century, European Parliament, Brussels, Belgium, September 18–20.

Fergus, L. 2005. Trafficking in women for sexual exploitation. Australian Centre for the Study of Sexual Assault. Briefing Paper no. 5, June. Melbourne.

Goodey, J. 2003. Recognizing organized crime's victims: The case of sex trafficking in the EU. In *Transnational organized crime: Perspectives on global security* ed. A. Edwards and P. Gill. New York and London: Routledge.

_____. 2004. Sex trafficking in women from Central and East European countries: Promoting a "victim-centred" and "woman-centred" approach to criminal justice intervention. *Feminist Review* 76:26–45.

Guiraudon, V. 2006. Trafficking and smuggling in France: Social problems as transnational security issues. In *Immigration and criminal law in the European Union: The legal measures and social consequences of criminal law in member states on trafficking and smuggling in human beings*, ed. E. Guild and P. Minderhoud. Leiden, Boston: Martinus Nijhoff.

Gulcur, L. and P. Ilkkaracan. 2002. The "Natasha" experience: Migrant sex workers from the former Soviet Union and Eastern Europe in Turkey. *Women's Studies International Forum* 25(4):411–21.

Hawkesworth, M. 1990. *Beyond oppression: Feminist theory and political strategy*. New York: Continuum.

Hughes, D. 2001. The "Natasha" trade: Transnational sex trafficking. *National Institute of Justice Journal* 246: 9–15.

IOM Counter-Trafficking Service. 2004. *Changing patterns and trends of trafficking in persons in the Balkan region*. Geneva: IOM. http://www.iom.hu/PDFs/Changing%20Patterns%20in%20Trafficking%20in%20Balkan%20region.pdf.

Jeffreys, S. 2002. Women trafficking and the Australian connection: Do legalised sex industries encourage the trafficking of women and children? Are they partly to blame for the explosion in this trade over the last decade? Whose needs are being served by the legitimation of sex work? *Arena Magazine* 58 April–May:44–48.

Kantola, J. and J. Squires. 2004. Discourses surrounding prostitution policies in the UK. *European Journal of Women's Studies* 11(1):77–101.

Kapur, R. 2002. The tragedy of victimization rhetoric: Resurrecting the "native" subject in international/post-colonial feminist legal politics. *Harvard Human Rights Journal* 15:1–37.

_____. 2005. Cross-border movements and the law: Renegotiating the boundaries of difference. In *Trafficking and prostitution reconsidered: New perspectives on migration, sex work, and human rights*, ed. K. Kempadoo, J. Sanghera, and B. Pattanaik. Boulder, CO: Paradigm.

Kelly, L. 2002. Journeys of jeopardy: A review of research on trafficking in women and children in Europe. *IOM Migration Research Series*, no. 11:1–71.

Kelly, R., J. Maghan,. and J. Serio. 2005. *Illicit trafficking: A reference handbook*. Santa Barbara, CA: ABC.

Kempadoo, K. 2005. From moral panic to global justice: Changing perspectives on trafficking. In *Trafficking and prostitution reconsidered: New perspectives on migration, sex work, and human rights*, ed. K. Kempadoo, J. Sanghera, and B. Pattanaik. Boulder, CO: Paradigm.

King, G. 2004. *Woman, child for sale: The new slave trade in the 21st century.* New York: Chamberlain Bros.

Kleimenov, M. and S. Shamkov. 2005. Criminal transportation of persons: Trends and recommendations. In *Human traffic and transnational crime: Eurasian and American perspectives,* ed. S. Stoecker and L. Shelley. Boulder, CO: Rowman and Littlefield.

Konrad, H. 2002. *Trafficking in human beings: The ugly face of Europe.* Paper presented to the EU/IOM STOP European Conference on Preventing and Combating Trafficking in Human Beings: A Global Challenge for the 21st Century, European Parliament, Brussels, Belgium, September 18–20.

Korn, A. and S. Efrat. 2004. The coverage of rape in the Israeli popular press. *Violence against Women* 10(9):1056–74.

Kwon, L. 2005. Raising awareness on the reality of human trafficking. *The Christian Post,* October 27. http://www.christianpost.com/article/20051027/21440_Raising_Awareness_on_the_Reality_of_Human_Trafficking.htm (accessed July 2, 2008).

Lamb, S. 1996. *The trouble with blame: Victims, perpetrators, and responsibility.* Cambridge, MA and London: Harvard University Press.

Lehti, M. and K. Aromaa. 2003. Trafficking in women and children in Europe. In *Organized crime, trafficking, drugs: Selected papers presented at the Annual Conference of the European Society of Criminology, Heuni, Helsinki,* ed. S. Nevala and K. Aromaa.

Lindstrom, N. 2004. Regional sex trafficking in the Balkans: Transnational networks in an enlarged Europe. *Problems of Post-Communism* 51(3):45–52.

Long, L. 2004. Anthropological perspectives on the trafficking of women for sexual exploitation. *International Migration* 42(1):5–31.

Lyons, H. 1999. *The representation of trafficking in persons in Asia: Orientalism and other perils.* Re/productions, http://www.hsph.harvard.edu/Organisations/healthnet/SAsia/repro2/issue2.htm (accessed July 20, 2006).

Mendelson, S. 2005. *Barracks and brothels: Peacekeepers and human trafficking in the Balkans.* Washington, DC: Centre for Strategic and International Studies.

Milivojevic, S. and S. Pickering. 2008. Football and sex: The 2006 FIFA World Cup and Sex Trafficking. *Temida* 11(2):21–47.

Miller, A. 2004. Sexuality, violence against women, and human rights: Women make demands and ladies get protection. *Health and Human Rights* 7(2):17–47.

Murray, A. 1998. Debt-bondage and trafficking: Don't believe the hype. In *Global sex workers: Rights, resistance, and redefinition,* ed. K. Kempadoo and J. Doezema. New York and London: Routledge.

Nikolic-Ristanovic, V. 2005a. What victims went through and how they survived. In *A life on one's own: Rehabilitation of victims of trafficking for sexual exploitation,* ed. L. Bjerkan. Oslo: Fafo.

Nikolic-Ristanovic, V. 2005b. Trgovina ljudima u Srbiji: izmedju moralne panike i društvene strategije. *Temida* 8(4):5–14.

Nikolic-Ristanovic, V., S. Ćopić, S. Milivojevic, B. Simeunovic-Patic, and B. Mihic. 2004. *Trafficking in people in Serbia.* Belgrade: OSCE.

Oberholer, R. 2003. To counter effectively organized crime involvement in irregular migration, people smuggling and human trafficking from the east. Europe's challenges today. In *Organized crime, trafficking, drugs: Selected papers presented* at the Annual Conference of the European Society of Criminology, Heuni, Helsinki, ed. S. Nevala and K. Aromaa.

O'Connell Davidson, J. 2006. Will the real sex slave please stand up? *Feminist Review* 83:4–22.

Petersen, K. 2001. Trafficking in women: The Danish construction of Baltic prostitution. *Cooperation and Conflict* 36(2):213–38.

Renzetti, C. 1999. The challenge to feminism posed by women's use of violence in intimate relationships. In *New versions of victims: Feminist struggle with the concept*, ed. S. Lamb. New York, London: New York University Press.

Rijken, C. 2003. *Trafficking in persons: Prosecution from a European perspective*. The Hague: Asser.

Roby, J. 2005. Women and children in the global sex trade: Toward more effective policy. *International Social Work* 48(2):136–47.

Sanghera, J. 2005. Unpacking the trafficking discourse. In *Trafficking and prostitution reconsidered: New perspectives on migration, sex work, and human rights*, ed. K. Kempadoo, J. Sanghera, and B. Pattanaik. Boulder, CO: Paradigm.

Saunders, and G. Soderlund. 2003. Threat or opportunity? Sexuality, gender and the ebb and flow of trafficking as discourse. *Canadian Woman Studies* 22(3-4):16–24.

Segrave, M. and S. Milivojevic, S. 2005. Sex trafficking: A new agenda. *Social Alternatives* 24(2):11–16.

Segrave, M., S. Milivojevic, and S. Pickering. 2009. *Sex trafficking: International context and response*. Cullompton, UK: Willan.

Simeunovic-Patic, B. 2005. Protection, assistance and support of trafficked persons: Current responses. In *A life on one's own: Rehabilitation of victims of trafficking for sexual exploitation*, ed. L. Bjerkan. Oslo: Fafo.

Spalek, B. 2006. *Crime victims: Theory, policy and practice*. New York: Palgrave Macmillan.

Stanko, E. 1982. Would you believe this woman? Prosecutorial screening for "credible" witnesses and a problem of justice. In *Judge lawyer victim thief: Women, gender roles, and criminal justice*, ed. N. H. Rafter and E. Stanko. Boston: Northeastern University Press.

———. 1985. *Intimate intrusions: Women's experience of male violence*. London: Unwin Hyman.

Stoecker, S. 2005. Human trafficking: A new challenge for Russia and United States. In *Human traffic and transnational crime: Eurasian and American perspective*, ed. S. Stoecker and L. Shelley. Lanham, MD: Rowman and Littlefield.

Sullivan, B. 2003. Trafficking in women: Feminism and new international law. *International Feminist Journal of Politics* 5(1):67–91.

Surtees, R. 2005. *Second annual report on victims of trafficking in South-Eastern Europe*. Geneva: IOM.

Truong, T. 2001. *Human trafficking and organized crime*. ORPAS Institute of Social Studies Working Paper no. 339, July. Rotterdam: ORPAS.

Tyldum, G., M. Tveit, and A. Brunovskis. 2005. *Taking stock: A review of existing research on trafficking for sexual exploitation*. Oslo: Fafo.

Ullman, S. and R. Knight. 1993. The efficacy of women's resistance strategies in rape situations. *Psychology of Women Quarterly* 17(1):23–39.

UN Office on Drugs and Crime. 2006. *Toolkit to combat trafficking in persons*. New York: United Nations.

U.S. Department of State. 2004. *Trafficking in persons report.* Washington, DC: U.S. Department of State. http://www.state.gov/g/tip/rls/tiprpt/2004/ (accessed July 2, 2008).

_____. 2005. *Trafficking in persons report.* Washington DC: U.S. Department of State. http://www.state.gov/g/tip/rls/tiprpt/2005/ (accessed July 2, 2008).

_____. 2006. *Trafficking in persons report.* Washington DC: U.S. Department of State. http://www.state.gov/g/tip/rls/tiprpt/2006/ (accessed July 2, 2008).

_____. 2008. *Trafficking in persons report.* Washington DC: U.S. Department of State. http://www.state.gov/g/tip/rls/tiprpt/2008/ (accessed July 2, 2008).

U.S. House of Representatives Subcommittee on Africa, Global Human Rights and International Operations. 2006. Modern day slavery: Spotlight on the 2006 Trafficking in Persons Report. *Forced labor, and sex trafficking at the World Cup.* Washington, DC: U.S. House of Representatives, http://www.internationalrelations.house.gov/archives/109/28104.PDF (accessed July 2, 2008).

van den Anker, C. 2004. Contemporary slavery, global justice and globalisation. In *The political economy of new slavery,* ed. C. van den Anker. Houndmills, UK: Palgrave Macmillan.

Vernier, J. 2006. French criminal and administrative law concerning smuggling of migrants and trafficking in human beings: Punishing trafficked people for their protection? In *Immigration and criminal law in the European Union: The legal measures and social consequences of criminal law in member states on trafficking and smuggling in human beings,* ed. E. Guild and P. Minderhond. Leiden, Boston: Martinus Nijhoff.

Ward, C. 1995. *Attitudes toward rape: Feminist and social psychological perspectives.* London: Sage.

Wijers, M. 2004. An exploration of the meaning of a human rights based approach to trafficking. *GAATW Alliance News* December 22.

Wijers, M. and M. van Doorninck. 2002. Only rights can stop wrongs: A critical assessment of anti-trafficking strategies. Paper presented to the EU/IOM STOP European Conference on Preventing and Combating Trafficking in Human Beings—A Global Challenge for the 21st Century, European Parliament, Brussels, Belgium, September 18–20.

Wonders, N. and R. Michalowski. 2001. Bodies, borders, and sex tourism in a globalized world: A tale of two cities—Amsterdam and Havana. *Social Problems* 48(4):545–71.

Zhao, G. M. 2003. Trafficking of women for marriage in China: Policy and practice. *Criminal Justice* 3(1):83–102.

Occupational Victimization

11

RICHARD LUSIGNAN AND
JACQUES D. MARLEAU

Contents

11.1 Introduction

Work is part of the lifestyle of the majority of individuals living around us and aged between 16 and 65 years, and constitutes one of the main activities we practice regularly, if not daily. Our occupation influences not only the premises (cities, districts, buildings) that we visit and the people we meet (general public, clients, suppliers) but also the frequency, itinerary, and schedule of our travels. In light of all this, the importance, both epidemiological and etiological, of studying the phenomenon of socioprofessional victimization is clear.

In the present chapter the term *socioprofessional victimization* will be used to describe the criminal victimization to which a group of individuals sharing an occupational practice is exposed. The victimization in question can occur in work settings or outside these settings but in relation to professional practice. What do victimological theories tell us about individuals who become victims through their occupational activities? What are their jobs? Their income level? Their place of practice? Even more important, which preventive strategies can be implemented to reduce the risks of aggression?

Very few authors have studied this specific aspect of victimization. The few studies of victimization-related components in work settings indicate that victimization is linked to (1) the performance of tasks requiring contact with clients with a potential for violence (e.g., adult offenders, juvenile delinquents), and (2) occupations characterized by the handling of valuables or money (Baril, 1984; Ellenberger, 1954). Is it possible to extend our knowledge to other types of workers? Let us begin by an overview of the main victimological theories.

11.2 Choosing an Explanatory Model

By taking a closer look at the theoretical explanations provided by victimology, we can appreciate each formal model's internal consistency, ability to explain specific phenomena, and potential for sustaining preventive practices.

A comparative reading highlights the use made by each theory of the concept of exposure. In addition, most of these theories are based on multiple elements—the exact nature of which varies from author to author—which facilitate or hinder the commission of criminal acts. In these analyses we will use the distinctions introduced by Cusson [1990] to clarify key notions:

- *Opportunity* is the union, at a given time in a given space, of material circumstances favorable to the success of an offense.
- *Vulnerability* is the sum of a target's characteristics that favors the commission of the offense or the impunity of the offender.

The relationships between the concepts comprising the four main theoretical models in victimology are presented in Table 11.1.

Each of these theories identifies predisposing factors for victimization, although the specific nature and contribution of these factors vary from theory to theory. For Hindelang et al. [1978], our occupational or recreational activities shape our lifestyle and directly influence exposure to crime. In their model, association with unknown individuals is another predisposing factor and exerts a more immediate influence. According to these authors, certain

Table 11.1 Links between Victimological Theories

	Lifestyle Model [Hindelang et al., 1978]	Routine Activity Model [Cohen and Felson, 1979]	Victimogenic Opportunities Model [Cohen et al., 1981]	Dutch Model [Van Dijk and Steinmetz, 1979]
Opportunities of victimization	Lifestyle (e.g., the pursuit of occupational and recreational activities) determines our exposure to places and times with high risks of victimization: direct incidence on victimization	Presence of potential offenders Multiple conditions that make targets vulnerable	Geographic proximity with potential offenders The degree of exposure, e.g., visibility and access to persons or goods yearned for Perceived attractiveness of the target, e.g., symbolic or material value, capacity to resist	Proximity: in relation both to space and social relationship, e.g., the amount of time devoted by teenagers and young adults to leisure activities, women's rights, urbanization Exposure, e.g., the opportunity to commit a crime when the offender comes into contact with his or her victim; combines both technical components (e.g., unlocked doors) and social aspects (neighborhood watch, police surveillance) Attraction aroused within the offender varies according to the type of offense planned
Factors of vulnerability	Lifestyle (e.g., the pursuit of occupational and recreational activities) determines the prevalence of our associations with potential offenders: point incidence of victimization	Absence of guardians able to protect the target	Presence of deterrent elements	

offenses (e.g., car theft) can be explained entirely—that is, independently of the presence of potential offenders—based on the probability of finding oneself in a high-risk place at a high-risk time. In addition, certain violent crimes can be explained by the prevalence of associations with unknown persons who share interests or leisure activities with the victim.

Dutch authors have also posited that exposure to crime, through technical and social victimogenic opportunities, is sufficient to explain victimization. For Van Dijk and Steinmetz [1979], proximity means sharing the same space but is also related to lifestyles and social roles (e.g., urbanization, women's rights) that favor a greater number of contacts with unknown people. In this context, exposure has two meanings: a technical meaning, for example, the locking or concealment of goods, and a social meaning related to police or neighborhood surveillance. Here, the attractiveness of the victim—for example, for the purposes of burglary—is evaluated through the lens of the offender's perceptions and the type of offense contemplated. The offender's perceptions constitute an important part of the victimization process.

Other victimological theories posit specific etiological contributions. According to Cohen and Felson [1979], exposure to crime can create an opportunity for crime. In a more recent publication, Cohen, Kluegel, and Land [1981] extended this analysis, with exposure seen as a predisposing factor consisting of a geographic component (proximity), visibility, access to targeted goods or persons, and the target's perceived attractiveness to the potential offender. On the other hand, victimization, as defined by these authors, comprises a vulnerability factor that triggers the infraction. In this respect, Cohen and Felson [1979] stress the importance of the absence of guardians able to protect the target, whereas Cohen et al. [1981] suggest factors that inhibit victimization. These factors include the presence of deterrent elements likely to protect the target and offense-specific characteristics (e.g., burglary requires more planning than does shoplifting) [Cohen et al., 1981].

Having identified the overall similarities and specificities of these theories, we will now review each of these models.

11.2.1 The Lifestyle Model

This model is based on the lifestyle of the victim and their sociodemographic characteristics, particularly (1) the expected behaviors of persons with various social roles; (2) the constraints to behavior attendant on economic status, education, and family obligations; and (3) the adaptation of individuals and their subcultures to behavioral and structural constraints.

This theory offers a general model of criminal victimization. According to Hindelang et al. [1978], each social actor has his or her own lifestyle based on his or her daily occupational or recreational activities.

Furthermore, these general conditions determine the degree of exposure to crime and the prevalence of associations, based on age and shared interests, with unknown people (including potential offenders). Here, the type of places (public or private), the time of the day (day, evening, or night), and the prevalence of contact with unknown people will present direct or ad hoc opportunities of victimization.

The extent to which a given lifestyle is victimogenic depends on the level of exposure of the victim and the degree to which potential victims associate with potential offenders. Thus, in a North American context, a white worker in his or her 40s who is married and living in the suburbs does not have the same risk of victimization as does an unemployed member of a visible minority who is in his or her 20s, single, and living downtown. Lifestyle—and especially employment status—has a major impact on the amount of time available for leisure activities. Exposure to high-risk places at high-risk times and the frequency of leisure activities all contribute to overall exposure to crime. Finally, the probability of meeting unknown people and potential offenders, itself influenced by age and shared interests, is also a determinant of the risk differential of the two profiles.

In addition, each actor has to adapt to expected roles and structural constraints, both as an individual and as a member of a group. This adaptation determines, among others, the individual's fear of crime and beliefs about the social reality of crime. These beliefs and attitudes later become part of the daily routine of the actor and the group to which he or she belongs.

Despite its limits, discussed below, this model has opened new avenues of research. The works of Hindelang, Gottfredson, and Garofalo set a trend since revisited by all victimologists [Van Dijk and Steinmetz, 1979; Cohen et al., 1981], who used empirical data gathered by victimization surveys in North America or Europe.

The contribution of Cohen and Felson [1979] is different from that of this first group because they were trying to understand the persistence of criminal activity in the midst of a decade of economic growth (1960–1968) and sustained educational and financial progress in all sectors of the American population. Their explanatory schema is based on the gradual transformation of common daily activities; this initial work was revised by Cohen et al. [1981] using data from victimization surveys.

11.2.2 The Routine Activity Model

Starting from different premises, Cohen and Felson's analysis of the evolution of goods, services, and social transformations (women's right, urbanization) leads them to propose an explanatory theory based on the modification of routine activities. In their view, the probability of victimization is linked to daily activities and routine behaviors. In this context, "routine activities" are important recurrent activities that contribute to the satisfaction of individual and collective needs. Bearing no relation to the cultural or racial origins of the individuals considered, these activities fashion everyday life. Such routine activities concern work; the search for food, shelter, and sexual partners; leisure activities; social interaction; personal education; and the education of children.

According to Cohen and Felson, structural changes in daily activities influence crime rates by modifying the convergence in space and time of the minimal defining elements of direct victimization. These elements create opportunities for victimization or contribute to the immediate vulnerability of targets. The presence of a potential offender and of targets that are desirable (because of their value, proximity, accessibility, or low capacity for defense) creates opportunities for victimization, whereas the absence of dissuasive factors (technical or human) has a direct impact on the vulnerability of victims or their belongings.

This theory encompasses the essential factors present in each incident of victimization. The underlying concepts are simple and can easily be used to shed new light on descriptive studies based on data closely related to particular settings. Although this theoretical vision can be qualified as minimalist, it can easily be transformed into a preventive intervention tool or be linked to concepts established by other victimologists, such as Van Dijk and Steinmetz [1979] or Cohen et al. [1981].

11.2.3 The Victimogenic Opportunities Model

In 1981, Cohen et al. published a study integrating explanations derived from the lifestyle and routine activity models. These authors identified five factors strongly related to opportunities for direct victimization: the degree of exposure (visibility and access to persons or goods), geographic proximity of potential offenders, presence of deterrent elements, perceived attractiveness of the target (e.g., symbolic or material value, capacity to resist), and characteristics of the offense that constrain its execution (inherent complexity of the planned offense).

Using bivariate and multivariate analysis, the authors meticulously investigated the impact of variables such as income, race, and age on the risks of victimization. Their results attest to the complex relationship between demographic variables and probabilities of victimization. For example, high income decreases (assault), increases (theft), or has a variable effect (burglary) on the possibilities of victimization (high probabilities for low and high incomes, lower probabilities for median incomes). These results highlight the multidimensional character of reality, as well as some pitfalls of victimological research.

11.2.4 The Dutch Model

The previous models shared American origins. However, there is a Dutch variant of these explanatory models. In a series of studies whose publication began in 1979, Van Dijk and Steinmetz analyzed victimization surveys conducted between 1974 and 1979. They observed a decisive effect on the risk of victimization when five factors are present simultaneously: proximity (geographic or social), exposure (technical or social), and attraction of the offender toward the crime he is planning to commit.

This concludes our overview of the theoretical explanations of victimization. In the next section, we examine empirical findings related to occupational victimization.

11.3 Occupational Victimization: The Global Picture

To proceed to the empirical measurement of this phenomenon, one has to resolve many different methodological issues. Specifically, a central issue is ensuring a sample of workers large enough to compensate for the low base rates of criminal victimization.

The study realized by Block, Felson, and Block [1985] uses samples gathered from a total of more than 2 million respondents over nine annual surveys of victimization [1973–1981]. From this master sample, the individuals holding a paid position at the time of their victimization were retained. These respondents represent 256 occupations; 120 other occupations each representing fewer than 50,000 workers were excluded from the analysis. The subgroup retained represents 40% (108,000/270,000) of the victimization events reported.

To our knowledge, this research was the first and only one to delve into socioprofessional victimization. The researchers reported the prevalence of victimized workers in specific given occupations, although, as in any victimization survey, the criminal acts reported by the respondents may have occurred in settings outside the workplace. Although the study by Block et al. [1985] does not answer all the questions raised in this chapter, it provides 1,230 occupation-specific victimization rates. This contribution to victimological knowledge is unique.

The results from this study allow us to draw an overall picture of occupational victimization by identifying occupations more or less at risk. After reviewing the overall findings, we will focus on the teaching profession as a detailed example of socioprofessional victimization.

The results obtained by Block et al. [1985] are presented in Table 11.2. We have codified the rates of occupational victimization reported by Block and his team and broken down these prevalences by the occupation of the

Table 11.2 Rates of Victimization by Occupation

	Robbery	Assault	Burglary	Larceny	Car Theft
Less-victimized workers	Opticians, stenographer, radio operators	Farmers, dentists, clergymen, secretaries, tool and die makers	Repairmen of farm implements, chemical engineers, telephone linemen	Barbers, repairmen of farm implements, data-processing equipment repairmen, dentists	Farm laborers, power linemen and cable men, millwrights
Annual rates of victimization per 1,000 workers	0	Between 6 and 12	Between 20 and 31	Between 107 and 121	2 or 3
Most-victimized workers	Busboys, recreation and amusement attendants, taxicab drivers, dishwashers	Sheriffs and bailiffs, police officers, recreation and amusement attendants, busboys	Recreation and amusement attendants, demonstrators, athletes	Recreation and amusement attendants, busboys, athletes	Demonstrators, hucksters and peddlers, athletes
Annual rates of victimization per 1,000 workers	Between 32 and 58	Between 316 and 346	Between 193 and 232	Between 783 and 1,331	Between 35 and 46
Annual median rate of victimization for 246 occupations	8	34	64	222	14

Source: Data from Block, R. et al., *Sociology and Social Research* 69(3):442–51, 1985.

respondent and the type of offense reported (robbery, assault, burglary, larceny, and car theft). We must also point out that these events were recorded regardless of whether the offense was actually attempted.

For each type of offense, the range of occupation-specific victimization rates is reported. For any given offense, the median rate of victimization is always lower than the mean rate, which clearly indicates distributions characterized by negative skews—indicating that a few occupations share the highest rates of victimization. Beyond these technical considerations, the analysis of the data reveals some characteristics shared by the occupations of the more victimized individuals that are not found within the occupations of respondents reporting lesser victimization rates.

11.3.1 Epidemiological Considerations

Workers who annually report the highest rates of robbery (between 3.2% and 5.8%) share occupations involving some kind of contact with the public. This type of contact—specific to restaurant staff, taxicab drivers, and attendants of recreational and amusement parks—can easily be associated with the concepts of exposure (visibility of and access to the targeted victim) and lack of dissuasive means, as described by Cohen and Felson [1979]. By contrast, opticians, stenographers, and radio operators all exhibit the lowest rates of victimization for robbery (0%). These latter occupations have in common work done alone or with a few collaborators. In this sense, the reduction of the probabilities of victimization appears to be at least partially dependent on the reduction of exposure to strangers.

Similar to robbery, the crime of assault appears linked to occupations in the service sector (attendants of recreational and amusement parks) and law enforcement and legal occupations (police officers, sheriffs, bailiffs). On an annual basis, between 31% and 34% of the individuals working in these types of occupations report events of victimization. Performing tasks related to the surveillance of goods or persons or to the application of penal or civil norms—in short, to assuming the role of a guardian (visible and accessible) or an agent of the judiciary system—increases the risks of physical assaults initiated by either the worker or an offender. These workers can also exert a symbolic attraction (the personification of the established order) for certain individuals. In contrast, farmers, dentists, clergymen, and secretaries all share the advantage of a much more peaceful work life and exhibit probabilities of violent victimization at the low end of the scale (0.6–1.2%). These workers have a limited network of collaborators and are not involved in the application of penal or judiciary norms.

For their part, offenses related to place of residence particularly affect people who are away from home for long periods, travel the country as attendants or representatives, or participate in sports-related events (professional athletes). These business trips probably involve personal vehicles because the occupations in question (including traveling salesmen) also share high rates of car theft.

In fact, professional athletes—who are absent from their residences while traveling and associate with unknown individuals in foreign places—appear to be frequent victims of various crimes against property. This victimization could be explained by the cumulative effects of exposure (access to their belongings while they are absent) and unfamiliar associations.

The workers reporting the least victimization related to crimes against property are characterized by the performance of solitary work or work involving a limited circle of collaborators (repairmen of farm implements or data-processing equipment, telephone linemen).

Another way to analyze the results of Block et al. [1985] is to calculate, for each type of offense, the ratio of each occupation's annual victimization rate to the median annual rate of victimization for all of the 246 workforce categories combined. This analysis reveals that the rates in most victimized occupations are 3 (car theft, burglary) to 10 times (assault) higher than the median rate for all occupations. By contrast, robberies and larceny present intermediate rates located between four and seven times the overall median.

These results tend to confirm the hypothesis of a close relationship between the type of work and violent victimization. For example, working with the public or in restaurants increases the probability of violent victimization by a factor of 10. In comparison, being away from one's residence (athletes, representatives of all kinds) has a lower impact (factor of 3) on the commission of crimes against property (burglary, car theft).

The relationship between occupational rates of victimization and the creation of specific etiological equations remains largely unexplored but is an interesting avenue for further research.

11.3.2 Etiological Considerations

From a victimological point of view, the occupation of park attendant at a recreational or amusement site is exceptional. This group of workers has one of the highest victimization rates in four of five offense categories (the exception being car theft). Our conception of this particular type of work involves the meeting of victims and offenders, each busily following their own course of activities until their paths overlap, as a result of sharing common spaces and time frames.

It could be interesting to further study the different types of workers gathered together under this umbrella designation. Many questions remain unanswered: Are the majority of workers in this category traveling fair workers? Are they guardians of urban theme parks? Or guardians of sport complexes? Are they seasonal nomads or municipal blue-collar workers?

Without minimizing the common association of teenagers and tourists with these work contexts, we are under the impression that the most victimized targets are seasonal nonunionized workers. Because they are not unionized, these workers have no means of negotiating additional security measures or obtaining other types of compensation (monetary or otherwise).

According to this perspective, victimized persons are characterized by the absence of means to prevent their victimization or to obtain compensation for its consequences. The time that these workers spend at work is entirely spent in public places and consists of the surveillance of properties belonging to their employer. This occurs in the context of leisure activities, festivities, and alcohol consumption (e.g., national holidays, regional fairs, sporting events).

This kind of context brings together many conditions related to victimization, both violent (robbery, assault) and nonviolent (burglary, larceny). Moreover, at the time of their victimization, these workers may be nomads or seasonal workers ("just passing through"): Their victimization does not mobilize local police departments or raise a commotion in the surrounding community.

For the remainder of this chapter, we will look at the victimization of teaching professionals from kindergarten through university level. As most readers have been in contact with teachers of different levels starting from a young age, we believe that this occupation can provide a good example of the application of victimology to the explanation and prevention of crime in work settings. Also, the time spent by students in school sometimes exceeds the time spent at home; therefore, some personal observations can add contextual knowledge to the situations described. This possibility would have been restricted for most readers had we chosen medical (e.g., hospital, day center) or correctional settings as detailed examples of this approach.

11.4 Victimization of Teachers

In the following pages we will try to answer two types of queries. First, what is the situation of teachers belonging to five different levels of teaching (kindergarten, elementary, high school, college/university, continuous/adult teaching)? The reference point is the incidence of victimization reported by Block et al. [1985]. Second, what hypotheses can explain the commission of different types of offenses (robbery, assault, burglary, larceny, car theft)? This analysis takes as its starting point the organizational characteristics of each occupation (e.g., sex ratio, times of the day at work, age, or type of students). Our general model of interpretation is the routine activity model as elaborated by Cohen and Felson [1979]: This model places daily activities (whether occupational or recreational) at the center of the risk of victimization.

Block et al.'s data on the teaching profession are presented in Table 11.3. These researchers collected information from both public and private sectors of education throughout the United States. At first glance, there are two high-risk zones of victimization for teachers compared with all 246 occupations. On the one hand, in the case of larceny, the rate for every level of teaching is higher than the global median, indicating the existence of a predilection toward the victimization of these professionals. On the other hand, college and university professors consistently exhibit higher rates of victimization compared with their colleagues at other levels, regardless of the type of offense. From these results, we deduce that teaching at the college/university level offers more opportunities (predisposing factors) for victimization and comprises more factors of vulnerability (triggering factors).

Finally, it is the convergence in space and time of three elements that constitute the victimogenic equation: a potential offender, a target coveted for different reasons (proximity, access, visibility, symbolic value, restraints relating to the type of offense planned), and the absence of dissuasive factors able to protect the target from victimization [Cohen and Felson, 1979].

We must immediately clarify that a given rate of victimization does not imply that the victim will be victimized by his or her own students. Rather, it means that the general constraints of the occupation (e.g., traveling time, location of school, location of parking lot, lighting system) bring workers into contact with potential and unknown offenders. Alternatively, we must also consider that the hours spent at the site of work can leave one's properties unguarded, which facilitates, for example, residential burglary during class hours on a school day.

Table 11.3   Teaching Level, Rates, and Types of Victimization

Rate per 1,000 Teachers	Robbery	Assault	Burglary	Larceny	Car Theft
College/ university	14	109	136	668	26
High school	3	34	46	240	10
Elementary school	2	20	54	238	10
Kindergarten	4	22	86	289	17
Adults/continuing education	7	28	62	253	5
Median victimization rate	8	34	64	222	14

Source: Data from Block, R. et al., *Sociology and Social Research* 69(3):442–51, 1985.

11.4.1 Robbery

By definition, this offense involves obtaining goods through the use of verbal threats or intimidation. University professors exhibit an annual victimization rate 1.75 times the general median for all occupations considered. The sex ratio in this group of teachers is probably close to one; thus, we must look for explanations other than the defensive capacity of the victims. Universities are public places where a high volume of students gather each day, work schedules are variable, changes of location are frequent, and alcohol may be consumed (e.g., either on campus or nearby in fraternity clubs, bars, pubs, carnivals). These teachers' work environment is accessible to the public 24 hours a day, 7 days a week. They leave or get to work according to highly personalized schedules, and they must travel from parking lots to offices, classrooms, or libraries. All these conditions define situations in which teachers can find themselves in isolated places where potential offenders await a victim.

11.4.2 Assault

The definition generally used of this offense in research is the striking of a victim with a part of the body (e.g., feet, fists, head). Again, university professors exhibit a rate higher (3.2 times) than the general median of all the occupations analyzed. The rate of aggression toward high school teachers is equal to the aforementioned median.

Adding to the elements previously described, we must consider the importance of issues related to obtaining good grades: the impact on students' short-, mid-, and long-term prospects; on obtaining a scholarship; or on idealized or material success, and the multiple cultural shades of failure (e.g., foreign students, national scholarship). In short, many underevaluated, because underrecognized, conflict-generating factors appear to be at play here.

11.4.3 Burglary

This offense is defined as the entry into the residence or workplace of a victim to steal his or her property. University professors hold first place, with a victimization rate of 2.1 times the median rate of all other occupations studied; they are followed by kindergarten teachers, who show a victimization rate 1.34 times the median norm.

The work schedule of university professors is generally more variable than that of other types of teachers. According to our explanatory hypotheses, this could prove a protective factor for residences or offices. During the fall and winter semester, time spent at the workplace is important but less predictable by a potential offender.

In contrast, during the summer semester, traveling out of the country (e.g., on annual vacations, on sabbatical leave, or while attending congresses outside the city, state, province, or country) can add to the risks of victimization by way of a burglary at the workplace or in the community.

11.4.4 Larceny

This criminal act refers to the unauthorized seizure of objects belonging to the victim. This type of offense, as mentioned earlier, is widespread in the general field of teaching. The respective annual rates of victimization reported by teachers of all levels are all superior to the general median; first place again goes to university professors, who have a 67% risk of being victims of larceny in any given year (3.01 times the median).

Here, the main explanation is related to the symbolic value of teachers' possessions. With regard to potential offenders, our suspicions center on the student population and on the ambivalent relationship some of them develop with their teachers. A pencil, a wallet, a handbag, a laptop ... each of these can embody the teacher and constitute a student's coveted target.

11.4.5 Car Theft

This category refers to a specific category of theft. University teachers exhibit an annual victimization rate 1.9 times the general median of all other occupations. Kindergarten teachers are also above the median by a factor of 1.2.

Our hypotheses are essentially the same as those advanced for larceny and burglary and are related to the duration of accessibility of cars in parking lots or at the victims' residences (including as a result of carpooling).

11.5 Discussion of the Application of Victimological Models to Work Settings

Theory building is still an ongoing process in the field of victimology. To successfully transfer our theoretical knowledge and assumptions to the real world, the preventionist in us has to deal successfully with different limits. First, one has to make use of studies published between 1950 and 1980, which rely heavily on demographic variables (age, race, level of income, civil status) as the basis for hypothetical lifestyles. By comparison, more recent publications use other, directly measurable, indicators, such as quantification of moments and activities of leisure [Miethe and Meier, 1990], presence of offending activities (violence, theft, vandalism), and alcohol consumption [Sampson and Lauritsen, 1990]. The turning point is located with the publication in

1981 of the works of Cohen and his collaborators: Their use of bivariate and multivariate analysis has led us to a world of finer nuances.

Second, we must consider the structure of the community in which victimization occurs. Smith and Jarjoura [1988] drew on research published in the 1930s and 1940s by Clifford R. Shaw and Henry D. McKay. This perspective emphasizes the notions of poverty, residential mobility, and racial heterogeneity. The results of Smith and Jarjoura demonstrate that social disorganization intervenes through a series of conditional relationships: Poverty is associated with violence but not with burglary, residential mobility affects violence and burglary, and racial heterogeneity is associated with burglary but not violence.

In general, researchers have found that replacing demographic indicators with more specific variables improves the understanding of victimization. Examples of such indicators include the proportion of single-parent families, numerical presence of the 12–20 age group, and population density [Smith and Jarjoura, 1988]. Lynch [1987] comes to similar conclusions about work victimization: Contact with the public, manipulation of valuables, and geographical mobility all improve our predictive capacities compared with reliance on sociodemographic factors.

We must also be aware that victimological models presume the stability of the criminal motivation of potential offenders. Victimization is presented as a linear result of routine activities and victimogenic opportunities that transform some individuals into vulnerable targets in the absence of protecting elements. In the same line of ideas, the role given to victims excludes the choices made by them in light of their own perceptions of the probability of victimization.

This rigid dichotomist conception of aggressor and victim does not incorporate the reversibility of the roles of offender and victim; this is true even though many studies have demonstrated an increase in the probability of victimization with the leading of a marginal or criminal lifestyle [Jensen and Brownfield, 1986; Sampson and Lauritsen, 1990; Fattah, 1991].

As we move closer to the occupational dimension of victimization, we realize that victimological models offer us rudimentary sketches of possible lifestyles: More work needs to be done to provide a larger and more thorough understanding of the relationships between lifestyles and work occupations.

11.6 Conclusion

Of a universe of 246 occupations studied by Block et al. [1985], we have identified some victimogenic trends and hypotheses related to work activity.

Above all, the present chapter has allowed us to underscore the importance of the socioprofessional perspective in victimology and the exceptional value of strategic analysis as applied to the workplace and beyond. We truly believe that it is possible to estimate the level and the type of criminal activities of a city district, a street, or a square by analyzing the ongoing occupations conducted on these premises. Furthermore, by improving our knowledge of occupational behaviors it becomes possible to develop specific prevention projects tailored to the specific risks and needs of different populations of workers.

References

Baril, M. 1984. *L'envers du crime. Les Cahiers de recherche criminologiques*, No 2. Montréal: Centre International de Criminologie Comparée.

Block, R., M. Felson, and C. R. Block. 1985. Crime victimization rates for incumbents of 246 occupations. *Sociology and Social Research* 69(3):442–51.

Cohen, L. E. and M. Felson. 1979. Social change and crime rate trends: A routine activity approach. *American Sociological Review* 44:588–608.

Cohen, L. E., J. R. Kluegel, and K. C. Land. 1981. Social inequality and predatory criminal victimization: An exposition and test of a formal theory. *American Sociological Review* 46:505–24.

Cusson, M. 1990. *Croissance et décroissance du crime*. Paris: Presses Universitaires de France.

Ellenberger, H. 1954. Relations psychologiques entre le criminel et la victim. *Revue Internationale de Criminologie et de Police Technique* 8:103–21.

Fattah, E. A. 1991. *Understanding criminal victimization*. Scarborough, ON: Prentice Hall.

Hindelang, M. J., M. R. Gottfredson, and J. Garofalo. 1978. *Victims of personal crimes: An empirical foundation for a theory of personal victimization*. Cambridge, MA: Ballinger.

Jensen, G. F. and D. Brownfield. 1986. Gender, lifestyles, and victimization: Beyond routine activity. *Violence and Victims* 1(2):85–99.

Lynch, J. P. 1987. Routine activity and victimization at work. *Journal of Quantitative Criminology* 3(4):283–300.

Miethe, T. D. and R. F. Meier. 1990. Opportunity, choice, and criminal victimization: A test of a theoretical model. *Journal of Research in Crime and Delinquency* 27:243–66.

Sampson, R. J. and J. L. Lauritsen. 1990. Deviant lifestyles, proximity to crime and the offender-victim link in personal violence. *Journal of Research in Crime and Delinquency* 27:110–39.

Smith, D. A. and G. R. Jarjoura. 1988. Social structure and criminal victimization. *Journal of Research in Crime and Delinquency* 25:27–52.

Van Dijk, J. J. M. and C. H. D. Steinmetz. 1982. *Victimization surveys: Beyond measuring the volume of crime*. The Hague: Research and Documentation Center of the Dutch Ministry of Justice.

Tourism and Victimization

12

ROB I. MAWBY, ELAINE BARCLAY,
AND CAROL JONES

Contents

12.1 Introduction

The 2004/2005 International Crime Victim Survey (ICVS) found that 15.7% of respondents had been the victim of at least one crime in the preceding year [van Dijk, van Kesteren, and Smit, 2008]. That is, the average member of the public could expect to experience at least one crime every 6 or 7 years. However, this average hides marked variations. Risk varies according to a number of variables: country of residence, where within a country one lives, age, gender, ethnicity, etc. To explain these patterns, victimologists have focused on citizens' behavior and the way that they spend their time as leading to an increase or decrease in risk of victimization. As travel and tourism become more significant features of modern-day living, it is therefore surprising that criminologists have largely ignored the relationship between tourism/travel and crime.* Unlike tourism researchers, for whom crime and deviance appear to hold considerable attraction [Ryan, 1993; Pizam and Mansfeld, 1996; Brunt and Hambly, 1999; Mansfeld and Pizam, 2006], criminologists have, with a few notable exceptions, avoided discussions of tourism as a crime generator. Even studies of antisocial behavior have tended to ignore tourists as offenders and tourist resorts as crime and disorder hotspots. True, a few victimologists have made reference to tourism in passing. For example, in the first edition of his text, Karmen [1984:66] noted that "tourists are notoriously vulnerable people," especially because they will be unwilling to return to give evidence should a case come to trial. By the third edition, he added that tourists' "less careful lifestyle," combined with general ignorance of risky locations, further explained their disproportionate risk [Karmen 1996:39].

This suggests that further consideration of the relationship between tourism and victimization is important for at least two reasons: first, because it can inform tourism academics and practitioners; and, second, because in identifying the various ways in which tourism impacts on risk, it can contribute to victimological theory. To this end, this chapter is divided into three key sections. In the first, we consider the ways in which victimologists have identified differential levels of risk, and we supplement these with findings on tourists as victims. Then, we describe how victimologists have attempted to explain these differential levels of risk and broaden these theories to apply them to tourists. Finally, we draw on four case studies to speculate and, to a limited extent, illustrate how the notion of the "average tourist" can be deconstructed, such that different levels of risk might be associated with different subgroups of tourists.

12.2 Identifying Differential Risk

In attempting to identify high-risk targets, researchers have adopted a variety of approaches. One involves asking known offenders to choose between potential targets and justify their choices. This approach, particularly common among burglary researchers, entails at least two disadvantages. First, most studies depend on interviews with arrested offenders, where it might be that more successful offenders (i.e., those who have not been caught) would reveal a different pattern, or with surrogates, such as students, who may make decisions on very different criteria. Second, subjects may not be

---

* There is considerable debate within the tourism literature over definitions of *tourism* and *tourist,* and whether, for example, those on business trips, visiting relatives, or attending mass events (such as the Football World Cup) should be classified as tourists. Here we use a broad definition, although clearly in some cases behavioral dimensions will vary.

entirely honest in their declarations, not necessarily because they set out to mislead the researcher but because they may exaggerate the extent to which they make rational and informed decisions. That said, research, particularly more recent studies using high-tech equipment [Lee and Lee, 2008], has much to offer theory.

The additional problem with applying this approach in the case of tourism, however, is that unlike, for example, burglary, it is difficult to identify a group of offenders who specialize in this offense. Consequently, researchers are reliant on the perspectives of offenders in general. That said, there is some limited evidence that tourists are considered worthwhile targets. Pickpocketing is a case in point. Inciardi [1976], for example, in an early study involving interviews with 20 pickpockets from Miami, noted that the professional pickpocket specifically targeted tourists, identified through their attitude, dress, and behavior. Similarly, Dusquesne's [1995] research on pickpocketing and purse snatching in France identified tourists as one of the targets of the thieves. Harper [2000, 2006], a tourism researcher, provides a similar picture vis-à-vis choice of targets by New Orleans' robbers.

Nevertheless, most research into differential risk focuses on data on crime victims. Traditionally, this relied on official statistics. However, as criminologists have demonstrated [Coleman and Moynihan, 1996], these data are clearly suspect, and some are more suspect than others. Whether a crime is recorded and subsequently becomes part of official statistics depends on the willingness of someone (usually the victim) to report it to the police and the willingness of the police to record incidents as crimes. Some property crimes, such as car thefts and successful burglaries, are likely to be reported in most cases. Violent offenses, particularly violent sex offenses, are subject to considerably more discretion and may remain unreported (by victims) or unrecorded (by police) and are thereby suspect, although in extreme cases data on crimes such as homicide provide valuable details about victims and their relationship with perpetrators [e.g., Karmen, 1996]. Moreover, if recorded crime patterns depend to some extent on the discretionary behavior of victims (to report) and police (to look for and record crime), individual and policy changes might have a considerable impact on crime statistics. For example, if the police respond to a perceived "crime problem" by cracking down on street crime, recorded crime may increase irrespective of any changes to actual crime levels. Alternatively, just as insurance requirements may be a major reason for reporting crime in general, so tourists may be influenced by whether they have travel insurance and different excess clauses.

Given the inherent weaknesses of police statistics, a more common approach is to compare police data with alternative sources. One popular alternative is to use victim surveys, such as the British Crime Survey (BCS) and the ICVS, which involve interviewing large samples of the public about crimes they have experienced. Crime data for England and Wales, for example, are now annually presented in a Home Office Statistical Bulletin. This confirms considerable variations in risk across the general population. For example, police records reveal marked regional differences, and BCS data show risks to be greater in urban than rural areas, and in the former to be highest in more deprived areas. On an individual level, the BCS also reveals distinct patterns: For example, victims of violent and sexual offenses are dispropor-tionately males, aged 16–24 years, nonwhite, single, and students or unem-ployed [Nicholas, Kershaw, and Walker, 2007].

Identifying the extent to which being a tourist is related to victimization is, however, even more problematic. Police data incorporate crimes committed by or against tourists but are unlikely to discriminate between these and more permanent residents. The police may use their discretion to record either the home or temporary address and do not routinely flag cases involving tourists. Even if they did, however, it would be difficult to quantify risk because figures on the numbers of tourists in an area, as well as their length of stay, are rarely available. There are exceptions. In the United States, for example, it is possible to get a fairly accurate picture of tourism in Florida because approximately 20,000 interviews are conducted annually at airports and on the highways with non-resident visitors before their departure [Schiebler, Crofts, and Hollinger, 1996]. Interviews cover details of each city or county in Florida visited, enabling the researcher to identify tourist concentrations. However, even here, because the length of time spent in each area does not appear to be recorded, it is impossible to construct victimization rates that are directly comparable with those of local residents. Yet if no count is made of the average number of tourists in an area in a specified period, crime rates will be exaggerated for the obvious reason that no account of numbers of tourists is built into the denominator.

Population surveys are even less likely to identify tourists. National or international surveys like the BCS and ICVS will generally capture crimes committed against respondents when on holiday but do not *distinguish* them as such. Local surveys, such as those carried out in England and Wales as part of the crime and disorder auditing process, tend to focus on local residents and exclude tourists altogether, effectively disenfranchising them [Mawby, 2008]. One option here is to interview tourists either during their holiday—raising difficulties associated with identifying tourists near the end of their vacation—or at their point of departure. The latter is in theory possible, if not straightforward, where there are a limited number of points of egress (e.g., airports, ferry terminals)* but less practical where tourists travel by car or do not have to cross border checkpoints, as on much of mainland Europe. An obvious alternative is to survey samples of the wider population about their previous holiday experiences. However, as Mawby, Brunt, and Hambly [1999]

---

* A method used successfully by Bellis et al. (2000, 2003) in surveys of the drug-taking habits of young tourists visiting Ibiza.

discovered, gaining access to sampling frames via tour operators can be difficult when companies are reluctant to acknowledge the negative aspects of tourism. Consequently, their research was based on *Holiday Which* readership, inevitably producing a rather skewed sample.

Bearing in mind these constraints, a number of researchers have considered crime in tourist resorts and against tourists. In the former case, research has been largely dependent on police data.

One common assumption is that crime will be more of a problem at the height of the tourist season and less evident in the low season. For example, in the British Isles, King's [1988] research demonstrated that on the island of Jersey crime increased during the summer, peak tourist months. Similar findings have been reported for the Isles of Scilly [Mawby, 2002]. In an earlier study in Miami, McPheters and Stronge [1974:290] compared tourism and crime patterns on a monthly basis between 1963 and 1966 and concluded that "major economic crimes (robbery, larceny, burglary) have a similar season to tourism, while crimes of passion (murder, rape and assault) have not." Walmsley et al. [1983], contrasting three tourist with three nontourist centers in New South Wales (NSW), also concluded that crime peaked in the tourist season in the former. Similar findings were reported by Fujii and Mak [1979] in Hawaii, Jud [1975] in Mexico, and Kelly [1993] in Queensland, Australia. However, not all research is as conclusive. For example, Walmsley et al. [1983] found little evidence of higher crime rates in the three tourist areas they covered compared with the nontourist centers, although offense patterns were different. Earlier research by Pizam [1982:7], considering the relationship between state crime rates and tourism and other social variables, concluded: "For five out of nine crimes tourism was not found to be a determinant at all. For the remaining four the magnitude of contribution was so low that it could be considered insubstantial." Pelfrey [1998] also found little evidence that tourist numbers increased the rates of violent crime in Honolulu and Las Vegas. Such studies raise the possibility that rates may vary for different types of tourism resorts, catering to different types of tourists.

Building on Kelly's [1993] earlier work, Prideaux [1996] considered these questions in relation to the three largest tourist destinations in Queensland, Australia: the Gold Coast, Cairns, and the Sunshine Coast. The three areas differed in a number of respects: For example, the Gold Coast had the most extensive tourist development, attracting predominantly interstate tourists; Cairns, a more urban location, attracted relatively more international tourists; and the Sunshine Coast, which is the least developed, accommodated the highest proportion of intrastate visitors. The areas also evidenced contrasting crime rates. In the Gold Coast and Cairns, where increased rates of crime had paralleled tourist development over a decade or more, crime was more common than in the Sunshine Coast and other, smaller tourism locations. Cairns, moreover, had an especially high rate of crimes against the person and public order offenses.

In stark contrast, little research has addressed the question of who are the victims of crime in resort areas. What there is, however, suggests that tourists face particularly high risks [Harper, 2001].

Perhaps the most useful comparison of tourist and resident victimization comes from an early study by Chesney-Lind and Lind [1986] in Hawaii. Having noted the difficulties experienced by earlier researchers in distinguishing between crimes against local residents and visitors, they used police data on the residential status of crime victims in two areas of Hawaii—Honolulu and Kauai County—during the late 1970s and early 1980s, and related these to the average daily tourist and resident subpopulations. They derived annual average crime rates per 100,000 population for residents and tourists in Honolulu (1981–1982) and Kauai (1978–1980) and demonstrated markedly higher rates for tourists in the former. For example, Honolulu had a burglary rate of 1,407 for residents and 2,045 for tourists, and 233 and 296, respectively, for violent crime. In Kauai, a less-developed tourist area, the pattern was rather different, with tourists experiencing less violent crime, auto theft, and burglary. Nevertheless, the authors concluded that tourists *were* more susceptible to crime than were local people. The rate of property crime against tourists in Honolulu, for example, was higher than the overall crime rate in all but one U.S. city with a population of 500,000–1,000,000, the exception, notably, being Orlando, itself a center of tourism. In a later study in Barbados, de Albuquerque and McElroy [1999] discovered that tourists had higher rates for acquisitive crime victimization but lower rates for nonacquisitive violent crimes. Most recently, Michalko [2003] noted the extent of crime against foreign tourists, especially Germans, in Hungary, with risk of property crime particularly high.

All these studies were dependent on police statistics. In one of the few victim surveys undertaken, Stangeland [1998] compared tourists interviewed at the end of their holiday with local residents of Málaga and foreign residents of properties on the Costa del Sol. He found that tourists' rates of victimization during a fortnight's (average) holiday were often not that much lower (and were sometimes higher) than those of the other groups over a whole year. For example, 4.3% of his Málaga sample and 1.1% of his Costa del Sol sample had experienced a robbery in the preceding year, whereas 1.4% of tourists had done so during their holiday. The figures for burglary were even starker: 2.3%, 2.3%, and 3.9%, respectively [Stangeland, 1998:66].

A survey of British holidaymakers questioned by Mawby et al. [1999; see also Brunt, Mawby, and Hambly, 2000; Mawby, 2000] also identified tourists as particularly at risk. Respondents were asked whether they had been the victim of any from a list of seven offenses while on their last holiday. Overall, 92 incidents were cited by 50 respondents. This translates to an approximate incidence rate* of 18% and a prevalence rate of 10%. The most common crime was burglary. At first sight this suggests that tourists rarely fall victim to crime while on holiday. However, the average length of holiday in this survey was 2 weeks; therefore, an approximate annual incidence rate would require us to multiply these figures by 26. Alternatively, this rate can be presented as a rate per 10,000 respondents/households per 2 weeks, and a crude comparison may be drawn with conventional victim survey data from the BCS [Mirrlees-Black, Mayhew, and Percy, 1996] by dividing the latter's incidence rates by 26.† This is, of course, only an approximation. However, the differences between traditional victim survey rates and these tourism victim survey rates are so great as to make such qualifications superfluous. The rate for burglary (excluding attempts), at 467 per 10,000 households, for example, far exceeded the BCS rate of 32 for burglary (including attempts). The unequivocal conclusion to be drawn from this is that people generally experience considerably more crime as tourists than they do while at home. Explaining this is the subject of the following section.

12.3 Explaining Differential Risk

One approach to explaining variations in risk is routine activity theory [Cohen and Felson, 1979; Felson and Cohen, 1980]. Routine activity theory attempts to explain the incidence and distribution of crime in terms of three sets of actors: potential victims, potential offenders, and law enforcement agencies and other "capable guardians." It has been used by tourism researchers to explain high victimization rates for tourists in general [Crotts, 1996] but may also be applied to different subgroups of tourists. Focusing on victim behavior, criminologists such as Cohen and Cantor [1981], Maxfield [1987], and Rountree and Land [1996] have demonstrated that lifestyle is closely associated with victimization. How we behave—how often and when we go out, what we do when out, and where we go—strongly influences the risk of crime. In this respect, the routine activities of victims interrelate with those of offenders and policing agents. In considering the relationship between tourists' behavior and victimization, we must therefore ask what it is that might put tourists in general at high risk, and why some might be even more likely to be victimized than others. Four aspects of lifestyle may be particularly important: rewards, justifiability of target, guardianship, and accessibility.

---

* Since people were only asked to record whether or not they had experienced any of the seven incidents, the incidence rate excludes cases where respondents suffered more than one crime from any one category.
† Data from the 1998 BCS are not strictly comparable, but rates were generally lower; therefore, the differences reported here would have been greater.

12.3.1 Rewards

All other things being equal, we might expect offenders to target affluent citizens rather than poorer people, at least for property offenses. Thus, in countries where tourists are affluent relative to the indigenous population, we might expect them to be especially at risk. More generally, tourists tend to have in their possession valuable and easily transportable items that might attract offenders, such as cash, credit cards, passports, or high-tech equipment.

12.3.2 Justifiability of Target

Tourists may be considered justifiable targets when offenders are able to neutralize the victim status of travelers. Crime can result from conflict between tourists and local residents. This conflict may stem from a clash of cultures and may include factors such as conflicting norms of dress, speech, and behavior. Such conflicts may cause tension between travelers and residents and resentment by local residents of the intrusive effects of tourism [Prideaux, 1995; Jobes, Barclay, and Donnermeyer, 2000]. Somewhat differently, the morals of tourists may be questioned by locals who see such matters as dress codes and interpersonal behavior as indicating that female travelers are "asking for it" and therefore not "real" victims. The rape and murder of Katherine Horton in 2006 in Thailand [Johns, 2007] are perhaps illustrative of this.

12.3.3 Guardianship

Third, we might expect tourists to be more at risk because of low levels of guardianship. This applies on at least three levels: self-guardianship, community guardianship, and formal (public or private) policing. In terms of self-guardianship, tourists in general display far less concern to minimize risk than they would at home, for example, displaying little anxiety about crime and spending more time on the streets after dark, leaving their accommodation unprotected. Indeed, a "culture of carelessness" might prevail [Ryan, 1993; Mawby, Brunt, and Hambly, 2000; Harper, 2006]. Alternatively, the ability of tourists to rely on others to provide guardianship and policing is restricted. On the one hand, a large number and high turnover of tourists within a resort will reduce the ability of neighbors to act as guardians and self-police their environment, a point stressed by Stangeland [1998]. On the other hand, tourists may be outside the routine policing arrangements adopted by the public police. Despite the introduction of specialist tourist police in some countries [Muehsam and Tarlow, 1995; Tarlow, 2000], elsewhere local police agencies may give low priority to crimes against tourists [Cohen, 1987, 1996]. Indeed, offenders may target tourists because the chance of a conviction is minimal [Inciardi, 1976]. Chesney-Lind and Lind [1986] noted that even when perpetrators of crimes against tourists were detained, they were likely to be released without charge, partly because of the reluctance of tourists to change their travel plans and make themselves available to appear as witnesses in court.

12.3.4 Accessibility

Accessibility refers to the extent to which the offender is afforded easy access. It may be physical (e.g., barriers restricting access) or social (e.g., offender lives some distance from potential target). Although this concept has traditionally been used in the context of burglary [Mawby, 2001], the accessibility levels relating to tourists are in stark contrast to those relating to the homeowner, who may deploy a range of social, physical, and technological forms of protection. Holiday accommodation may not incorporate safes or security locks on doors, and where this prompts tourists to carry valuables on their person, their risk of street crimes increases. Moreover, tourists may be more accessible targets because their routine activities bring them into crime hotspots [Sherman, Gartin, and Buerger, 1989] and/or into close proximity to offenders. To a large extent, this may be a matter of choice: prioritization of leisure facilities and the nighttime economy or the desire to purchase alcohol or drugs. Lack of awareness is an additional factor. Tourists are often unaware of the predatory hot spots for crime and may undertake risky activities such as frequenting night clubs and bars at late hours or accidentally venturing into unknown parts of the community that locals consider "unsafe." In this context, for example, Gallivan [1994:42] interviewed a Miami police officer who claimed that much crime was the result of new arrivals to the country who were reluctant to pay road tolls, subsequently driving off the toll road and ending up in a high-crime "zone of body shops, used car lots and working-class housing."

These four aspects of lifestyle may be particularly important in explaining why tourists are a high-risk group. However, as already noted there are a variety of subgroups of tourists, the variations between which equate to the differing lifestyles of citizens in general. Despite this, with few exceptions [see especially Cohen, 1972, 1987] crime risk has not been tied to any tourist typology. In the following section, therefore, we revisit our discussion of the extent and reasons for tourist victimization by focusing on four case studies. The first two relate to tourist groups, respectively, organized youth holidays packaged around sun, alcohol, and sex, and backpacking. In these cases, there is no established research on victimization, and our argument is largely speculative. The next two relate to tourist accommodation, respectively, hotels and caravan/camp parks, where there is more research evidence available.

12.4 Case Studies

12.4.1 Teens and 20s Holidays

The image of British "lager louts" abroad surfaced in the late 1980s in Spain, with reports of excessive drinking among (predominantly) young, male holidaymakers culminating in public disturbances and aggressive, noisy, and violent behavior [Ryan, 1991:159–60]. Ryan concluded that the problem stemmed from a combination of four factors:

- A background culture that emphasized group cohesiveness, ethnocentricism, and what has subsequently been described as "laddish" behavior
- The freedom of being away from home with its conventional constraints
- Expectations of a "good time" fueled by images produced by both advertising and returning holidaymakers
- Mass tourism where the resort aims to create "England abroad"

Since then, the proliferation of a tourist market from operators like Club Med and Club 18–30, aimed at "young singles," with the promise of sun, alcohol, and sex, has provided the basis for episodic media exposés in Ayia Napa (Cyprus), Newquay (England), and Faliraki (Rhodes). A Foreign and Commonwealth Office (FCO) report in 2005 underlined this by suggesting that "clubbing," involving alcohol, drugs, and sex, was the main focus for young British holidaymakers abroad.* Nor is this an exclusively British phenomenon, as the example of "schoolie" celebrations in Australia illustrate, with the end of the school year seeing thousands of school leavers ("schoolies") descending on coastal resorts to celebrate.† Gold Coast resorts like Surfers Paradise are particularly favored and indeed to a large extent promote themselves as catering to young singles [Homel et al., 1997].

However, although the limited academic interest in the topic almost exclusively focuses on the crime and disorder problems *created* by young tourists, it is arguable that such tourists are also at high risk of victimization themselves, whether from other tourists or local offenders. Our

---

* www.travelmole.com/stories/104313.php. And see FCO [2007] British Behaviour Abroad report at www.fco.gov.uk/servlet/Front? pagename=OpenMarket/Xcelerate/ShowPage&c =Page&cid=1007029391638&a=KArticle&aid=1184757793657.
† See for example:
http://entertainment.news.com.au/common/printPage/0,6164,5517703%5E7485%5E%5 Enbv,00.html,
www.themercury.news.com.au/common/story_page/0,5936,5544472%255E421,00.html, http://townsvillebulletin.news.com.au/printpage/0,5942,5438850,00.html, and http://www.goldcoast.qld.gov.au/t_news_item.asp?PID=2303&status=Archived.

research in Cornwall, for example, showed that Newquay, the place in the United Kingdom where teenagers are allegedly most likely to go for their first holiday without their parents [Mawby, 2007], was a hotspot for crimes *against (particularly young) tourists*. Faliraki, on the Greek island of Rhodes, is another case in point. In 2002, the *Guardian* featured under the headline "Erotic Emma: Drunk and at Risk" a story about the risk of rape in Faliraki, repeating a Home Office warning to females holiday-ing there alone [Gillan, 2002]. Rapes, involving both British and Greek perpetrators, appeared to have been relatively common, if rarely reported and even less commonly recorded [Gillan, 2002; McVeigh, 2003]. Then, in 2003, 17-year-old Patrick Doran was fatally stabbed with a broken bottle in a nightclub brawl, leading to a plethora of media exposés [Brunt and Davies, 2006].

Nevertheless, these stories are a rarity, with most of the emphasis placed on young tourists as the problem rather than the victims. However, when comparing them with tourists in general, there are good grounds for speculating that Emma and Patrick are not atypical. Although the valuables carried or brought by young tourists might not be excessive, on the other criteria we identified they score highly. Thus, their unruly or seemingly amoral behavior might help define them as justifiable targets, while they score low on guardianship and high on accessibility.

In terms of self-guardianship, they spend considerable time out after dark, leaving hotel rooms unprotected, and their high alcohol consumption makes them easy prey for robbery and sexual offenses. The fact that their peers are behaving in a similar fashion makes community guardianship unlikely, and their behavior means they will be afforded low priority for pro-tection by the police.

In terms of accessibility, they are likely to stay in poor-quality accommo-dation, where it is easy to force access, and where safes are a rarity. Finally, the focus on drink and sex means they spend considerable time in nightlife areas, where they are likely to cross the paths of offenders attracted there by their presence or also there to party. For example, it had become com-mon practice for holiday reps in Faliraki to organize bar crawls, billed as nights out to introduce newly arrived tourists to the local "attractions." These involved tourists paying in advance for the night and being taken to about 10 pubs and clubs, where the drinks were provided "free." This puts young tourists at their most vulnerable in crime hotspots.

12.4.2 Backpacking

Backpacking is an expanding phenomenon among young people in Britain and other Western societies, identified by some as epitomizing "post-modern" tourism [Cohen, 2003]. Backpackers provide a consistent and reliable clientele to many rural and remote areas often bypassed by conventional tourists. They also provide a highly valued source of labor for seasonal, short-term work in these regions. In addition, during the past decade a flourishing industry of hostels, restaurants, cafes, clubs, outdoor equipment shops, and magazines has emerged to cater to their requirements [Israel, 1999].

At the same time a number of high-profile homicide cases have raised fears over the safety of young independent travelers. These include the recent rape and murder of 21-year-old Welsh backpacker Katherine Horton in Thailand. However, similar crimes occurring in Australia stretch back at least to the early 1990s, when seven backpackers perished at the hands of serial killer Ivan Milat in NSW. More recently, after a prolonged police investigation and trial, Bradley Murdoch was found guilty of the murder of Peter Falconio, at the time traveling through the Northern Territory with girlfriend Joanne Lees.

In the light of such concerns, it is perhaps surprising that research into backpackers is both limited and of recent origin [Loker-Murphy and Pearce, 1995; O'Reilly, 1997; Ross, 1997; Uriely, Yonay, and Simchai, 2002; Cohen, 2003] and that little has addressed safety issues [Israel, 1999].

Precise definitions of backpacking have proved elusive [Pearce, 1990; McCulloch, 1991; O'Reilly, 1997; Uriely et al., 2002; Cohen, 2003], not least because there is a disparity between backpackers' ideologies and practices. However, backpackers may be broadly described in terms of who they are, what they do, and why they choose to travel in the way they do. Thus, they tend to be young people from relatively middle-class backgrounds who, in the transition period between education and career,* opt to travel widely for significant periods, away from mainstream tourist routes/resorts, generally on a limited budget, with the aim of experiencing authenticity and freedom away from the "tourism bubble." According to Cohen [2003], they are a postmodern remolding of the "drifters" he described in his seminal work on tourist subgroups [Cohen, 1972, 1973]. However, there are considerable subcategories of backpackers, according to, among other things, age, length of trip, extent to which the trip is preplanned, subcultural affiliation, interaction with other backpackers, and motivation for traveling in this way. Although these variables may themselves be associated with risk of victimization, there has been little research on the crime concerns and experiences of backpackers. Cohen [1987] did suggest that his "drifter" subgroup was more at risk of victimization than were conventional tourists, but other than this, Israel's [1999] brief discussion paper is the only published source to date to concentrate on the victimization of backpackers. However, backpackers seem to fit all four criteria we identified earlier.

---

* Or, in the case of Israelis, those completing military service [Uriely, Yonay, and Simchai, 2002].

First, in terms of rewards, backpackers frequently visit poorer countries where they appear affluent relative to the indigenous population. Moreover, there is considerable evidence that, despite a focus on minimizing expenditure, backpackers carry with them considerable wealth in the form of cash and high-tech equipment. Second, backpackers may be considered justifiable targets, where they are seen as symbols of Western capitalist values, especially where their moral values are questioned.

Third, we might expect backpackers to be more at risk because of low levels of guardianship. Thus, the guardianship levels available to or adopted by the backpacker are in stark contrast to those of the homeowner, who may deploy a range of social, physical, and technological forms of protection. Backpackers often cannot or choose not to take safer options. Hitchhiking or opting for cheaper travel and accommodation leaves backpackers exposed to the least desirable aspects of society. Moreover, what gives backpacking its appeal also makes it hazardous [Cohen, 1987; Israel, 1999; Elsrud, 2001]. Both Thoms [2002] and Moshin and Ryan [2003] found that almost half of backpackers traveled alone. Independence allows more interactions with locals and other travelers and more opportunities for free travel or accommodation, but it also means that backpackers lack the protection that travel packages offer. In Cohen's terms, they exist outside the "tourist bubble" that surrounds conventional tourists. They need to carry their possessions with them or leave them in insecure locations, and they adopt vulnerable strategies for carrying and securing possessions. Backpacker hostels provide little by way of security and also accommodate seasonal workers, unemployed persons, and others seeking cheap accommodation, who may also be the perpetrators of crime [Jobes et al., 2000]. Although the wider literature suggests that tourists in general display far less concern to minimize risk than they would at home, for example, displaying little anxiety about crime and spending more time on the streets after dark [Mawby et al., 2000], this may be even more the case among backpackers, albeit some authors have concluded that safety is a salient issue among backpackers [Ross, 1997], especially among women [Mohsin and Ryan, 2003]. Drug and alcohol use also means that the capability of self-guardianship is reduced.

Alternatively, the ability of backpackers to rely on others to provide guardianship and policing is restricted. On the one hand, a large number and high turnover of backpackers within a hostel will reduce the ability of backpackers to act as guardians and self-police their environment. On the other hand, backpackers may be outside the routine policing arrangements adopted by tour companies/reps and the public police. Local police agencies may, moreover, give low priority to crimes against tourists [Cohen, 1996] and especially nonconventional tourists [Cohen, 1987].

Fourth, backpackers may be highly accessible targets. To a large extent, this may be a matter of choice: prioritization of leisure facilities and the nighttime economy, the desire to purchase alcohol or drugs, and the prospect of sexual liaisons with strangers may put backpackers at increased risk [Allen, 1999; Israel, 1999]. Lack of awareness is an additional factor, although it is likely that backpackers are more aware of unsafe locations through their communication with other backpackers, either in person or through the Internet.

12.4.3 Hotel Crime

There has been relatively little research on hotel crime, much less hotel crime in tourist areas. However, in one notable early exception, Gill, Salmon, and Hill [1993] suggested that hotels in tourist areas experienced high levels of crime, and that although many of these involved offenses committed by guests against the hotels, others involved guests as victims. Also in the United Kingdom, Jones and Groenenboom [2002] argued that crime is a significant problem for prestigious London hotels, exacerbated by the nature of the hospitality industry and the design and location of hotels. The extent of crime taking place in hotels in one British city, or at least in specific hotels, was illustrated in a 2006 news feature on the Adelphi Hotel in Liverpool, the site of—allegedly—81% of all hotel room burglaries in the city center in the previous 12 months.*

Although in the United States, Huang, Kwag, and Streib [1998] concluded that crime was not common in hotels,† this is the exception, with Zhao and Ho [2006] identifying hotel crime as common in Florida, and Ho, Zhao, and Brown [2009] similarly reporting high rates of hotel crime in Miami Beach. Hotel security has been the subject of extensive discussion in the United States [Hinz, 1985; Smith, 1993; Beaudry, 1996], with high-profile legal cases underlining the need for increased security [Palmer, 1989; Prestia, 1993; Bach, 1996; LeBruto, 1996]. The extent of crime against hotel guests in tourist areas is unsurprising. Research on commercial crime suggests that it is far more common than crime against households and householders [Mawby, 2006]. Similarly, in a survey of business people from the United States, Berger [1992] found that hotel burglary was the most common crime cited.

Our own research [e.g., Mawby and Jones, 2007] focused on hotel crime in two tourist districts in the southwest of England, which we called Sunnybay and Funland. In both districts hotels were predominantly located in a coastal environment, with tourists the predominant clientele. Most were accessed

---

* http://icliverpool.icnetwork.co.uk/0100news/0100regionalnews/tm_objectid=17452044
  &method=full&siteid=50061&page=1&headline=adelphi-crimewave-name_page.html.
† However, they based their rates of crime against hotels on the average number of guest rooms, producing a far lower rate than one using the number of hotels as the denominator.

directly from the street,* with about one-third accessed via a private driveway. Most had private car parks,† although some acknowledged that guests often had to park in the streets.

Police crime data for Sunnybay and Funland were analyzed for a 3-year period, April 1999 to March 2002. All crimes that were coded as taking place in hotels, guesthouses, etc., as well as their grounds, were included. As Table 12.1 indicates, over the 3 years 1,226 hotel-based offenses were recorded in Sunnybay and 726 in Funland, that is, approaching one recorded offense per hotel per annum. Of the recorded offenses in Sunnybay hotels, 50.2% were classified as burglary and more than one-quarter as "other theft." In Funland the proportion of offenses classified as burglaries was slightly lower, at 43.1% with proportionally more thefts (other).

Repeat burglaries are particularly common against commercial targets [Mawby, 2006], and, as the Adelphi example illustrates, hotels are no exception. For burglary, no fewer than 17 hotels in Sunnybay were targeted on at least 10 occasions over the 3 years. Put another way, 37.2% of all burglaries occurred at 17 hotels. In Funland repeat burglary was also common.

Interviews with 120 hoteliers in Sunnybay and 84 in Funland, not surprisingly, indicated considerably more crime against hotels and their guests than were recorded in police statistics, but—partly as a result—a lower proportion of it involved more serious offenses such as burglary. Nevertheless, 22.1% of respondents from Sunnybay and 23.2% of those from Funland said that in the 12 months up to March 2002, they had experienced burglary/theft of guest property, and the corresponding figures for burglary/theft of hotel property were even higher, at 34.6% and 45.8%, respectively.‡ Larger hotels were more likely to experience crime than smaller hotels and boarding houses [Jones and Mawby, 2005].

Thus, our research confirms that of other studies in identifying hotels in tourist areas as crime hotspots. In explaining this, justifiability of targets seems unimportant. However, revisiting the other three criteria—rewards, guardianship, and accessibility—is helpful:

- Rewards: Although tourists staying in hotels may bring with them easily transportable valuable items, equally they are likely to leave many of these in their hotel room during the day.
- Guardianship: Guardianship applies at both the level of the hotel itself and the room. Hotels need to be consumer friendly and accessible. Consequently, security staff members tend to be low key, and even where other staff members are given a security responsibility,

---

* 67.1% in Sunnybay; 57.1% in Funland.
† 89.3% in Sunnybay; 90.5% in Funland.
‡ These categories are not, of course, mutually exclusive: In some cases, a burglary might have involved theft of both hotel and guest property.

Table 12.1   Percentage of Different Offenses Recorded as Taking
Place in Hotels, Sunnybay and Funland, 1999–2002

	Sunnybay ($n = 1226$)	Funland ($n = 726$)
Common assault	2.0	3.0
Other violence	2.0	1.9
Sexual offenses	0.7	0.8
Robbery	0.0	0.1
Theft of vehicle	0.1	0.3
Taking (vehicle) without owner's consent	0.0	0.3
Theft from vehicle	2.6	2.3
Criminal damage to vehicle	0.8	1.7
Vehicle interference	0.3	0.0
Cycle theft	1.1	0.7
Burglary (dwelling)	6.2	5.5
Burglary (other)	44.0	37.6
Check/credit card fraud	2.8	1.9
Forgery/other fraud	3.8	4.1
Handling	0.6	0.1
Drug offenses	1.3	1.7
Other criminal damage	5.5	8.4
Theft from shop	0.1	0.0
Other theft	25.6	29.2
Other offenses	0.5	0.3

the transience of hotel populations makes security problematic. As
with tourists in general, hotel guests tend to spend relatively long
periods out of their accommodation, during which time their rooms
are left unguarded. In this sense, we might speculate that risk would
be greater than for those in self-catering apartments, which are
designed to be used in the evenings, for meals, etc. Moreover, the
ways in which hotels are managed to a greater or lesser extent adver-
tise lack of self-guardianship. For example, if conventional room
keys are used and hung in a visible place in the hotel lobby, potential
burglars may be able to identify empty rooms. Although many hotels
have improved security by using keycards or keeping keys hidden
from public display, most still operate a system whereby guests display a notice to inform staff that their room is unoccupied and can
be serviced, conveniently alerting the potential offender that their
room is unguarded and open to a burglary. Nevertheless, the capacity for and emphasis on guardianship might be expected to vary. The
fact that smaller hotels, for example, experienced less crime may be
explained in terms of ease of guardianship.

- Accessibility: Again, accessibility applies to both the hotel and the individual guest room. Because hotels, as semiprivate spaces, need to be easily accessible, access to the guest rooms is relatively unproblematic. Rooms are rarely alarmed, and door locks are no challenge to a relatively proficient burglar. Safes are becoming more common, but our research indicated that only about one-half of hotels in Sunnybay and Funland had hotel safes available to guests, and few had room safes. Indeed, as Table 12.2 indicates, in general, guardianship levels were low and accessibility levels high.

In conclusion, the rewards available to offenders combined with poor guardianship and easy accessibility make hotel crime a relatively common phenomenon.

12.4.4 Camp/Caravan Parks

Crime victimization within caravan parks is an issue that has not been previously discussed within criminology. In one exception, Mawby and Gorgenyi's [1997] research on burglary in the Hungarian town of Miskolc

Table 12.2   Percentage of Hotels with the Following Security Measures at the Time of Interview

	Sunnybay	Funland
Guest room keys	95.7	91.7
Window locks in guest rooms	62.9	70.2
Window locks on other windows	54.3	66.7
Central safe for guest use	47.9	59.5
Keys secured out of sight in public areas	37.1	64.3
Closed-circuit television (CCTV) in reception area	33.6	33.3
Security information for guests	30.0	46.4
CCTV in public areas	25.0	22.6
Centralized alarm system	22.1	16.7
CCTV in car park	16.4	15.5
Hotel security staff	14.3	13.1
Slot in reception for returned keys	13.6	28.6
CCTV in external property	11.4	20.2
Stand-alone alarm system	10.0	7.1
Bolts on room doors	7.1	0.0
Guest room electronic door cards	2.1	1.2
Safes in guests rooms	2.1	10.7
Spy holes in guest room doors	2.1	1.2
Panic chains	2.1	4.8

identified second homes, located in parks on the city perimeter, as particularly vulnerable to burglary. However, the fact that this research covered
domestic burglary in general, and only incidentally unearthed high levels of
second- home burglary, illustrates some of the research difficulties involved.
For example, victim surveys normally exclude caravan parks from the sample
of addresses surveyed, and police statistics rarely identify park site crime in
a way that makes it easily accessible to researchers. However, more detailed
analysis of police crime data may enable us to distinguish location according to whether park sites or caravans were targeted. In Australia, research
by Barclay and Mawby [2006] addressed park crime in NSW and Western
Australia (WA), while in England work is currently ongoing in two districts
of Cornwall [Mawby, Mcintosh, and Barclay, 2008].

The findings from these studies are ambiguous. On the one hand, there
is mixed evidence that caravan parks in general are hotspots of crime and
disorder, or that visitors perceive them to be unsafe. On the other hand, there
are marked differences between sites.

In terms of crime on caravan parks in general, Barclay and Mawby's
[2006] research in NSW and WA found relatively low levels of park crime.
Indeed, secondary analysis of police statistics suggested that caravans were
more at risk off site than on, illustrating perhaps the possibility of parks
adopting some of the guardianship qualities associated with gated communities [Low, 2004; Vesselinov, Cazessus, and Falk, 2007; Waszkiewicz, 2007].
Similarly, interviews with tourists staying on parks indicated that crime was
not generally considered a problem and that direct personal experience of
crime while staying on parks was minimal. In contrast, Mcintosh's research
in Cornwall, England, found crime in holiday parks to be more common.
Taking 16 park sites that primarily catered to tourists, 193 crimes were
recorded by the police in 2006 and 2007, including 47 burglaries, 11 cycle
thefts, 8 thefts from vehicles, and 39 other thefts. Not surprisingly, interviews
with a sample of tourists staying at these sites revealed considerably higher
levels of victimization. Thus, although they had on average only been away
from home for 7–8 days, no fewer than 13.8% of respondents said they had
been the victim of a crime during this holiday [Mawby et al., 2008]. Despite
these differences, both studies found considerable variations in crime rates
between different park sites. In Cornwall, for example, 2 of the 16 sites registered only one recorded crime each over the 2 years (at rates of 0.7 and
0.9 per 100 pitches). At the other extreme, three sites registered more than
10 crimes per 100 pitches. Interviews with tourists at the different sites
revealed a broadly parallel pattern.

In explaining these differences, the importance of guardianship and
accessibility seemed crucial. Guardianship is important on a number of levels. For example, in Australia, Barclay and Mawby [2006] found that caravan parks with fewer crime and disorder problems tended to have deployed

in-house security or had forged good relationships with local police, who as a result provided a greater policing presence. Interestingly, guardianship potential was also increased where tourists were staying on parks that also catered to permanent residents, whose knowledge of the park and different lifestyle afforded them a greater ability to provide informal guardianship within the site. Self-guardianship was also important. Thus, in Cornwall, those going out in the evening more often and those leaving their accommodation empty for at least two evenings per week were most likely to have experienced crime, especially crimes committed on the park site and around their accommodation. The fact that, in line with earlier research [Mawby et al., 2000], caravan park users considered their security on holiday of less concern than when they were at home meant that they afforded low priority to protecting their property or person. Different accessibility levels also helped account for differences both between and within parks. For example, in Australia, parks located in towns and park homes nearer to towns and pubs tended to experience greater risk. On the other hand, in both countries parks with more secure perimeter fencing experienced less crime. Within the parks, tourists were also more vulnerable where they left possessions outside their temporary homes. In England there was also some evidence that tents, which were more accessible than caravans, were targeted. Finally, it is worth stressing that access is facilitated when offenders are themselves tourists staying on the park. Whereas in Australia the impression was that most offenses were committed by local residents rather than those staying on the parks, in Cornwall it seemed that many offenses were committed by fellow tourists. Park sites that catered to and were marketed at younger tourists, at the cheaper end of the market, correspondingly experienced more crime.

This may, to some extent, explain why caravan parks are not necessarily crime and disorder hotspots. As with tourist areas in general, the way that sites are marketed attracts distinctive groups of holidaymakers, some of whom may commit crime, although the behavior patterns of the majority may or may not increase their risk of victimization. Reward also importantly affects risk. On the second-home sites described by Mawby and Gorgenyi [1997], owners, who generally lived in small urban apartments, tended to store goods throughout the year, making them attractive targets when not occupied. In contrast, caravans in England and Australia are rarely furnished with goods attractive to a thief. Rather, it is the goods that tourists bring on holiday with them that make them desirable targets, and the fact that tourists (and their possessions) change regularly means the rewards are constantly replenished. In this sense, the attraction of goods worth stealing (rewards) appears more important than ease of access or lack of guardianship. Whether there are, equally, differences—between Australia and England or between park sites—in the value of goods that tourists take on holiday and leave in their tent or caravan is a question that has not been addressed. Discussions with local police in Cornwall, however, suggest that some groups of tourists who stay on parks and spend their evenings "out on the town" bring with them valuables, including expensive clothing and jewelry, that are left unprotected in their park homes while they spend the daytime on the local beaches.

Thus, although there is no strong evidence that caravan parks are inevitably crime and disorder hotspots, the concepts of reward, guardianship, and accessibility are useful in suggesting why some sites, and correspondingly some tourists, are more at risk than others.

12.5 Discussion

There has been little research on the relationship between tourism and crime, even less on tourists as victims, and that which has been carried out is largely the work of tourism researchers rather than criminologists. This may, to some extent, be because both official crime statistics and victim surveys rarely allow one to distinguish between tourists and local people, but it is probably more because criminologists and victimologists have rarely considered this an interesting topic. This is regrettable, not least because the evidence suggests that tourists are at considerable risk of victimization but paradoxically worry little about issues of insecurity and danger, even post 9/11. This poses considerable challenges for crime reduction policies in tourist resorts.

Furthermore, just as criminologists make use of lifestyle factors in explaining different levels of risk among the conventional population, so we can explain high levels of victimization among tourists in terms of the distinctive ways they behave when on holiday and the nature of their accommodation. At least four aspects of lifestyle seem to be important: rewards, justifiability of target, guardianship, and accessibility. Tourists experience higher levels of risk where they offer potentially higher rewards to the offender, where their victim status can be discounted, where guardianship of their person and property is limited, and where accessibility is relatively easy. This chapter has described research to support this. However, it is equally likely that the same factors can be used to explain why particular subgroups of tourists will experience different levels of risk, and here there is an even greater paucity of research. Few tourist researchers have focused on differences between subgroups of tourists, much less the extent to which such differences impact on risk. We would suggest that this is a fertile area for future research.

As a starting point, we have identified four case studies. The first two relate to specific categories of tourist, respectively, young people who prioritize sun, alcohol, and sex, and those backpacking. Here there has been little criminological research, and the discussion is largely speculative. Nevertheless, we would suggest that backpackers and—especially—youths whose holiday priorities center around alcohol consumption are at particularly high risk of victimization. The next two relate to tourist accommodation, respectively, hotels and caravan/camp parks. Here there is some research evidence available. This demonstrates that hotels, and at least some caravan parks, are crime hotspots. In attempting to explain these patterns we have suggested that all four case studies demonstrate poor guardianship and high accessibility (see Table 12.3), although in the case of caravan and camp parks there are marked differences that might explain differential levels of risk. The explanatory power of rewards is more varied. Generally it seems that although not all the tourist groups considered are wealthy, albeit backpackers may be wealthy relative to local people, in most cases a higher proportion of their wealth is accessible. For example, credit cards, cash, and jewelry may be either carried on the person or left in insecure accommodation. Additionally, it might explain why caravan park crime occurs when parks are relatively full, rather than empty and poorly guarded. Finally, in the case of holidaymakers in their teens and 20s and backpackers in particular, the fact that they are outsiders, their behavior, and what that behavior is thought to symbolize may mean that they, and not local people, are targeted.

The fact that theories that explain victimization among the general population can be applied to tourists is scarcely surprising. After all, the test of a good theory is its broader applicability. What is more surprising is that criminologists and victimologists have largely ignored the topic, leaving it to tourism academics. The aim of this chapter, consequently, is not only to review the literature but also to introduce criminologists to an area that has received so little attention from their peers, but is a fertile area for research.

Table 12.3   Aspects of Lifestyle Related to Risk for the Four Case Studies

	Rewards	Justifiability of Targets	Guardianship	Accessibility
Teens and 20s holidays		Generally; especially sexual offenses	Overall low	In terms of accommodation and outside space
Backpacking	Relative to locals High proportion accessible	Symbolic of Western values	Overall low	In terms of accommodation and outside space
Hotel crime	High proportion of accessible hotels and rooms		Poor but variable	Relatively easy
Caravan/camp parks	Targeted when in use High proportion accessible		Variable	Variable

References

Albuquerque, K. de and J. McElroy. 1999. Tourism and crime in the Caribbean. *Annals of Tourism Research* 26(4):968–84.

Allen, J. 1999. Crime against international tourists. NSW Bureau of Crime Statistics and Research, contemporary issues in crime and justice, 43. www.bocsar. nsw.gov.au/lawlink/bocsar/ll_bocsar.nsf/vwFiles/cjb43.pdf/$file/cjb43.pdf (accessed July 1, 2008).

Bach, S. 1996. Tourist-related crime and the hotel industry: A review of the literature and related materials. In *Tourism, crime and international security issues*, ed. A. Pizam and Y. Mansfeld, 281–96. Chichester, UK: Wiley.

Barclay, E. and R. I. Mawby. 2006. *Crime and caravan parks: A report to the Western Australian office of crime prevention*. Perth, Australia: Western Australian Office of Crime Prevention.

Beaudry, M. H. 1996. *Contemporary lodging security*. Woburn, MA: Butterworth-Heinemann.

Bellis, M. A., G. Hale, A. Bennett, M. Chaudry, and M. Kilfoyle. 2000. Ibiza uncovered: Changes in substance use and sexual behaviour among young people visiting an international night-life resort. *The International Journal of Drug Policy* 11:235–44.

Bellis, M. A., K. Hughes, A. Bennett, and R. Thomson. 2003. Role of an international nightlife resort in the proliferation of recreational drugs. *Addiction* 98(12): 1713–21.

Berger, L. 1992. Hotel crime: Are you as safe as you think? *Corporate Travel* November: 26–29.

Brunt, P. and C. Davis. 2006. The nature of British media reporting of hedonistic tourism. *Crime Prevention and Community Safety: An International Journal* 8(1):30–49.

Brunt, P. and Z. Hambly. 1999. Tourism and crime: A review. *Crime Prevention and Community Safety: An International Journal* 1(2):25–36.

Brunt, P., R. I. Mawby, and Z. Hambly. 2000. Tourist victimisation and the fear of crime on holiday. *Tourism Management* 21:417–24.

Chesney-Lind, M. and I. Y. Lind. 1986. Visitors as victims: Crimes against tourists in Hawaii. *Annals of Tourism Research* 13:167–91.

Cohen, E. 1972. Towards a sociology of international tourism. *Social Research* 39(1):64–82.

———. 1973. Nomads from affluence: Notes on the phenomenon of drifter-tourism. *International Journal of Comparative Sociology* 14:89–103.

———. 1987. The tourist as victim and protege of law enforcement agencies. *Leisure Studies* 6(2):181–98.

———. 1996. Touting tourists in Thailand: Tourist oriented crime and social structure. In *Tourism, crime and international security issues*, ed. A. Pizam and Y. Mansfeld, 77–90. Chichester, UK: Wiley.

———. 2003. Backpacking: Diversity and change. *Tourism and Cultural Change* 1(2):95–110.

Cohen, L. and D. Cantor. 1981. Residential burglary in the United States: Life-style and demographic factors associated with the probability of victimization. *Journal of Research in Crime and Delinquency* 18:113–27.

Cohen, L. and M. Felson. 1979. Social change and crime rate trends: A routine activities approach. *American Sociological Review* 44(4):588–608.

Coleman, C. and J. Moynihan. 1996. *Understanding crime data*. Buckingham, UK: Open University Press.

Crotts, J. C. 1996. Theoretical perspectives on tourist criminal victimization. *The Journal of Tourism Studies* 7(1):2–9.

Dusquesne, V. 1995. *Les vols à la tire*. Paris: Institut des Hautes Études de la Sécurité Inteneur.

Elsrud, T. 2001. Risk creation in travelling: Backpacker adventure narration. *Annals of Tourism Research* 28(3):597–617.

Felson, M. and L. E. Cohen. 1980. Human ecology and crime: A routine activity approach. *Human Ecology* 8(4):389–405.

Fujii, E. T. and J. Mak. 1979. The impact of alternative regional development strategies on crime rates: Tourism vs agriculture in Hawaii. *Annals of Regional Science* 13(3):42–56.

Gallivan, J. 1994. Looking for trouble with the Miami police department. *The Guardian* January 22:42.

Gill, M., M. Salmon, and J. Hill. 1993. *Crime on holiday. Studies in crime, order and policing*. Research paper no. 1. Leicester, UK: University of Leicester.

Gillan, A. 2002. Erotic Emma: Drunk and at risk. *The Guardian* June 22:13.

Gottfredson, M. 1984. *Victims of crime: The dimensions of risk*. Home Office Research study no. 81. London: HMSO.

Harper, D. W. 2000. Planning in tourist robbery. *Annals of Tourism Research* 27(2):517–20.

_____. 2001. Comparing tourists crime victimization. *Annals of Tourism Research* 28(4):1053–56.

_____. 2006. The tourist and his criminal: Patterns in street robbery. In *Tourism, security and safety: From theory to practice*, ed. Y. Mansfeld and A. Pizam, 125–37. Oxford: Butterworth-Heinemann.

Hinz, W. 1985. Sanibel police undercover county-wide "Carnie" operation. *Florida Police Chief* 11(1):69–75.

Ho, T., J. Zhao, and M. P. Brown. 2009. Examining hotel crimes from police crime reports. *Crime Prevention and Community Safety: An International Journal* 11(1):21–33.

Homel, R., et al. 1997. Preventing drunkenness and violence around nightclubs in a tourist resort. In *Situational crime prevention: Successful case studies*, ed. R. V. Clarke, 263–82, 2nd ed. Guilderland, NY: Harrow and Heston.

Huang, W. S. W., M. Kwag, and G. Streib. 1998. Exploring the relationship between hotel characteristics and crime. *FIU Hospitality Review* 16(1):81–93.

Inciardi, J. A. 1976. The pickpocket and his victim. *Victimology* 1(3):446–53.

Israel, M. 1999. The victimisation of backpackers. *Alternative Law Journal* 24(5):229–32.

Jobes, P. C., E. Barclay, and J. F. Donnermeyer. 2000. *A qualitative and quantitative analysis of the relationship between community cohesiveness and rural crime, part 2*. Armidale, Australia: Institute for Rural Futures, University of New England.

Johns, N. 2007. Tourism and sentencing: Establishing status privileges. *International Journal of the Sociology of Law* 35(2):63–74.

Jones, C. and R. I. Mawby. 2005. Hotel crime: Who cares? *Crime Prevention and Community Safety: An International Journal* 7(3):19–35.

Jones, P. and K. Groenenboom. 2002. Crime in London hotels. *Tourism and Hospitality Research* 4(1):21–35.

Jud, G. D. 1975. Tourism and crime in Mexico. *Social Science Quarterly* 56:324–30.

Karmen, A. 1984. *Crime victims: An introduction to victimology*. Monterey, CA: Brooks/Cole.

_____. 1996. *Crime victims: An introduction to victimology*. Belmont, CA: Wadsworth.

Kelly, I. 1993. Tourist destination crime rates: An examination of Cairns and the Gold Coast, Australia. *Journal of Tourism Studies* 4(2):2–11.

King, D. A. 1988. Summertime crime in Jersey with particular reference to visitors to the island. PhD diss., University of Southampton.

LeBruto, S. M. 1996. Legal aspects of tourism and violence. In *Tourism, crime and international security issues*, ed. A. Pizam and Y. Mansfeld, 297–310. Chichester, UK: Wiley.

Lee, K-H. and J-Y. Lee. 2008. Cross-cultural analysis of perceptions of environmental characteristics in the target selection process for residential burglary. *Crime Prevention and Community Safety: An International Journal* 10(1):19–35.

Loker-Murphy, L. and P. L. Pearce. 1995. Young budget travelers: Backpackers in Australia. *Annals of Tourism Research* 22(4):819–43.

Low, S. 2004. *Behind the gates: Life, security and the pursuit of happiness in fortress America*. New York: Routledge.

Mansfeld, Y. and A. Pizam. 2006. *Tourism, security and safety: From theory to practice*. Burlington, MA: Butterworth-Heinemann.

Mawby, R. I. 2000. Tourists' perceptions of security: The risk-fear paradox. *Tourism Economics* 6(2):109–21.

_____. 2001. *Burglary*. Cullompton, UK: Willan.

_____. 2002. The land that crime forgot? Auditing the Isles of Scilly. *Crime Prevention and Community Safety: An International Journal* 4(2):39–53.

_____. 2006. Commercial burglary. In *The handbook of security*, ed. M. Gill, 430–63. London: Macmillan/Pergamon.

_____. 2007. Crime, place and explaining rural hotspots. *International Journal of Rural Crime* 1:21–43. www.ruralfutures.une.edu.au/rurcrime/ijrc.htm (accessed July 1, 2008).

_____. 2008. Understanding and responding to crime and disorder: Ensuring a local dimension. *Crime Prevention and Community Safety: An International Journal* 10(3):158–73.

Mawby, R. I., P. Brunt, and Z. Hambly. 1999. Victimisation on holiday: A British survey. *International Review of Victimology* 6:201–11.

_____. 2000. Fear of crime among British holidaymakers. *British Journal of Criminology* 40(3):468–79.

Mawby, R. I. and I. Gorgenyi. 1997. Break-ins to weekend homes: Research in a Hungarian city. In *Crime and criminology at the end of the century*, ed. E. Raska and J. Saar, 120–32. Tallinn, Estonia: Estonian National Defense and Public Service Academy.

Mawby, R. I. and C. Jones. 2007. Attempting to reduce hotel burglary: Implementation failure in a multi-agency context. *Crime Prevention and Community Safety: An International Journal* 9(3):145–66.

Mawby, R. I., W. Mcintosh, and E. Barclay. 2008. *Burglary geographies: Applying theories from domestic burglary to caravan park crime.* Paper presented at the British Society of Criminology Conference, Huddersfield.

Maxfield, M. G. 1987. Household composition, routine activity and victimization: A comparative analysis. *Journal of Quantitative Criminology* 3(4): 301–20.

McCulloch, J. 1991. *Backpackers: The growth sector of Australian tourism.* Brisbane: Queensland Parliamentary Library.

McPeters, L. R. and W. B. Stronge. 1974. Crime as an environmental externality of tourism: Miami, Florida. *Land Economics* 50:359–81.

McVeigh, K. 2003. Faliraki: A Greek tragedy. *The Scotsman*, August 23.

Michalko, G. 2004. Tourism eclipsed by crime: The vulnerability of foreign tourists in Hungary. *Journal of Travel and Tourism Marketing* 15(2–3):159–72.

Milman, A. and A. Pizam. 1988. Social impacts of tourism on Central Florida. *Annals of Tourism Research* 15:191–204.

Mirrlees-Black, C., P. Mayhew, and A. Percy. 1996. *The 1996 British crime survey: England and Wales.* HO Statistical Bulletin 19/96. London: HMSO.

Mohsin, A. and C. Ryan. 2003. Backpackers in the Northern Territory of Australia: Motives, behaviours and satisfactions. *The International Journal of Tourism Research* 5(2):113–31.

Muehsam, M. J. and P. E. Tarlow. 1995. Involving the police in tourism. *Tourism Management* 16(1):9–14.

Nicholas, S., C. Kershaw, and A. Walker. 2007. *Crime in England and Wales 2006/07.* HO Statistical Bulletin 11/07. London: Home Office. www.homeoffice.gov.uk/rds/pdfs07/hosb1107.pdf (accessed July 1, 2008).

O'Reilly, C. C. 1997. From drifter to gap year: Mainstreaming the backpacker experience. MA thesis, University of Surrey, Roehampton.

Palmer, R. A. 1989. The hospitality customer as crime victim: Recent legal research. *Hospitality Education and Research Journal* 13(3):225–29.

Pearce, P. L. 1990. *The backpacker phenomenon: Preliminary answers to basic questions.* Townsville, Australia: Department of Tourism, James Cook University.

Pelfrey, W. V. 1998. Tourism and crime: A preliminary assessment of the relationship of crime to the number of visitors at selected sites. *International Journal of Comparative and Applied Criminology* 22(1–2):293–304.

Pizam, A. 1982. Tourism and crime: Is there a relationship? *Journal of Travel Research* 20(3):7–10.

Pizam, A. and V. Mansfeld. 1996. *Tourism, crime and international security issues.* Chichester, UK: Wiley.

Prestia, K. L. 1993. *Chocolates for the pillows nightmares for the guests: The failure of the hotel industry to protect the public from violent crime.* Silver Spring, MD: Bartleby.

Prideaux, B. 1995. *Mass tourism and crime: Is there a connection? A study of crime in major Queensland tourism destinations.* Proceedings of the Australian National Tourism Research and Education conferences 1994, Bureau of Tourism Research, Canberra, 251–60.

———. 1996. The tourism crime cycle: A beach destination case study. In *Tourism, crime and international security issues*, ed. A. Pizam and Y. Mansfeld, 59–76. Chichester, UK: Wiley.

Ross, G. F. 1997. Backpacker achievement and environment controllability as visitor motivators. *Journal of Travel and Tourism Marketing* 6(6):69–82.

Rountree, P. W. and K. C. Land. 1996 Burglary victimization, perceptions of crime risk, and routine activities: A multilevel analysis across Seattle neighborhoods and census tracts. *Journal of Research in Crime and Delinquency* 33(2):147–80.

Ryan, C. 1991. *Recreational tourism: A social science perspective.* London: Routledge.

——. 1993. Crime, violence, terrorism and tourism: An accident or intrinsic relationship. *Tourism Management* 14(3):173–83.

Schiebler, S. A., J. C. Crotts, and R. C. Hollinger. 1996. Florida tourists' vulnerability to crime. In *Tourism, crime and international security issues*, ed. A. Pizam and Y. Mansfeld, 37–50. Chichester, UK: Wiley.

Sherman, L. W., P. R. Gartin, and M. E. Buerger. 1989. Hot spots of predatory crime: Routine activities and the criminology of place. *Criminology* 27(1):27–55.

Smith, H. 1993. *Hotel security.* Springfield, IL: Charles C. Thomas.

Stangeland, P. 1998. Other targets or other locations? An analysts of opportunity structures. *British Journal of Criminology* 38(1):61–77.

Tarlow, P. 2000. Letter from America: A short history of tourism oriented policing services. *Crime Prevention and Community Safety: An International Journal* 2(1):55–58.

Thoms, C. 2002. *Backpackers in Australia, 1999.* BTR Niche Market Report 1. Canberra: Bureau of Tourism Research.

Uriely, N., Y. Yonay, and D. Simchai. 2002. Backpacking experiences: A type and form analysis. *Annals of Tourism Research* 29(2):520–38.

van Dijk, J., J. van Kesteren, and P. Smit. 2008. *Criminal victimisation in international perspective: Key findings from the 2004-2005 ICVS and EU ICS.* The Hague: Boom Legal. http://rechten.uvt.nl/icvs/pdffiles/ICVS2004_05.pdf (accessed July 1, 2008).

Vesselinov, E., M. Cazessus, and W. Falk. 2007. Gated communities and spatial inequality. *Journal of Urban Affairs* 29(2):109–27.

Walmsley, D. J., R. M. Boskovic, and J. J. Pigram. 1983. Tourism and crime: An Australian perspective. *Journal of Leisure Research* 15(2):136–55.

Waszkiewicz, P. 2007. Gated communities: Effect of fear of crime. Paper presented at the 7th Annual Conference of the European Society of Criminology, Bologna.

Zhao, J. and T. Ho. 2006. Are foreign visitors more likely victimized in hotels? Policy implications. *Security Journal* 19(1):33–44.

Responses to Criminal Victimization

IV

Victims and Criminal Justice in Europe

13

JOANNA SHAPLAND

Contents

13.1 Introduction

Although victim participation is essential for the smooth working of criminal justice, the relationship between victims and criminal justice, in modern times in Western societies, has been a relatively fraught one. The increasing use of state prosecutors, rather than individual private prosecutions by victims, has tended to minimize perceptions of the necessity and importance of all lay witnesses, and particularly victims. Criminal justice has become seen, by many professionals in criminal justice, as primarily a matter between the state and the offender. Some theorists, such as Christie [1977], have argued that this is an inevitable consequence, with the state and its professionals increasingly "stealing" the original conflict (the crime) and its resolution from the victim and offender. Christie suggests that there is little possibility of reform, with the participants needing to find any support necessary from outside criminal justice, in civil justice (compensation or mediation procedures) or in victim assistance and support. Others are not so pessimistic, although appreciating the difficulty in carving out an appropriate place for victims in criminal justice, amid the plethora of

347

official agencies now involved (e.g., police, prosecution, judiciary, and probation services). Shapland [1988] has referred to these agencies as fiefdoms, proud of their own territory and prepared to repulse anyone encroaching on it, such as, potentially, victims. Certainly, the history of criminal justice reform in Europe in relation to victims is a history of slow progress and considerable difficulties.

The difficulties seem to be somewhat greater in common law, Anglo-Saxon jurisdictions (such as England and Wales, the United States, and Australia) than they do in mainland European countries, whose legal systems are based on Napoleonic or Roman law principles (such as France or the Netherlands). In common law countries, procedure has reduced to being a process between state agencies (in court represented by the prosecutor) and the offender (represented by a defense legal representative), with, effectively, an umpiring role for the judge. In mainland European countries, although procedures in different countries vary, more emphasis is placed on building a file (the dossier) setting out the evidence—which aims to contain all relevant material—and less on oral evidence. Victim claims (e.g., for compensation) and victim statements about what happened and the effects of the offense can often form part of the file. In several countries, this has given rise to the possibility of the victim joining his or her civil claim for compensation to the criminal case (*partie civile*) and so becoming a party to the case, required to be notified of its progress.

Throughout Europe, there has been a gradual and growing appreciation of the effects of the crime and the criminal justice process on victims and of the need to ameliorate the process to meet some of victims' justified criticisms. Victim support and assistance programs exist in all countries, although their scope, coverage, and services vary considerably. Some attention has been paid to the need to inform victims of the progress of the criminal case. Certain special measures have been taken to allow some greater participation, particularly for vulnerable witnesses, in some countries. However, given the recommendations of the Council of Europe Recommendation on the Position of the Victim in Criminal Justice (in 1985) and the framework decision of the European Commission in 2001, progress is slow. The chapter will concentrate on progress in England and Wales but will also look at the separate jurisdictions of Scotland and Northern Ireland, as well as make comparisons, where possible, with mainland European countries, given their different legal framework. In this, it is important to consider not only legislative change but also what has occurred in practice (often a very different matter). The difficulty is that the tradition of evaluation of criminal justice initiatives is very variable throughout Europe. Most substantial changes in England and Wales have been evaluated, and the results published. In other countries, information is patchier. There is a very good review of the position in 2000 by Brienen and Hoegen [2000] covering many European countries, but an update on this is only now being undertaken.*

The first question to consider, however, is the extent to which offenses—and victims—actually come into contact with criminal justice and so the extent to which provisions for victims in criminal justice impact on victims.

13.2 Do Victims Interact with Criminal Justice?

Although the words *victim* and *criminal justice* are often heard in the same breath, it is not automatic for victims to become involved with criminal justice. For the criminal justice process to start, normally with the police, the offense has to be reported to the criminal justice authorities. Most commonly, this is done by victims themselves or by witnesses acting on their behalf. If the assault was in a bar, the bartender will ring the police—or if the theft took place in the university, the university security staff will ring the police if the victim requests it. However, the victim may not wish to inform the police and have the incident recorded as a crime [Ericson, 1982], and it is unlikely that the police will come across offenses themselves [Hough and Clarke, 1980]. Maguire and Bennett [1982], for example, found that the vast majority of the house burglaries he studied in England and Wales were reported by victims.

The formal legal position when an offense becomes known to the police varies for different countries in Europe. In England and Wales, for example, the police have discretion as to whether to record an offense as a crime, although they would normally do so if the victim wished it and will certainly do so for all serious offenses for which there is sufficient evidence that a criminal offense has occurred. For less serious offenses, however, it can be a negotiation between victim and police as to whether an offense should be recorded as a crime and the offender pursued and prosecuted, or whether the police should treat the offense in a more informal way, or whether they should merely record it as intelligence about what is happening in the area, with little attempt to find the perpetrator [Shapland and Vagg, 1988]. Different outcomes are likely depending on whether the offenders are known, whether they are young, whether they are local, and whether this is likely to be a one-off, minor incident.

In Germany, in contrast, the formal position is that the police must record any offense they consider a crime and investigate it, with the likelihood of prosecuting any offender who is caught. Other European countries have formal positions between those of Germany and England and Wales

---

* Tilburg University's INTERVICT Institute is carrying out an evaluation of the progress of countries toward the 2001 European Union's Framework Decision's provisions, with the Portuguese victim assistance society. This should be published in 2009.

[Brienen and Hoegen, 2000]. Everywhere, however, the amount of investigative effort put into a particular offense is likely to depend on the likelihood of
catching the offender, given the evidence, and the seriousness of the offense,
which includes the emphasis given to it by the victim and the effects on the
victim.

The likelihood of an offense being reported to the police in each country
is not necessarily high. Crime surveys, such as the British Crime Survey
(BCS) [Moley, 2008] and the International Crime Victims Survey (ICVS)
[van Dijk et al., 2007], show that:

> The frequency with which victims (or relatives and friends on their behalf)
> report offences to the police is strongly related to the type of offence involved.
> In most countries, almost all cars and motorcycles stolen were reported, as
> well as 75 per cent of burglaries with entry. About two-thirds of thefts from
> cars were reported, and rather more than half of bicycle thefts and robberies.
> Only about a third of all assaults and threats were drawn to the attention of the
> police, although the figure was higher for assaults with force than for threats.
> Sexual incidents mentioned to interviewers were least frequently reported
> (on average 15%). Where sexual assault was mentioned, though, 28 per cent
> of incidents were reported; where offensive behaviour was involved, only
> 10 per cent were drawn to police attention. [van Dijk et al., 2007:109]

On average, across the 30 countries studied in the 2004–2005 ICVS, 41%
of these crimes were reported to the police—so a majority never came to the
attention of the police. The highest reporting rates in Europe were in Austria
(70%), Belgium (68%), Sweden (64%), and Switzerland (63%), whereas low
rates were found in Bulgaria, Iceland, Estonia, and Poland—although these
were nothing like the low reporting rates found in developing countries in
other parts of the world.

If the offense is not reported to the police and does not come to police
attention, then necessarily the victim does not have any interaction with the
criminal justice system. This means that the victim also will not be able to
benefit from any victim assistance whose gateways are via criminal justice
system personnel (police, prosecutors, courts). We know that the effects of
the offense on the victim are generally less serious in offenses not reported
to the police—but this does not mean that all victims whose cases are not
reported suffer no effects—far from it. Just one example are the cases of rape
and child abuse that may not come to light for many years.

Some have argued that too much attention has been focused on victims
who have contact with criminal justice and that it would be better to turn
from a crime-focused approach to a harm-focused approach, where priorities for action (meaning governmental action) would be set by the amount
of harm experienced by individual victims and society [Garside, 2006]. Part
of the rationale for this approach is the fact that a majority of "traditional"

crimes are not reported to criminal justice, as we saw above, hence little is offered to the majority of victims. Part is an appreciation that some criminal offenses, such as health and safety offenses or environmental crimes, can cause serious harm to both individuals and communities but are rarely dealt with through traditional criminal justice means [Tombs and Whyte, 2004]. Although these are serious arguments, they do not seem to me to lay aside the importance of criminal justice. Where victims do report offenses to the police, it is clear that they have considerable expectations of what the criminal justice system will do about those offenses, as has been shown in all empirical studies of victims from the beginning of victimology empirical research in Europe in the 1980s [Maguire and Bennett, 1982; Shapland et al., 1985].

13.2.1 Victims' Reactions to Crime

Before discussing the reactions of victims to criminal justice and the initiatives that have been taken by criminal justice in the past 20 or so years, it is important to explore victims' initial reactions to crime. From victims' reactions to crime come victims' needs for assistance and victims' expectations of criminal justice—and hence their reactions to what criminal justice personnel do.

In Europe, we are faced with considerable challenges in trying to meet victims' needs. The challenges stem from the fact that, for most victims, crime is not normal. It is not expected; it is a shock. From that stems the feelings of disruption, of the bubble of our normal lives being punctured, and of guilt as to how it happened to me, which are reported by many victims of crime [Shapland et al., 1985; Shapland and Hall, 2007]. The exception to this is of course where victimization is repeated again and again and becomes a feared but expected part of people's lives, which is why child abuse, domestic violence, and racial harassment are so terrible and why we see them as so serious.

But for most victims of burglary, theft, damage, or assault in the developed world, crime is not expected. Given that crime rates, particularly property crime rates, have been decreasing over the past several years by a very considerable amount in many countries in Europe [van Dijk et al., 2007], crime is becoming even more unexpected. The reaction of people to becoming a victim is, therefore, normally one of shock. Indeed, when people are burgled, have goods stolen, or are assaulted, they are not normally in a very good state to think clearly and rationally about exactly where to go for help. The emergency health system is likely to function about exactly as it would if any injuries were caused through an accident. But criminal justice is not prioritized around meeting victim needs—and does not seem to have changed very substantially in this respect in the past 20 years. It is because the priority of policing is not crime victims but catching offenders, investigating offenses, and keeping the peace/preventing further offenses.

Early research on victim expectations in England and Wales when they reported offenses to the police emphasized that what was important was not only efficiency (the police come; the police come quickly; police officers ask the right questions to catch the offender) but also the manner of the police: that the police should show interest, should take account of the shocked state of the victim, and should either refer people to victim assistance or give them information about it [Shapland et al., 1985].

In England and Wales, the government has set Victim's Charter Standards—four of them for the police. Ringham and Salisbury [2004], using BCS responses, set out to see to what extent victims felt the police were meeting those standards. They found the police were seen as providing a good response in terms of efficiency and showing interest in the crime, but, after the initial encounter, feedback was clearly not sufficient:

- Seventy-three percent of victims felt they did not have to wait or waited a reasonable amount of time for the police response.
- Sixty-five percent said the police showed enough interest in their crime, and 60% said the police showed enough effort.
- BUT only 51% said the police gave them a phone number to contact the officer or crime desk responsible for their case.
- Forty-six percent said the police provided the "Victims of Crime" leaflet.
- Just 34% of victims felt they had been kept very or fairly informed by the police about the progress of the investigation.

The BCS interviews a sample of the general public, asking everyone who has been a victim in the past 12 months about their experiences with the police and criminal justice system. Hence the results above show the experiences of all those who have had any dealings with the police as a victim. The Witness and Victim Experience Survey (WAVES) [Moore and Blakeborough, 2008] deals only with victims and witnesses in cases in which the offender is caught and is charged—that is, victims whose cases have proceeded further into the criminal justice system.[*] The Code of Practice for Victims of Crime [Office for Criminal Justice Reform, 2005a] says that all victims must be provided by the police with the leaflet "Victims of Crime," which tells them what is likely to happen next and gives them information about victim assistance. Moore and Blakeborough [2008] found that 74% of victims recalled being given such a leaflet. This is much higher than the BCS findings above and suggests that the police may be targeting information and help on particular kinds of victims, particularly burglary victims and victims of more serious crimes.

---

[*] The offenses covered by the WAVES are violence against the person, robbery, burglary, theft and handling stolen goods, and criminal damage.

A recent review of the needs of victims in the Netherlands has shown a very similar pattern of needs in relation to criminal justice: Victims need help in contacting the police; the police should arrive quickly; and victims should be treated as interested parties. Victims should be kept informed and, where relevant, consulted [Boom et al., 2008]. Some other European countries have institutionalized some information to victims. For example, in France, the police or prosecutor will provide victims with a copy of their report to the criminal justice authorities on the spot—but requirements to notify the victim thereafter are the responsibility of the prosecutor, so it is rare that the police will keep victims informed [Brienen and Hoegen, 2000]. Similarly, in France, concise information leaflets for victims exist—but they are rarely to be found in police stations; rather, they are in courts and prosecutors' offices, town halls, and victim support centers. There is a disjunction between where victims report and where duties to support victims lie. There are no automatic referral systems to victim assistance services, unlike in the United Kingdom. The position is similar in Germany, with only victims who have an active role as a party in the criminal case (an auxiliary prosecutor or claiming compensation) being considered as in need of information [Brienen and Hoegen, 2000]. In contrast, in the Netherlands, there are automated computerized procedures for the police to record victim wishes about referral to victim assistance and to be kept informed, although it is doubtful that these are used in every case [Brienen and Hoegen, 2000].

13.3 The Subsequent Progress of the Case and Decisions to Prosecute

What happens after this first encounter with the police? The early English research, which interviewed victims of violent crime who had reported to the police and whose offenders had been caught, found that, after the initial encounter, when three-quarters of victims were satisfied with what the police had done, satisfaction started dropping markedly [Shapland et al., 1985]. The prime reason was lack of feedback on what was happening with the case and consequent perceptions that the police were not doing much, were not interested, and did not seem to care. That research, which has been widely publicized, was done some 30 years ago. It is dispiriting that, despite feedback to victims becoming an important part of policy responses, similar results exist today.

So, for example, the WAVES found, for England and Wales, that although 61% of victims were recontacted about their case within 1 month, 1 in 10 victims claimed that they did not hear anything further from the criminal justice authorities at all [Moore and Blakeborough, 2008]. However, the Code of Practice states that victims should be kept informed of case progress at least monthly. If victims are not themselves contacted by the police to say what is happening, then many victims will try to contact the police. The question then is whether they are facilitated to do so. The "No Witness, No Justice" initiative by the government in England and Wales states that victims and witnesses should have a nominated key contact person [Cabinet Office, 2005]. The WAVES found that 74% of victims reported they had been provided with a contact—but that means one-quarter of victims had not. The response of the criminal justice authorities is patchy.

Most of the responsibility in England and Wales for notifying victims is placed on the police, not the prosecutor. Only the prosecutor, however, can provide reasons why the charge a suspect faces has been changed or why the prosecution of the case has been discontinued by the prosecutor. There has been considerable negotiation with the Crown Prosecution Service (CPS) since their formation about the response they would be able to make to victims. The most recent initiative is that Witness Care Units have been set up in each area in England and Wales, staffed by CPS staff and police personnel (but not necessarily prosecutors or police officers) [CPS, 2008]. The CPS Code of Practice came into force in 2006 and indicates that vulnerable or intimidated witnesses should be notified within 1 working day if there is insufficient evidence to charge the offender* and within 5 working days for all other victims. If this is happening, it would show very substantially improved standards of service. The One Stop Shop pilot [Hoyle et al., 1998], which aimed to provide information at all stages to victims of serious crimes, fell down largely because of lack of information received from the CPS and the higher courts (Crown Court).

In France, the public prosecutor has a formal obligation to inform the victim about the final decision regarding prosecution (if, of course, a suspect has been apprehended). This includes any decision as to whether to attempt mediation between victim and offender [Brienen and Hoegen, 2000]. Brienen and Hoegen comment, however, that in practice many victims are not informed. The particular need in France to inform victims expeditiously is because victims have the right to pursue a claim for compensation alongside the criminal prosecution but need to lodge that claim in good time. In Germany, there is a similar duty on the prosecutor if the prosecutor intends to drop the prosecution—but no provision to tell victims that the case is going ahead. The Netherlands have set up service desks to provide information to victims about the case. This provides a more automatic system that is likely to be more effective in practice, but it means that, except in serious cases, there is likely to be less contact with the public prosecutor [Brienen and

---

* See below for the definition and provisions relating to vulnerable and intimidated witnesses.

Hoegen, 2000]. It is clear that there is no one uniform system for interaction between police, prosecution, and victim across Europe—and that no system is currently working in a foolproof way.

13.4 At Court

Few victims attend court—because only a relatively low proportion of offenders are caught; because many offenders plead guilty and so witnesses are not required; or because, in civil law countries on the European mainland, hearing witnesses orally is rare—rather, statements are taken from witnesses and put together in a dossier laid by the prosecution before the court.

Nonetheless, where witnesses do appear at court, their evidence is vital for the outcome of the trial. In common law countries (such as England and Wales and the United States), there is a tradition of oral evidence and, if the offender does not plead guilty, then the victim is highly likely to need to testify in court.

Previous research evidence about victims' own views of testifying has produced mixed findings. Early British evidence indicated that victims did not necessarily find the process traumatic if they were well supported [Shapland et al., 1985]—but it is clear that victims of sexual abuse or assault have very different reactions, both in the United Kingdom and in the United States [Holmstrom and Burgess, 1978; Shapland et al., 1985]. This is because of aggressive and intrusive cross-examination by defense lawyers that may probe into intimate details and also may explore the victim's previous sexual history. In England and Wales, legal moves have been made to prohibit such questioning, such that judges can intervene— but they are discretionary on the judge. Jennifer Temkin's research [1987; Temkin and Krahé, 2007] has shown that judges are very loath to intervene and that the experience of giving evidence as a sexual assault victim remains problematic.

Paralleling the development of initiatives in the United States—where witness care programs were some of the earliest initiatives to support victims and help them to testify—major initiatives have been taken in England and Wales (and are being implemented in the rest of the United Kingdom as well) to support witnesses at court. We need to notice that these are initiatives for all witnesses (although they tend to be dominated by prosecution witnesses) and are not restricted to victims. It is clear that the dominant philosophy behind these initiatives is to aid criminal justice, rather than to support victims especially. Nonetheless, they have been among the more successful initiatives in the area of victim services.

An early initiative in England and Wales was the development of the Witness Service. Initially provided at the higher courts, it was then rolled out to magistrates' courts. It is run by Victim Support[*] through the provision of a separate grant from government. The Witness Service:

- Staffs reception desks or helps to staff reception desks.
- Has a room in which witnesses can wait, with comfortable furniture, away from the other party.
- Will provide a visit to the court to look around the courtroom before the trial (a familiarization visit)—although only 60% of those eligible for such a visit in a recent survey were offered one [Moore and Blakeborough, 2008].
- Will provide help with expense forms and any other bureaucracy.
- Provides support through volunteer staff, although staff are not counselors or legally trained and so can only give a listening ear [Victim Support, 2008].

These are many of the services highlighted by surveys of courts in England and Wales as being very variable before the advent of the Witness Service [Shapland and Cohen, 1987; Shapland and Bell, 1998]. Earlier research paints a picture of intimidation by offenders, lack of facilities (including such basic facilities as refreshments and lavatories), lack of signage to courts, and a general view that courts were being run for the benefit of the professionals working at the courthouse, rather than the witnesses attending to give evidence [Shapland and Cohen, 1987; Rock, 1993]. By 2002, 81% of witnesses had contact with the Witness Service, a considerable expansion since the equivalent 2000 survey, when only 51% had contact [Angle et al., 2003]. This was because of the expansion of the Witness Service to all courts in England and Wales.

However, a minority of witnesses still feel intimidated at court. The 2002 survey found that 26% felt intimidated by an individual, whereas 21% felt intimidated by the process of giving evidence or by the court environment itself [Angle et al., 2003]. The strongest predictors of dissatisfaction among witnesses were feeling they were taken for granted at court and feeling intimidated by the process or the court environment. Clearly, although there have been significant improvements, there is still more work to do. This has led to the special provisions for vulnerable and intimidated witnesses in England and Wales, as described below.

The Witness Service's work primarily kicks in when they are notified that the witness will be attending court. The problem is that there are still difficulties with notification of hearings and information about victim/witness needs before this. The One Stop Shop pilot was an attempt to address these barriers to information flowing through the criminal justice process, by providing

---

[*] In England and Wales—and by Victim Support Scotland as a free service at all courts in Scotland.

one information point (at the level of the police) through which victims could be notified, for serious crime offenses only [Hoyle et al., 1998]. Dates of court hearings were one of the most important expectations victims had from the One Stop Shop (together with being informed of the verdict and sentence). Just over one-fifth said they had not been told about the date of trial (or the verdict or sentence). Most of those who were told were informed by the One Stop Shop personnel—but just less than one-half were in fact informed by other people, primarily other police personnel. Clearly, even when a special initiative was mounted, there were still difficulties getting information to all victims, even the relatively small category of victims of serious crimes.

Similar findings occur for other European countries. In France, information about the date and location of the hearing should be provided to the victim who reported the crime—and any victim who has also joined their civil claim for compensation through the *partie civile* procedure will be summonsed to court [Brienen and Hoegen, 2000]. However, Brienen and Hoegen comment that it is common for victims who are not civil claimants not to be informed, often contacting victim assistance organizations or the prosecution, only to find that their case has already been heard. This is particularly true where "speedy justice" measures are being used, whereby the offender may be tried and sentenced within 1 day. In Germany, the dominance of the system itself is even more marked. The victim needs only to receive information about the date and place of the hearing if he or she has an active role to play in those proceedings (as a witness or as an auxiliary prosecutor pursuing a civil claim for compensation alongside the criminal trial in a similar form of *partie civile* as in France) [Brienen and Hoegen, 2000]. The Netherlands places more duties on the prosecution than do France or Germany. The prosecution service should inform victims as soon as possible of the date and place of the trial and of any change of date. Although information about the initial trial date seems mostly to occur, postponements are more rarely notified, with the accompanying danger that victims will come to court, only to find that the case has been put over to another date [Brienen and Hoegen, 2000].

13.4.1 Initiatives in Relation to Vulnerable and Intimidated Witnesses

A major series of initiatives in England and Wales, which are being adopted subsequently in Scotland and in Northern Ireland, concern special provisions for vulnerable witnesses called to give evidence at court. The idea that some witnesses need special treatment so that they are enabled to give their best evidence is an old one. Children who testify have been treated differently in relation to oaths and to how they were questioned for many years. Particular provisions for children giving evidence were discussed in the Pigot report

[1989], which recommended that evidence from children might be allowed in court even though taken on video much earlier. This was followed by provisions to allow judges to remove wigs and gowns when dealing with child witnesses and oral evidence at the trial, where necessary via a remote television link, and so forth.

These provisions became standard practice in relation to child witnesses, particularly for child abuse cases. Social workers and police officers became used to working together to interview children where abuse was suspected, using videotaped interviews undertaken in comfortable surroundings. Such evidence became routinely used at court. Where children were required also to give oral testimony, this was often from a different room in the court house, using a live television link, so that the child could only see the judge or the lawyer questioning him or her, rather than the whole courtroom (and hence the suspect). The court participants could, however, see the child.

More controversial were suggestions that these kinds of provisions should be extended to other witnesses who might be particularly vulnerable. Research by Sanders et al. [1997] showed that adult victims with learning disabilities had very similar difficulties to those of children and indicated strongly that they should receive the benefit of similar measures in the courtroom. The Home Office report, *Speaking Up for Justice*, in 1998 proposed a much wider category of vulnerable witnesses to include both witnesses who were intrinsically vulnerable (such as child witnesses, witnesses with learning disabilities, and witnesses with other disabilities) and also witnesses who were vulnerable because of potential intimidation or because of the nature of the offense itself. The prime example of the last were victims of sexual assault, both adult and child victims. The Criminal Justice and Youth Evidence Act in 1999, which followed closely on the report, expanded the "special provisions" originally introduced for child witnesses to all vulnerable witnesses, and they now include giving evidence via a television link, prerecorded examination in chief and cross-examination, screening off witnesses from the defendants, clearing the public gallery of the court, the removal of lawyers' wigs and gowns in the Crown Court, and giving evidence through intermediaries.

The possibility of using each of these provisions needs to be discussed in a pretrial hearing, at which the CPS is supposed to bring forward any need for such measures. Their use is at the discretion of the judge, providing the witness falls within the definition of a vulnerable witness as noted in the 1999 Act. The categories of persons eligible for special measures are children aged less than 17 years, witnesses under a physical disability or physical disorder, witnesses with a learning disability or mental disorder, and witnesses likely to suffer particular distress, including victims of sexual offenses and witnesses who fear or suffer intimidation.

The use of these special measures and witnesses' reactions to them have been analyzed using the WAVES [Hamlyn et al., 2004]. This is a survey of witnesses aged 16 years and over who give evidence at court in cases where an adult offender has been charged. Therefore, it includes victims and other prosecution witnesses, although not police officers or expert witnesses. It does not include sexual or domestic violence, crimes involving a fatality, or any crime where the defendant was a family member or a member of the household, but covers a wide range of offenses, including violence, burglary, theft, and criminal damage.

Hamlyn et al. [2004] interviewed 569 witnesses, of whom 42% were aged less than 17 years; and 13% reported a disability that limited daily activities, 70% reported either fearing or experiencing intimidation, and 15% were victims of a sexual offense. It is clear from this that the different categories of vulnerable and intimidated witnesses (VIW) overlap—many witnesses who are vulnerable for other reasons also fear intimidation.

Compared with all witnesses, VIW were less satisfied with their overall experience. Overall 69% were very or fairly satisfied with their treatment compared with 78% of all witnesses [Angle et al., 2003]. Child witnesses (those aged less than 17 years) tended to be more satisfied than adults, and people who had experienced or feared intimidation tended to be less satisfied than those who had not. However, as we shall see, the use of special measures did seem to have a major positive effect on witnesses.

By 2004, video-recorded evidence-in-chief was used by 42% of child witnesses, a live television link for giving evidence for 83% of child witnesses (i.e., the vast majority), and removal of wigs and gowns at the Crown Court by 15% of Crown Court witnesses. Rates for adult witnesses were much lower (e.g., only 15% of adult VIW were offered a live link). Other forms of assistance, including pagers, escorts, and intermediaries, were used only rarely among VIW.

Witnesses using special measures rated them very highly. As Hamlyn et al. [2004:xii] said:

> For example nine in ten witnesses using the live TV link found this helpful, and a similar proportion found using video-recorded evidence-in-chief useful. The importance of special measures is further vindicated by the finding that 33 per cent of witnesses using any special measure said that they would not have been willing and able to give evidence without this.

In addition, witnesses using special measures were less likely to be anxious, less likely to experience cross-examination as very upsetting, and more likely to have a favorable opinion of the criminal justice system. It is clear that the use of special measures and the provisions of the Act are one of the rare success stories of the criminal justice system in relation to witnesses (and victims).

Unfortunately, however, other aspects of criminal justice services to victims seemed still to be lacking, even among these VIW. Just more than one-third of VIW said that they had not been kept informed at all about the progress of the case (36%) (a little more than one-quarter of VIW said that they had been kept regularly informed [32%], and the remaining 37% said that they had been informed occasionally). Pretrial familiarization visits to the court seemed, however, to have been implemented. Twenty-nine percent of VIW had visited the court before the trial to familiarize themselves. This increased to 68% for victims of sexual offenses. But nearly half of VIW stated that the original date set for the court hearing had been changed, with this occurring in almost half of cases on the day of the trial (35%) or the day before (10%). This clearly caused upset and anxiety.

While giving evidence, most VIW felt they could understand the questions put, but there was a minority who found it difficult, who did not feel they could ask for a break in questioning, or who felt overawed and unable to communicate their difficulties.

VIW are supposed, under the legislation, to be consulted about the possible use of special measures (usually by the police acting on behalf of the CPS). However, Hamlyn et al. [2004] found that only 32% had been consulted (although when they were, the vast majority felt their input had been effective). This ties in with the chief drawback in the way in which the special measures have been enacted—whether it is thought to raise the possibility of their use in a pretrial hearing. The problem is that unless the prosecution (police, prosecutor) think about it during their perusal of the file, it is highly likely that such a hearing will not consider special measures. If, for example, there is no clear note on the file about the advisability of measures, and if the prosecutor receives the file close to the time of the hearing, then no one may raise the issue. Clearly, as the use of special measures has become more widespread, then prosecutors, etc., are likely to think about them when the witness falls into an obvious category (e.g., child witness). However, adults with disabilities may not be obvious until they reach court. This was the finding of Burton et al. [2006], who estimated, in a qualitative study, that there are considerable gaps. They considered that 24% of witnesses in their sample were potentially vulnerable or intimidated compared with 9% actually identified by agencies for their sample and the 7–10% envisaged by *Speaking Up for Justice* [Home Office, 1998].

Readers will have noticed that in this section, I have been speaking of "witnesses" rather than "victims." The provisions for VIW are of course for all prosecution witnesses, which are likely to include victims. However, some victims are not called to give evidence, although there may be testimony from other prosecution witnesses.* Equally, many cases do not proceed to an active trial with oral evidence because the offender pleads guilty. In both

---

* The evidence from the victim may be agreed by the defense, for example, if the victim was not present at a burglary and was merely giving evidence about damage caused and property taken.

these examples, the VIW provisions do not apply to victims—and there will not necessarily be any provisions for victims. It is clear that this radical action in England and Wales on behalf of witnesses has been taken because they are witnesses, and so the progress of the prosecution and trial depends on them. It is reminiscent of the early U.S. provisions to get witnesses to court in the 1970s and 1980s (e.g., witness warning programs, familiarization visits). The priority is criminal justice, not victims. Nonetheless, the measures have proved very beneficial to those victims (and other witnesses) who have used them. Equivalent provisions do not yet seem to have been introduced on a statutory basis in other parts of Europe.

13.5 A Role for Victims in Sentencing?

One of the most debated potential reforms in relation to victims in England and Wales has been their potential role in sentencing. Here, I am referring to sentencing within the standard criminal justice system for adult offenders. Restorative justice has become a mainstream option for young offenders in England and Wales,* and youth conferencing is now the mainstream stat-utory requirements in Northern Ireland [Campbell et al., 2006]. For adult offenders, however, most lawyers have been very loathe to permit any victim input during the phase between conviction and sentencing. They have been afraid that sentencing might become driven by vindictive victims[†] or judges overly affected by a recital of the effects of the offense on victims. Essentially, they have argued that sentencing is a matter for the state and the offender and that the victim should have no role.

This is despite two developments: the increasing use of compensation as part of the sentence, and the case law requiring judges to be aware of the effects of the offense on victims when sentencing. Compensation orders (payments by the offender to the victim as part of the sentence of the court) were introduced in England and Wales in 1972, and by 1988 through the Criminal Justice Act, judges were not only required to consider one in any case where there is an identifiable victim and loss, injury, or damage, but also to give reasons why they did not use a compensation order were they to decide not to make one. Clearly, judges cannot consider compensation to the victim without knowing the extent of loss, injury, etc., and they are required to inform themselves on this. Compensation orders were also introduced in

---

* Through the use of referral orders (trained members of the community sitting on panels to decide on the form of the sentence—attendance at programs, supervision, etc.—for first offenders sentenced by the court to a referral order, victims may be present at such panels [Crawford and Newburn, 2003]), reparation orders, compensation orders, etc.
† Although all the evidence suggests that victims in England and Wales and in Northern Ireland are very rarely vindictive [Dignan, 2005; Doak and O'Mahony, 2006].

Scotland and the Netherlands in the early 1980s and into Northern Ireland somewhat later.

The case law on sentencing and victim effects in England and Wales has been driven by the effects of sexual assault offenses on victims and in particular the need for judges to take account of the serious and long-lasting effects on victims of rape [Shapland and Hall, forthcoming]. The position is that judges should be aware of the effects on victims, and any information necessary for sentencing can be admitted in evidence during a hearing before sentencing. Information concerning the mental and psychological effects on victims (particularly for sexual assaults or violent crime), information that the victim wishes particularly to convey his or her forgiveness of the offender, and information in relation to losses (to consider the making of a compensation order) are particularly relevant.

Hence it becomes very important that judges should receive accurate information on the effects of the offense on the victim. However, means to ensure this occurs have been slow to be implemented. In the 1980s, information about losses was so rarely presented that the best predictor of whether a compensation order would be made was whether anyone mentioned the word *compensation* in any context during the case [Shapland et al., 1985]. The position has improved. Judges would now routinely consider financial losses (damage, theft) in a case where a compensation order is a possibility (i.e., the offender is not going to be given a prison sentence). However, information on the psychological and social effects of the offense is still not routinely available.

The first government initiative in England and Wales to create reliable possibilities for this information to reach the judge was the Victim Statement pilot, part of the One Stop Shop initiative for victims of serious crime [Hoyle et al., 1998]. They found that around 30% of victims wished to make a statement to the police detailing the effects of the offense on them.[*] The researchers judged that most of these statements did add additional material to the victim's evidential statement to the police, mostly about the emotional effect of the offense. Statements did not exaggerate effects—if anything, they tended to underplay them. For the majority of victims, the process of making such a victim personal statement was helpful. However, approximately 90% of victims did not know what use had been made of their statement in the criminal justice process. They hoped it had been taken into account by the prosecution and the judge, but they did not know.

---

[*] Victim statements about the effects of the offense on them have been called by various terms in England and Wales but are generally known as *victim personal statements* (sometimes as victim effect statements, or, for homicide cases, family impact statements). In the United States, they would be called victim impact statements. Several states in the United States allow victims to give their opinion on sentencing in such a statement.

Subsequent research interviewed professionals working in criminal justice to see what use was being made of these victim statements [Morgan and Sanders, 1999]. They found that most of the magistrates' court officials and some of the Crown Court judges in the areas were aware of the pilot victim statement projects. Judges welcomed the idea of victim statements in principle, primarily because they provided additional information on the effects on the victim, but could be dubious as to whether victim statements should influence sentence. Victim statements were usually in the prosecution file but might not be read in court or given to the judge, depending on the prosecutor's view of their veracity or usefulness. It seems, therefore, that whether victim statements were used varied according to the views of professionals. Sentencers found it impossible to recall whether the statement had actually affected sentence. This finding is not surprising. Sentencing is a habitual decision, taken after perusal of numerous documents and hearing views from several people (e.g., probation service or mitigation by the defense lawyer). It is very difficult for professional decision makers to recall exactly which element affected the sentence in which way.

The legal position in England and Wales is that victim personal statements may contain evidence as to the effects of the offense on the victim but should not include any opinion by the victim as to what the sentence should be [Practice Direction, 2001, 4 All ER 640]. If they do contain any such opinion, then the court should ignore this. Given that victim personal statements are normally taken by the police, they rarely contain opinions and tend to be restricted to bare facts.

Victim personal statements were supposed to be rolled out nationally in England and Wales in October 2001, but their implementation has been acknowledged as very patchy [Graham et al., 2004; Office for Criminal Justice Reform, 2005b]. New efforts have been made through Local Criminal Justice Boards in the past few years to try to encourage police officers to remember to offer the possibility of making a victim personal statement to victims. There remain problems, however. Police officers may not remember or have time to take such a statement. Victims are asked to make the statement at the same time as they have made their statement of evidence about the crime itself, which is normally very soon after the offense, when effects have not yet become clear. Although victim personal statements can be updated, in practice it is not clear that victims are taking or being offered the opportunity to do so. The statement is taken by a police officer, even though it is evidence from the victim—and it is often put in the police officer's words. This can lead to challenges later in court but also is less likely to convey to judges exactly what the victim wishes to say.

The most recent evaluation of the extent to which victims are offered the opportunity to make a victim personal statement and whether they are taking this opportunity is provided by the WAVES [Moore and Blakeborough, 2008].

The survey found that only just more than one-third of victims interviewed recalled being given the opportunity to make a victim personal statement, whereas 53% said they had not been given the opportunity. More victims of violent crime recalled it being suggested by the police than victims of theft and handling—suggesting that police officers' views on when such statements might be useful continue to play a part. The authors conclude:

> There is some evidence that standards highlighted in the Victim and Witness Delivery Plan are not being met. Most noteworthy is the severe lack of availability of the Victim Personal Statement. With more than half of victims not recalling having been offered the opportunity to make such a statement, there is a need for the CJS [Criminal Justice System] agencies to revisit the use and promotion of this intervention. [ibid.:v]

It is clear that professionals in the criminal justice system, including judges, are ambivalent about the need to collect and make regularly available to sentencers information about the effects of the offense on victims. Because such statements are taken by the police and collected in the prosecution file, police and prosecution views also come into play. However, the case law indicates strongly that judges should be aware of effects on victims and, where necessary, seek out such information. It is a mark of the ambivalence of legal professionals toward victims and toward any input from victims at sentence that the provisions are not currently universally effective.

Because of the lack of effectiveness, there has been considerable pressure from victims groups representing victims of homicide (death by dangerous driving, as well as murder and manslaughter) to allow relatives of homicide victims to make oral statements in court about the effects of the offense and their loss before sentence. A consultation document, *Hearing the Relatives of Murder and Manslaughter Victims* [Department for Constitutional Affairs, 2005], led to a proposal for a pilot scheme to test what became called a *family impact statement*—a statement to the court by the bereaved family in homicide cases that could be made orally or in writing to the court about the effect of the crime on their family. The statement could be given by a lawyer (including the prosecutor), the family themselves, or a layperson. The pilots were at five Crown Court centers (Manchester, London, Birmingham, Cardiff, and Winchester) and ran between April 2006 and April 2008. The pilots were evaluated together with two other initiatives for bereaved families: the opportunity to meet with the prosecutor, and up to 15 hours of free legal advice to the family on social and personal matters arising from the death [Sweeting et al., 2008].

Overall, the possibility of making a family impact statement was welcomed by the family of the homicide victim. Some families wanted to give the court a better appreciation of the victim's character, whereas others wanted the defendant to understand the impact of what had been done. Of 392 eligible families, 316 took part in the pilots, and in 124 a family impact statement was delivered at court [Sweeting et al., 2008]. Some families did not wish to make a statement, sometimes because they did not think it would have an effect on sentencing, and sometimes because they feared the emotional strain. Families often chose prosecuting counsel to make the statement, and few took up the option of an independent advocate— although I would suggest that this might be different in rare cases where the family might think there was state involvement in the victim's death. Families welcomed the family impact statement because it created a sense of active involvement in the trial—perhaps very different from what they may have experienced in relation to coroners' proceedings. If, however, the family was denied an opportunity to make the statement, if it was edited, or if the statement seemed to have no impact on the judge, then there was distress.

Practitioners, including the judiciary, had mixed views. Although statements were seen to provide a voice for families and this was helpful for them, some strongly opposed the statement, especially oral delivery in court, because they felt that it introduced victims' views and also unwelcome emotion into court. These views replicate those of some members of the judiciary and prosecutors to (written) victim personal statements, discussed above. They seem to me to reflect a worrying view of the court and its role in criminal justice. If the court is to be the community forum for dealing with serious breaches of the criminal law, including deliberate hurt caused by one citizen to another, then that court will need to deal with and reflect societal disquiet about that event. If it does not, then it could be argued as having failed in one of its major roles and having compromised its legitimacy. Major harm caused to one citizen will cause emotion, and it is important that that emotion should be able to be expressed (within limits, so that proceedings can continue). In my view, lawyers who are against any expression of emotion in court are confusing the role of the judge (to be impartial, calm and calming, presiding over proceedings) with the role of the court. They may also be reflecting concern over judges' (or their own) potential ability to deal with proceedings if emotion is expressed. Banning emotion, however, is removing expressions of societal disquiet from the court as a forum, leaving it, potentially, to the media or to informal justice (e.g., lynch mobs). If that were to occur, it would seem to work against the rule of law.

The other two elements of the pilot scheme were contact with prosecutors, including a meeting, and legal assistance. The pretrial support and meeting were welcomed, as would be expected from the findings of previous research (see above). However, take-up of the meeting varied across sites, with families not always seeing the purpose of the meeting or that it was relevant to them. For some families, support from police family liaison officers (assigned to every family where there is a homicide) may have been sufficient, without a further need for meeting the prosecutor. The CPS has decided to roll out the pretrial support scheme nationally from October 2007, together with the making of a family impact statement and the prosecutor reading it at court at all Crown Court centers. The initial focus of the scheme on murder and manslaughter has been widened to include death by dangerous driving and driving while unfit through drink or drugs.

Take-up of legal assistance was very limited (only 21 families used this possibility), possibly because of a lack of awareness and understanding of this element among both families and practitioners. These results can be seen as emphasizing the need to explain services, especially new services, to victims. In Western countries, victimization, especially serious victimization, is rare and comes as a shock. Citizens are unlikely to have much knowledge of victim services before they become a victim—and so there is a task of outreach and explanation.

13.6 During Sentence

In 1990 in England and Wales, the Victim's Charter [Home Office, 1990] announced that, for the first time, victims would be consulted before offenders were released from life sentences. Their wishes and interests would be taken into account during the parole board decision-making process. The National Probation Service was tasked with visiting such victims and ascertaining their views (e.g., about the dangers of revictimization if offenders were to be released into the same area), and as a result the Probation Service started Victim Liaison Units in each of its areas. In 1995 the provisions were extended to cover victims of serious sexual or violent offenses where the term of imprisonment was 4 years or more (whose offenders would fall under the Parole Board's provisions), and in 2001 there was a further substantial increase to such offenses where imprisonment was for 1 year or more.

This was a major new responsibility for the National Probation Service, which previously had only been concerned with offenders. Unfortunately, initially it was not accompanied by any funding. Victim liaison officers were supposed to contact victims within 2 months of sentencing and provide information about what would happen during the offender's sentence and ask if victims wished to opt in to the consultation. If victims wanted to opt in, they were then to return to consult with victims during the process of considering the offender's release. They soon found, first, that the victims they visited at the first stage had not necessarily been informed about the sentence (or the charge/conviction) by anyone else earlier because of the failures in providing information discussed above. Thus, probation officers bore the brunt of victims' displeasure at others' failings. Crawford and Enterkin

[2001], evaluating the early period of the scheme, found that indeed receiving information was victims' main reason for opting in.

Second, the status of the report written by the probation officer as a result of the consultation at the second visit was relatively unclear. As it might impact on the offender's release, for human rights reasons, it had to be made available to the offender and his or her legal representative. The parole board might well make use of the report to put additional license requirements on any parole license if victims were afraid of further intimidation—but the risk victims took was that their concerns about the release would be known by the offender, which might itself lead to intimidation. More recently, funding has been made available to the probation service to carry out the task of victim liaison in serious cases. Victim liaison officers emphasize the importance of making contact with victims after sentence, rather than leaving contact to just before potential release. They have become inured to sometimes becoming the first ones to talk to the victim and let the victim know about the progress of the case. The difficulties over the status of victim views as quoted in reports by victim liaison officers in relation to parole and release and the potential for intimidation of victims by offenders as a result have not, however, been solved.

13.7 The Changing Conceptions of Victims in Criminal Justice

Dignan [2005:63] has referred to the years up to around 2000 in England and Wales as "Victim neglect during the 'era of disenfranchisement'." Its origin was professional criminal justice agencies, particularly the police and prosecution, taking over primary responsibility for prosecuting the offender. It has been a long and slow process to start re-enfranchising victims so that they can have consideration, respect, and dignity during a criminal justice process that they feel is trying "their" crime. Many would argue that, despite governmental rhetoric in England and Wales—the government announced in 2002 that it would be putting victims "at the heart of criminal justice"— actual progress has been halting, patchy, and far from complete.

It is certainly true that, in England and Wales, court surroundings have been made far more human for victims (and other witnesses and laypeople) attending court. There are separate waiting rooms; there are reception points; there are signposting, refreshments, and Witness Support. Moreover, there have been major legislative changes to help vulnerable and intimidated witnesses to give their "best" evidence and schemes to help families of homicide victims. However, these initiatives have largely been peripheral to the court proceedings themselves and their view of the victim.

In terms of receiving information and being consulted, there has been partial enfranchisement in England and Wales. The CPS has acknowledged it should consult with victims before making decisions to drop a case or change charges. Police are supposed to inform victims of the result of the case. Victims are consulted by the National Probation Service before offenders are released from prison on life licenses or on parole. However, these communication channels, as Dignan [2005] comments, are often one way. They inform victims of what the system has done, and they acquire information for use in the system's decisions, but they do not allow most victims to present their information (e.g., about the effects of the offense) to the system. There is little opportunity to engage in dialogue with criminal justice. There is certainly very little opportunity to engage in dialogue with the offender because restorative justice is only a mainstream option for young offenders.

The position, as far as it can be judged, in other jurisdictions in Europe, is also one of a will to try to meet victim needs but not at the cost of significant change to the existing criminal justice system. Victim services tend to be just that—victim services—rather than rights. There is very considerable resistance from practitioners to any major change in the role or status of victims. Provisions tend to be about information (Do victims get informed as to what is happening? Can they take up their existing rights, e.g., for *partie civile* compensation claims?) and assistance at court to give evidence. Progress is often slow and halting, and established interests among practitioners have the power to reverse or take over more controversial provisions. An example is the transformation of the decentralized *maisons de justice* in France, which originally housed prosecutors, as well as mediators, to provide local delivery of criminal justice services, into advice centers to advise citizens on how to approach civil and criminal justice [Wyvekens, 2008]. Mediators' work has now often been merged with that of the new auxiliary prosecutors, who are often former criminal justice practitioners. Mediation—and decentralized criminal justice services—are being absorbed back into more mainstream criminal justice culture.

Some, however, would argue that a focus on meeting victim needs within criminal justice is misplaced because few victims have much contact with criminal justice. They argue that we should not try to change victims' roles in relation to prosecution or the court because these attempts are often sabotaged by criminal justice and twisted toward criminal justice systemic ends, rather than really benefiting victims. Instead, we should put resources into victim assistance and support or develop civil justice means (such as compensation claims or community mediation) because these measures directly benefit victims.

My own view is that reform needs to take into account both victims' own views about where they see the various systems as failing them, as well as the role and purpose of justice. There is no doubt that victims appreciate victim assistance and support—but they also clearly appreciate a more sensitive, informative, and consultative approach from criminal justice, as the evaluations described above have demonstrated.

A long time ago, van Dijk [1983] classified the different types of response to victims according to their ideological remit:

- Care or welfare for victims (because victims have been hurt—just as others in society have been hurt through illness, accident, or poverty; this is the welfare state approach, and examples in relation to victims include criminal injuries compensation schemes).
- Resocializing offenders (using victims in the service of offenders, e.g., to make offenders more aware of the harm they have caused, thereby promoting rehabilitation; examples include some reparation initiatives and victim impact offender behavior programs).
- Radical or anticriminal justice (advocating a civil justice response because criminal justice will never change; examples include the use of community restorative justice in place of criminal justice or restorative justice within criminal justice; victim assistance schemes run outside of criminal justice).
- Retributive or criminal justice.

When asked, victims themselves have seen the last ideology—the criminal justice ideology—as most appropriate for offenses that victims themselves see as against the criminal law (i.e., they are victims of a *crime*). It is a prime reason why victims continue to report offenses to criminal justice authorities, such as the police (in the United Kingdom) or prosecutors (in mainland European countries). If those criminal justice authorities become hostile or uncaring in terms of the ways in which victims can approach them or victims are dealt with by them, then it would not be surprising if those same authorities become seen as less legitimate. A way in which this can be expressed is as a lack of confidence in criminal justice by citizens, a matter which is now being regarded as of some concern to states [Criminal Justice Review Group, 2000; Hough and Roberts, 2004].

Creating a criminal justice system more attuned to the ways in which victims (and witnesses) are able to deal with it in today's insecure world is clearly difficult. The history of evaluation of criminal justice initiatives is that reform is slow, sometimes patchy, and sometimes resisted by other interests. That seems to be the case across countries in Europe, whether they come from a common law or Napoleonic legal tradition. The precise form of the initiative clearly needs to be attuned to the local legal culture and in line, as far as possible, with both practitioner and public expectations. But the lessons of attempting reform to meet victim needs are that progress will be slow, wherever it is attempted. It needs considerable government will and a lengthy pilot period to mitigate practitioner fears. However, giving up the attempt

International Handbook of Victimology

can have serious effects on how criminal justice itself is perceived—and that is one of the integral tasks of government itself.

References

Angle, H., S. Malam, and C. Carey. 2003. *Key findings from the witness satisfaction survey.* Home Office Research Findings No.189. London: Home Office.

Boom, A. ten, K. F. Kuijpers, and M. Moene. 2008. *Behoeften van slachtoffers van delicten: Een systematische literatuurstudie naar behoeften zoals door slachtoffers zelf geuit.* The Hague: Boom.

Brienen, M. and E. Hoegen. 2000. *Victims of crime in 22 European criminal justice systems.* Nijmegen, the Netherlands: Wolf Legal.

Burton, M., R. Evans, and A. Sanders. 2006. Are special measures for vulnerable and intimidated witnesses working? Evidence from the criminal justice agencies. Online Report 01/06. London: Home Office at http://www.homeoffice.gov.uk/rds (accessed November 1, 2008).

Cabinet Office. 2005. *No witness no justice.* London: Cabinet Office at http://archive.cabinetoffice.gov.uk/opsr/local_service_projects/criminal_justice/no_witness/index.asp (accessed November 1, 2008).

Campbell, C., R. Devlin, D. O'Mahony, et al. 2006. Evaluation of the Northern Ireland Youth Conferencing Service. NIO Research and Statistical Series Report No. 12. Belfast: NIO. http://www.nio.gov.uk/evaluation_of_the_northern_ireland_youth_conference_service.pdf (accessed November 1, 2008).

Christie, N. 1977. Conflicts as property. *British Journal of Criminology* 17:1–15.

Council of Europe. 1985. *Recommendation No. R (85) 11 on the position of the victim in the framework of criminal law and procedure.* Strasbourg, France: Council of Europe.

Crawford, A. and J. Enterkin. 2001. *Victim contact work in the probation service: A study of service delivery and impact.* Leeds, UK: CCJS.

Crawford, A. and T. Newburn. 2003. *Youth offending and restorative justice.* Cullompton, UK: Willan.

Criminal Justice Review Group. 2000. *Report of the review of criminal justice in Northern Ireland.* Belfast: HMSO.

Crown Prosecution Service. 2008. Your CPS. http://www.cps.gov.uk/yourcps.html (accessed November 1, 2008).

Department for Constitutional Affairs. 2005. *Hearing the relatives of murder and manslaughter victims.* London: Department for Constitutional Affairs.

Dignan, J. 2005. *Understanding victims and restorative justice.* Milton Keynes, UK: Open University Press.

Doak, J. and D. O'Mahony. 2006. The vengeful victim? Assessing the attitudes of victims participating in restorative youth conferencing. *International Review of Victimology* 13:157–78.

Ericson, R. V. 1982. *Reproducing order: A study of police patrol work.* Toronto: University of Toronto Press.

European Commission. 2001. *Council Framework Decision of 15 March 2001 on the standing of victims in criminal proceedings (2001/220/JHA).* Brussels: European Commission.

Garside, R. 2006. *Right for the wrong reasons: Making sense of criminal justice failure.* Crime and Society Foundation monograph 2. London: Crime and Society Foundation at http://www.crimeandjustice.org.uk/opus293/RFWR.pdf (accessed November 1, 2008).

Graham, J., K. Woodfield, M. Tibble, and S. Kitchen. 2004. *Testaments of harm: A qualitative evaluation of the victim personal statements scheme.* London: National Centre.

Hamlyn, B., A. Phelps, J. Turtle, and G. Sattar. 2004. *Are special measures working? Evidence from a survey of vulnerable and intimidated witnesses.* Home Office Research Study 283. London: Home Office.

Holmstrom, L. L. and A. W. Burgess. 1978. *The victim of rape: Institutional reactions.* Chichester, UK: John Wiley.

Home Office. 1990. *Victim's charter: A statement of the rights of victims of crime.* London: HMSO.

_____. 1998. *Speaking up for justice: Report of the interdepartmental working group on the treatment of vulnerable or intimidated witnesses in the criminal justice system.* London: Home Office.

Hough, J. M. and R. V. G. Clarke. 1980. *The effectiveness of policing,* Introduction: 1–16. Aldershot, UK: Gower.

Hough, M. and J. Roberts. 2004. *Confidence in justice: An international review.* Home Office Research Findings 243. London: Home Office. http://rds.homeoffice.gov.uk/rds/pdfs04/r243.pdf (accessed November 1, 2008).

Hoyle, C., E. Cape, R. Morgan, and A. Sanders. 1998. Evaluation of the "One Stop Shop" and victim statement pilot projects. Home Office Occasional Paper 07/08. London: Home Office. http://www.homeoffice.gov.uk/rds/pdfs/occ-one.pdf (accessed on November 1, 2008).

Kershaw, C., S. Nicholas, and A. Walker. 2008. *Crime in England and Wales 2007/08.* Home Office Statistical Bulletin. London: Home Office.

Maguire, E. M. W. and T. Bennett. 1982. *Burglary in a dwelling: The offence, the offender and the victim.* London: Heinemann.

Moley, S. 2008. Public perceptions. In *Crime in England and Wales 2007/08,* ed. C. Kershaw, S. Nicholas, and A. Walker, 117–29. Home Office Statistical Bulletin 07/08. London: Home Office http://www.homeoffice.gov.uk/rds/pdfs08/hosb0708.pdf (accessed November 1, 2008).

Moore, L. and L. Blakeborough. 2008. *Early findings from WAVES: Information and service provision.* Ministry of Justice Research Series 11/08. London: Ministry of Justice.

Morgan, R. and A. Sanders. 1999. The uses of victim statements. Home Office Occasional Paper. London: Home Office. http://www.homeoffice.gov.uk/rds/pdfs/occ-vicstats.pdf (accessed November 1, 2008).

Office for Criminal Justice Reform. 2005a. *The code of practice for victims of crime.* London: Office for Criminal Justice Reform. http://www.cjsonline.gov.uk/downloads/application/pdf/Victims%20Code%20of%20Practice.pdf (accessed November 1, 2008).

_____. 2005b. *Local criminal justice board victim and witness delivery toolkit 4: Taking victims' views into account.* Victim Personal Statements. London: OCJR.

Pigot Report. 1989. *Report of the advisory group on video evidence.* London: Home Office.

Ringham, L. and H. Salisbury. 2004. Support for victims of crime: Findings from the 2002/2003 British Crime Survey. Home Office Online Report 31:04. London: Home Office. http://rds.homeoffice.gov.uk/rds/pdfs04/rdsolr3104.pdf (accessed November 1, 2008).

Rock, P. 1993. *The social world of an English Crown Court: Witnesses and professionals in the Crown Court Centre at Wood Green*. Oxford: Clarendon.

Sanders, A., J. Creaton, S. Bird, and L. Weber. 1997. *Victims with learning disabilities: Negotiating the criminal justice system*. Centre for Criminological Research Occasional Paper no. 17. Oxford: Oxford University Centre for Criminological Research.

Shapland, J. 1988. Fiefs and peasants: Accomplishing change for victims in the criminal justice system. In *Victims of crime: A new deal?*, ed. M. Maguire and J. Pointing. Reprinted in 1994 in *A reader on criminal justice*, ed. N. Lacey. Oxford: Oxford University Press.

Shapland, J. and E. Bell. 1998. Victims in the magistrates' courts and Crown Court. *Criminal Law Review* August:537–46.

Shapland, J. and D. Cohen. 1987. Facilities for victims: The role of the police and the courts. *Criminal Law Review* January:28–38.

Shapland, J. and M. Hall. 2007. What do we know about the effects of crime on victims? *International Review of Victimology* 13:175–218.

_____. Forthcoming. Victims at court: Necessary accessories or centre stage? In *Victims in contemporary criminal justice*, ed. A. E. Bottoms and J. Roberts. Cullompton, UK: Willan.

Shapland, J. and J. Vagg. 1988. *Policing by the public*. London: Routledge & Kegan Paul.

Shapland, J., J. Willmore, and P. Duff. 1985. *Victims in the criminal justice system*. Aldershot, UK: Gower.

Sweeting, A., R. Owen, C. Turley, P. Rock, M. Garcia-Sanche, L. Wilson, and U. Khan. 2008. *Evaluation of the victims' advocate scheme pilots*. Ministry of Justice Research Series 17/08. London: Ministry of Justice.

Temkin, J. 1987. *Rape and the legal process*. London: Sweet & Maxwell.

Temkin, J. and B. Krahé. 2007. *Sexual assault and the justice gap: A question of attitude*. Oxford: Hart Publishing.

Tombs, S. and D. Whyte. 2004. *Safety crimes*. Cullompton, UK: Willan.

van Dijk, J. J. M. 1983. Victimologie in theorie en praktijk; een kritische reflectie op de bestaande en nog te creëen voorzieningen voor slachtoffers van delichten. *Justitiële verkenningen* 6:5–35.

van Dijk, J. J. M., J. van Kesteren, and P. Smit. 2007. *Criminal victimization in international perspective: Key findings from the 2004–2005 ICVS and EU ICS*. Tilburg, the Netherlands: Tilburg University INTERVICT.

Victim Support. 2008. Help for witnesses. http://www.victimsupport.org.uk/vs_england_wales/services/witness_services.php (accessed November 1, 2008).

Wyvekens, A. 2008. "Proximity justice" in France: Anything but "justice and community"? In *Justice, community and civil society*, ed. J. Shapland. Cullompton, UK: Willan.

Lobbying for Rights
Crime Victims in Israel

14

URI YANAY AND TALI GAL

Contents

14.1 Introduction

This article discusses the process underlying the enactment of the Rights of Crime Victims Law, 2001, in Israel. Since Israel gained its statehood in 1948, crime has never been considered a pressing social problem.* Neither

---

* In recent years, crime rates have risen. According to Israel Police statistics, each day about 50 people of different age groups and genders seek medical care in hospital emergency rooms because of criminal assault [Israel Police Statistics, 2005].

have crime victims, who were assumed to be looked after by their immediate and extended families or by members of the community. Only in serious cases, or when no family was available, would welfare and rehabilitation services provide help and cover costs on a one-time, discretionary basis.

However, faced with the ongoing Middle East crisis, with its immense human and economic costs, Israel's legislature, the Knesset, has acknowledged public responsibility for victims of hostile (terrorist) acts. Victims' right to long-term support and benefits has been secured under the Victims of Hostile Acts (Pensions) Law, 1970. The provisions of this law do not involve means tests or discretion. By enacting this law, the Knesset made a clear distinction between victims of hostile ("terrorist") acts and victims of "common," criminal acts. Victims of terrorist acts were acknowledged and formally supported, whereas those suffering criminal injury were not entitled to specific support or compensation. This distinction has engendered growing dissatisfaction and criticism among crime victims and their families, by professionals, and the public.

Indeed, the 1985 United Nations (UN) Declaration of Basic Principles of Justice for Victims of Crime and Abuse of Power had never been at the center of Israeli public discourse, more pressing social issues superseding it. To put victims' rights on the public agenda, to help bring up crime victims as a social problem, and to enhance their sociolegal rights, crime victims and other concerned individuals and social groups gathered into a coalition. Encouraged by academics and supported by other professionals, including civil servants from the Ministry of Justice, this coalition has achieved growing recognition from members of the Knesset. In 2001, a new Rights of Crime Victims Law was enacted. Enactment of this law, only 3 years after the founding of the victims' rights lobby, may be proof of its significant role. This article describes the legislative process leading to the Rights of Crime Victims Act and analyzes the forces that contributed to its enactment.

This article comprises five parts. The first focuses on the construction of social problems and lawmaking. The second part discusses the rights of crime victims in Israel before the new law, and the third part deals with the formation of a coalition for victims' rights in Israel. The fourth part marks the birth of the Rights of Crime Victims Law. The fifth, and final, part discusses the lessons to be drawn from these developments.

14.2 Social Problems and Lawmaking

Laws deal with real-life situations [Zander, 1994]. Situations are associated with people, individuals, and groups that confront social conditions, some of which are deemed "social problems." Merton [1966] argues, in his "objectively given" approach to social problems [Goode and Ben Yehuda, 1994], that to construct a life situation as a "social problem," several conditions must be met. First, there must be a clearly perceived gap or discrepancy between norms and existing social reality. Second, the discrepancy must prove to be socially and hence politically disturbing. The more disturbing the situation, the more attention it will receive. Finally, a clear solution that deals with the situation must be presented.

Social problems do not emerge by themselves. Putting a social problem on the public agenda involves a distinct claim-making process [Spector and Kitsuse, 1977]. To be effective, the process must be directed at a powerful, influential audience. The higher the audience in the social hierarchy, the easier it will be able to lead and introduce social change by legislation.

Legislators constantly negotiate claims coming from all walks of life, and if they perceive a given life situation as a social problem, they are in a pivotal position to make a difference [Evan, 1980]. Furthermore, legislators are in the best position to negotiate the necessary resources required to meet the desired end [Chambliss, 1976, 1993]. Enacting a law and budgeting its administration can make a significant change and help solve any situation seen as a social problem [Holstein and Miller, 1990].

To overcome the gap between norms and facts, Habermas [Payrow-Shabani, 1998] appeals to the medium of law, which gives legitimacy to the political order and provides the system with its binding force. Legitimate lawmaking itself is generated through a procedure of public opinion and will formation that produces "communicative power," which in turn impacts and shapes the process of social institutionalization.

Some view crime victim policy in light of cultures of control and punishment across neoliberal societies [Garland, 2001]. Others pursue victims' rights focusing on the victims, victimology, and human rights. Elias [1986:228] highlights this point with the claim that "as we continue exploring these relationships, we may find that victimology and human rights converge." In discussing the politics of helplessness, misery, and disenchantment, Elias [1986:230] focuses on the traditional politics of victimization, arguing: "Victims ... have not yet shaken their second class status. When victimized, they lack confidence in receiving the aid they need, and for a good reason—they often must tolerate inadequate services, cultural insensitivity, political insignificance, and official maltreatment."

Campaigns on behalf of crime victims have been launched on the international level [Bassiouni, 1988]. However, in most industrialized Western countries, victims' needs and rights are associated with the pioneering work of local lobbying groups termed *crime victim movements* [Sebba, 1996]. Among such groups are the National Organization for Victim Assistance (NOVA) in the United States, Victim Support in the United Kingdom, Canadian Organization for Victim Assistance (COVA) in Canada, the Weisser Ring in Germany, and the National Institute for Assistance for Victims (INVAVEM) in France [Sebba, 1996].

Motivated by "bottom up" victim advocacy initiatives and becoming aware of the social problem that they reflect, New Zealand was the first country to take legislative measures, with its 1963 Criminal Injuries Compensation Act [Rock, 1990], providing compensation for innocent people injured by crime and the dependants of murder victims. In England, crime victims' rights have been associated with the work of a number of dedicated reformers [Fry, 1959] and working parties [Home Office, 1959, 1961]. The Criminal Injuries Compensation Scheme in the United Kingdom [Greer, 1996] was established in 1964 by a written answer to a parliamentary question [House of Commons Debates, Vol. 697, June 24, 1964; Home Office, 1964]. For more than 30 years, commencing on August 1, 1964, this Scheme made more than half a million *ex gratia*, discretionary payments to people who suffered criminal injuries. The Scheme "emphasized a doctrinal analogy with common law concepts and remedies" [Miers, 1997:4].

In his analysis, Rock [1984] attributes much of the attention paid to crime victims in England to the work of the National Association of Victim Support Schemes, later known as Victim Support. In addition to serving crime victims in the community, this voluntary organization has put victim interests on the public-political agenda. Much of the antioffender rhetoric was transformed into victim rights and victim service agendas [Henderson, 1985:937]. Miers suggests that in some parts of the world, this process marks the "politicization of the experience of personal victimization," in line with conservative penal values [Miers, 1997:10]. Furthermore, Miers argues that a Home Office White Paper [1959] adumbrated many of the penal reforms of the 1960s and turned them into victims' rights [Miers, 1997:10]. In England, the pendulum of rights moved toward crime victims.

Indeed, the victim movement in England managed to put the rights of crime victims on the political agenda. As a result, in the mid-1990s, Victim Support ceased being *ex gratia* and became law. From 1996, crime victims in Great Britain could claim the right to criminal injury compensation, rather than merely ask for it [Duff, 1998].

In the United States, California was the first to follow the innovative outlook of New Zealand and Great Britain, introducing a victim support and compensation program in 1965. Over the following years, federal legislation on crime victims had been on the Congressional agenda but with meager results [McGillis and Smith, 1983:31]. Although crime and "law and order" issues are prominent features of U.S. public and political debate, victims' rights and services, paradoxically, had escaped the American social agenda.

In 1967, President Johnson established the President's Commission on Law Enforcement and Administration of Justice to examine crime and criminal justice and identify possible solutions to increasingly pressing issues involving urban riots and crime victims. However, it was only in the 1970s that a victim movement emerged in the United States. The American victim movement was formed by many different groups, among them the National Coalition against Sexual Assault, the National Coalition against Domestic Violence, and the Victims' Assistance Legal Organization, joined soon thereafter by Mothers Against Drunk Driving and the National Center for Victims of Crime (formerly the National Victim Center) [Carrington and Nicholson, 1984].

In 1982, President Reagan appointed a task force, headed by Lois H. Herrington, to study the needs of crime victims and the problematic nature of their interface with police, prosecutors, the judiciary, and parole boards. This was a formal attempt to define the needs of crime victims and ensure that such needs were attended to, as part of other state provisions [President's Task Force, 1982]. To consider the work of this task force, one must keep in mind the prominence of the victims' movement as a social-political force, with several specific victim groups represented [Sebba, 1996]. To deal with victims' needs, the President's Task Force made major recommendations to hospitals, the clergy, the bar, schools, and others.

In the United States, the Victims of Crime Act of 1984 (VOCA) established a crime victim fund to support federal and state victim compensation and assistance programs [Tobolowsky, 2001:10]. In line with the President's Task Force, the federal government and the majority of the states have enacted constitutional or legislative provisions requiring victim notification of important events and actions in the criminal justice process, and to varying degrees permitted crime victim presence at critical stages of the criminal justice process [Tobolowsky, 2001:11].

The victim movement did not bypass continental Europe, where the major thrust has occurred only since 1985, encouraged by a number of international initiatives [Maguire and Shapland, 1990:206]. In addition to these initiatives, it was also "public reaction against increasing crime rates combined with increasingly impersonal, uncaring and ineffective criminal justice systems and growing awareness of the serious impact of crime on individuals" [Maguire and Shapland, 1990:206]. However, unlike the United States, where voluntary organizations emphasize victims' rights, the Europeans called for better services for victims [Maguire and Shapland, 1990:207]. Specifically, the Council of Europe adopted the 1983 European Convention on the Compensation of Victims of Violent Crimes, the 1985 Recommendation on the Position of the Victim within the Framework of Criminal Law and Procedure, and the 1987 Recommendation on Assistance to Victims and the Prevention of Victimization.

Indeed, legislation involves a network of informal understandings rooted in social interaction. Concerning crime, the "vertical interaction thesis" involves reciprocity between citizens as individuals or organized by victim movements, lawmaking, and law-enforcing officials. The "congruence thesis" holds that the underlying social interaction becomes possible if legal norms are broadly congruent with formal and informal social practices and conventions [Postema, 1994].

Despite the UN Declaration and the examples of European and other countries, Israel enacted a law and designed a program for victims of hostile acts only. Crime victims were not viewed as a "social problem," and their personal and legal needs were not attended to. To advance the victims' agenda and enact the Rights of Crime Victims Law, intense interaction was needed, involving crime victims, voluntary victims' services, civil servants, lawmakers, and others in the legal and academic communities. This interaction led to the construction of a new set of norms, congruent with international standards regarding victims' rights.

14.3 The Rights of Crime Victims in Israel

In Israel, both local and foreign victims of terrorist acts are entitled to broad state assistance and compensation, under the 1970 Hostile Acts (Pensions) Law, funded by the state. This law covers victims of terrorism only. Victims of common law crimes have come to realize that their urgent needs are processed through the lengthy "normal" channels of municipal services offices, the National Insurance Institute (Israel's Social Security), or voluntary organizations [Yanay, 2005a]. There had never been specific state services designed to meet the needs of crime victims.

In recent years, however, several laws have been enacted giving crime victims some indirect recognition but no legal "rights." They are encapsulated in the Basic Law: Human Dignity and Liberty; in the Evidence Law; and in some participation rights prescribed either by law or by State Attorney guidelines. These legal provisions are described below.

14.3.1 Basic Law: Human Dignity and Liberty

Although Israel has no formal constitution, several basic laws are considered to have quasi-constitutional status. The Basic Law: Human Dignity and Liberty, enacted in 1992, provides that "Every person is entitled to the protection of his life, personal security, and dignity."* Because of its broad language, this basic law is open to interpretation and development by the Supreme Court. Indeed, in several decisions, the Supreme Court has ruled that this applies to crime victims, not just offenders. Former Chief Justice M. Shamgar stated the matter, thus:

> In our times it is more than once forgotten that the right to one's dignity is not only the defendant's dignity but also the dignity of the complainant, the witness, the victim. [DNP 3750/94]

---

* Public Law 1391, 1982, p. 150.

14.3.2 Evidence Law

Israeli legislators have shown notable compassion to specific, vulnerable groups, such as young children, victims of intrafamily abuse, and victims of sexual offenses, in the area of evidence law. As early as 1955, the Knesset enacted the Evidence Amendment (Child Protection) Law, which empowered professionally trained child investigators to have extensive authority in cases involving victims or witnesses of intrafamily or sexual offenses, who are under the age of 14. Such children may not be called to testify without a child investigator's permission, and as a rule may be interviewed only by the child investigator [Evidence Amendment (Child Protection) Law, 1955, Articles 2(a), 4]. If the child investigator permits the child to give testimony in court, it must be *in camera*, with only the prosecutor, the defendant, the defense attorney, and the child investigator present, unless the court grants special permission for others (Article 2b). The law also authorizes the court to decide, in cases involving severe intrafamily sexual abuse, to exclude the parent-defendant from the courtroom, leaving the defense attorney to represent him or her during the child's testimony, to prevent any emotional damage to the child (Article 2a). If the child investigator does not permit the child to testify in court, then the investigator him- or herself may testify on what the child has said in a forensic interview and may then present a report of the forensic interview as evidence (Article 9). This is a unique exception to the rule against hearsay evidence; there must be corroborative evidence to obtain a verdict of guilty (Article 11).

The Evidence Amendment (Child Protection) Law, however, is not the only law protecting victims in their role as witnesses. Under the leadership of women's rights [Strum, 1989] and children's rights activists, and with the support of some officials at the Israeli Ministry of Justice, several law amendments were enacted in the 1990s to protect victims of sexual assaults from various aspects of potential revictimization during courtroom testimony.

The Criminal Procedure Amendment (Sexual Offenses Testimony) Law, 1996, allows witnesses in sexual abuse trials to testify through a closed-circuit video system in cases in which testifying in the presence of the defendant may constitute abuse of the victim or harm the victim's testimony. This law also provides a "rape shield" protection, prohibiting the investigation of a victim of sexual assault about his or her sexual history, unless such investigation is needed to prevent a perversion of justice.

The Evidence Ordinance (New Version), 1971, permits children to testify against their parents when they have been subjected to sexual or physical abuse or when parents have violated protection orders aimed at child protection. In any other type of criminal proceeding, children's testimony against parents is inadmissible.

14.3.3 Privacy

Before enactment in 2001 of the Rights of Crime Victims Law, Israeli law did not provide a general right of crime victims to privacy; instead, individual provisions of various laws provided privacy to victims and witnesses under certain circumstances, mainly to children and victims of sexual offenses.

The Youth Law, 1960, provides the main protection of the privacy of child victims. The law makes it a criminal offense to disseminate any information that may identify a child as someone whose case has been brought to court or to a welfare officer for intervention; as someone who has attempted or committed suicide; as a delinquent or immoral person; as a relative of a criminal; as a victim of intrafamily abuse or a sexual or physical assault; or as one who has undergone psychiatric tests, treatment, hospitalization, or even an HIV test (Article 24). The consent of the child or the child's caretaker for the dissemination of such information is irrelevant and does not protect the disseminator from criminal charges. The maximum penalty for such dissemination is 1-year of imprisonment (Article 11).*

The Evidence Amendment (Child Protection) Law, 1955, prohibits dissemination of information identifying a child who has testified in a sexual abuse case. The maximum penalty for disseminating such information is 6 months of imprisonment and a fine (Article 6). This provision relates only to children who have been investigated or interviewed.

The Penal Law, 1977, provides, with regard to sex offenses, that it is illegal to publish the name or other identifying information of a person as a victim of a sexual assault, unless the victim has given his or her consent for such publication. The penalty for such unlawful publication is 1-year of imprisonment (Article 352).

Finally, the Courts Law (Consolidated Version), 1984, states in Article 68 the principle of an open court, or the right of the public to attend court hearings. However, several exceptions are included, aimed at protecting a victims' privacy. First, the court may decide to conduct a hearing *in camera*, in the best interests of a child. Second, the court may make such decision for the best interest of a victim or defendant in a sexual offense case (Article 68a[4] and 68a[5]). Third, the court may also decide to conduct a hearing *in camera* if public attendance would discourage a witness from giving full testimony. These decisions depend, however, on the discretion of the court. The law also prohibits any publication of a name, picture,

---

* The provisions regarding confidentiality of child victimization, HIV tests, and mental health proceedings were added in 1998 with the active involvement of children's rights advocates.

or any identifying information of a child who is a defendant or witness in any criminal case, and of a victim of a sexual offense, except with the permission of the court (Article 70c). Moreover, publication of court proceedings conducted *in camera* is forbidden without special permission of the court.

14.3.4 Participation Rights

The right of crime victims to take part in the decision-making process in the criminal justice system has become a topic of public discussion only in recent years. The involvement of crime victims in the different stages of the criminal process had been extremely limited before the 2001 reform, although isolated provisions did allow crime victims some degree of input, as outlined below.

Under the Criminal Procedure Law (Consolidated Version), 1982 (hereinafter, the Criminal Procedure Law), a complainant has the right to receive notification of a decision by the state prosecutor not to file charges. The notification must include the reasons for the decision. On receiving the notification, the complainant is entitled to file an administrative appeal before the Attorney General, who reviews the prosecutor's decision (Articles 63 and 64).

The Criminal Procedure Law also allows victims to initiate and lead private prosecutions in a number of offenses listed in the law (Article 62 and Second Annex). In such cases, the private prosecution is under the sole responsibility of the victim, but the public prosecution may take over a privately initiated prosecution. When victims have the right to file a private prosecution, they do not have the right to file an appeal on the public prosecutor's decision not to prosecute. In other words, following a decision of the public prosecutor to close a case, victims have only one alternative—to either file an administrative appeal or prosecute privately—depending on the nature of the offense and its severity.

In 1995, a provision was added to the Criminal Procedure Law (paragraph 187b) in sexual offense cases, giving criminal courts the power to request a Victim Impact Statement (VIS) after conviction and before sentencing. The VIS, prepared by a social worker, includes a description of the condition of the victim and the damage caused by the offense.

14.3.5 State Attorney Guidelines

The 1990 State Attorney Guidelines for treating crime victims reflect a relatively sensitive approach. Directed at district attorneys, the Guidelines did not have the power of legislation and could not be enforced; the Guidelines were, however, in the public domain and had at least a declarative value. Crime victims and victims' advocates could surely use them as an instrument for claiming their rights.[*]

Although the Guidelines afforded crime victims several hitherto nonexistent rights, such as the right to receive case-related information and notification, they did not grant victims any right to express their views or have any influence on the decision-making process. Clearly, not only were the Guidelines insufficient because of their weak normative status, but they were also insufficient in substance. The State Attorney Guidelines were, nevertheless, an important starting point in the process of victim rights advocacy.

14.4 Forming a Partnership for Crime Victims

Before the 2001 Rights of Crime Victims Law, a number of voluntary organizations were involved in crime victim issues, mainly on behalf of victims of violent crime. The most noteworthy among them were volunteer services designed for women and children who feared, or suffered, criminal victimization. Such nongovernmental organizations (NGOs) joined forces with other service providers and human rights activists to lobby for and promote victims' rights in Israel. The most important organizations have been:

> *The Israel Women's Network:* The principal women's rights lobby in Israel. The Israel Women's Network has been successful in putting the feminist issue on the public agenda through highly publicized litigation, legislative work, and continuous work with the media.

---

[*] The following rights were provided for crime victims in the Guidelines:
  a. The victim's right to obtain, on request, a notice regarding filing charges against the defendant and the defendant's arrest and release.
  b. The victim's right to review the indictment and photocopy it.
  c. The victim's right to receive notice of the date for the arraignment, of any change in the scheduled court hearings that may influence the victim's attendance, and the date for sentencing.
  d. The victim's right to obtain the verdict and sentence, including the expected release date.
  e. The victim's right to receive information regarding various decisions made by the prosecutor, such as changes in the charges, termination or delaying of the prosecution process, any plea bargain, and the prosecutor's recommendation for the sentence.
  f. The prosecutor's duty to consult with an expert or welfare officer concerning a child victim before entering a plea bargain.

The Association of Rape Crisis Centers in Israel (ARCCI): In conjunction with the Israel Women's Network, in 1996 ARCCI founded a victim/witness assistance program for victims of sexual assault in Israel. Under the project, which enjoys the support of several district prosecutors' offices in Israel, a volunteer escorts the victim throughout the criminal justice process, commencing with the report made to the police, on to the police investigation, communication with the prosecutor, court testimony, and finally the court decision. The volunteer functions as a liaison between the victim and the public agencies, provides support and encouragement to the victim, refers her to appropriate social services in the community, and advocates her rights throughout the criminal justice process.

The National Council for the Child (NCC): The largest advocacy organization in Israel promoting children's rights. Its ombudsmen deals each year with thousands of calls made with regard to the violation of children's rights. In 1998, because of the large number of calls received on behalf of child crime victims, the NCC founded the Child Victim Assistance Project. Through the project, child victims and their supporting family members receive information, support, and advocacy services throughout the criminal justice process. The Child Victims Assistance Project is managed by a lawyer and staffs volunteer law students, with the support and guidance of a social worker. Concurrently, severely victimized children who need mental health support are referred to the appropriate community medical and social services.

Families of Murdered Children: On September 17, 1997, Tamar Brez, in her 20s, was brutally murdered on the roof of a large hardware store near Tel Aviv. In addition to the horrible trauma connected with the cruel and highly publicized murder itself, her mother, Ora Brez, went through a series of additional traumas following her encounters with the law enforcement agencies throughout the criminal justice process. Together with Lara Tzinman, mother to another murder victim, and other bereaved parents, Ms. Brez organized a group with the twin goals of serving as a support network for bereaved families and lobbying for their rights during the criminal justice process. The group's primary activity has been bringing their ordeal to the forefront of the news.

B'zchut: the Center for the Rights of People with Disabilities: Founded by the Association for Civil Rights in Israel, B'zchut acts as the leading organization lobbying for the rights of all people with disabilities in Israel. It promotes the integration of people with disabilities in the community through accommodation, employment, and accessibility to public areas. Understanding the unique difficulties that people with disabilities who were criminally victimized endure, B'zchut has become involved in victims' rights advocacy.

Forum for Directors of Battered Women's Shelters: Acting as the umbrella organization for all refuges for battered women in Israel, the Forum identifies policy issues that arise from everyday shelter work. Many of the women residing in shelters are involved in criminal processes following their victimization and lack adequate means to meet their needs. Thus, the Forum has decided to participate in activities designed to promote reform in the criminal justice system in Israel, which would help to ensure victims' rights.

14.5 Turning a Partnership into a Coalition

Apparently the strongest catalyst for action in the victims' rights area has been the loud outcry for change coming from those involved in the field. All the above organizations have been dealing with various aspects of support for crime victims. Despite their different target populations, similarities between them are immense. All victims' advocates had to deal with similar obstacles, such as lack of legal standing for crime victims in the criminal justice process, lack of authorized representation in the criminal justice system relating to the needs and predicaments of the criminally victimized, to their pain and suffering. Above all, these groups have had to deal with a system that is rather suspicious of outside intervention and reluctant to make change in favor of victims.

The idea to create a coalition came from the three nongovernmental, voluntary organizations serving crime victims: the Women's Network and the ARCCI, which together founded the Victim Witness Assistance Program; and the NCC, which founded the Child Victim Assistance Project. The growing awareness of the three organizations of the difficulties that crime victims and their advocates endure, as well as the fact that at least two of them, the Women's Network and the NCC, are advocacy organizations striving to promote women's and children's rights, respectively, at the macro level, led them to join forces to engender reform in the victims' rights field. A decision was reached to create a coalition that would promote solutions for the difficulties that all victims—women, children, and others—share when they find themselves involved in the criminal justice system. The fact that each population group had its specific problems, although not an obstacle, was not ignored; the Coalition was created based on an understanding that although each organization had a different agenda, all had an underlying, unifying mission—the promotion of victims' rights.

14.5.1 Stage 1: Setting the Mission

In February 1998, a first meeting of the project directors and legal advisors of the three organizations was held.[*] It was decided to join hands to promote victims' rights legislation and to call on other organizations involved in victim-related issues to join the Coalition. The general consensus was that the partnership should be as broad as possible and could include organizations representing any group because any person could become a victim. It was also decided that Coalition members approach academics involved in victim policy and services.[†] Furthermore, from that point and onward, members of the Coalition received recognition and substantial assistance from a handful of Ministry of Justice officials.[‡]

At their second meeting, the participants decided on the goal of the Coalition: establishing a legal basis for crime victims' rights. The means to achieve that goal were raising public awareness to the issue, conducting a comparative study of international developments in the field, and drafting a legislative proposal. At subsequent meetings, the Coalition members took on themselves substantive tasks, such as contacting academics, preparing a comparative study into victims' rights, and preparing a large public conference.

Later, other groups joined the Coalition, among them representatives of B'zchut, Families of Murdered Children, and the Forum of Directors of Battered Women's Shelters. Other organizations active in various human right areas stressed their support for the Coalition's work but did not take an active part in it, mainly because they had their own agendas.

14.5.2 Stage 2: Formalizing the Coalition

After several months, it became clear that the Coalition would face serious difficulties in moving ahead without technical assistance. Coalition leaders, all of whom held important positions in their own organizations, had to struggle to find time to promote Coalition objectives, in addition to their own organizations' tasks. In October 1998, Coalition leadership

---

[*] The facts related to the coalition are based on the coalition's protocols, available at the offices of coalition members, and the authors' recollections.

[†] Among them were Professor Uri Yanay, School of Social Work, Hebrew University; Professor Leslie Sebba, Center for Criminology, Hebrew University; Professor Emanuel Gross, Haifa University Law School; and Dr. Sara Ben-David, Department of Criminology, Bar Ilan University.

[‡] First and foremost, Yehudit Karp, the then Deputy Legal Advisor for the Government, who acted diligently on the subject from the 1980s, and encouraged the coalition's work from the outset. Another close ally of the coalition was Ido Druyan, then a prosecutor at the Tel Aviv District Attorney's Office.

contacted Shatil* and requested support in coordinating the Coalition. Shatil's director agreed and appointed one of its own staff members as Coalition coordinator. The Coalition's leadership was now free to concentrate on its mission.

Individuals with personal experiences as victims joined the Coalition around the same time: a rape victim and a victim of continued stalking and, some months later, the grandmother of a 7-year-old girl who had been sexually assaulted. The combination of the professional representatives of the human rights organizations, mostly lawyers, and the victims themselves (Families of Murdered Children included) significantly contributed to the work of the Coalition, while also causing its members some frustration. An example is disagreements regarding the definition of *crime victim* in the legislative proposal that later became the Victims' Rights Bill. To include the families of murdered children in the bill, the definition was drafted to include "first degree relatives of those who died as a result of the crime." This formulation was criticized by the families because it did not explicitly mention the word *murder*—an omission that, in their opinion, minimized the gravity of the offenses. The lawyers in the Coalition thought, on the other hand, that the definition would secure rights to more families because it would also include the families of those who were killed by unpremeditated murder or even manslaughter.

14.5.3 Stage 3: Marketing the Mission

In June 1999, the Coalition held its first conference on victims' rights at Tel Aviv University.[†] The keynote speaker was Dame Helen Reeves, founder and chief executive of Victim Support, United Kingdom. The program of the conference was diverse, including scholars from different disciplines, distinguished officials from the Ministry of Justice, the Public Attorney's Office, Public Defender's Office, the police, a judge, and members of the Coalition. Each representative had, undoubtedly, a different goal in mind, but victims' rights were clearly seen as the common denominator.

Yehudit Karp, at the time the Deputy Legal Advisor to the Israeli government and the most persistent civil servant striving for victims' rights since the 1980s, was waiting for a public initiative to arise. The "bottom-up"

---

[*] An NGO established by the New Israel Fund to provide technical assistance to human rights organizations in Israel.
[†] The Coalition managed to produce the event thanks to the financial aid of Ahsalim— Association for Planning and Development of Services for Children and Youth at Risk and their Families, the British Council, and the Minerva Center for Human Rights at the Hebrew University. The schools of Social Work at both Tel Aviv University and The Hebrew University of Jerusalem provided the academic auspices for the conference.

Coalition became her ally, and the conference was a significant first step in enacting a victims' rights law, which she fully supported.

Notwithstanding the staff's empathy with victims, at the organizational level, the police and the Public Attorney's Office were both very skeptical of the call for victims' rights. Both institutions had always operated according to adversarial system principles. These principles are based on the axiom that the two parties to the criminal justice procedure are the State, represented by the police or prosecution, and the defendant. The introduction of the victim as a third party was a new, intimidating idea, both in terms of procedural burden and the substantive definition of the role of the public authorities. However, perhaps those representatives preferred to take part in a process of policy change, rather than being left out of it.

The Public Defender's Office had a clearer view: Its leaders were against the new concept, as it represented a concrete threat to defendants' rights. Apparently, they accepted the Coalition's invitation to speak at the conference because they considered it a platform to have their side heard.

Undoubtedly, the highlights of the conference were the personal testimonies of a mother of a murdered victim and of a young woman who had survived a brutal gang rape. Both women spoke not only about their loss and trauma but also particularly about the second trauma that they had both suffered following the encounter with law enforcement agencies. As members of the Coalition, these women spoke about their personal pain, knowing that their presentations might make a difference in someone's mind and open some hearts for change.

The conference was an important event, bringing the subject to the attention of both its own participants and the general public. The unique encounter between governmental officials, NGO representatives, and crime victims and their families created an opportunity for dialogue and cooperation.

On the following day, the Coalition and Ministry of Justice held a round-table discussion with the participation of Dame Helen and senior officials from all governmental, academic, and nongovernmental bodies involved in victims' issues. The discussion concerned the critical dilemmas connected with victims' rights legislation, as such dilemmas became apparent from the Coalition research and drafting work. This was a first event in which representatives from many different disciplines met and exchanged views. The personal testimony of a young woman who had been sexually abused demonstrated how legal barriers, such as the statute of limitations and other evidentiary rules, made it impossible to bring the perpetrator, her uncle, to justice. As with the public event the previous day, the emotional and academic aspects made a very powerful combination.

The two-day event was the public launching of the Coalition in its efforts to promote victims' rights in Israel. During the conference, Coalition members distributed a short statement of opinion, which identified the main rights that must be provided for victims. Many participants of both events expressed support, understanding, and encouragement for the Coalition in promoting its agenda.

14.6 The Knesset: Private and Government Bills

During the following months, Coalition members strived to conclude the drafting of the legislative proposal and plan the campaign for "marketing" it to the Knesset.* The decision was that it would be desirable to have a large and heterogeneous list of Knesset members serve as sponsors of the bill, including both men and women, religious and secular, and members from across the political spectrum. The Coalition "lobbying group" held numerous meetings and discussions with Knesset members. Moreover, the Coalition "press liaison group" brought the subject to media attention and published coverage of any event connected with criminal victimization. The assumption was that the greater the media exposure, the more Knesset members would be interested in sponsoring it.

Eventually, on October 5, 1999, 17 Knesset members from across the political spectrum, led by Yael Dayan, submitted the bill to the Knesset. The date was set to allow the bill to be brought before the plenum on November 11, Antiviolence Day.

The Victims' Rights bill included the full range of rights that Coalition members had hoped to promote based on a comparison with existing legislation in other parts of the world. Following a general statement concerning the victim's right to dignity, safety, and equality, the bill included three types of rights. The first type included rights connected with protecting victims from further victimization, either by the offender or by the criminal justice process itself. This category of rights included protecting the victim from additional harm from the offender or the offender's surrogates, and the victim's right not to be investigated before his or her safety is secured. Furthermore, the bill included the right to privacy and confidentiality of the victim's personal information, the right to have the proceedings managed within a reasonable time frame, to be escorted with a person of the victim's choice during the criminal proceedings, and not to have the victim's sexual history investigated.

The second group of rights may be called "participation" rights, indicating that the crime victim is a partner to the criminal justice process. The bill included the right of any victim to be informed of developments in the criminal process, to be heard by any decision maker before any decision making throughout the criminal proceedings, and to have access to the investigation file in cases where a decision not to prosecute has been made.

---

* For this goal, Shatil provided a lobbyist who coordinated the campaign.

Lobbying for Rights   389

The third category of rights included in the bill consisted of "social rights," such as the right of any victim to receive aid, support, and advocacy services funded by the government, and the right to state compensation for being victimized.

Presented to the Knesset, the bill faced strong objection from the Government Legislation Committee, which held up the bill because the related costs were not estimated and thought to be high. To continue the process, Member of Knesset (MK) Yael Dayan reached a compromise with the Committee, under which the "social" chapter of the bill was excluded, for the time being. Additionally, some changes were made in the definition of crimes included in the bill, which resulted in a narrower application. The parties agreed that the bill would not be promoted before June 2000 to provide the Ministry of Justice some time to draft its own bill. Following the compromise, the Government Legislation Committee gave its approval, and the amended bill was presented to the Knesset plenum. The bill passed a first reading on December 12, 1999.[*]

14.6.1 The Government Bill

Aware of the initiatives and public processes that were widely reported in the media, the Ministry of Justice did pick up the gauntlet and started to work on the drafting task. An interministerial committee headed by Yehudit Karp was formed; at its first meeting, on February 2, 2000, it decided to invite both Coalition members and academic experts to take part in its work. The committee was subsequently divided into three subcommittees. One subcommittee focused on drafting a victim assistance scheme; another focused on planning a victim's compensation mechanism; the third focused on planning a model for child-victim services.

The drafting work of the governmental bill was slow, as most broad-forum projects tend to be. First draft for comments was distributed to the Coalition in June 2000, but the draft did not include the victim assistance and the compensation chapters. In December 2000, the interministerial committee held a general meeting in which two of the subcommittees, those on victim compensation and the child victim assistance model, presented their proposals. The compensation subcommittee suggested a victim benefit program through the National Insurance Institute, a social security scheme identical to the workers' compensation program. The other subcommittee proposed a three-level model for child victim assistance. The first level would involve regional assistance centers for providing all necessary "first-aid" services to child victims under one roof; the second would coordinate support and rehabilitation services that already exist in the community, which would

[*] The bill was adopted unanimously, with 20 votes in favor and none against.

be broadened and upgraded. The third level would be a new national authority that would develop guidelines for treating child victims and supervising
the other services. The contribution of Coalition members to the work of the
committee was critical. However, both subcommittees were asked to incorporate comments made by interministerial committee members; to date, neither subcommittee has finalized its report. The compensation subcommittee
confronted strong objections from the Ministry of Finance and awaited a
research evaluation of victims' financial needs, which was barred by bureaucratic obstacles. The child victims' assistance subcommittee did not finalize
its task because of substantial questions that arose while formulating its recommendations into a legislative proposal.

Meanwhile, MK Yael Dayan lost her patience, after having postponed
submission of her private member's bill for more than a year. On February
15, 2001, the Knesset Committee on Constitution, Legislation, and Law held
a meeting to prepare the bill for the crucial second and third readings in the
Knesset plenum. Before that meeting, Coalition members informed Dayan
that they would fully support her bill and provided her with some suggestions for improving its wording. At the meeting, Yehudit Karp expressed
her general support for Dayan's bill but suggested including some provisions from the government's bill. However, the concrete wording of the bill
was not discussed at the meeting. It was completed during many informal
discussions between Coalition representatives, Ms. Karp, and MK Dayan.
Another party to the negotiations was the Public Defender's office, which
raised many concrete objections. In its next meeting held on February 27, the
Knesset Committee on Constitution, Legislation, and Law endorsed the bill,
article by article. The revised bill, approved by the Public Defender's Office,
the Ministry of Finance, and the Ministry of Justice, now included many
articles adopted from the government's proposal, which in part broadened
its application to its original purpose.

14.7 Claims Accepted: The Birth of the Victims' Rights Law

On March 6, 2001, the Knesset passed second and third readings of the
Rights of Crime Victims bill, making it law. For the first time, crime victims
in Israel had procedural and substantial rights. The law made a distinction
between victims of violent and sexual assaults and other victims, providing
the former with a broader scope of rights, stipulating that:

> The victim's entitlement is that any right granted in the law shall be provided
> with consideration to his or her needs, dignity and privacy, and within a
> reasonable time frame. Victims of sexual and violent crimes are further

provided with the right to have the criminal process completed within a reasonable time frame, to prevent any injustice.

Minor victims are entitled to have their rights ensured, with adjustments according to the circumstances, in accordance with the principles of the UN Convention on the Rights of the Child, and the child's age. Victims with disabilities are entitled to have their rights provided, assured in accordance with the People with Disabilities Rights Law, 1998.

Victims have the right to protection from their offender or the offender's surrogates, including protection in court. Victims have the right to receive information regarding alternative measures of protection. Such information must be provided to victims in a language they understand.

The authorities are prohibited from providing the personal information of the victim to any person and are mandated to keep such data in separate files.

The law stipulates that crime victims are entitled to information about their legal rights, about existing victim assistance services, and about the criminal justice process in general. Furthermore, crime victims are entitled to receive, on request, information about the progress of their case; finally, victims who have requested so in advance have the right to be immediately updated with important developments in their case (as detailed in the Second and Third Annexes to the law), without the victims' need to initiate repeated enquiries. The Fourth Annex includes the right of the victim to information concerning developments in the detention of the accused in cases of sexual and violent crimes. With certain exceptions, crime victims are entitled to a copy of the indictment.

Victims of sexual and violent crimes have the right to be interviewed by the police in a manner that does not prejudice their dignity and privacy. Moreover, investigation of the victim's sexual history, excluding questions regarding past sexual contact with the suspect, is prohibited. Victims of sexual or violent crimes are further entitled to be escorted, by a person of their choice, to police investigations and court hearings, including those held *in camera*. Victims of sexual and violent crimes have the right to express their views whenever the authorities consider to withhold the criminal process ("close the case"), to accept a plea bargain, to release the accused from jail, or to pardon the accused. Moreover, the victim of any crime may submit a written statement to the police, to be handed to the court in the presentencing stage, detailing the harm caused by the offense. All rights provided under the law to crime victims shall be granted, in cases of death, to the victim's next of kin.

The law further provides that both the Public Attorney's Office and the police shall establish special units to address the rights provided to victims by the law.

To enable the authorities to prepare for full application of the law, gradual time frames were set. Some of the provisions entered into force 3 months after the law's enactment (i.e., in June 2001); other provisions were scheduled to enter into force 18 months after enactment (in September 2002); the remaining provisions were to come into force 30 months after enactment the law (in September 2003).*

14.8 Discussion

The Rights of Crime Victims Law, 2001, has been the result of a long process, at the center of which has been the experiences of people who were criminally victimized. Their situation reflects a social problem and a perceived need for public recognition, support, compensation, and a formal legal standing in the criminal process system. Victims were not alone in this process. Others supported the process by acknowledging victims' experiences, as well as the predicaments and exigencies attendant on criminal victimization.

Indeed, three main actors were involved in this process. The first was the State, represented by the Ministries of Justice and Finance. The second actor was crime victims, represented by various nongovernment victim support organizations. The third was the Israeli legislature, the Knesset. If crime victims' lack of status is acknowledged as a genuine, pressing social problem, the Knesset could enact a new law, intended to secure and regulate victims' rights in the criminal process, to provide victims adequate, professional support, and even state compensation.

As illustrated in this chapter, the state was ambivalent about the Rights of Crime Victims Law, 2001. On the one hand, the Ministry of Justice was convinced that Israel must have a crime victim support and compensation law, as most Western, industrialized countries do. The Ministry of Justice argued that without such a law, Israel, as a state, did not conduct its social policy in accordance with the provisions of the UN Declaration of Basic Principles of Justice for Victims of Crime and Abuse of Power [1985]. However, the Ministry of Finance claimed that it could not cover the administrative and operative costs of such a law, the costs of which were not at first assessed, and opposed the initiative. It was clear that without the requisite funding and the consent of the Treasury, victims' needs would not be acknowledged. After all, the Ministry of Finance is under pressure to acknowledge and support an endless number of pressing problems—why accept this one? It was up to the second "actor," crime victims, to make its case.

The second actor was the Coalition, which in Israel is similar to those in other countries, including the United States. Therefore, it had the opportunity to borrow a set of "off-the-peg" models and analysis for action. It consisted of the so-called "angry victims," whose victimization is not only enduring

---

* Since the writing of this chapter, several amendments have been made to the law, most of which either postponed or narrowed its application. The main provisions, however, remain largely unchanged.

and scarring but also frequently lodged in an already lively politics of gender [Yanay, 2005b]. The coalition consisted principally of advocacy organizations for women and children, as well as individual victims of sexual and violent crimes. In a way, male victims, victims of property crimes, victims of fraud and white collar crime, elderly victims, and many others, amounting to the vast majority of crime victims, were not part of the Coalition. However, the Coalition and the other actors in the process still attempted to promote the interests of all victims, according to universal standards set up by international human rights documents. Indeed, the Crime Victims' Rights Law applies to all victims of crimes regarded as misdemeanors or worse.

Indeed, individual crime victims, their families, and voluntary victim support organizations joined together in an attempt to lobby for their "rights." These organizations created the Coalition. The power of this Coalition can be attributed to three different sources. First, no one can argue with individual crime victims or with a group of parents of murdered children. The experiences of victims or parents who lost their loved ones in a criminal act are not negotiable. When such victims describe their painful ordeal and need for rights and services, it is difficult to stop them, let alone argue with their experiences.

Second, the Coalition brought together crime victims, voluntary victim services, victim advocates, and human rights activists whose joint mission was to secure the rights of crime victims (mainly those of violent crimes) and their need for support. Despite their different, sometime conflicting, agendas, these organizations have joined hands to create an effective alliance. Finally, members of the academic community, mainly in the fields of social work, law, and criminology supported the Coalition. Their independent, profound knowledge of victim policies in Israel and elsewhere reinforced the Coalition and gave it powerful backing. They argued that Israel is not in line with UN international declarations, and that helping victims of hostile (terrorist) acts only is not right because crime victims share similar needs and predicaments and deserve to be fairly and equally treated.

The third actor was the Knesset. Engaging in victims' rights and laws was not only a respectful, honorable topic to deal with but also could give any member of the Knesset a positive image in the public eye. Several members of the Knesset were ready to support a private bill. These MKs, headed by Yael Dayan, supported the bill prepared by the Coalition. Faced with this private initiative, the Ministry of Justice could not ignore an issue that became a challenge. Therefore, parallel to the private MK's bill, a government bill was submitted, and the only question left was which of the two bills would win the race, knowing that the Ministry of Finance opposed both.

Both the Ministry of Justice and the supportive legislators needed Coalition knowledge and expertise. They also needed the public pressure put by the Coalition against the Treasury, demanding that all resources necessary for the law be secured.

The Coalition, on the other hand, depended on the Knesset members to enact the bill and on the governmental officials to give their approval to the related reform. While striving to achieve such cooperation, Coalition members had to endure the slow bureaucratic pace of governmental committees and, more importantly, to settle for Dayan's consent to vote for a narrower version of the bill.

As in all negotiations, compromise is the feasible optimum one may wish for. Indeed, the compromise was simple: The law was to be enacted if it bore little or no cost. The compromise was that all the bill's clauses that cost no money would be approved, whereas those provisions with a price tag would be postponed.

As a result, the law is not identical to the proposed bill. All the "social" (support and compensation) rights were removed from the law and will not be provided for in the foreseeable future. Indeed, the law does include many "procedural rights," such as the right for information, the right to be heard before important decisions are made, and the right to be present in all court hearings. However, several clauses in the new law cost money. For example, according to the law, crime victims are entitled to state protection, mainly from those against whom they lodged a criminal complaint. Protecting victims costs money, especially if there is a need for alternative housing, such as a hotel room or refuge. Moreover, each police station has to appoint an officer to liaise with crime victims, provide information, and answer questions that relate to their cases. These things cost money too and will only be gradually provided.

No victim can sue an agency for failure to fulfill its obligations under the law. In a way, the law reflects symbolic recognition (which is undoubtedly important); the nature of the rights bestowed on victims appears to be "aspirational" rather than "justiciable." A more prominent discourse on rights might induce agencies to change their behavior.

The Coalition is not satisfied with any of the compromises made because many of the basic underlying problems have not been solved. At the same time, the Coalition managed to introduce a change: It succeeded in putting victims' rights on the social-political agenda by making politically acceptable claims. The Coalition also succeeded in presenting the fate of crime victims and their lack of rights—and turned it into a publicly acknowledged social problem. This problem reflects the needs and predicaments of many who were criminally victimized, but have no one, and nowhere, to turn to. A combination of cooperation between various enthusiastic actors and unique political circumstances led to a revolutionary law that, for the first time in Israel, acknowledges crime victims as participants in the criminal process pursuant to their victimization. It is up to the Coalition, human rights organizations, and the academic community to continue the initial "push" that characterized the first phase of the Coalition's efforts, to close ranks and prepare for the second round of legislation, a round that might be more difficult, and expensive, but also justified if victims' welfare is to be fully pursued.

References

Bassiouni, M. C. 1988. *International protection of victims*. International Association of Penal Law. Toulouse: Eres.

Chambliss, W. J. 1976. The state and criminal law. In *Whose law? What order?* ed. W. J. Chambliss and M. Mankoff, 66–106. New York: Wiley.

_____. 1993. On lawmaking. In *Making law: The state, the law, and structural contradictions*, ed. W. J Chambliss and M. S. Zatz, 3–33. Bloomington: Indiana University Press.

Carrington, F. C. and G. Nicholson. 1984. The victim movement: An idea whose time has come. *Pepperdine Law Review* 1:1–13.

DNP 3750/94. *Plonny v. State of Israel*, PD 48(4) 621.

Duff, P. 1998. The measure of criminal injuries compensation: Political pragmatism or dog's dinner? *Oxford Journal of Legal Studies* 18:105–42.

Elias, R. 1986. *The Politics of victimization: Victims, victimology and human rights*. New York: Oxford University Press.

Evan, W. M. 1980. Law as an instrument of social change. In *The sociology of law: A social–structural perspective*, ed. W. M. Evan, 554–62. New York: Free Press.

Fry, M. 1959. Justice for victims. *Journal of Public Law* 8:191–94.

Fuller, R. C., and R. R. Myers. 1941. The natural history of a social problem. *American Sociological Review* 6:320–29.

Garland, D. (2001). *The culture of control: Crime and social order in late modernity*. Oxford: Clarendon.

Goode, E., and N. Ben-Yehuda (1994). *Moral panics: The social construction of deviance*. Oxford: Blackwell.

Greer, D. (1996) United Kingdom: Great Britain. In *Compensating Crime Victims—A European Survey*, ed D. Greer, 573–638. Frieburg im Breisgau, Germany: Max Planck Institute.

Henderson, L. 1985. The wrongs of victims' rights. *Stanford Law Review* 37:937.

Holstein, J. A., and G. Miller. 1990. Rethinking victimization: An interactional approach to victimology. *Symbolic Interaction* 13:103–22.

Home Office. 1959. *Penal practice in a changing society*. Cmnd 645 (White paper). London: HMSO.

_____. 1961. *Compensation for victims of crime of violence*. Cmnd 1406. London: HSMO.

_____. 1964. House of Commons Debates, Vol. 697, June 24, 1964.

Israel Police. 2003. *Crime in Israel*. Jerusalem: Israel Police, Statistical Division.

Maguire, Mike, and J. Shapland. 1990. The victim movement in Europe. In *Victims of crime-problems, politics and programs*, ed. A. J. Lurigio, W. G. Skogan, and R. C. Davis, 205–25. Newbury Park, CA: Sage.

McGillis, D. and P. Smith. 1983. *Compensating victims of crime: An analysis of American programs*. Washington, DC: U.S. Department of Justice.

Merton, R. K. 1966. Social problems and sociological theory. In *Contemporary social problems*, ed. R. K. Merton, and R. A. Nisbet. New York: Harcourt Brace Jovanovich.

Miers, D. 1997. *State compensation for criminal injuries.* London: Blackstone.

Oestreich, J. E. 1999. Liberal theory and minority group rights. *Human Rights Quarterly* 21:108–32.

Office for Victims of Crime, The. 2000. *A voice for victims: Report on victim services in Ontario.* Ontario: Canada.

Postema, G. J. 1994. "Implicit law." *Law and Philosophy: An International Journal of Jurisprudence and Philosophy of Law* 13:361–87.

Payrow-Shabani, A. 1998. Discourse ethics, legitimacy, and power. *Contemporary Philosophy* 20:24–31.

Rock, P. 1986. *A view from the shadows: The Ministry of the Solicitor General of Canada and the making of justice for victims of crime initiative.* Oxford: Clarendon.

_____. 1990. *Helping victims of crime.* Oxford: Clarendon.

Sebba, L. 1996. *Third parties, victims and the criminal justice system.* Columbus: Ohio State University Press.

_____. 1999. The creation and evolution of criminal law in colonial and post-colonial societies. *Crime History and Societies* 3:71–91.

Spector, M., and J. I. Kitsuse. 1977. *Constructing social problems.* Menlo Park, CA: Cummings.

Strum, P. 1989. Women and the politics of religion in Israel. *Human Rights Quarterly* 11:483–503.

Tobolowski, P. M. 2001. *Crime victim rights and remedies.* Durham, NC: Carolina Academic Press.

United Nations. 1985. *Declaration of basic principles of justice for victims of crime and abuse of power.* New York: United Nations.

U.S. Government. 1982. *President's task force on victim of crime: Final report.* Washington, DC: Office of Justice Publications.

Yanay, U. 2005a. *Victims of violent crimes: Assistance provided by local welfare bureaus—A research report.* Jerusalem: Hebrew University.

_____. 2005b. Women refuges in Israel: From voluntary initiative to a government partnership (in Hebrew). *Social Security* 70:77–109.

Zander, M. 1994. *The law making process,* 4th ed. London: Butterworths.

Victim Services in the United States

15

BERNADETTE T. MUSCAT

Contents

15.1 Introduction

This chapter highlights the history of victim services in the United States from the mid-1970s until the present day. The chapter focuses on the major types of services that are available to assist victims of intimate partner violence, sexual assault, elder abuse, and child abuse. This is not the totality of individuals who are victimized nor is this representative of the full array of services that are available. The next section addresses crisis intervention and counseling options for victims. This is followed by a discussion of the roles and responsibilities of the victim advocate as he or she works in the community and with the criminal justice system. Finally, the chapter concludes with victim advocacy coalitions, some major policies addressing victims and victim service provision, and victims' rights. A fine balance was reached in presenting breadth and depth throughout this chapter. To the seasoned practitioner, much is absent. However, to the novice, an array of topics is presented with the intention of whetting one's appetite to learn more regarding victim services in the United States.

15.2 History of Victim Services in the United States

Up until the 1970s, victims had few options available to assist in the aftermath of a crime. The first responders were law enforcement, and, if needed, victims received medical attention. If a referral was given by a medical practitioner, some may have received counseling, but beyond those few things, victims were largely on their own. The myriad of feelings associated with victimization were exacerbated when the victim interacted with the criminal justice system. This system was not only confusing but also filled with various players who had no victim-specific training. Law enforcement officers were primarily concerned with apprehending the offender. This often meant relentless and repeated questioning to gather facts for the investigation. The courts proved to be a frightening and confusing prospect for victims who were unsure of the process, the status of their case, and what role they should play. Many victims also feared the offender and the outcome of testifying. The fear of reprisals contributed to many victims' unwillingness to testify, and cases were dismissed. The combination of factors was conducive neither to solving, prosecuting, or punishing the crime, nor in helping victims to cope, recover, and heal [Ennis, 1967; U.S. Law Enforcement Assistance Administration, 1976; Lowenberg, 1980; Bureau of Justice Statistics, 1994; Tomz and McGillis, 1997].

The 1970s was a period when many groups began to clamor for change, insisting that more must be done to reduce the psychological and financial consequences of victimization. Women's advocacy groups were particularly vocal about the treatment of rape and domestic violence victims, noting that the criminal justice system's insensitivity further revictimized, rather than helped, victims. Another problem stemmed from the lack of available services. By 1972 only three victim assistance programs—Aid for Victims of Crime (St. Louis, Missouri), Bay Area Women Against Rape (San Francisco, California), and the Rape Crisis Center (Washington, D.C.)—existed in the United States* [Walker and Kilpatrick, 2002]. By the mid-1970s, there were only a handful of programs nationwide that provided services to rape and domestic violence victims. Women's advocacy groups recognized that more must be done to help victims. This call was heard in 1974 by the Law Enforcement Assistance Administration (LEAA) of the U.S. Department of Justice, which provided initial funding to eight victim assistance programs nationwide [Tomz and McGillis, 1997].

By the early 1980s, LEAA was terminated but not without having contributed $50 million to the development of victim assistance programs [Tomz and McGillis, 1997]. With limited federal funding, organizations had to rely on local monies and alternate sources of income to continue service provision. Some were forced to restrict services to the neediest victims (e.g., children and elderly persons), and others had to close their doors. In 1980, California was the first state to respond to the lack of funding by providing statewide monies for victim services. Most states did not follow suit for several years [Tomz and McGillis, 1997].

As the victim services movement continued its expansion with greater service provision, increased funding, and the passage of victim-oriented

---

* As of 2008, each of these organizations remains operational.

policies, attention turned toward and continues to be placed on professionalizing the field. This includes expanding expertise and training with a multidisciplinary approach to understanding social, psychological, and legal principles. Many universities now offer a class or classes that focus on victim-related issues (e.g., Victimology, Family Violence, Child Abuse, and Violence against Women), and a few universities offer academic certificates, minors, and majors focusing on victimology. Regardless of the expansion of training and academic offerings, the victim services field continues to debate about certification, credentialing, and requiring formal education in a particular academic discipline(s). These issues will remain part of the field's ongoing discussion and identity formation. The end result of professionalizing the field will bring with it acceptance by other professionals, greater respect for those who work with victims, and professional level salaries [Walker and Kilpatrick, 2002].

The future of the victim services movement will see a continued expansion of services, greater attention paid to traditionally marginalized victims (e.g., victims with disabilities; lesbian, gay, bisexual, transgender, and questioning [LGBTQ] victims; immigrant victims) and the identification of new victims requiring services (e.g., identity theft, cyber crimes). The field will continue to fight for greater funding, crime victims' rights, and legislation to further assist victims.

15.3 Intimate Partner Violence Services

15.3.1 Shelters and Transitional Housing

One of the first types of victim services provided shelter for victims of intimate partner violence. Shelters first opened in the mid-1970s and continue to exist today. Shelters provide a place for battered women to have temporary housing when escaping a violent relationship. This is particularly important for women with few financial resources and limited social networks to turn to for assistance. Often battered women are turned away by family and friends who do not want to get involved, are fearful for their own safety, and/ or are frustrated by the repeated abuse and continued reunions with the batterer. Inevitably the abuse will continue, and the victim will need sanctuary. Shelters provide an alternative for battered women and their children, but bed space is limited, and they are frequently filled to capacity. The need for shelter is great given that an estimated 1.3 million women are battered each year, and more than half of the cities in the United States noted that intimate partner violence was a primary cause of homelessness [National Coalition Against Domestic Violence, 2007].

In 2006, an estimated 29% of requests for shelter were denied because of a lack of resources [U.S. Conference of Mayors, 2006]. According to the

National Network to End Domestic Violence, each day there are approximately 1,700 women who are denied shelter access because of a lack of space [National Network to End Domestic Violence, 2007].

Shelters provide immediate temporary housing and a safe place to stay for battered women and their children. Shelters give women some time to heal and to determine options for the future. The amount of time that a victim may use shelter services varies from state to state, but it is typically anywhere from 30 to 90 days [Humphreys and Lee, 2005]. The shelter is typically a large home in a residential neighborhood that houses up to 25 people. Most states require that shelters remain private, and, as such, there are usually no identifiable markers to indicate that the home is a shelter for battered women. The victim can access the shelter by contacting the police or by calling the shelter's hotline. If the latter is called, then the hotline worker will contact the police who will often drive the victim to the undisclosed shelter location [Shostack, 2001].

Once at the shelter, an advocate will determine the victim's and children's needs. This occurs through an intake process where individuals are screened for mental illness, substance abuse problems, anger management concerns, suicidal tendencies, and the like. If the person is identified as having any of these issues or if she is deemed to be a danger to herself or others, she is not permitted access. In many cases, shelters also will deny access to any male children who are more than 16 years old. To reside at the shelter, the victim and children must participate in counseling sessions and actively work toward living outside the shelter. Often shelters will assist women with identifying legal, medical, social, housing, education, employment, and child care options. If they meet the requirements of participating in counseling sessions and actively working toward living outside the shelter, women may stay at the shelter until they have secured alternate housing (e.g., with a family/friend, an apartment, or transitional housing) [Shostack, 2001].

Transitional housing is a long-term program that is available for victims of intimate partner violence, sexual assault, and stalking to help them move into a permanent residence. This housing option is similar to shelters in that individualized services such as counseling/support groups, safety planning, and victim advocates are available to residents. Transitional housing usually provides assistance with employment, transportation, child care, and referrals. This setting affords victims greater independence than a shelter but also provides the support needed to help the victim live a life free from violence. The cost of transitional housing varies, but typically the victim pays a nominal amount. Rent is based on a sliding fee scale, which increases over time, commensurate with her employment and ability to pay. The lower rent gives the victim ample opportunity to save money for a security deposit when she moves into permanent housing. Transitional housing is available for anywhere from 3 months to 2 years [Office on Violence Against Women, 2008].

15.3.2 Rape Crisis Programs and Sexual Assault
Nurse Examiner Programs

In 1972, the first two grassroots rape crisis centers opened their doors in San Francisco (Bay Area Women Against Rape) and Washington, D.C. (D.C. Rape Crisis Center). These and later centers focused on educating communities about the prevalence of rape, changing societal attitudes that perpetuated rape myths and blamed the victim, preventing rape, and providing crisis intervention and treatment. Rape crisis centers also offer advocacy services in the aftermath of an assault. The range of services includes determining the victim's safety and medical needs, advising the victim about options (e.g., forensic medical exam, reporting), ensuring that physical evidence is preserved (e.g., not bathing, removing clothes, brushing teeth, or other activities that may alter the victim's body), assisting with transportation to the hospital, and dispatching a victim advocate to the victim.

The advocate is instrumental in providing crisis intervention, empowering the victim to make informed decisions, making appropriate referrals for counseling and community services, and completing victim compensation forms. At the victim's request, the advocate can be present during the forensic medical exam or remain in the hospital while the exam takes place. The rape crisis advocate is trained to understand victim response and plays a vital role in reminding the victim that the rape is not her fault. If the case goes through the criminal justice system, the advocate can serve as a liaison with law enforcement and prosecutors to help the victim with reporting, adjudication, and sentencing. If this is a high-profile case, the advocate can serve as the victim's spokesperson to ensure the victim's anonymity. The advocate's primary concern should always be focused on helping and empowering victims to heal and recover [Kilpatrick, Whalley, and Edmunds, 2002].

A Sexual Assault Nurse Examiner (SANE) program creates a special environment in which the forensic medical exam can take place. In the early 1990s, the first SANE programs began to appear, and currently there are several hundred operational programs throughout the United States. The majority of these are located in emergency room settings in urban and suburban settings with very limited offerings in rural areas. West Virginia has a mobile SANE program that travels throughout the state to go to the victim, rather than having the victim travel hours, to complete an evidentiary exam [Office for Victims of Crime, 2008]. The SANE program room is usually part of, and yet separated from, the hospital or clinic. In some locales, the SANE program is a stand-alone facility. In many cases, victims can enter and leave through a private entrance that provides a greater sense of personal safety. Most SANE programs have a nurse examiner on call 24 hours a day, 7 days a week. These specialized programs help to decrease the amount of time that a victim has to wait to obtain medical care and can streamline the process for payment for the evidentiary exam* [Kilpatrick et al., 2002].

Once in the SANE program area, a nurse examiner will use state-of-the-art technology to collect physical evidence and handle the evidentiary aspects of a sexual assault. The nurse examiner will explain the victim's options in addressing sexually transmitted diseases and pregnancy. The nurse examiner's education and training ensure thorough evidence collection while also treating victims with dignity and compassion during the evidentiary exam. The testimony provided by SANE has helped prosecutors to increase the conviction rates for sexual assaults [Kilpatrick et al., 2002; Office for Victims of Crime, 2008].

15.3.3 Hotlines

Most local and national victim service agencies provide a telephone crisis hotline 24 hours a day, 7 days a week. Hotlines provide immediate short-term counseling to help the person get through the crisis. They do not provide long-term or ongoing counseling or treatment. If long-term mental health treatment is needed, the hotline worker, who is trained in crisis intervention and victim services, will provide a referral to the appropriate community agency. Most people think that crisis hotlines provide assistance to the victims of intimate partner violence and sexual assault or to those contemplating suicide. In reality, anyone may call the hotline to talk about a victimization; to get information and resources; to get assistance with safety planning, transportation, or medical care; and/or to determine legal options for protective orders, reporting crimes, and the like. The goal of the hotline worker is to ensure that the victim is safe while providing sensitive and compassionate care [Kilpatrick et al., 2002; Bennett et al., 2004].

15.4 Services for Older Adults

The demographics of older adults indicate that those over the age of 65 are one of the fastest-growing sectors in the United States. As such, elder abuse and crimes against older adults are receiving greater attention. Older adults bring unique challenges to victim services because of their reluctance to report crimes, fear of retaliation for reporting, and shame of reporting when the abuser is a family member. As a result, there are specific victim service programs that exist to help older adults who are victimized

---

* State monies are available through STOP Violence Against Women formula grant funds to pay the full out-of-pocket expense for sexual assault evidentiary exams.

[Tomz and McGillis, 1997]. This section will focus on only two of the many programs that exist: Adult Protective Services (APS) and TRIADs.

15.4.1 Adult Protective Services

APS is an organization that is responsible for investigating and providing services for older and dependent adults who are being mistreated as a result of neglect, exploitation, and physical/sexual abuse. APS will conduct investigations in-home and in institutional settings (e.g., state-operated care homes, institutional settings, schools, and adult foster homes) to determine whether abuse is taking place and the extent of the abuse. Once a full assessment is completed and the abuse is confirmed, the APS case worker will determine the root cause of the problem and the appropriate intervention services needed to end the abuse. The APS caseworker can help the victim access services (e.g., financial assistance, guardianship services), arrange transportation, make immediate emergency decisions regarding medical care and/ or removal from a facility, and make referrals to community social service organizations for long-term care. Adults have several rights when interacting with APS. A few of these rights include the right to refuse protective services unless the adult is suffering from abuse, neglect, or exploitation and if he or she lacks the capacity to consent to APS services. Another right is that adults must be given the opportunity to participate in and be consulted regarding all decisions made on their behalf. Adults also have the right to a court-appointed attorney *ad litem* to represent the adult's interests in any court proceedings. The goal of APS is to ensure that older and dependent adults are able to live a life free from maltreatment and abuse [Texas Department of Family and Protective Services, 2008].

15.4.2 TRIADs

A TRIAD is a collaborative effort among law enforcement, those who work with older adults, and community senior citizen groups (e.g., the American Association of Retired Persons [AARP] and Area Agency on Aging [AAA]). First created in 1987, the goal of a TRIAD is to reduce and prevent crime, decrease the fear of victimization, and improve services for older adults. The original intention was to increase law enforcement response to crime, enhance law enforcement services and interactions, and prevent crime of older adults [U.S. Department of Justice, 1998].

     Since their inception, TRIADs have expanded to include representatives from district attorney's offices and victim service organizations. Together they also work with other TRIAD members to raise awareness about safety issues facing older adults. This awareness includes information about specific crimes and victimization, identifying strategies to reduce vulnerabilities to crime, community resources, and ways to improve the quality of life for older adults. TRIADs are tailored to addressing the unique needs and concerns of the community in which they reside. As such, a TRIAD will work on local concerns, rather than broader state or national issues. The TRIAD listens to older adults in that community and then works collaboratively to address these issues and find solutions [U.S. Department of Justice, 1998].

15.5 VINE: Victim Information and Notification Everyday

One of the fundamental rights for crime victims is the right to information and notification. The telephonically and Internet-based Victim Information and Notification Everyday (VINE) program was implemented in 1998 to ensure that these two rights are provided to crime victims. VINE is available in most states and provides victims with a toll-free number to receive information regarding the status of criminal cases and pertinent information regarding an incarcerated offender (e.g., the location of the offenders, or custody changes) [Young and Stein, 2004]. The victim also can register to be notified when an inmate is released. The VINE system will call registered victims repeatedly for 48 hours or until contact is made. The victim is given a personal identification number (PIN) that must be entered to ensure verification that the appropriate person received the information. Services are available in English and Spanish, and live operators are available 24 hours a day, 7 days a week throughout the year to provide information [Tomz and McGillis, 1997].

15.6 Financial Remedies

The costs of being a victim do not stop with the emotional and physical pain. The financial burdens associated with victimization are high. According to one estimate, the cost of personal crime alone is approximately $105 billion each year in health care costs, lost earnings, and funding for victim services [Miller et al., 1996; Gaboury and Edmunds, 2002]. According to the Bureau of Justice Statistics, in 2004 the total economic loss to victims was $1.1 billion for violent crime and almost $15 billion for property crimes [Bureau of Justice Statistics, 2006]. To help offset the financial costs to victims, two programs will be highlighted here—victim compensation and restitution.

15.6.1 Victim Compensation

In 1965, California was the first state to enact a crime victim compensation program. Today victim compensation programs are available in all states, the District of Columbia, the U.S. Virgin Islands, Guam, and Puerto Rico [Young and Stein, 2004]. These programs reimburse victims for crime-related expenses, including medical and mental health care, funeral costs, and lost wages. Victim compensation programs are governed by state laws, but most states have comparable eligibility requirements and benefits. Victim compensation is funded by offender fees and fines and the federal Victims of Crime Act (VOCA) fund. Compensation is paid to the victim when all other financial resources, insurance, and restitution monies are exhausted. Each year approximately $450 million is administered to 200,000 crime victims, which amounts to approximately $10,000–25,000 per victim [National Association of Crime Victim Compensation Boards, 2008].

To be eligible to receive compensation, one must be a primary victim of a violent personal crime, including child abuse, drunk driving, elder abuse, intimate partner violence, and sexual assault. Homicide survivors are also eligible to receive compensation. Those who are victims of property crimes are not covered under most victim compensation programs. To receive compensation, the victim must apply for compensation in the state where the crime occurred, not in the state in which he or she resides, if these are different. The victim must report the crime to law enforcement officers and file a compensation claim within a set period (typically within 1 year after the crime occurred). The victim must be innocent of all wrongdoing and did not contribute to the crime for which he or she is seeking compensation. The victim must cooperate with law enforcement and prosecution, but the offender does not have to be apprehended or convicted for victims to receive com-pensation [Office for Victims of Crime, 2004].

15.6.2 Restitution

Restitution is a court order that requires an offender to make a monetary payment to the victim as a result of the crime committed against the person. Restitution is set during the sentencing phase. Each state has statutory guidelines outlining the amount to be awarded and collection mechanisms. Restitution is collected by probation, departments of corrections, parole, or private collection agencies and then disbursed to the victims. If an offender willfully fails to pay restitution, his or her probation or parole can be revoked. Some courts also play a role in collecting restitution by thoroughly investigating all of the offender's assets, preserving those assets, and garnishing income (e.g., wages, lottery winnings, inmate wages, trust accounts, and civil lawsuits). Despite these efforts, many victims never receive the full amount of restitution that has been awarded [Office for Victims of Crime, 2002].

15.7 Restorative Justice

Restorative justice brings together victims, offenders, and the community to determine an appropriate response to the crime committed. Unlike the criminal justice system, which is based on retribution, restorative justice is based on the philosophy of repairing the wrongs associated with the crime. Restorative justice is used extensively throughout the world but remains relatively new in the United States, where it has largely been reserved as an option for juvenile offenders and postsentencing. The idea behind both is that young people should have an opportunity to be rehabilitated and that restorative justice should not replace criminal sanctions. One of the components used in the United States is the victim-offender reconciliation program (VORP), also known as victim-offender mediation. VORP is a type of restorative justice because it provides a forum for victims and offenders to talk about the impact that the crime has had on the victim. Unlike traditional mediation options, VORP does not allow the two parties to reach a mutual agreement. Instead, the offender learns about how the crime affected the victim and listens to the victim's proposed options for remedying the harm caused. Restorative justice requires a community component (e.g., the victim's family and friends, concerned citizens, victims' advocates, law enforcement) to be present in victim-offender interactions to ensure that the offender is held accountable for his or her actions, including following through with the victim's requested remedies. The latter is a key component of the principles of restorative justice because the remedies help the victim to regain his or her life, to repair the harm caused by the crime, and to become whole again [Tomz and McGillis, 1997].

15.8 Services for Child Victims

Annually the Bureau of Justice Statistics (BJS) provides data on a variety of different types of crimes, criminal sanctions, and victim and offender characteristics. According to BJS, 67% of all reported victims of sexual assault were aged less than 18 years, and 34% were not yet teenagers. One of every seven child victims of sexual assault was not even 6 years old [U.S. Department of Justice, 2008]. BJS also notes that approximately 60,000 incarcerated offenders have victims aged less than 18 years. Bringing this figure closer to home, that means that one of every five violent offenders in state prison is incarcerated for abusing a child. More than half of the incarcerated offenders committed crimes against victims aged less than 12 years, and 70% of the offenders were incarcerated for sexually assaulting a child [Greenfeld, 1996]. These statistics represent only a fraction of the crimes against children because these data are based on reported crimes and those where the offender was convicted.

There are numerous cases that do not fit into either of these categories. Although there are several victim services available to the youngest victims, this section will focus on only a few—Child Protective Services (CPS), Court-Appointed Special Advocates (CASA), Multidisciplinary Interview Centers (MDICs), and mandatory reporting laws.

15.8.1 Child Protective Services

CPS is an organization that investigates allegations of child neglect, maltreatment, exploitation, and physical/sexual abuse. There are several options when a case is investigated by a CPS caseworker. The case could be unfounded (i.e., not enough evidence indicative of abuse), and the files are closed with no further action taken. Another option is that the caseworker has a suspicion of abuse but not enough concrete evidence to know that abuse occurred. When this happens, the case is pending and will require a follow-up investigation. If no further abuse or suspicions of abuse linger, the case is closed. The final category occurs when abuse is "founded" or when there is enough evidence to indicate that there is abuse. At this point, a CPS caseworker or a representative of the criminal justice system will handle the case. If the abuse or neglect is simply a matter of parents or guardians not having enough money to properly feed, clothe, or shelter the children, then a CPS caseworker will help the family to identify community food banks, rental subsidies, and/or other resources to assist with the care and maintenance of the family. Likewise, if the parents or caretakers are mentally, emotionally, and/or physically unable to care for the children, then community referrals are provided as assistance. The intention is to help the families stay together by providing appropriate referrals and resources. On the other hand, if it is a case of willful abuse or neglect and the child is not in immediate danger, CPS will work with the family to resolve problems and reduce the stress that is contributing to the abuse. CPS will create a contract with the family whereby the parent or guardian must successfully complete parenting classes, anger management programs, drug/alcohol treatment, mental health counseling, and educational/vocational/employment training to keep the children. CPS will continue to conduct home visits during this time of contractual obligation. If the parent or guardian does not abide by the contract, the conditions of the contract will be increased, and the time that the family is monitored will be extended. If during the second phase of the contract the family is still not meeting the requirements of the contract, then the children will be removed and either be placed with a family member or friend. If this option is unavailable, then the children will be placed in the foster care system until the parent or guardian fulfills his or her part of the contract. Typically, this is a temporary placement, but sometimes foster care becomes a permanent placement. The goal of CPS is to work with the family first before removing the child and placing him or her in another home. The process of removing a child from his or her family is traumatic, and this is meant as a last resort unless the child is in immediate danger. CPS will work with the children and families to end the abuse and neglect, to ensure that appropriate services are received, and to reunify the family if a family or foster care placement is needed [Whitcomb, Hook, and Alexander, 2002].

15.8.2 Court-Appointed Special Advocates

CASA is an organization that is composed of individuals who volunteer to be a guardian *ad litem* (GAL) for a child. The idea was conceived in 1977 by a Seattle judge who saw the need for children to have an advocate in court proceedings. The idea spread to other courtrooms around the United States. The CASA will conduct an independent investigation of the child's circumstances to determine his or her needs. To accomplish this, the CASA will meet with the child, the family and/or foster care family, the school, and other individuals who are part of the child's life. The volunteer will remain with the case for approximately 2 years or until the child is placed in a home that is permanent and safe [Whitcomb et al., 2002]. By 1990, the U.S. Congress passed the Victims of Child Abuse Act, which called for an expansion of CASA programs throughout the United States. By 2007, there were more than 900 local programs with more than 50,000 CASA volunteers serving 225,000 abused and neglected children nationwide [National Court-Appointed Special Advocates (NCASA), 2008].

15.9 Multidisciplinary Interview Center

An MDIC is a program that coordinates the interviewing efforts of law enforcement, prosecutors, and defense attorneys who may have to interview a victim of a sensitive violent crime (e.g., child abuse, elder abuse, abuse of victims with disabilities). The interview center allows all the parties to meet in a centralized location to interview the victim at single time. This process means that the victim retells the crime once without having to repeat it multiple times, in different locations, and to different people.

The center is typically located in a homelike setting to ease the interviewing process for the victim. The center is divided in two with one room used as an interview room, which is subdivided from the waiting room by a two-way mirror. Sometimes the interview room is filled with toys to help young victims feel more comfortable. The waiting room allows the multiple interviewers to sit and watch the interview as it is taking place. A single interviewer who is in the interview room with the victim will ask the questions. The single interviewer will receive questions from all parties before the interview begins. The single interviewer is wired to be able to hear if the others who are behind the two-way mirror have additional questions for the victim. Any further questions are fed to the interviewer through the earpiece that transmits sound only in his or her ear. Once the interviewer hears the question, he or she will inquire or prompt the victim for more information. In addition to the earpiece used to relay questions to the single interview, the room is wired with state-of-the art technology that allows the interview to be videotaped [U.S. Department of Justice, 1998].

15.10 Mandatory Reporting Laws

The mandatory reporting law was established in 1974 under the Child Abuse Prevention and Treatment Act (CAPTA) and has since been amended several times. In the late 1990s, all 50 states extended mandatory reporting requirements to include older and dependent adults because of the vulnerability of these two groups to abuse and neglect. Mandatory reporting laws require that any individual who as part of their profession has regular contact with a child and/or older/dependent adult must report any reasonable suspicions of physical/sexual abuse and/or neglect to the proper authorities (e.g., law enforcement or child/adult protective services). Mandated reporters include, but are not limited to, health care practitioners, law enforcement officers, school personnel, day care providers, spiritual leaders, social workers, mental health care practitioners, medical examiners and coroners, and lawyers. If a mandated reporter fails to report an allegation of abuse or neglect, that person is subject to the sanctions as specified by state laws (e.g., civil liability, loss of licensure). Mandatory reporting laws also specify to whom the report should be made, the timeliness of the report, and the consequences for failure to report [Whitcomb et al., 2002]. After the investigation, if no abuse or neglect is founded, the mandated reporter is immune from liability because the report was made with a reasonable suspicion of abuse and in "good faith" [Child Welfare Information Gateway, 2008].

15.11 Therapy and Recovery

In recent years, there has been greater recognition that victims' responses are not the same for the same type of crime. In fact, a single victim may have different reactions to multiple crimes. Just as all people are different, so too are the reactions that they experience to a traumatic event. Given this understanding, there are multiple types of therapeutic models available to victims. This section focuses on only a few—crisis intervention, individual counseling, relationship counseling, family counseling, and peer-support and group counseling. The section concludes with a brief description of the victim-counselor privilege laws.

15.11.1 Crisis Intervention

Crisis intervention refers to providing immediate assistance to an individual after a traumatic event. The type of intervention provided is based on the victim's needs and can include responding to a crime scene, transporting a person to a hospital or shelter, providing medical assistance, helping a victim to locate a missing loved one, or providing a shoulder to cry on. Victims have varying and unpredictable responses to a crisis, which necessitates a crisis intervention that is tailored to the specific needs of the person at the time of the crisis. The important part of crisis intervention is being there for the victim and asking what he or she wants and needs at that traumatic moment. It is equally important to not make assumptions about what is in the victim's best interest. Instead, crisis intervention involves providing options and letting the victim make the decision. These early decisions can be very helpful as the victim sorts through the crime and its aftermath [Alexander, 2005]. Effective crisis intervention is dependent on accurately assessing the situation, defusing any volatile situations, working with the victim to determine immediate needs, developing a plan of action, providing options, making referrals for short- and long-term resources, and providing information regarding what will happen next and why [Tomz and McGillis, 1997; Myer and Conte, 2006].

15.11.2 Individual Counseling

Individual counseling is a one-on-one session between the victim and a mental health care provider. Many victims choose this type of counseling because it affords them a sense of privacy in discussing difficult and traumatic events that may also be embarrassing, humiliating, or shameful. Given the diversity of victims and their responses to trauma, individual counseling allows for a personalized session to focus on the issues that are most important (e.g., fears for personal safety, problems in the immediate and/or extended family, feelings of anxiety/depression). The individual attention is important for a victim to sort through and find guidance on his or her concerns without having to share time with others. Individual counseling sessions can help victims to express their feelings, cope with vulnerabilities, avoid self-blame and doubt, and rebuild their lives. Counseling can also help victims to participate in the criminal justice system [Tomz and McGillis, 1997].

15.11.3 Relationship Counseling

Relationship counseling or couples counseling is an option for couples who are having difficulty coping with a victimization that may threaten their relationship. For example, if the couple's child was murdered, they may experience problems communicating or interacting with one another. They may also have different means of coping with the loss of their child. One parent may become overprotective of the other children, whereas another feels the need to disengage from the family. As a result, couples counseling could assist them in reconnecting with one another as a couple or as parents to their remaining children. In other situations, one member of the couple may have been victimized, and the other partner is unable to cope. An example of this is when one partner is sexually assaulted by a stranger. It is difficult for the victim to be intimate with a loved one and may also be difficult to talk about what he or she is feeling. The victim may not want to be touched and/or may feel intense fear associated with being touched even by someone the victim knows loves him or her. Couples counseling can give both partners an opportunity to discuss these feelings, thoughts, emotions, and fears in a way that they may not be able to do in the absence of a trained counselor.

Couples counseling should not be used when there is violence in the relationship (e.g., intimate partner violence and sexual assault) because of the power differential between the couple. In other words, the batterer controls the relationship through threats, intimidation, coercion, and fear. These tactics can be very subtle, such as "a look" that may be used to control the victim but may go undetected in a therapeutic environment. Couples counseling should also not be used for couples with abusive relationships because the goal of this type of counseling is to renew and restore the relationship. This could be very dangerous and put the victim's safety at risk. As such, victims and batterers should go to individual or group counseling but not attend counseling together [McWhirter, 2006].

15.11.4 Family Counseling

Family counseling enables all family members to come together to discuss problems within the familial unit. This type of counseling is an opportunity for the family to communicate, listen, and work together to resolve issues that affect the entire family. Family counseling is typically used to help parents work better with at-risk or delinquent youth, while helping the child explore why he or she is acting out in antisocial ways. In other situations, it is used to help the family cope with the loss of a loved one or to address addictions. Sometimes, family counseling is used to help women and children cope with intimate partner abuse and leaving the batterer. In this circumstance, it is appropriate for the abused parent and child to openly communicate about their thoughts, feelings, and emotions. It is also a good idea for both the victim and the children to go to counseling separately to discuss age-appropriate concerns and fears with a third party. Much like relationship counseling, family counseling should not be used to bring abusive adults together for the purpose of reconciliation. Instead, each person in the couple should seek counseling separately before considering therapy together as a couple or as a family [McWhirter, 2006].

15.11.5 Peer Support and Group Counseling

Group therapy provides an opportunity for those who share a common event, such as a victimization, to reflect and to learn from another's experiences. Group therapy is used for survivors of intimate partner violence, child abuse, sexual abuse, and homicide, to name a few. Members benefit from the support of those who understand, and together they can work through issues of fear, depression, shame, isolation, and helplessness associated with the crime [Wanlass, Moreno, and Thomson, 2006]. In addition to working on recovering from the victimization, the group will also work on self-esteem, functional relationships, and developing communication, decision-making, and living skills. The goals of the group involve sharing, learning from one another, and moving toward recovery.

This type of therapy is often used in conjunction with individual counseling as an added source of support for the victim. Some group meetings are voluntary, which means that members may vary from one time to another. Other groups have more stable membership between sessions. In most cases, groups meet on a weekly basis for 1–2 hours. Groups tend to be small, with 5–10 people, because it is easier to share sensitive matters in front of a few people rather than a large group. This type of therapy requires a skilled practitioner who can manage a group setting with multiple responses, varying defense mechanisms, intense reactions, and different communication styles.

Group therapy can be an effective tool for recovery because it provides a safe environment for building social networks, increased social stability, and interpersonal support. This is particularly important for victims who are often isolated or lack functional relationships for positive interactions [McWhirter, 2006].

15.11.6 Victim-Counselor Privilege Law

Many types of communication are protected from being disclosed in court, including doctor-patient, attorney-client, husband-wife, clergy-parishioner, and therapist-patient. In recent years, some states have considered extending nondisclosure rights to the communication between a nonlicensed counselor and a victim. These states argue that nonlicensed counselors are often employed at publicly funded organizations, such as domestic violence shelters and rape crisis centers. Many women would go without counseling services if they had to pay for them out of pocket. In the interest of providing counseling services and in fairness to all victims regardless of socioeconomic status, victim service providers advocate that the right to nondisclosure should be extended to counselors and victims. These laws allow the victim to speak freely to the counselor without fear that the professional will be required to testify as a witness. In some locales, the nondisclosure extends to written counseling records and reports. There are three types of victim-counselor privilege laws—absolute (no disclosure of any confidential counseling records or communication without the victim's consent), semiabsolute (disclosure in limited situations when the disclosure is in the public interest, such as mandatory reporting), and qualified (the courts determine whether the victim's confidentiality outweighs the value of the evidence to the defendant's case). The extension of victim-counselor privilege laws throughout all 50 states is a hope for the future [Office for Victims of Crime, 2002].

15.12 The Role of the Victim Advocate

The role of the victim advocate is very diverse and depends on the type of organization within which the advocate is working and the type of victim with whom the advocate interacts. Some victim advocates work for nonprofit community-based organizations, whereas others work with the criminal justice system, local or state agencies, and advocacy coalitions. The role of the victim advocate ranges from crisis intervention, referrals, victim accompaniments (e.g., to the hospital, courts), community education, political advocacy, training for those who work with victims (e.g., law enforcement, prosecutors, human service providers, medical and mental health personnel), and many other activities. This section will highlight some of the many different roles played by victim advocates as they provide system-based services, working with the media, and death notifications. This section also addresses ethics and the vicarious trauma that victim advocates experience when working with crime victims.

15.12.1 Victim Advocates

The role of victim advocates are varied and have traditionally only focused on the primary crime victim. In recent years, advocates have begun to provide services to secondary and tertiary victims. The services provided by victim advocates can be broken down into four broad categories. First, advocates provide emergency services, including crisis intervention, shelter, food, clothing, access to medical and mental health services, and relocation. When the person is a victim of a property crime, the advocate can provide a security survey to help the victim determine appropriate and affordable security mechanisms to ensure greater safety. The next major service provided by victim advocates is emergency financial assistance. This can include money for transportation, food, shelter, toiletries and personal items, phone calls, and other emergency items that the victim may need. These emergency funds are usually made available through a petty cash fund that the advocate must receive authorization to use. A program director or supervisor is able to authorize and disburse the emergency funds for the victim. Emergency funds are based on need, the victim reporting the crime to the police in a timely manner, and participation with the criminal justice system. Another major service provided by victim advocates includes transportation to a shelter, to the hospital, to court, and to access community services. Many times transportation is provided through vouchers to allow victims to use public transportation, shuttles, and/or taxi services at no cost. Finally, advocates provide advocacy and support services at the scene of the crime, at the victim service organization, and/or by conducting home visits after the crime. The intention is to provide immediate crisis intervention, determine needs, and provide assistance and referrals. The advocate can also help the victim to file victim compensation claims, court-related services, and assistance with writing or presenting victim impact statements (VIS). Victim advocates can provide assistance with every aspect of the criminal justice system [Tomz and McGillis, 1997].

15.12.2 System-Based Services

In recent years the criminal justice system is taking a more proactive role in working with and providing assistance for victims. In some circumstances, this means greater collaboration with community-based victim service programs and victim advocates. In other situations, the criminal justice system has hired victim advocates to be part of law enforcement departments, district attorney's offices, and correctional institutions. This section highlights the different roles and responsibilities of victim advocates as they work with the criminal justice system.

15.12.2.1 Law Enforcement

Victim advocates work with law enforcement officers throughout the United States in a variety of capacities. Sometimes, victim advocates serve as a liaison between a community-based victim service program and the law enforcement department. Other times, the victim advocate is hired by the police department. In either situation, the victim advocate can go on ride-alongs, which can be mutually beneficial. It provides advocates with an opportunity to interact one on one with officers and to serve victim's immediate crisis intervention needs—a job that law enforcement typically prefers not to do. Ride-alongs also allow both law enforcement and advocates to learn about the challenges of each other's job. Once a collaborative relationship is established between advocates and law enforcement departments, then together they can determine opportunities for cross-training and joint orientations to ensure that the two groups know about and work together from the outset. The training can include information regarding the role of the victim advocate, when the advocate should be contacted, and how the advocate can assist law enforcement. This type of training can highlight victim sensitivity, awareness of victim dynamics, and the importance of victim advocates in helping victims to cooperate with police. Advocates and law enforcement can also work on guidelines for sharing arrest reports, interviewing, and crisis intervention to help streamline the process and better serve victims' needs [Tomz and McGillis, 1997].

15.12.2.2 The Courts

Victim advocates work with the various courtroom participants, including prosecutors and judges. Sometimes advocates work directly in the district attorney's offices, whereas other times they serve as a liaison between community victim service organizations and the courts. In either situation, they have various roles in the courtroom.

One of the most important aspects of a victim advocate in the courtroom is to explain the process to victims and witnesses. Often victims and witnesses do not understand court proceedings and/or are fearful of being in the same room with the offender. The advocate can address these concerns by answering all questions before, during, and after an interaction with the court; he or she can explain what will happen next and why, and determine the next step(s) for the victims or witnesses. This is very important because court can be confusing; it can be difficult to hear; and the rulings may be unclear to victims or witnesses who are unfamiliar with legal jargon. The advocate can also provide timely notifications to victims or witnesses regarding upcoming court appearances and the expectations for being in court, including being on time and the likelihood of a continuance. If needed, the advocate works with the victim or witness regarding transportation or travel to the courthouse, overnight accommodations, appropriate demeanor and dress, safely entering and exiting the courthouse and courtroom, and securing child care. Once in the courtroom, the advocate can provide much-needed support, a shoulder to cry on, some tissues if testimony becomes emotional, and water. The advocate can even prepare the victims or witnesses for potentially difficult, embarrassing, or uncomfortable questions that may arise while testifying. Once the advocate is able to allay some of the victims' and witnesses' fears and anxieties, then the prosecutor can focus on providing good evidence and a strong case [Tomz and McGillis, 1997].

Victim advocates can also help judges by working with victims who become emotional on the stand or while waiting in the courtroom. Often judges do not like the disruptions caused by victims or witnesses who become distraught or who have outbursts that may slow down courtroom proceedings. A victim advocate can help with this process by providing the much-needed emotional support that can help to calm victims or witnesses.

Victim advocates can also assist victims and witnesses to prepare, write, and/or present a VIS and restitution recommendations. Both the support and the assistance with VIS can help judges by keeping the court running smoothly with few interruptions [Tomz and McGillis, 1997].

15.12.2.3 Corrections

Traditionally victim advocates have not had a role to play within corrections because this system's sole focus has been punishing and rehabilitating the offender. Since the 1990s, correctional institutions have gained a greater appreciation for the need to keep victims abreast of the offender's whereabouts within the system, notification of release, the types of rehabilitative programs offered to offenders while incarcerated, and parole conditions. Often victims have a myriad of questions regarding corrections, including delineating between probation or parole and jail or prison, why the offender is in a community correctional institution rather than being "locked up," and "What is early release, and when and why does it happen?" A victim advocate can answer these and other questions, explain correctional institutions, and help victims to know and understand their rights. Victim advocates can also help victims use the VINE or other notification systems to determine the status of the offender while incarcerated. In some states, the victim advocate will work with correctional institutions to set up a payment schedule and to withhold earnings to ensure that restitution is paid. The advocate can collect and disburse those monies without the offender ever knowing the victim's whereabouts. In a correctional setting, victim advocates can also create a fact or information sheet with pertinent information about referrals for victim and community service organizations. Another important role for advocates is to provide support to victims during parole and other hearings. The advocate can ensure that the victim has a separate waiting area to minimize victim-offender contact and can assist the victim in writing and/or presenting a VIS. For those victims who may want to interact with the offender through victim-offender mediation, VORP, or restorative justice, the victim advocate can help facilitate these programs. This includes preparing the victim for what he or she might expect in interacting with the offender and ensuring the victim's safety during the process. If the advocate is not a trained mediator, then he or she will contact someone with this expertise. Finally, victim advocates provide victim impact classes and panels for offenders. During these classes, victims speak directly to offenders about how the crime has impacted their lives. The hope is that impact classes will help offenders to see the pain caused and knowing the impact will help deter future crimes [Monsey, 1994; Umbreit, 1994; Tomz and McGillis, 1997].

15.12.3 Death Notification

One of the most difficult aspects of being a victim advocate is giving a death notification to surviving family members. It is essential that advocates are sensitive, compassionate, timely, and accurate in delivering the notification. Mothers Against Drunk Driving (MADD) developed and refined a curriculum to train advocates to give death notifications. The core elements of a death notification include selecting the right person (e.g., one who is calm and confident rather than someone who is stressed) to deliver the notification and ensuring that he or she understands what the impact will be on the surviving victims. The factors that influence the intensity of the death notification include the suddenness of the death, the severity of the death, the surviving victims' ability to understand what happened, and the overall familial stability at the time of the death. The shock of the event is very difficult on victims and their ability to understand what has happened. The surviving victims' ability to cope will depend on their physical, mental, emotional, and spiritual health, which varies greatly with each survivor. At this critical time, it is important for the victim advocate to provide survivors with the opportunity to express emotions freely, to provide calm reassurance, to help the survivor regain control, and to provide assistance with future preparations. Another core component of a death notification is to be certain of the victim's identity, how and where the death occurred, where the deceased is now, and the contact information for any law enforcement officer(s) who might have been involved in the case. A third component is to conduct the death notification in person, preferably with another person, not over the phone or through writing. The assistance of a second person can be helpful if there are multiple family members or a large group together at the time of the notification. The advocate should have credentials or identification to ensure that he or she is allowed entry into the survivor's home. A notification should not be given at the door or in the doorway. Instead, the advocate and the survivor(s) should sit down. The advocate should be very specific about identifying the victim and the survivor's relationship to the victim (e.g., "Are you the parents of Michael Jones?"). A notification should be given to parents or spouses before siblings and never to a child alone because this puts the burden on the child to notify the remaining family members. The notification should be simple, direct, and informal while also providing warmth, compassion, and support at a difficult time. It is important to use common language, avoid jargon, and answer questions honestly. The advocate can also offer to help with securing child care, calling others, making funeral arrangements, and/or transporting the family to identify the victim. Finally, the family should be notified before the media when there is media interest in the story [Ellis and Lord, 2002].

15.12.4 Working with the Media

The news media play a significant role in public safety by providing important information about the nature and extent of crime occurring in communities and efforts to prevent crime and assist victims. However, this coverage sometimes raises legitimate concerns about the victim's rights to privacy in the vulnerable aftermath of victimization. In some cases, victims perceive aggressive, insensitive reporting as a direct threat to their ability to grieve with dignity and to their personal safety. Victim advocates can help in this process by assisting victims to work with the media in high-profile cases. The advocate's role is to determine the victim's needs and to follow through. Some victims do not want to speak to the media and will ask the victim advocate to speak on their behalf. Other victims want to speak to the media, and the advocate can help set up these interviews at a neutral location (e.g., victim service provider's office) rather than at the victim's home. The advocate can also create media access areas for press releases, updates, and photos. These areas are usually close to a place that a victim may frequent (e.g., police department or courthouse) but are separate enough that the victim can pass easily without being mobbed by media inquiries. The victim advocate can also help a homicide survivor or parents or guardians whose child has been kidnapped to select their loved one's photo for presentation in media outlets [Seymour, 2002].

15.12.5 Vicarious Trauma

Vicarious trauma refers to the psychological distress experienced by those who work with someone who experienced a traumatic event. The distress can take many forms, including stress, burnout, fatigue, low empathy, and/or losing boundaries whereby the person too closely relates to the victim's suffering. When someone experiences vicarious trauma, he or she may have feelings that are very similar to the one's the victim is feeling, including nightmares, avoidance, and hypersensitivity. The person suffering from vicarious trauma may use alcohol and/or other substances as a coping mechanism [Palm et al., 2004].

Vicarious trauma may be exacerbated by having intimate knowledge about the details of the crime and/or if he or she has experienced trauma in his or her own life. In either situation, the advocate may experience difficulty working with the victim. This is problematic on two levels—for the victim because he or she is not likely receiving the best, most objective services available, and for the service provider who is suffering along with the victim with few outlets for addressing the symptoms of vicarious trauma [Adams et al., 2006]. Research on vicarious trauma is inconclusive as to why some people experience vicarious trauma and others do not, and why the extent, severity, or length of time that one experiences vicarious trauma differs so much between individuals. Organizations can respond to vicarious trauma by providing a quiet room for employees to relax, providing or extending the number of personal days off, allowing more time off, and ensuring the availability of counseling. In combination, such practices can provide short- and long-term assistance for those experiencing vicarious trauma [Seymour and Edmunds, 2002].

15.12.6 Ethics

The field of victim services is very broad, and this diversity has contributed to the lack of a professional organization of victim service providers. As a result, there are no standardized guidelines for ethical behavior for victim service providers. Instead, there are several guiding principles that victim service providers generally adhere to as appropriate for interacting with victims. The guidelines are broken down into four areas: scope of services, coordinating within the community, direct services, and administration and evaluation.

Scope of services suggests that victim service providers represent themselves and their services accurately and act professionally when interacting with others. In addition, service providers should have a high level of professional competence, which includes understanding their legal responsibilities and obligations and performing all duties in accordance with governmental and organizational laws, regulations, policies, and procedures.

The second overarching principle of ethical behavior involves collaboration and cooperation among colleagues and professionals to evaluate, enhance, and improve the effective service provision. Next, victim service providers are to protect the victim's civil rights, which include the right to not be discriminated against while receiving services. Confidentiality of one's personal information and records should also be protected. In the event that confidentiality cannot be protected (e.g., state or federal laws that require open records), then the victim should be notified immediately. Another related ethical guideline is that victim service providers should not engage in actions, behaviors, or styles of communicating that are victim blaming. Victim service providers should interact professionally and objectively by treating all victims equally, not exploiting the victim's trust, disclosing any potential conflicts of interest, and terminating the professional relationship when the victim is not likely to benefit from continued services. Finally, services should be available for colleagues who need assistance when they are traumatized by a criminal event or through interactions with a victim.

The final ethical guideline requires administrators and supervisors to monitor and report any employee who mistreats victims or otherwise does not follow the principles outlined here. The report can be made to a professional or organizational board, a governmental compliance agency, funding sources, or other entity that is responsible for adoption of these ethical guidelines [Standards for Victim Assistance Providers and Programs, 2003]. As the victim services field evolves, it is likely that these and other ethical guidelines will be standardized and legalized in the future.

15.13 Advocacy for Change: Coalitions, Policy, and Crime Victims' Rights

One of the most critical aspects of victim services is the creation of advocacy coalitions, the expansion of policies to address victimization and increase funding for service provision, and the promotion and enforcement of crime victims' rights. This section provides a brief overview of each of these topics. There are a plethora of coalitions and policies that currently exist in the United States, but given the parameters of this chapter only a few are highlighted. The paucity of information provided here should not be misconstrued as a lack of effort in the United States. Instead, the content of this section could easily fill several chapters.

15.13.1 Advocacy Coalitions

The victim services movement has a variety of coalitions that work on specific types of crimes to advocate for policy changes and increased funding, to raise awareness, and to ensure more effective service provision for victims of these crimes. Victim service coalitions began in 1974 with the founding of Families and Friends of Missing Persons in Washington. By 1980, two other coalitions formed: Parents of Murdered Children (1978) and MADD (1980). All of these coalitions continue to exist today. The genesis of these coalitions was to serve as a support group for those who were traumatized by the crime, but later each added political advocacy to their repertoire. Many coalitions began as grassroots movements because a single person and/or family was impacted by a crime and felt that something must be done to ensure that others did not suffer in the same way [Young and Stein, 2002]. These coalitions worked to raise awareness, to set the political agenda for legislative change, to increase funding for nonprofit member service provider organizations, to expand the training and professional development available to victim advocates and allied professionals, and to fight for increased rights for crime victims [Walker and Kilpatrick, 2002].

The mid-1970s also ushered in a period that necessitated these disparate victim service programs to meet, discuss common concerns, learn from each other, and advocate for change. Two main events furthered these goals. The initial effort occurred in 1976 when Fresno, California, became the host site of the first National Organization of Victim Assistance (NOVA) meeting. NOVA provided a forum to unite social service providers and criminal justice personnel. The goal of this meeting was to foster a more victim-oriented perspective throughout the criminal justice process. This initial meeting and later ones served as a catalyst to identify and address victims' needs, including increasing victim services and funding, implementing and enhancing

victim compensation and restitution options, and developing creative programs to address individual, family, and community disputes (e.g., mediation, conflict resolution) [Tomz and McGillis, 1997].

The second uniting event occurred in 1978 when the existing crime
victim assistance programs worked to create NCASA and the National
Coalition Against Domestic Violence (NCADV). These coalitions worked to
address funding, to create more services to reach more victims, and to implement more victim-centered legislation to address these crimes [Young, 1986;
Walker and Kilpatrick, 2002].

Victim service organizations and coalitions pushed for legislative reforms
and increased political attention focused on crime victims. By 1981, President
Ronald Reagan proclaimed Crime Victims' Week, and the Attorney General's
Task Force on Violent Crime issued its inaugural report calling for the creation of a distinct Task Force whose sole focus was to consider victims' issues.
This group was created and became the President's Task Force on Victims of
Crime. Within 1 year of formation, the President's Task Force issued 68 recommendations targeting both the public and private sectors and the crimi-
nal justice system to do more to improve the treatment of crime victims. One
of the recommendations included an amendment to the U.S. Constitution
to include victims' rights—a recommendation that remains unfulfilled. In
1983, the U.S. Department of Justice created the Office for Victims of Crime
(OVC) to implement the 68 recommendations of the President's Task Force
[President's Task Force on Victims of Crime, 1982; Tomz and McGillis, 1997;
Walker and Kilpatrick, 2002].

In the absence of a U.S. Constitutional amendment to address victims'
rights, Congress passed the Federal Victim and Witness Protection Act
(1983) to provide witness protection, restitution, and fair treatment of
federal victims and witnesses of violent crimes. The federal initiative led
to a rippling effect with states passing victims' bills of rights and increased
funding for program expansion, training, and professional development. In
1984, the federal government passed VOCA, which established the Crime
Victims Fund. This fund, comprising federal criminal fines, penalties, and
bond forfeitures, provided monies for local victim service organizations,
state victim compensation programs, and research. The combination of
heightened public awareness and political support contributed to the
expansion of victim service funding, greater emphasis placed on law
and order, and more attention focused on victims' rights [Walker and
Kilpatrick, 2002].

The late 1980s through the 1990s saw many sweeping legislative changes,
including the reauthorization of VOCA, the expansion of crime victim compensation programs to all 50 states, states' adoption of victims' bills of rights,
state constitutional amendments, and specific laws to address campus security; child abuse, neglect, and kidnapping; gun control; hate crimes; sexual

assault; and violence against women. During this time, the U.S. Supreme Court also upheld the right of victims to give an impact statement in capital cases. This period included an influx of research focusing on prevalence of victimization; trauma response, mental health concerns, and recovery; program and policy evaluation; and identifying promising practices. This research, coupled with increased funding and legislative advances, laid the foundation for the provision of better and more effective service provision [Walker and Kilpatrick, 2002].

15.13.2 Victims of Crime Act

One of the consequences of the President's Task Force on Victims was to enact the VOCA of 1984, which created the OVC as part of the U.S. Department of Justice and created a Crime Victims Fund as part of the U.S. Department of Treasury. The fund amasses revenues from fines placed on those convicted of federal offenses, from forfeited bail bonds, and other assessments. OVC uses these funds to provide state governments with support for victim assistance and prevention programs, state compensation programs, training and technical assistance, and grants. Each state must determine a statewide funding plan for the allocated monies.

VOCA specifies the types of services that can receive these funds, including crisis intervention, medical and mental health care, hotline services, emergency living services (e.g., food, clothing, transportation, and shelter), legal assistance and criminal justice advocacy, the enforcement of victims' rights, and other services that provide coping, stabilizing, and safety assistance to primary and secondary crime victims. VOCA funding priorities include providing programs and services to victims of intimate partner violence, sexual assault, child abuse, and to those who have been traditionally underserved (e.g., elder abuse, victims with a disability). Since 1988, separate funds are available from the Assistance for Victims of Federal Crime in Indian Country grant program to create programs and services for American Indians. Since its inception, VOCA has provided more than $1 billion to approximately 3,000 victim assistance organizations and allied professionals serving more than 2 million victims each year [Tomz and McGillis, 1997].

15.13.3 Violence Against Women Act

In 1994, Congress enacted the Violence Against Women Act (VAWA) to address the victimization of women and children from intimate partner violence, sexual assault, and stalking in the United States. The U.S. Department of Justice created the Violence Against Women Program Office to administer the provisions of the Act. The Act provides funding to expand intervention and prevention services/programs; increase identification, investigation, and prosecution of crimes; ensure victim safety and offender accountability; expand legal remedies; and improve the response and effectiveness of those department and organizations that work to address violence against women [Tomz and McGillis, 1997]. In addition to victim assistance organizations, monies are also allocated to local, state, and tribal governments; law enforcement departments; district attorney's offices; and all nonprofit organizations that assist victims of the VAWA-specified crimes. VAWA provides funding to ensure that organizations work collaboratively to end the victimization of women and children [Seymour et al., 2002]. In 2005, President Bush signed VAWA 2005 into law, which provides $3.3 billion over 5 years to assist with violence against women [NCADV, 2008].

15.13.4 Crime Victims' Rights

The call for a federal constitutional amendment to include crime victims' rights began in the mid-1980s. Since then, every state has adopted some legal rights for crime victims either through a victims' bill of rights or via a state constitutional amendment. The rights that are granted victims vary from state to state, but there are certain provisions that can be generalized to most locales. Victims have several rights; among these are:

- The right to reasonable safety and protection from the accused
- The right to accurate and timely notification of the offender's status while incarcerated or on release and court proceedings related to the crime
- The right to consultation with an attorney before a case is dismissed and/or plea agreement is reached
- The right to a speedy trial
- The right to be present at all public criminal justice proceedings
- The right to be heard by making a statement regarding plea bargains, sentencing, parole, and release hearings
- The right to confidentiality regarding the victim or witnesses' contact information
- The right to receive full and timely restitution as ordered
- The right to be treated with fairness, respect, and dignity [National Center for Victims of Crime, 2004

These rights were extended to victims of federal crimes through the passage of the Justice for All Act of 2004. The act consists of a few major components that include protecting and enforcing crime victims' rights in federal criminal proceedings; eliminating substantial backlogs of DNA samples collected at crime scenes and from convicted offenders; and improving and expanding the ability of local, state, and federal crime labs to test DNA. The Act authorizes the distribution of grant monies to develop, establish, and maintain programs to provide services and enforce victims' rights; for training and technical assistance; and to enhance victim notification systems. The Act also requires that the Department of Justice receive and investigate all complaints regarding violations of victims' rights. The victim or the government can enforce these rights by filing a petition with the court of appeals, which must issue a decision within 72 hours of the filing. If the file is denied, the court must clearly provide a reason in writing that is placed on the record. If there is a violation of the victim's rights, the Department of Justice is responsible for creating appropriate disciplinary sanctions. Finally, the Act calls for an expansion of training regarding crime victims' rights. As of 2008, funding for the Justice for All Act has not yet been appropriated by Congress [Office for Victims of Crime, 2006].

15.14 Conclusions

This chapter is not meant to be an exhaustive examination of victim services in the United States but rather a broad overview of what is available to crime victims. The victim service movement has seen tremendous growth during the past 30 years from just a few organizations to what is now several thousands of organizations strong. During this period, the laws, policies, and funding opportunities for victim services have all expanded to address more victimizations and to help more victims. Crime victims' rights now exist, and continued efforts are underway to ensure that the U.S. Constitution is amended to include these rights. Despite these advances, more has yet to be accomplished to effectively serve crime victims. The hope is that the future will see a continued expansion in funding for service provision, training for criminal justice officials and allied professionals, the enforcement of victims' rights, and more policies that help victims. The goals for the future are straightforward—to ensure that victims receive services, that policies are in place to right the wrongs of a crime, and that victims are treated with sensitivity, dignity, and respect to foster healing and long-term recovery.

References

Adams, R. E., J. A. Boscarino, and C. R. Figley. 2006. Compassion fatigue and psychological distress among social workers: A validation study. *American Journal of Orthopsychiatry* 76(1):103–108.

Alexander, D. A. 2005. Early mental health intervention after disasters. *Advances in Psychiatric Treatment* 11:12–18.

Anonymous. 1998. *New directions from the field: Victims' rights and services for the 21st century*. Washington, DC: U.S. Department of Justice, Office of Justice Programs, Office for Victims of Crime.

Anonymous. 2002. *Privacy of victims' counseling communications*. Legal Series Bulletin 8. Washington, DC: U.S. Department of Justice, Office for Victims of Crime.

Bureau of Justice Statistics. 1992. *Criminal victimization in the United States*. Washington, DC: U.S. Department of Justice, Bureau of Justice Statistics.

———. 2006. *Criminal victimization in the United States, 2004: Statistical tables*. Table 81, Washington, DC: Bureau of Justice Statistics. http://www.ojp. usdoj.gov/bjs/pub/pdf/cvus04.pdf (accessed September 19, 2006).

Carroll, A. E. and J. Lord. 2002. *Homicide*. National Victim Assistance Academy, Office for Victims of Crime. http://www.ojp.usdoj.gov/ovc/assist/nvaa2002/chapter12. html (accessed June 15, 2008).

Child Welfare Information Gateway. http://www.childwelfare.gov (accessed April 30, 2008).

Ennis, P. H. 1967. *Criminal victimization in the United States: A report of a national survey*. Washington, DC: U.S. Department of Justice Law Enforcement Assistance Administration, United States. http://www.ncjrs.gov/App/Publications/abstract. aspx?ID=620 (accessed June 20, 2008).

Gaboury, M. and C. Edmunds. 2002. *Financial assistance for victims of crime: Civil remedies*. Office for Victims of Crime, National Victim Assistance Academy textbook. http://www.ovc.gov/assist/nvaa2002/chapter5_1.html#1 (accessed June 14, 2008).

Greenfeld, L. A. 1996. *Child victimizers: Violent offenders and their victims*. Bureau of Justice Statistics, Office of Justice Programs (March 1996, NCJ-158625). http://www.ojp.usdoj.gov/bjs/pub/pdf/cvvoatvx.pdf (accessed July 10, 2008).

Humphreys, J. and K. Lee. 2005. Sleep disturbance in battered women living in transitional housing. *Journal of Mental Health Nursing* 26:771–80.

Kilpatrick, D. G., A. Whalley, and C. Edmunds. 2002. *Sexual assault*. National Victim Assistance Academy, Office for Victims of Crime. http://www.ojp.usdoj.gov/ovc/assist/nvaa2002/chapter10.html (accessed June 22, 2008).

Lowenberg, D. A. 1980. Your clients will be there next year. Will you? In *Victim/witness programs: Human services of the 80s*, ed. E. C. Viano, 404–10. Washington, DC: Visage.

McWhirter, P. T. 2006. Community therapeutic intervention for women healing from trauma. *The Journal for Specialists in Group Work* 31(4):339–51.

Miller, T., M. Cohen, and B. Wiersema. 1996. *Victim costs and consequences: A new look*. Washington, DC: U.S. Department of Justice, National Institute of Justice.

Myer, R. A. and C. Conte. 2006. Assessment for crisis intervention. *Journal of Clinical Psychology: In Session* 62(8):959–70.

National Association of Crime Victim Compensation Boards. 2008. *Crime victim compensation: Resources for recovery*. http://www.nacvcb.org/documents/Fact%20 sheet.doc (accessed June 5, 2008).

National Center for Victims of Crime. 2004. *Issues: Victims' bill of rights*. http://www. ncvc.org/ncvc/main.aspx?dbName=DocumentViewer&DocumentID=32697 (accessed July 4, 2008).

National Coalition Against Domestic Violence. 2008. *Violence against women act (VAWA) appropriations*. National Coalition Against Domestic Violence. http:// www.ncadv.org/files/2008vawa.pdf (accessed June 10, 2008).

_____. N.d. *Domestic violence and housing.* http://www.ncadv.org/files/Housing_.pdf (accessed June 13, 2008).

National Coalition for the Homeless. 2007. *Domestic violence and homelessness, NCH Fact Sheet #7.* http://www.nationalhomeless.org/publications/facts/domestic. pdf (accessed July 1, 2008).

National Court Appointed Special Advocates (NCASA). 2008. *Overview.* http://www. nationalcasa.org (accessed May 2, 2008).

National Network to End Domestic Violence. 2007. *Domestic violence counts: A 24-hour census of domestic violence shelters and services across the United States.* Washington, DC: National Network to End Domestic Violence.

National Public Radio. 2008. *Housing first: A special report.* National Public Radio, July 31, 2008. http:www.npr.org/news/specials/housingfirst/whoneeds/abuse. html (accessed June 13, 2008).

Newmark, L. and R. Allen. 2003. *Standards for victim assistance providers and programs, National Victim Assistance Consortium.* Columbia, SC: National Criminal Justice Reference Service.

Office for Victims of Crime. 1992. Ordering restitution to the crime victim. *Legal Series Bulletin* 6. Washington, DC: Office for Victims of Crime. U.S. Department of Justice, Office of Justice Programs.

_____. 2004. *State crime victim compensation and assistance grant programs.* Washington, DC: Office for Victims of Crime. http://www.ojp.usdoj.gov/ ovc/publications/factshts/compandassist/welcome.html (accessed June 25, 2008).

_____. 2008. *Implementing SANE programs in rural communities: The West Virginia model.* Washington, DC: Office for Victims of Crime. http://www.ojp.usdoj.gov/ ovc/publications/infores/WVA_Mobile_SANE_guide/welcome.html (accessed June 10, 2008).

Office on Violence Against Women. 2008. *Transitional housing assistance grants programs.* Washington, DC: Office on Violence Against Women, U.S. Department of Justice. http://www.ovw.usdoj.gov/thousing_grant_desc.htm (accessed July 3, 2008).

Palm, K. M., M. A. Polusny, and V. M. Follette. 2004. Vicarious traumatization: Potential hazards and interventions for disaster and trauma workers. *Prehospital and Disaster Medicine* 19(1):73–78.

Seymour, A. 2002. *The news media's coverage of crime and victimization.* National Victim Assistance Academy, training manual. Washington, DC: Office for victims of crime.

Seymour, A. and C. Edmunds. 2002. *Mental health needs, section 2, stress management.* National Victim Assistance Academy, training manual. Washington, DC: Office for Victims of Crime.

Seymour, A., J. Sigmon, and E. Smith. 2002. *Special topics: Funding for victim services.* National Victim Assistance Academy, Chapter 22, Office for Victims of Crime. http://www.ojp.usdoj.gov/ovc/assist/nvaa2002/chapter22_8.html (accessed June 22, 2008).

Shostack, A. L. 2001. *Shelters for battered women and their children: A comprehensive guide to planning and operating safe and caring residential programs.* Springfield, IL: Charles C. Thomas.

Texas Department of Family and Protective Services. *About adult protective ser-vices.* http://www.dfps.state.tx.us/Adult_Protection/About_Adult_Protective_Services/ (accessed June 23, 2008).

Tomz, J. E. and D. McGillis, 1997. *Serving crime victims and witnesses,* 2nd ed. Washington, DC: U.S. Department of Justice.

Umbreit, M. 1994. *Victim meets offender: The impact of restorative justice and media-tion.* Monsey, NY: Willow Tree.

U.S. Conference of Mayors. 2006. *A status report on hunger and homelessness in America's cities: 2006.* Washington, DC: U.S. Conference of Mayors.

U.S. Department of Justice, Office of Justice Programs, Office for Victims of Crime. 1998. *New directions from the field: Victims' rights and services for the 21st cen-tury.* Washington, DC: U.S. Department of Justice, Office of Justice Programs, Office for Victims of Crime.

U.S. Law Enforcement Assistance Administration. 1976. *Criminal victimization in the United States: A comparison of the 1973 and 1974 Findings,* 40–41. Washington, DC: U.S. Department of Justice, Law Enforcement Assistance Administration.

Walker, S. D. and D. G. Kilpatrick. 2002. *Scope of crime/historical review of the vic-tims' rights discipline.* National Victim Assistance Academy textbook, Office for Victims of Crime. http://www.ojp.usdoj.gov/ovc/assist/nvaa2002/chapter1.html (accessed July 3, 2008).

Wanlass, J., J. K. Moreno, and H. M. Thomson. 2006. Group therapy for abused and neglected youth: Therapeutic and child advocacy challenges. *The Journal for Specialists in Group Work* 31(4):337–47.

Whitcomb, D., M. Hook, and E. Alexander. 2002. *Child victimization.* National Victim Assistance Academy, Office for Victims of Crime. http://www.ojp.usdoj.gov/ovc/assist/nvaa2002/chapter11.html (accessed June 10, 2008).

Young, M. 1986. History of the victims' movement. In *Victims of violence,* ed. F. Ochberg, 311–21. Washington, DC: National Center for Victims of Crime.

Young, M. and J. Stein. 2004. *A component of the office for victims of crime oral history project.* Office for Victims of Crime: 2002-VF-GX009. http://www.ojp.usdoj.gov/ovc/ncvrw/2005/pg4c.html (accessed June 10, 2008).

Fear of Crime in the Republic of Ireland

Understanding Its Origins and Consequences

16

MICHELLE BUTLER AND
PAUL CUNNINGHAM

Contents

16.1 Introduction

Although individuals have been concerned about crime for centuries, "fear of crime" is a relatively recent concept. The expression *fear of crime* first began to appear in American newspapers during the 1930s and was used to explain the public's reaction to criminal behavior. However, the term *fear of crime* was not used in Europe until the early 1960s. It was during this time that the development of victim surveys and improvements in information-gathering technologies made data collection more manageable and the measurement of fear of crime* possible [see Emsley, 1987; Lee, 2007]. In this chapter, the level of fear of crime in Ireland is explored, as well as its impact on quality of life. First, the concept of fear of crime is examined before moving on to discuss how fear of crime became an area of public concern in Ireland. Next, the methods used to assess fear of crime in Ireland are described, and the factors predicting fear of crime and its impact on quality of life are identified. Last, the potential relationship between victimization and fear of crime is examined, and the implications arising from the research findings are explored.

16.2 Defining Fear of Crime

Fear of crime is difficult to define because it can refer to a range of thoughts, emotions, and beliefs regarding an individual's vulnerability and that of his or her loved ones and the wider community [Ferraro, 1995]. For example, fear of crime is usually taken to mean an individual's fear of becoming a victim of crime [Maxfield, 1984; John Howard Society of Alberta, 1999; Gabriel and Greve, 2003]. However, it can also refer to people's concern about general crime levels, their beliefs regarding their risk of victimization and that of their loved ones, as well as an apprehension about the possible consequences of victimization [Warr, 1984; Skogan, 1987; Box, Hale, and Andrews, 1988; Carrach and Mukherjee, 1999]. This diversity has resulted in fear of crime

---

* Any measurement of fear of crime depends on individuals accurately acknowledging and reporting their fears. As such, these measurements tend to assess an individual's reported fear of crime and may not take account of unconscious feelings of fear. For this reason, the use of the term *fear of crime* in this chapter refers to an individual's acknowledged and reported fear of crime.

being defined as "an emotional response of dread or anxiety to crime or symbols that a person associates with crime" [Ferraro, 1995:4].

There are many factors that are believed to contribute to a fear of crime [see Ferraro, 1995; Hale, 1996; Lee, 2007]. These include personal attributes, previous experience of victimization, characteristics of the environment, and wider social influences such as the media. Personal characteristics, such as age, gender, ethnicity, geographical location, and education, have all been found to be related to fear of crime [Clemente and Kleiman, 1976; Box et al., 1988; Hough, 1995; Chadee and Ditton, 2003]. Specifically, females, older adults, ethnic minority groups, and individuals from urban locations tend to report a greater fear of crime than others [Box et al., 1988; Ferraro, 1995; Hale, 1996].

An individual's perception of crime as a frequent occurrence may also result in feelings of fear as individuals believe they are at an increased risk of being victimized [Warr and Stafford, 1983; Ferraro, 1995]. In particular, past experience of being a victim of crime may increase an individual's perception of being at risk of future victimization [Skogan, 1987; Box et al., 1988]. However, the relationship between fear of crime and victimization is not always straightforward. For example, while having been a victim of crime may increase an individual's belief of being at risk of further victimization, it may also reduce the perceived seriousness of being victimized [see Agnew, 1985; Winkel, 1998]. In this way, variations between individuals' perceptions of the frequency and seriousness of criminal behavior may explain differences in their levels of fear.

In addition, research indicates that fear of crime can be influenced by characteristics of the environment and wider social processes [Heath and Petraitis, 1987; Ferraro, 1995]. Skogan [1986, 1990] suggests that a location's reputation for being crime prone depends on the amount of criminal activity in it and on various "signs of crime." Signs of crime are features of the environment that increase an individual's perceived risk of victimization [Skogan and Maxfield, 1981; Skogan, 1990]. Broken windows, graffiti, burned-out houses and/or cars, homelessness, beggars, and "rowdy" youths can act as signs of crime [Wilson, 1968; Wilson and Kelling, 1985; Ferraro, 1995]. Such signs of crime, combined with an area's reputation for being crime prone, are believed to indirectly influence fear of crime by heightening an individual's perceived risk of being victimized [LaGrange et al., 1992].

Further, wider social processes can also shape an individual's perceptions of crime, sense of vulnerability, and of the consequences associated with victimization. For example, a growth in media technologies is believed to have facilitated a greater awareness of crime, as well as a greater awareness of "risk" among the public [Beck, 1992; Furedi, 2002; Lyng, 2005]. Such awareness of being "at risk" is believed to have contributed to a culture of fear that encourages feelings of uncertainty and anxiety among the population [see Furedi, 2002]. As such, fear of crime appears to be located within, and linked to, wider fears about such matters as employment, the family, security, health, finances, and the state of the government [Taylor, 1996; Ewald, 2000; Tulloch and Lupton, 2003; Walklate and Mythen, 2008]. Consequently, Hollway and Jefferson [1997] suggest that some individuals may project their fears about wider, more difficult to control issues onto crime, as crime appears actionable and potentially controllable. Accordingly, some individuals may report a fear of crime that stems from wider anxieties and/or feelings of vulnerability rather than their risk of being victimized or their previous experience of victimization.

16.3 Fear of Crime in the Republic of Ireland

In Ireland, the past few decades have seen increasing attention being paid to crime and the impact of crime on Irish citizens. This, in turn, has prompted a greater awareness of crime and its effect among the general population [see Kilcommins et al., 2004]. In particular, a combination of factors in the 1980s and mid-1990s provided the catalyst for widespread public anxiety about crime and crime control, which resulted in a greater attentiveness to issues such as fear of crime and its impact on quality of life.

In the early 1980s, Ireland experienced an economic recession that contributed to high levels of unemployment, emigration, and poverty [see Laver et al., 1987]. The recession, combined with the Troubles in Northern Ireland, caused individuals to be more concerned with unemployment, inflation, and Northern Ireland than with domestic crime and crime control, despite increasing crime figures [see Kilcommins et al., 2004]. This led some commentators to state that Ireland remained a nation curiously unconcerned by crime despite an unprecedented increase in official crime statistics [O'Donnell and O'Sullivan, 2003].

The majority of the Irish public seemed to remain unconcerned about crime until a series of events in the 1980s and mid-1990s. During the late 1970s and 1980s, Ireland experienced an increase in the number of people using drugs, especially heroin, to such an extent that Dublin (the capital of Ireland) was believed to be experiencing an "opiate epidemic" [see Dean et al., 1985; O'Mahony, 1993]. Official crime statistics indicate that the number of burglaries, robberies, and thefts increased significantly during this period; commentators suggested that these increases were associated with the growing number of drug addicts in Ireland and their need to fund their habit [see O'Mahony and Guilmore, 1983; Charleton, 1995]. This led to feelings of disquiet among those living in urban locations, particularly Dublin, about the harm caused by drug use, as well as the lavish lifestyles of criminals involved in supplying drugs [see Kilcommins et al., 2004; O'Donnell, 2007].

Such feelings of disquiet led to a number of protest marches in which community members demanded that drug dealers leave their local communities [see
Charleton, 1995; Kilcommins et al., 2004; Lyder, 2005; O'Donnell, 2007]. This
increase in drug abuse prompted a general feeling of unease, against which
events in the mid-1990s led to widespread concern about crime and lawlessness amongst the Irish public [Kilcommins et al., 2004; O'Donnell, 2007].

In the mid-1990s, the economic recession began to ease, and a number
of high-profile killings occurred, demonstrating that crime is a problem not
only for deprived urban areas but also for rural locations [see McCullagh, 1999;
Kilcommins et al., 2004]. In particular, two high-profile killings led to a public
outcry throughout Ireland. In June 1996, a member of An Garda Síochána,*
Detective Gerry McCabe, was shot dead during an attempted robbery in
Adare, County Limerick. Two weeks later, Veronica Guerin, an investigative
journalist with the *Sunday Independent*, was murdered. These events prompted public apprehensiveness about lawlessness; it was in this context that issues
of crime and the public's fear of crime began to receive special attention [see
Kilcommins et al., 2004; O'Donnell, 2007; Coulter, 2008].

These killings also served to trigger widespread media coverage of crime
and its impact [see Kilcommins et al., 2004; O'Donnell, 2007; Coulter, 2008]. In
particular, it was during this time that the media coverage of crime became more
widespread and intense, providing more colorful descriptions of criminal behavior than had been provided previously [see O'Connell, 1999, 2002; O'Donnell
and O'Sullivan, 2003; Coulter, 2008]. This led some to suggest that the media's
portrayal of crime encouraged a fear of crime by contributing to an impression
that crime had increased significantly during the previous decade [see Kerrigan
and Shaw, 1985; McCullagh, 1996; Brown, 2007, 2008; Coulter, 2008]. Indeed, a
study of the Irish media's portrayal of crime found that the Irish public's perceptions of crime were not linked to official crime statistics but were rather associated with age, sex, and newspaper readership [O'Connell and Whelan, 1996].
Hence this media coverage of crime served to reflect and reinforce the public's
concern about criminal activities and prompted the government to focus anew
on criminal justice matters [see Kilcommins et al., 2004; O'Donnell, 2007].

This renewed focus on criminal justice matters also led to a number of
national surveys examining the nature and extent of crime, victimization,
and fear of crime in Ireland [see Central Statistics Office, 1999; Watson, 2000;
Garda Research Unit, 2002].

16.3.1 Fear of Crime and Victimization

Fear of crime is usually measured through survey research. In Ireland, the
Central Statistics Office's (CSO) Crime and Victimisation Surveys and Garda

---

* An Garda Síochána is the Irish Police Force.

Public Attitudes Surveys are used to measure the level of fear and victimization experienced by the public. Figures from the Crime and Victimisation Survey 2006 indicate that levels of fear among the Irish public remained relatively stable in the previous decade. The Crime and Victimisation Survey is part of the Quarterly National Household Survey that surveys 39,000 Irish households quarterly. A special module on Crime and Victimisation was included in the 1998, 2003, and 2006 Quarterly National Household Surveys. Based on the results of these surveys, approximately 25% of the Irish public was found to feel either unsafe or very unsafe walking alone in their neighborhood after dark, and 7% felt unsafe or very unsafe in their home alone at night [see CSO, 1999, 2004, 2007].

Similar figures were also observed in the Garda Public Attitudes Surveys. The Garda Public Attitudes Survey is a nationwide survey investigating respondents' attitudes and experiences of An Garda Síochána, crime, fear of crime, and the criminal justice system more generally. Since 2002, the Garda Public Attitudes Surveys have been conducted annually and, from 2005 onward, they have consisted of a nationally representative sample of approximately 10,000 respondents [see O'Dwyer et al., 2005; Kennedy and Browne, 2006, 2007]. Results for the Garda Public Attitudes Surveys 2002–2006 indicate that between 24% and 29% of respondents felt either unsafe or very unsafe walking alone in their neighborhood after dark, whereas 41–54% were worried about becoming a victim of crime [see Garda Research Unit, 2002; Sarma, 2003; Sarma and O'Dwyer, 2004; O'Dwyer et al., 2005; Kennedy and Browne, 2006, 2007].

As in other countries, females, older age groups, and ethnic minorities tended to be more worried about becoming a victim of crime and to report feeling less safe than males or younger adults [see Sarma and O'Dwyer, 2004; O'Dwyer et al., 2005; Kennedy and Browne, 2006, 2007; Walker, 2007]. In addition, respondents from urban areas (other than Dublin) also tended to report lower feelings of safety walking alone in their neighborhood after dark than those from more rural locations [see Kennedy and Browne, 2006, 2007].

These figures compare favorably with feelings of safety and fear of crime internationally. However, in two recent international surveys, the Irish public's risk of victimization was judged to be higher than that of most countries surveyed [see Van Dijk et al., 2006; Van Dijk, Van Kesteren, and Smit, 2007]. This suggests that the relationship between the experience of victimization and fear of crime is not straightforward.

Research in Ireland indicates that approximately 6% of respondents aged 18 or more have been victimized in the previous year [see Kennedy and Browne, 2007]. These victims were predominately male and in the 25–44 age category. The majority (84%) were the victim of one crime, with domestic burglary, criminal damage, and physical assault—excluding domestic and/ or sexual assault—being the most common [see Kennedy and Browne, 2007].

Nevertheless, those most at risk of victimization appear to be the least concerned about becoming a victim of crime.

Figures from the Crime and Victimisation Surveys indicate that those most at risk of crime (i.e., young adult males) tend to be the least likely to report a fear of crime. Instead, women and older age groups tend to acknowledge a greater fear of crime than men or respondents from younger age categories [see Watson, 2000; CSO, 2007]. This may be because of the limitations involved in the use of survey research to measure fear of crime and/or reluctance by male respondents to appear "unmanly" by admitting feelings of vulnerability [see Goodey, 1997; Sutton and Farrall, 2005]. However, it is also possible that a fear of crime may reduce an individual's probability of becoming a victim of crime by encouraging individuals to avoid risky situations [see Dubow, McCabe, and Kaplan, 1979; Ferraro, 1995; Boroorah and Carcarch, 1997; Watson, 2000]. As such, it is unclear whether individuals who fear crime experience less victimization as a result of the constrained lifestyles they adopt or whether they are less likely to become a victim of crime regardless of whether they adopt a constrained lifestyle.

Research suggests that being a victim of crime in Ireland is associated with reduced feelings of safety [see CSO, 1999, 2004, 2007; Watson, 2000]. In her research, Watson [2000] found that being a victim of crime can result in a number of physical, financial, and psychological effects. In particular, the experience of victimization can result in increased feelings of anxiety, loss of sleep, difficulty concentrating, and a restriction of activities. Being a victim of crime may also influence an individual's perception of crime as a social problem. According to Watson [2000], victims of crime tend to perceive the level of crime to be greater than the general population, with victims more likely to perceive drug use, teenagers hanging around in the streets, and rubbish and litter to be very common problems. Being a victim of crime may, therefore, not only decrease feelings of safety but also lead to a reduction in quality of life as individuals attempt to restrict their activities to reduce their probability of being victimized.

Fear of crime can also affect quality of life. Quality of life can be both positively and negatively affected by fear of crime [Garofalo, 1981; Ferraro, 1995; Holloway and Jefferson, 1997; Patsios, 1999; Seefelt et al., 2002]. Positive consequences include encouraging individuals to engage in behaviors that attempt to reduce their risk of victimization, increase their resistance to being victimized, and minimize the potential costs of victimization [see DuBow et al., 1979; Garofalo, 1981; Ferraro, 1995]. In contrast, fear of crime may negatively affect quality of life by prompting individuals to severely restrict their activities, potentially reducing their physical, social, and emotional well-being [see Holloway and Jefferson, 1997; Patsios, 1999; Seefelt et al., 2002]. However, the potential impact of fear of crime on quality of life can vary depending on an individual's age, gender, and social circumstances [see Garofalo, 1981; Ferraro, 1995].

16.4 The Present Study: Purpose and Methodology

The purpose of the present research was to investigate the level of fear of crime in Ireland and its impact on quality of life. More specifically, the aims and objectives of this study were to:

- Examine the level of fear of crime in Ireland
- Investigate the factors that influence stated levels of fear
- Assess the reported impact of fear of crime on quality of life
- Identify the factors influencing the effect of fear of crime on quality of life
- Advance recommendations for the development of strategies and/or initiatives aimed at reducing fear of crime and its consequences

The methods used to investigate fear of crime in Ireland and the research findings are presented in the following sections.

16.4.1 Methodology

Secondary data analysis of the 2007 Garda Public Attitudes Survey was conducted to identify the factors predicting fear of crime in Ireland and its impact on quality of life. The raw data for the 2007 Garda Public Attitudes Survey were examined because the Garda Public Attitudes Surveys are con-ducted annually and the 2007 data were the most up-to-date data available.

16.4.1.1 The Statistical Sample

The 2007 Garda Public Attitudes Survey consisted of a nationally represen-tative sample of 10,067 respondents. Respondents were voluntarily recruited across the Republic of Ireland using a random cluster sampling framework. Of these respondents, 4,916 (48.8%) were male and 5,151 (51.2%) were female. Respondents ranged in age from 18 years to more than 65 years and came from a range of both urban and rural locations. Respondents were predominantly of Irish nationality with a working or lower middle socioeconomic status, some form of secondary school education, and who were employed or in further education or training at the time of completing the survey (see Table 16.1).

16.4.1.2 Measurement

Similar to other surveys, fear of crime was measured in the 2007 Garda Public Attitudes Survey by asking respondents whether they were worried about becoming a victim of crime and to rate how safe they felt in their neighbor-hood and at home alone after dark. However, as questions about how safe participants feel in their home or neighborhood after dark have been criticized for exaggerating levels of fear [see Hale, 1996; Farrall et al., 1997; Farrall and

Table 16.1   Garda Public Attitudes Survey 2007 Sample Demographics

Demographics	Number	Percentage
Age group:		
18–24 yrs.	1,402	13.9
25–44 yrs.	4,154	41.3
45–64 yrs.	3,045	30.2
65+ yrs.	1,458	14.5
Unknown	8	0.1
Nationality:		
Irish	9,225	91.6
English/British	286	2.8
Other EU	304	3.0
Non-EU	238	2.4
Unknown	14	0.1
Education:		
No education/primary only	933	
Secondary education	6,157	61.1
Nondegree qualification	842	8.4
Primary degree or higher	2,005	19.9
Unknown	130	1.3
Socioeconomic status:		
Upper middle/middle	805	8.0
Lower middle	3,051	30.3
Skilled working	2,277	22.6
Other working	2,191	21.8
Lowest subsistence level	105	1.0
Farmer >50 acres	554	5.5
Farmer <50 acres	230	2.3
Unknown	855	8.4
Employment status:		
Unemployed/not working	582	5.8
Domestic duties	1,244	12.4
Further education/training	601	6.0
Working part-time	981	9.7
Working full-time	5,298	52.6
Retired	1,267	12.6
Unknown	94	0.9
Locality:		
Dublin city	2,035	20.2
Other city (Cork, Galway, Limerick, Waterford)	935	9.3
Town (10,000–40,000 population)	1,112	11.0
Town (1,000–10,000 population)	1,636	16.3
Village/rural/open country	3,901	38.8
Unknown	448	4.5

Gadd, 2003; Sutton and Farrall, 2005], fear of crime was measured solely on the extent to which respondents reported a fear of becoming a victim of crime.

Respondents were asked "Do you worry that you might become a victim of crime?" to which they responded either "Yes" or "No." If they responded Yes, they were then asked to state which of the following crimes they were worried about: rape, being mugged or robbed, physical attack by a stranger, being pestered or insulted in a public place, being subjected to a racist attack, burglary, car theft, having items stolen from their car, and having their property vandalized.

Respondents were also asked to rate how much their fear of crime affected their quality of life on a 5-point Likert scale ranging from "greatly reduced quality of life" to "no effect on quality of life."

16.4.1.3 Data Analysis

Frequency and percentage tables were used to explore the extent to which respondents reported being worried about becoming a victim of crime, the type of crimes they feared, and the impact of this fear on their quality of life.

Following on from this, a multinomial logistic regression analysis was used to investigate the factors associated with individuals experiencing a fear of crime and the impact of this fear on their quality of life. The extent to which respondents feared crime and its impact on their quality of life was divided into three categories: do not fear crime (63.5%), fear crime but it does not affect quality of life (21.5%), and fear crime to an extent that moderately, significantly, or greatly reduces quality of life (15%). Multinomial regression analysis was used as it is a form of regression analysis that is specifically designed for use with a nominal or ordinal dependent variable that contains more than two categories. In the multinomial regression analysis, the impact of the following factors was explored: demographic information, official burglary crime rates by Garda division,* perceptions of crime in the local area, previous experience of victimization, and satisfaction with An Garda Síochána. The regression results presented in this chapter are based on the final regression model from which all nonsignificant factors have been removed.

16.4.2 Fear of Crime and Its Impact on Quality of Life

Approximately 36.5% of respondents ($n = 3,671$) stated they were worried about becoming a victim of crime. In particular, they were worried about

---

* In 2007, there were 25 different Garda divisions within An Garda Síochána. The official crime rates for a number of different crimes were highly correlated ($r = 0.7$ and above), and, for this reason, only the crime rate for burglary is included in the analysis so as to avoid multicollinearity. The crime rates per 1,000 population were obtained from the CSO [2008].

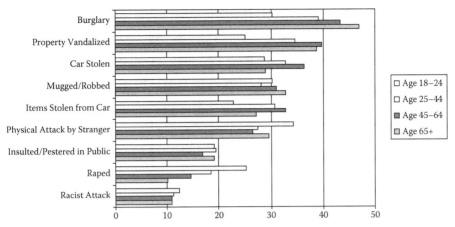

Figure 16.1 Percentage fearing crime by age group and crime type.

burglary (89%), being mugged or robbed (82.3%), having their property van-dalized (82%), being physically attacked by a stranger (78.8%), having their car stolen (74.5%), and having items stolen from their car (71.9%).

These individuals seemed to be less concerned about being pestered or insulted in a public place (52.6%), rape (43.1%), or racist attacks (26.1%). However, these figures may underestimate minority communities' concerns about racist attacks because the majority of respondents were Irish nationals and, as such, are less likely to become victims of a racist attack. Among non-Irish and non-British respondents, 54% feared being the victim of a racist attack.[*]

The age and gender of respondents also appeared to influence the types of crimes they feared because more females were worried about rape (23.8% compared with 4% of males), whereas older respondents were worried about property crime, and younger respondents were worried about violent crime (see Figure 16.1).

This implies that variables such as age and gender may influence the extent to which individuals fear crime in Ireland.

16.4.2.1 Impact on Quality of Life

Of those who feared crime, 70.5% ($n = 2,588$) stated that their fear of crime affected their quality of life. Responses to this question were measured on a 5-point Likert scale ranging from "no effect on quality of life" to "greatly reduced quality of life." These responses were recategorized into two groups consisting of those whose quality of life was moderately, significantly, or greatly reduced by their fear of crime and those whose fear of crime had no effect on their quality of life or reduced their quality of life a little. Among those reporting a fear of crime, 41.1% stated that their fear of crime mod-erately, significantly, or greatly reduced their fear of crime, whereas 55.4%

---

[*] Respondents' ethnicity was not recorded in the 2007 Garda Public Attitudes Survey. Hence nationality is used as a proxy measure of ethnicity.

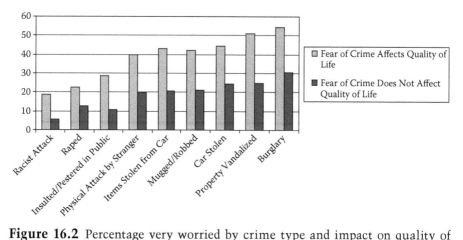

Figure 16.2 Percentage very worried by crime type and impact on quality of life.

felt that their quality of life was not reduced or only reduced a little. The remainder did not know how much their fear of crime affected their quality of life. Accordingly, 63.5% of all respondents did not fear crime, whereas 21.5% feared crime but it did not affect their quality of life, and 15% feared crime that moderately, significantly, or greatly reduced their quality of life.

Among those who reported a reduced quality of life, almost twice as many individuals reported being very worried about several types of crime compared with those whose fear of crime did not affect their quality of life (see Figure 16.2).

In addition, of those who feared crime, fear of crime appeared to have a greater impact on quality of life for females compared with males, with, among those who reported being worried about becoming a victim of crime, 42.4% of females stating that their quality of life was moderately, significantly, or greatly reduced compared with 38.9% of males. Similarly, fear of crime appeared to have a greater impact on quality of life for respondents aged 65 or more than respondents aged 18–24, as 47.6% of those aged 65 or more stated that their quality of life was moderately, significantly, or greatly reduced compared with 34% of those aged 18–24.

As with fear of crime, these findings suggest that variables such as age and gender can influence the extent to which individuals fear crime and its effect on their quality of life.

16.4.3 Factors Predicting Fear of Crime and a Reduced Quality of Life

To identify the factors influencing fear of crime and the impact of this fear on quality of life, a multinomial regression analysis was used. As previously mentioned, respondents were divided into three groups: those who did not fear crime; those who feared crime but it did not affect their quality of life; and those whose fear of crime moderately, significantly, or greatly reduced their quality of life. The reference group for the multinomial logistic regression analysis was those respondents who did not fear of crime. The results presented in this section are based on the final regression model that was found to significantly predict fear of crime ($p < .001$) and had a pseudo r^2 value of 20.2%.

A number of factors were identified as significantly predicting fear of crime and its impact on quality of life, including demographic variables, official burglary crime rates by Garda Division, perceptions of local criminal activity, previous experience of victimization, and satisfaction with An Garda Síochána (see Table 16.2).

A number of factors appeared to increase an individual's probability of experiencing fear of crime, including their gender, age, perceptions of local criminality, history of victimization, and satisfaction with An Garda Síochána. However, there were also a number of factors that seemed to distinguish between those whose fear of crime affected their quality of life and those whose fear of crime did not moderately, significantly, or greatly reduce their quality of life.

16.4.4 Demographic Information

Based on the regression results, a number of demographic factors influenced the extent to which individuals feared crime and the impact of this fear on their quality of life. For example, females and those aged 65 or more were more likely to fear crime compared with males and those aged 25–44 (odds ratio of 1.81 and 1.35, respectively). In contrast, other EU and non-EU nationals were less likely to report a fear of crime compared with Irish nationals while controlling for personal victimization (odds ratio of 0.66 and 0.48, respectively). However, caution may be required in interpreting this result because the small number of other EU and non-EU respondents ($n = 590$) may have biased the result, particularly as the regression results indicate that being the victim of a racist attack is associated with both fearing crime and a reduction in quality of life. Therefore, demographic information, such as age, gender, and nationality, may play an important role in influencing an individual's probability of experiencing a fear of crime and/or a reduced quality of life.

An individual's socioeconomic status and marital status also appeared to influence the extent to which individuals feared crime and the effect of this fear on their quality of life. Individuals from an upper middle/middle socioeconomic status were less likely to state that their quality of life was affected by their fear of crime, whereas other working socioeconomic status respondents were less likely to be in the group whose fear of crime did not affect their quality of life (odds ratio of 0.74 and 0.85, respectively). In addition, those whose socioeconomic status was unknown seemed to be less

Table 16.2   Odds Ratios for Fear of Crime and Impact on Quality of Life

Variable	Fear Crime but Does Not Affect Quality of Life	Fear Crime and Affects Quality of Life
Gender (reference = male)		
Female	1.81[a]	2.39[a]
Age (reference = 25–44 years)		
18–24	0.97	0.66[a]
45–64	1.10	1.06
65+	1.35[b]	1.54[a]
Nationality (reference = Irish)		
British	0.78	0.86
Other EU	0.66[c]	0.89
Non-EU	0.48[a]	1.09
Socioeconomic status (reference = lower middle)		
Upper middle/middle	1.05	0.74[c]
Skilled working	0.93	1.11
Other working	0.85[c]	1.02
Lowest subsistence level	0.66	0.81
Farmer	0.80	0.78
Missing	0.78[c]	0.71[c]
Marital status (reference = married/cohabitating)		
Single	0.86[c]	1.07
Separated/divorced	1.13	1.17
Widowed	0.88	1.41[b]
Education (reference = upper secondary)		
No qualifications/primary only	1.16	1.44[b]
Lower secondary	0.92	1.23[c]
Nondegree qualification	1.20	0.83
Degree or higher	1.18[c]	1.01
Employment status (reference = working full-time)		
Unemployed/not working	1.14	1.33[c]
Domestic duties	1.18	1.19
Further education/training	1.33[c]	1.21
Working part-time	1.26[c]	0.99
Retired	1.05	1.32[c]
Locality (reference = town 10,000–40,000 population)		
Dublin city	0.66[a]	0.90
Other city	1.19	1.29[c]
Town (1,000–10,000 population)	0.73[b]	0.88
Village/countryside	0.91	1.09
Crime rates by Garda division		
Burglary per 1,000 population	0.96[a]	0.98[c]

Table 16.2 (continued)

Variable	Fear Crime but Does Not Affect Quality of Life	Fear Crime and Affects Quality of Life
Perceived change in crime (reference = staying the same/decreasing)		
Increasing	1.53[a]	3.27[a]
Perceive youth crime as problem (reference = no)		
Yes	1.13	1.34[b]
Perceive public nuisance as problem (reference = no)		
Yes	1.07	1.40[a]
Perceive property crime as problem (reference = no)		
Yes	1.24[a]	1.39[a]
Victim of a racist attack (reference = no)		
Yes	2.23[a]	2.95[a]
Recent victim of a crime (reference = no)		
Personal victimization	1.47[a]	2.41[a]
Household victimization	1.52[b]	2.04[a]
Both	1.71	3.46[a]
Satisfaction with Garda visibility (reference = very satisfied/satisfied)		
Dissatisfied/very dissatisfied	1.48[a]	1.72[a]
Garda satisfaction overall (reference = very satisfied/satisfied)		
Dissatisfied/very dissatisfied	1.33[a]	1.88[a]

[a] $p < .001$.
[b] $p < .01$.
[c] $p < .05$.

likely to fear crime (odds ratio of 0.78) or to experience a reduced quality of life (odds ratio of 0.71). Those who were widowed were also more likely to report that their fear of crime affected their quality of life (odds ratio of 1.41), whereas single respondents were less likely to be in the "fear crime but does not affect quality of life" category (odds ratio of 0.86). Accordingly, widowed individuals, regardless of their socioeconomic status, were more likely to report a reduced quality of life, whereas those of an upper-middle or middle socioeconomic status were less likely to state that their fear of crime affected their quality of life.

Similarly, education level and employment status were also associated with fear of crime and a reduced quality of life. Individuals with no formal or primary or a lower secondary education were more likely to report that their quality of life was reduced by their fear of crime (odds ratio of 1.44 and 1.23, respectively). In contrast, those educated to degree level or higher were more likely to report that their quality of life was not affected by their fear of crime (odds ratio of 1.18). Unemployed or not working respondents were also more likely to report that their quality of life was affected by their fear of crime, as were those who were retired (odds ratio of 1.33 and 1.32, respectively). In comparison, those engaged in further education or training and/or working part-time were more likely to fear crime but to state that this fear did not affect their quality of life (odds ratio of 1.33 and 1.26, respectively). Hence unemployed, not working, and retired individuals were more likely to experience a reduced quality of life, whereas those educated to degree level, engaged in further education or training, and working part-time were more likely to fear crime but state that this fear did not affect their quality of life.

Further, the type of area in which the individual resided seemed to affect his or her probability of reporting a fear of crime and/or a reduced quality of life. Individuals living in Dublin city and smaller towns (population between 1,000 and 10,000) appeared to be less likely to fear crime (odds ratio of 0.66 and 0.73, respectively), whereas those living in cities other than Dublin were more likely to report that their fear of crime affected their quality of life (odds ratio of 1.29).

These findings suggest that demographic information, such as age, gender, and socioeconomic status, can be used to identify individuals at risk of experiencing a fear of crime, as well as those whose fear of crime moderately, significantly, or greatly reduced their quality of life.

16.4.5 Crime in Local Area

Official crime rates and perceptions of local criminal activity also influenced fear of crime and its impact on quality of life. The official burglary crime rate per 1,000 population was found to significantly influence both the extent to which individuals feared crime and the effects of this fear on their quality of life (odds ratio of 0.96 and 0.98, respectively). Only the official crime rate for burglary was included in this analysis because the official crime rates for murder, theft, drug offenses, burglary, and assault were highly correlated ($r = 0.7$ or greater). Intriguingly, as burglary crime rates increased, an individuals' probability of experiencing fear of crime slightly decreased, suggesting that living in an area with a high crime rate for burglary may lead to a perceived normalization of crime. Consequently, living in an area with a high crime rate for burglary may lead to a perception that crime is a normal occurrence and, in this way, reduce an individual's fear of crime.

Interestingly, however, the results of the regression analysis suggest that people's perceptions of crime do not necessarily correspond to official crime statistics. Whereas individuals living in an area with a high crime rate for burglary may be less likely to fear crime, individuals who believed that property crime is a problem in their local area, regardless of official crime statistics, were more likely to fear crime and to report a reduced quality of life (odds ratio of 1.24 and 1.39, respectively). Similarly, those who believed that the level of crime in their locality had increased were more likely to fear crime and to report that this fear affected their quality of life (odds ratio of 1.53 and 3.27, respectively). Consequently, an individual's perception that crime had increased in their locality, as well as their perception that property crime was a problem in their local area, increased their probability of developing a fear of crime and experiencing a reduced quality of life even while controlling for official crime statistics.

In addition, perceptions of local youth crime and public nuisance appeared to differ between those whose fear of crime did not affect their quality of life and those whose quality of life was reduced by their fear of crime. Individuals believing that youth crime and public nuisance were a problem where they lived were more likely to report that their fear of crime affected their quality of life than those who did not (odds ratio of 1.34 and 1.40, respectively).

These findings indicate that perceptions of crime in one's local area, as well as official crime rates, can influence fear of crime and its impact on quality of life. However, it is difficult to determine whether perceptions of crime as a problem in one's locality cause fear of crime or whether individuals who are afraid of crime pay more attention to potential criminal activities in their area than those who do not fear crime.

16.4.6 Experience of Victimization

Another factor found to significantly predict the extent to which individuals feared crime and the impact of this fear on their quality of life was their previous experience of victimization.

Individuals who had been the victim of a crime in the past year were more likely to fear crime and were especially at risk of reporting a reduced quality of life (odds ratio of 1.47 and 2.41, respectively). Similarly, individuals stating that a member of their household had been victimized were also more likely to fear crime and to state that this fear had affected their quality of life (odds ratio of 1.52 and 2.04, respectively). However, individuals who had previous experience of both personal victimization and household victimization were almost 3.5 times more likely to report that their fear of crime moderately, significantly or greatly reduced their quality of life (odds ratio of 3.46). Further, individuals who had been the victim of a racist attack were also more likely to fear crime and to report that their quality of life was affected by this fear (odds ratio of 2.23 and 2.95, respectively).

Therefore, previous experience of a racist incident, personal victimization, household victimization, and/or both personal victimization and household victimization are associated with individuals experiencing a fear of crime and a reduced quality of life.

16.4.7 Satisfaction with An Garda Síochána

Last, respondents' level of satisfaction with An Garda Síochána was also found to significantly predict whether they feared crime and the effect of this fear on their quality of life.

Compared with those who were satisfied or very satisfied with the level of visibility provided by An Garda Síochána, individuals who were dissatisfied or very dissatisfied were more likely to fear crime and to state that this fear reduced their quality of life (odds ratio of 1.48 and 1.72, respectively). Similarly, those who were dissatisfied or very dissatisfied with the overall performance of An Garda Síochána were more likely to fear crime and to report that this fear of crime affected their quality of life compared with those who were satisfied or very satisfied with the overall performance of An Garda Síochána (odds ratio of 1.33 and 1.88, respectively).

Accordingly, feelings of satisfaction with Garda visibility and performance are associated with a lower probability of experiencing a fear of crime, whereas feelings of dissatisfaction are associated with a higher probability of experiencing a fear of crime and a reduced quality of life. However, as before, the causal relationship between satisfaction with An Garda Síochána and fear of crime remains unclear because individuals who are afraid of crime may pay more attention to policing issues than those who are not afraid of crime.

Therefore, it appears that females, individuals aged 65 or more, victims of crime and racist attacks, those dissatisfied with An Garda Síochána, and individuals perceiving property crime to be a problem in their area are more likely to experience a fear of crime and reduced quality of life. In addition, the results indicate that widows and widowers, and individuals with no formal or primary or a lower secondary-level education, are especially at risk of having their quality of life affected by their fear of crime, as are those who are unemployed or not working, retired, and living in a city other than Dublin. Individuals who perceive youth crime and public nuisance to be a problem in their locality are also more likely to report a reduced quality of life than those who do not. In contrast, individuals living in an area with a higher official crime rate for burglary, Dublin city, and/or smaller towns were less likely to fear crime, whereas upper-middle or middle socioeconomic status individuals and those with a degree or higher qualification were less likely to report that their quality of life was affected by their fear of crime.

16.5 Discussion

Although international research suggests that there are a number of factors associated with individuals experiencing a fear of crime, the exact origins of this fear remain unknown. Some researchers suggest that a fear of crime can arise as vulnerable groups project their fears about wider, more difficult to control issues onto crime because crime appears actionable and controllable [see Hollway and Jefferson, 1997]. Others argue that it is the experience of victimization and an individual's perceived risk of being victimized that result in a fear of crime [Box et al., 1988; LaGrange et al., 1992; Ferraro, 1995]. The purpose of this chapter was to examine the factors associated with fear of crime and a reduction in quality of life and to identify the possible origins and consequences of fear of crime in Ireland.

Based on the regression results, whether individuals reported a fear of crime and a reduced quality of life appeared to depend on three underlying processes: previous experience of victimization, feelings of personal vulnerability, and a normalization of crime. These processes are explored further in the following sections.

16.5.1 Previous Experience of Victimization

As in other countries [see Skogan, 1987; Box et al., 1988], a history of victimization was associated with individuals reporting a fear of crime in Ireland such that individuals with a previous experience of victimization are more likely to fear crime than those who have not been victimized. Unlike those who suggest that the relationship between victimization and fear of crime is not straightforward [see Agnew, 1985; Winkel, 1998], the experience of victimization in Ireland appears to be directly related to individuals reporting a fear of crime and a reduced quality of life. In particular, individuals who have experienced both personal victimization and household victimization are almost 3.5 times more likely to report that their quality of life has been moderately, significantly, or greatly reduced by their fear of crime. In addition, victims of a racist attack are also more likely to be afraid of crime and for this fear to affect their quality of life. This suggests that individuals who have experienced victimization are especially at risk of developing a fear of crime and for this fear to reduce their quality of life.

This finding corresponds to previous research in Ireland that found that being a victim of crime is associated with reduced feelings of safety and may also lead to a reduction in quality of life [see CSO, 1999, 2004, 2007; Watson, 2000]. In particular, there are a number of physical, financial, and psychological costs associated with victimization in Ireland [see Watson, 2000], which, if ameliorated, may mitigate the effects of victimization on fear of crime and quality of life. This implies that if the experience of victimization could be reduced and/or the negative costs of victimization lessened, an individual's probability of fearing crime and it negatively affecting their quality of life may also be reduced.

16.5.1.1 Personal Vulnerability

Individuals' feelings of personal vulnerability also appeared to influence their fear of crime and the effect of this fear on their quality of life. Similar to other countries, age, gender, socioeconomic status, education, and employment status were found to influence fear of crime and its impact on quality of life [see Box et al., 1988; Hale, 1996; Mirrlees-Black and Allen, 1998; Stafford et al., 2007]. In particular, females and those aged 65 or more were more likely to fear crime and to report a reduced quality of life than males and those aged 24–45.

Numerous international studies have found that older adults tend to report a greater fear of crime than younger age groups despite being at a lesser risk of victimization [Clemente and Kleiman, 1976; Box et al., 1988; Hale, 1996]. This has become known as the fear/risk paradox and has led some researchers to question the "rationality" of this fear, implying that fear of crime is more of a "problem" for older adults than crime itself [Clemente and Kleiman, 1976; Jaycox, 1978; Lindquist and Duke, 1982]. However, older adults may be more likely to fear crime because the potential physical, psychological, and economic consequences associated with crime may be more serious for older adults than younger adults. Similarly, individuals aged 18–24 may be less likely to report that their quality of life is affected by their fear of crime as a result of a sense of invulnerability frequently associated with youth [see Elkind, 1967] and/or because the consequences of crime may be less serious for younger people. For example, younger people may have fewer material possessions (e.g., such as a house, car) that can be damaged or stolen, and they may also be less concerned about their ability to deal with criminal situations because of their youth, agility, and sense of invulnerability. This suggests that older adults may be more likely to fear crime and for this fear to reduce their quality of life because of concerns about their physical, financial, and psychological ability to cope with offenders and/or the experience of victimization.

Females and widowed individuals were also more likely to fear crime and to experience a reduction in their quality of life. Females may be more likely to fear crime and experience a reduced quality of life as a result of feelings of personal vulnerability heightened by concerns about being sexually assaulted and/or abused by a loved one [see Warr, 1984; Killias, 1990; Ferraro, 1995; Stanko, 1997]. These concerns are believed to heighten females' fears about other types of crimes by decreasing feelings of safety [Ferraro, 1995; Stanko, 1997]. Widowed individuals are also more likely than married or cohabiting individuals to report that their quality of life is affected by their fear of crime. This may be because of feelings of vulnerability arising from feelings of loneliness and/or a limited support network. However, individuals may also experience feelings of personal vulnerability as a result of their ability to cope with the financial costs of victimization.

In particular, individuals with no formal or primary education or lower secondary education and individuals who are unemployed, not working, or retired may feel especially vulnerable to the effects of victimization. These individuals may experience a reduced quality of life because victimization may have a greater impact on their quality of life than others, particularly if they are unable to financially cope with the costs and/or repercussions associated with being a victim of crime. In contrast, upper-middle and middle socioeconomic status respondents may be less likely to report a reduced quality of life because the consequences of crime may be lessened for these individuals by insurance, crime prevention measures, and/or their ability to financially cope with the costs associated with victimization. Individuals educated to degree level or higher, working part-time, or in further education or training were also more likely to fear crime but to report that this fear did not affect their quality of life. This may be because of the limited resources available to them to replace stolen or damaged possessions, which may mean that, although they fear crime, this fear does not affect their quality of life. Accordingly, further research is needed to clarify how feelings of personal vulnerability may increase fear of crime and the effect of this fear of quality of life.

Individuals can also feel vulnerable if they feel "at risk." Furedi [2002] suggests that, because of a growth in media technologies, there is now a greater awareness of crime among the public, as well as a greater sense of being "at risk." For example, although individuals aged 65 or more are less likely to be victimized, media coverage of stories in which older adults are physically attacked may increase their perceptions of being at risk and, in this way, increase their fear of crime. In this research, perceptions of crime as increasing in one's local area were related to an individual fearing crime and this fear reducing their quality of life. Perceptions of property crime, youth crime, and public nuisance as a problem in one's locality were also related to individuals experiencing a reduced quality of life because of their fear of crime. This implies that perceptions of crime as a problem in one's locality can lead individuals to feel "at risk." Similarly, dissatisfaction with Garda performance and visibility may also lead individuals to feel "at risk." However, as previously stated, the causal relationship between these perceptions and fear of crime remains unclear because individuals who fear crime may be more attentive to policing and crime issues than those who do not fear crime. Accordingly, by addressing feelings of risk and vulnerability, it may be possible to lessen the impact of fear of crime on quality of life.

It has also been argued that the growth in media technologies has not only contributed to a greater awareness of being at risk of crime but also more generalized feelings of unease and uncertainty as people become aware of their risk of ill health, unemployment, financial instability, and family instability [see Beck, 1992; Furedi, 2002; Lyng, 2005]. This has led some researchers to suggest that individuals may project their fears about wider more difficult to control issues onto crime because crime appears actionable and potentially controllable [see Holloway and Jefferson, 1997]. This implies that some individuals may experience a fear of crime that appears to be disproportionate to their environment, previous experience of victimization, and/or probability of being victimized but which is related to their wider fears and anxieties. Therefore, a greater awareness of how an individual's fear of crime may be related to wider feelings of anxiety and/or vulnerability may be required when attempting to lessen an individual's fear of crime and its impact on quality of life.

16.5.1.2 Normalization of Crime

Interestingly, the relationship between official crime rates and fear of crime appeared to be somewhat more complex. As official crime rates for burglary increased, an individual's probability of experiencing a fear of crime decreased slightly. In addition, their probability of experiencing a reduced quality of life also decreased slightly as burglary crime rates increased. This suggests that individuals living in an area in which burglary is more prevalent may be more likely to perceive burglary and crime as a normal occurrence and, as a result, be less fearful. However, as the experience of victimization is associated with an increased probability of fearing crime and experiencing a reduced quality of life, living in a high-crime area may lead to normalization of crime, if the individual or his or her household has not been victimized. These findings indicate that although living in an area with a high crime rate for burglary may lead to normalization of crime for those who have not yet been victimized, fear of crime and its impact on quality of life may be increased for those who have been victimized.

Differences were also observed between those whose quality of life was affected by their fear of crime and those whose quality of life was not affected based on their location. Individuals residing in a city other than Dublin were more likely to experience a reduced quality of life. This corresponds to findings from the Garda Public Attitudes Surveys, which found that respondents from urban areas (other than Dublin) tend to report feeling less safe walking around their neighborhood after dark [see Kennedy and Browne, 2006, 2007]. In particular, residents of urban areas are believed to experience a fear of crime because of lower feelings of safety arising from a transient population and low community cohesion [see Skogan, 1986, 1990; Ferraro, 1995]. Although this may explain why individuals living in cities other than Dublin may experience a reduced quality of life, it does not explain why residents of Dublin city are not equally affected. Based on the regression results, residents of Dublin city and smaller towns are less likely to fear crime. In the case of smaller towns, community cohesion may be higher, increasing feelings of safety. With regard to Dublin, it is possible that the high rates of criminal activity observed in the city [see CSO, 2008] may lead to a perceived normalization of crime for those who have not been victimized. It is also possible that the wide range of services available in Dublin may mitigate some concerns regarding victimization and/or feelings of personal vulnerability. However, further research is required to identify why residents of smaller towns and Dublin city may be less likely to fear crime but residents of cities other than Dublin are more likely to experience a reduced quality of life.

16.5.1.3 Reducing Fear of Crime and Its Impact on Quality of Life

Based on these findings, a number of recommendations for strategies and/or initiatives aimed at reducing fear of crime and its impact on quality of life can be made. These include reducing victimization, improving services for victims of crime, providing supports for vulnerable and/or disadvantaged groups, and addressing local perceptions of crime and policing. There are also a number of areas worthy of further investigation to examine how some individuals come to experience a greater reduction in their quality of life than others.

16.5.2 Reducing Victimization

Because victimization is related to fear of crime and a reduction in quality of life, reducing victimization should reduce fear of crime and its impact on quality of life. Measures to reduce victimization may include reducing crime levels, reducing the opportunities for criminal activity to occur, and empowering individuals so that they are aware of the techniques they can use to reduce their probability of being victimized, as well as what they should do if victimized. Providing individuals with information about crime prevention measures, information on techniques to design out opportunities for crime, as well as providing information on crime hotspots and the types of crime individuals may be likely to experience can assist in reducing victimization. However, unless the underlying causes of criminal behavior are addressed, these measures are unlikely to substantially reduce crime and, consequently, victimization. Therefore, it is the provision of services to those who have been victimized that may play a central role in ameliorating fear of crime and its effect on quality of life.

16.5.3 Provision of Services to Victims

Because victims of crime are more likely to fear crime and experience a reduced quality of life, adequate support services are required to mitigate the effects (physical, financial, emotional, and psychological) of this experience on their quality of life. Particular attention should be paid to those victims who have had both a personal experience of victimization and whose household has been victimized because these individuals, as well as victims of racist attacks, are especially at risk of experiencing a reduced quality of life. When reporting a crime, individuals who have been victimized should receive information about local services available to them to assist them with the physical, financial, and psychological consequences of victimization. However, as victims of crime may not always report their victimization to the police, community and voluntary organizations should also be able to provide individuals with information about local services available to assist them, where required, in dealing with the effects of victimization.

16.5.3.1 Supports for Vulnerable Individuals

The results of this analysis also demonstrate that fear of crime, as well as its impact on quality of life, is not evenly distributed throughout society. Therefore, support services should be targeted at vulnerable groups who are most at risk of experiencing a reduced quality of life.

The regression results reveal that vulnerable groups, such as widows and widowers, those aged 65 or more, retired individuals, those who are unemployed or not working, and those with no formal, primary, or lower secondary level education are more likely to have their quality of life affected by their fear of crime. This suggests that interventions should be focused on specific groups, such as elderly persons, widows and widowers, retired individuals, and those experiencing educational and economic disadvantage, if the effects of fear of crime on quality of life are to be reduced. In particular, community and voluntary groups may assist in reducing fear of crime and its impact on quality of life by informally engaging with individuals to reduce their feelings of vulnerability. Because feelings of vulnerability may also be related to wider anxieties, individuals dealing with these vulnerable groups may need to be aware of how wider anxieties can impact on fear of crime and, consequently, quality of life.

It is also worth noting that the higher levels of fear of crime and reduced quality of life experienced by these groups may be the result of their more vulnerable position within society. Accordingly, more general measures toward increasing social inclusion may reduce fear of crime and its effect on quality of life.

16.5.4 Perceptions of Local Crime and Policing

Another method of influencing individuals' fear of crime and their quality of life is to examine their perceptions of crime and policing. Although it is unclear whether these perceptions cause fear of crime or fear of crime causes these perceptions, it may nonetheless be possible to influence fear of crime and its effect on quality of life by engaging with, and addressing, local communities' concerns about crime and/or policing.

Because dissatisfaction with the overall performance and level of visibility provided by An Garda Síochána was associated with fear of crime and a reduction in quality of life, improving satisfaction levels may decrease fear of crime and its impact on quality of life. In Ireland, the use of community policing and joint policing committees can play an important role in this regard. Through their involvement in these activities, An Garda Síochána attempt to address local communities' concerns about criminal activity and endeavor to tailor their response to crime to the needs of the local community [An Garda Síochána, 2007]. Therefore, the use of joint policing committees and community policing to engage with the community can provide a means by which feelings of dissatisfaction can be addressed, as well as local perceptions of crime.

The media also have a role to play in influencing the public's perception of crime and, consequently, their fear of crime and its impact on quality of life. By being aware that perceptions of crime can increase fear of crime and its effect on quality of life, the media should endeavor to ensure that stories of crime accurately reflect the nature and extent of their true occurrence. By highlighting potentially problematic criminal activities, media stories can encourage individuals to engage in precautionary measures but may also inflate fear of crime levels if they do not accurately portray the true prevalence of these activities [see Brown, 2007, 2008; Coulter, 2008]. In this way, responsible journalism can inform and encourage individuals to engage in crime prevention measures without unnecessarily inflating fear of crime and affecting quality of life.

16.5.5 Further Research

The results of this analysis also indicate that there are a number of areas worthy of further investigation to broaden our understanding of fear of crime and its impact on quality of life. For example, further research could be used to clarify the relationship between gender, locality, and fear of crime to identify how females come to be more likely to fear crime, whereas residents living in Dublin city and smaller towns are less likely to fear crime. Similarly, further research could be used to examine why older adults are more likely to fear crime despite their lower risk of victimization. In particular, the effect of perceived vulnerability and the normalization of crime should be examined to explore how, and in what circumstances, these processes influence fear of crime and its impact on quality of life.

In conclusion, although this research revealed that, as in other countries, some segments of the population are more at risk of experiencing a fear of crime and reduced quality of life than others, further research is needed to clarify why this is so.

References

Agnew, R. S. 1985. Neutralizing the impact of crime. *Criminal Justice and Behavior* 12(2):221–39.

Beck, U. 1992. *The risk society*. London: Sage.

Borooah, V. K. and C. A. Carcach. 1997. Crime and fear: Evidence from Australia. *The British Journal of Criminology* 37(4):635–57.

Box, S., C. Hale, and G. Andrews. 1988. Explaining the fear of crime. *British Journal of Criminology* 28(3):340–56.

Brown, V. 2007. RTE going over the top on crime. *Irish Times*, November 7.

_____. 2008. Sensationalist coverage is a crime in itself. *Sunday Business Post*, February 24.

Carrach, C. and S. Mukherjee. 1999. Women's fear of violence in the community. In *Trends and issues in crime and criminal justice*, ed. A. Graycar. Canberra: Australian Institute of Criminology.

Central Statistics Office. 1999. *Quarterly national household survey, crime and victimisation: September–November 1998*. Dublin: The Stationery Office.

_____. 2004. *Quarterly national household survey, crime and victimisation: September–Quarter 4, 1998 and 2003*. Dublin: The Stationery Office.

_____. 2007. *Crime and victimisation: Quarterly national household survey 2006*. Dublin: The Stationery Office.

_____. 2008. *Garda recorded crime statistics 2003–2006*. Dublin: The Stationery Office.

Chadee, D. and J. Ditton. 2003. Are older people most afraid of crime? Revisiting Ferraro and LaGrange in Trinidad. *British Journal of Criminology* 43(3): 417–33.

Charleton, P. 1995. Drugs and crime—making the connection: A discussion paper. *Irish Criminal Law Journal* 5(2):220–40.

Clemente, F. and M. Kleiman. 1976. Fear of crime among the aged. *Gerontologist* 16:207–10.

Coulter, C. 2008a. The media and criminal justice policy-making. Paper presented at the North-South Criminology Conference, Dublin.

Coulter, C. 2008b. Media must act to ensure crime reporting is fair and balanced. *The Irish Times*, July 7.

Dean, G., A. O'Hare, A. O'Connor, M. Kelly, and G. Kelly. 1985. The opiate epidemic in Dublin 1979–83: Are we over the worst? *Irish Medical Journal* 80(5):139–42.

DuBow, F., E. McCabe, and G. Kaplan. 1979. *Reactions to crime: A critical review of the literature*. Washington, DC: U.S. Department of Justice, Law Enforcement Assistance Administration.

Elkind, D. 1967. Egocentrism in adolescence. *Child Development* 38:1025–34.

Emsley, C. 1987. *Crime and society in England, 1750–1900*. New York: Longman.

Ewald, U. 2000. Criminal victimisation and social adaptation in modernity. In *Crime, risk and insecurity*, ed. T. Hope and R. Sparks. London: Routledge.

Farrall, S., J. Bannister, J. Ditton, and E. Gilchrist. 1997. Questioning the measurement of the "fear of crime": Findings from a major methodological study. *British Journal of Criminology* 37(4):658–79.

Farrall, S. and D. Gadd. 2003. Fear today, gone tomorrow: Do surveys overstate fear levels? http://www.istat.it/istat/eventi/perunasocieta/relazioni/Farral_abs.pdf (accessed May 9, 2008).

Ferraro, K. 1995. *Fear of crime: Interpreting victimization risk*. Albany: State University of New York Press.

Furedi, F. 2002. *Culture of fear*. London: Continuum.

Gabriel, U. and W. Greve. 2003. The psychology of fear of crime: Conceptual and methodological perspectives. *British Journal of Criminology* 43(3):600–14.

Garda Research Unit. 2002. *Garda public attitudes survey 2002*. Templemore, Ireland: Garda Research Unit.

Garofalo, J. 1981. The fear of crime: Causes and consequences. *The Journal of Criminal Law and Criminology* 72(2):839–57.

Goodey, J. 1997. Boys don't cry: Masculinities, fear of crime and fearlessness. *British Journal of Criminology* 36:401–71.

Hale, C. 1996. Fear of crime: A review of the literature. *International Review of Victimology* 4:79–150.

Heath, L. and J. Petraitis. 1987. Television viewing and fear of crime: Where is the mean world? In *The fear of crime*, ed. S. J. Ditton and S. Farrall. Aldershot, UK: Ashgate Dartmouth.

Hollway, W. and T. Jefferson. 1997. The risk society in an age of anxiety: Situating fear of crime. *The British Journal of Sociology* 48(2):255–66.

Hough, M. 1995. *Anxiety about crime: Findings from the 1994 British Crime Survey*. London: Home Office Research and Statistics Directorate.

Jaycox, V. 1978. The elderly's fear of crime: Rational or irrational. *Victimology* 3:329–34.

John Howard Society of Alberta. 1999. *Fear of crime*. Alberta, Canada: John Howard Society of Alberta.

Kennedy, P. and C. Browne. 2006. *Garda public attitudes survey 2006*. Templemore, Ireland: Garda Research Unit.

_____. 2007. *Garda public attitudes survey 2007*. Templemore, Ireland: Garda Research Unit.

Kerrigan, G. and H. Shaw. 1985. Crime hysteria. *Magill*, April 18.

Kilcommins, S., I. O'Donnell, E. O'Sullivan, and B. Vaughan. 2004. *Crime, punishment and the search for order in Ireland*. Dublin: Institute of Public Administration.

Killias, M. 1990. Vulnerability: Towards a better understanding of a key variable in the genesis of fear of crime. *Violence and Victims* 5(2):97–108.

LaGrange, R. L., K. F. Ferraro, and M. Supancic. 1992. Perceived risk and fear of crime: Role of social and physical incivilities. *Journal of Research in Crime and Delinquency* 29:311–34.

Laver, M., P. Mair, and R. Sinnott. 1987. *How Ireland voted: The Irish general election of 1987*. Dublin: Poolbeg.

Lee, M. 2007. *Inventing fear of crime: Criminology and the politics of anxiety*. Cullompton, UK: Willan.

Lindquist, J. H. and J. M. Duke. 1982. The elderly victim at risk: Explaining the fear-victimization paradox. *Criminology* 20:115–26.

Lyder, A. 2005. *Pusher's out: The inside story of Dublin's anti-drug movement*. Bloomington, IN: Trafford.

Lyng, S. 2005. *Edgework: The sociology of risk-taking*. London: Routledge.

Maxfield, M. G. 1984. *Fear of crime in England and Wales*. London: Her Majesty's Stationery Office.

McCullagh, C. 1996. *Crime in Ireland: A sociological introduction*. Cork: Cork University Press.

_____. 1999. Rural crime in the republic of Ireland. In *Crime and conflict in the countryside*, ed. G. Dingwall and S. R. Moody. Cardiff: University of Wales Press.

Mirrlees-Black, C. and J. Allen. 1998. *Concern about crime: Findings from the 1998 British crime survey*. Research findings no. 83. London: Home Office Research Development and Statistics Directorate.

O'Connell, M. 1999. Is Irish public opinion towards crime distorted by media bias? *European Journal of Communication* 14:191–212.

_____. 2002. The portrayal of crime in the media—Does it matter? In *Criminal justice in Ireland*, ed. P. O'Mahony. Dublin: Institute of Public Administration.

O'Connell, M. and A. Whelan. 1996. The public perception of crime prevalence, newspaper readership and "Mean World" attitudes. *Legal and Criminological Psychology* 3:29–57.

O'Donnell, I. 2007. Crime and its consequences. In *Best of times? The social impact of the Celtic tiger*, ed. T. Fahey, H. Russell and C. T. Whelan. Dublin: Institute of Public Administration.

O'Donnell, I. and E. O'Sullivan. 2003. The politics of intolerance—Irish style. *British Journal of Criminology* 43(3):253–66.

O'Dwyer, K., P. Kennedy, and W. Ryan. 2005. *Garda public attitudes survey 2005*. Templemore, Ireland: Garda Research Unit.

O'Mahony, P. 1993. *Crime and punishment in Ireland*. Dublin: Round Hall.

O'Mahony, P. and T. Guilmore. 1983. *Drug abusers in the Dublin committal prisons: A survey*. Dublin: The Stationery Office.

Patsios, D. 1999. Poverty and social exclusion amongst the elderly. *Working paper 20, Poverty and social exclusion survey of Britain, 1999*. Bristol, UK: Townsend Centre of International Poverty Research, University of Bristol.

Sarma, K. 2003. *Garda public attitudes survey 2003*. Templemore, Ireland: Garda Research Unit.

Sarma, K. and K. O'Dwyer. 2004. *Garda public attitudes survey 2004*. Templemore, Ireland: Garda Research Unit.

Seefelt, V., R. M. Malina, and M. A. Clark. 2002. Factors affecting levels of physical activity in adults. *Sports Medicine* 32:143–68.

Skogan, W.G. 1986. The fear of crime and its behavioural implications. In *From crime policy to victim policy*, ed. E. A. Fattah. London: Macmillan.

_____. 1987. The impact of victimization on fear. *Crime & Delinquency* 33:135–54.

_____. 1990. *Disorder and decline: Crime and the spiral of decay in American neighbourhoods*. New York: Free.

Skogan, W. G. and M. G. Maxfield. 1981. *Coping with crime: Individual and neighborhood reactions*. Beverly Hills, CA: Sage.

Stafford, M., T. Chandola, and M. Marmot. 2007. Association between fear of crime and mental health and physical functioning. *American Journal of Public Health* 97(11):2076–81.

Stanko, E. A. 1997. Safety talk: Conceptualising women's risk assessment as a technology of the soul. *Theoretical Criminology* 1:53–76.

Sutton, R. M. and S. Farrall. 2005. Gender, socially desirable responding and the fear of crime: Are women really more anxious about crime. *British Journal of Criminology* 2:212–24.

Taylor, I. 1996. Fear of crime, urban fortunes and suburban social movements: Some reflections on Manchester. *Sociology* 30:317–37.

Tulloch, J. and D. Lupton. 2003. *Risk and everyday life.* London: Sage.

Van Dijk, J., R. Manchin, J. Van Kesteren, S. Nevala, and G. Hideg. 2006. The burden of crime in the EU. *Research report: A comparative analysis of the European crime and safety survey (EU ICS) 2005.* Brussels: EUICS Consortium.

Van Dijk, J., J. Van Kesteren, and P. Smit. 2007. *Criminal victimisation in International perspective: Key findings from the 2004–2005 ICVS and EU ISC.* The Hague: WODC.

Walker, M. 2007. *Travellers/ethnic minority communities' attitudes towards an Garda Síochána.* Templemore, Ireland: Garda Research Unit.

Walklate, S. and G. Mythen. 2008. How scared are we? *British Journal of Criminology* 48(2):209–25.

Warr, M. 1984. Fear of victimization: Why are women and the elderly more afraid? *Social Science Quarterly* 65(3):681–702.

Warr, M. and N. Stafford. 1983. Fear of victimization: A look at the proximate causes. *Social Forces* 61:1033–43.

Watson, D. 2000. *Victims of recorded crime in Ireland: Results from the 1996 survey.* Dublin: Oak Tree.

Wilson, J. Q. 1968. The urban unease: Community vs. city. *The Public Interest* 12:25–39.

Wilson, J. Q. and G. Kelling. 1985. Broken windows: The police and neighborhood safety. In *The ambivalent force*, ed. A. Blumberg and E. Niederhoffer. New York: Holt, Rinehart and Winston.

Winkel, F. W. 1998. Fear of crime and criminal victimisation: Testing a theory of psychological incapacitation of the 'Stressor' based on downward comparison processes. *British Journal of Criminology* 38(3):473–84.

Restorative Justice

V

When Prisoners Leave
Victim–Offender Relationships in a Transitions Context

17

ROB WHITE

Contents

17.1 Introduction

The aim of this chapter is to consider broad questions regarding prisoner transitions from prison to community, as well as victims' rights in the course of these transitions. The three main themes of the chapter are:

- That we have to live with those we punish (so how do, or should, we prepare prisoners for release back into the community?)

- That we have to support those who have been harmed by crime (so how do, or should, we involve victims in the criminal justice system?)
- That victims and offenders have different rights, needs, and responsibilities (so how do, or should, these interact in relation to specific issues, such as release and the conditions of release?)

The chapter is intended to clarify issues and to stimulate informed discussion of issues relating to victim–offender relations.

The original impetus for this discussion was periodic media stories that tended to present a negative account of prisoner leave programs in Tasmania, Australia. On several occasions, prisoners who were on day release or on short-term release had chanced on former victims on the street or received publicity from the local newspaper for being out and about in the community. The press and electronic media tended to sensationalize these events, usually from the point of view of how awful it is for victims to unexpectedly run into offenders who had harmed them or their families. In one example, a female prisoner who was serving time for murder was photographed in a video shop, selecting videos to take back for viewing with her fellow inmates at the prison.

This kind of media coverage is damaging in at least two different ways. First, it tends to undermine the idea of community-based release programs for prisoners. As will be seen, such programs are essential if a smooth transition from prison to community is to be possible. Second, the coverage tends to stir up raw emotions and vindictive feelings among direct victims, secondary victims, and the general public. It makes victims feel badly; it makes them feel angry; and it makes them feel afraid. Except for calls to lock up prisoners until their sentence is served, there is nothing positive—for victims, or for offenders—to improve the existing situation. Some victims are retraumatized, as the media explicitly recount over and over again the harms they had suffered. Their subjective state is harnessed to the agenda of the tabloid presenter, their pain used instrumentally to sell television programs and newspapers. It is a lose–lose situation for victim and offender alike.

However, victim concerns and interests are important to the success of transition schemes. How and why this is the case are the substantive concern of this chapter.

17.2 Release Programs: Living with Those We Punish

The importance of bringing offenders back into the discussion of victims (in the same way that we need to make sure that victims are never omitted from discussions concerning offenders) is that offenders who are prosecuted and convicted are more often than not likely to reoffend. Especially for offenders who have served time in prison, the odds are that they will victimize someone at some stage after their release. In other words, one of the biggest predictors of recidivism is imprisonment itself. This is because of a number of reasons, including preprison factors (such as poor literacy, unemployment, and mental illness) and factors stemming from incarceration itself (such as the influence of criminal culture in prison and the stigma associated with having served time in prison). Finding work and employment postrelease is difficult in the best of times. For many, the solution resides in going back to the familiar: crime and reliance on illegal means to make a living.

Thus, prevention of reoffending is simultaneously prevention of victimization. Analysis of how we might actually achieve this suggests novel ways in which to engage prisoners in a victim–offender relationship. This section provides an overview of interventions related to offenders, particularly early release options and community-based programs.

17.2.1 Offender Re-entry

Integrating offenders into mainstream society is a huge task, one that ultimately requires a communal commitment. Victims, too, are important to this task.

> The successful re-entry of offenders into the community is neither a linear process nor one that can be accomplished by a single agency. It requires collaboration and commitment from literally anyone concerned about public safety, as well as commitment to ensuring that victims' rights are consistently enforced and victim services are consistently provided. It requires communities—including crime victims—to be open to, and involved in, partnerships that provide a wide range of opportunities for offenders to return to the community as focal members who, given the chance, can be held accountable for their actions, as well as be monitored and provided with supportive services to reduce their chance of recidivism, to become productive and responsible members of society. [Seymour, 2001:2]

For the present purposes, our concern is not with release from prison as such. Rather, the focus is on early release, which provides the best chance to guide the process of offender integration and/or reintegration. There are various conditions of release, among them:

- Temporary absence—for special purposes, such as family, work, sport, and education
- Transitional release—probation and parole
- Alternatives to prison—special types of release

In institutional or operational terms, the movement away from prison involves varying forms of release and decarceration. These are summarized in Figure 17.1.

Parole—This is where an offender serving time in detention can serve part of the sentence in the community under the supervision of parole officers and under certain restrictive behavior conditions.

Day-leave schemes—This is where the prisoner is allowed to take advantage of educational or work-related activities while still serving a sentence in some type of secure custody.

Conditional release order—Where certain prisoners deemed amenable to, and who would benefit from, a community-based program, especially educational and vocational programs, are granted leave to live in the general community under close supervision and with appropriate counseling.

Camps—Where the offender is placed in a wilderness or boot camp of some kind, with the proviso that they are expected to learn self-discipline, be rehabilitated and subjected to a rigorous schedule of activities. There are specialized camps for specific categories of offender (e.g., young people and/or indigenous people), as well as postrelease camps that attempt to develop offender skills, knowledge, and confidence after they have served their sentence.

Home detention—This can take several forms, involving in some cases electronic tracking devices or, in other cases, unpredictable phone or in-person checks from the appropriate correctional authority. The offender is restricted in movement and is, in effect, a prisoner at home, rather than in a secure, mass correctional facility.

Periodic detention—This allows a sentenced prisoner to be at liberty in the community on a defined basis. Prisoners are held in custody on a part-time basis only, usually consisting of two consecutive days in a 1-week period (such as the weekend).

Figure 17.1 Types of release and decarceration.

There are then different kinds of release available to inmates, some of which are tied to temporary absence (e.g., for funerals of family members) and others which constitute transitions toward reintegration back into the community (e.g., structured prerelease programs). Access to different forms of early release varies across state and international jurisdictions.

For example, in Queensland, the use of a *halfway house* was initiated in the early 1990s as one possible way of dealing with increasing prison populations. The idea behind such facilities is provision of a quasi-normal community setting that recognizes the varying risk levels that inmates present to the community, and that contribute to their reintegration.

> In effect, the various facilities proposed would operate as a stepped security system involving self-contained accommodation units with prisoners remaining on the premises, except when engaged in approved activities (e.g., work, medical, special purpose courses). At the same time while in the facilities, inmates would be obliged to voluntarily participate in self-management and discipline exercises involving cleaning, cooking, budgeting, education, self-esteem, and other such programs of self-development. [Begg, 1991:274]

The halfway house is designed for those inmates who are low to medium risk offenders. It is meant to provide a cost-efficient yet proactive response to reducing recidivism rates by assisting prisoners in breaking the cycle of their offending behavior.

In Canada, there are a number of different systems of early release in which inmates are moved into community settings. For example, *day parole* is the earliest form of conditional release, which is accompanied by strict conditions that dictate where the candidate will live (e.g., an approved community correctional center), the type of treatment or vocational and educational facilities candidates may attend, and adherence to strict curfews [Grant and Gillis, 1999:1].

The relationship between temporary release and parole, and temporary release and recidivism, is important. For example, Ellis and Marshall [2000] have given weight to the importance of these relationships in a study that compared reconviction rates for paroled and nonparoled inmates in the United Kingdom. Generally, the findings indicate that the use of supervised release has a positive effect on the reduction of recidivism [Ellis and Marshall, 2000:304]. In similar research, Grant and Gillis [1998] studied the impact of the day parole program on federal inmates in Canada. Day parole is a program designed to introduce inmates to the outside world before their ability to apply for full parole. The program allows an inmate to move into a community housing setting and to attend educational, vocational, or treatment programs but requires the inmate to return at a set time [Grant and Gillis, 1998:1]. The study found a significant relationship between the use of the day release programs and the successful completion of full parole [Grant and Gillis, 1998:45]. Indeed, 85% of inmates who successfully completed day parole went on to fulfill the full parole obligations without any intervention from the criminal justice system [Grant and Gillis, 1998:45].

The issue of permitting inmates to re-enter the community in controlled conditions, such as day release, has had considerable debate within the community in Australia and elsewhere. Much of the argument has been based on the issue of having convicted offenders being able to access the general community before their full sentence has been completed, or before they are eligible for full parole. Many such day release schemes involve allowing inmates to attend educational and vocational training that is not supplied by the prison authorities or in the prison environment. In a study by the Correctional Service of Canada, Grant and Gillis [1998:49] concluded that day release does not substantially increase the risk to the community. Furthermore, they argued that the goal of corrections is to reintegrate the offender in the community, and that having some of the sentence completed in the community setting is useful. Such programs also have implications with regard to possible employment connections for offenders in the transition from prison to community.

Reviews of the system of classification of prisoners in Tasmania and the administration of the prisoner leave program agree that such programs are considered an essential part of the transition process. For example, the Honourable F. M. Neasey commented in 1993 that:

The Tasmanian prison system is on the whole a very safe, small, quiet, prudently conducted system. But we are more conservative than practically all other Australian regimes are in the extent to which we take (or fail to take) measures to try to prepare long-term prisoners for anticipated release and re-integration into the community, and to enable them to keep their family ties together while they are in prison. Both of these are desirable objectives to be pursued in the cause of conducting a humane and just prison system, and also improving the chances of prisoners staying free of crime when released. [Neasey, 1993:40]

Although observers have periodically noted administrative problems in the delivery of prisoner leave programs [Neasey, 1993; Leggat and Baohm, 1999], there has largely been no questioning of the strategic value of such programs in preparing prisoners for life on the outside. Expert criticism has generally been directed at policy and procedural issues. These have included, for example, issues relating to clarification of the purpose and objective of each category of leave, as well as explicit and detailed listing of the criteria for eligibility for each category of leave [e.g., Leggat and Baohm, 1999].

By way of contrast, and as recognized in professional literature on parole and prerelease issues [Nelson and Trone, 2000], there is often negative media when (1) certain classes of prisoners are publicly exposed as being on certain leave programs, and (2) particular victims are accorded considerable attention in voicing their objections to the release of "their" prisoner. The net result of sensationalized media treatment that focuses on these types of issues is the potential delegitimation of such programs. This is problematic for a number of reasons, ranging from their destructive impact on socially useful prisoner transition processes, through to the undermining of newly created procedures designed to enhance victims' rights in general. Some of these issues are explored below.

17.2.2 The Importance of Prerelease Programs

Part of the impetus for prerelease and parole programs is the sheer number of people entering, as well as leaving, the prison systems. With major increases in prison populations in places such as Australia, the United States, and the United Kingdom [Walmsley, 2007], increasing concern and attention has been directed at what happens to inmates once they have been released [Petersillia, 2001a&b]. Thus, "If even a modest proportion of those returning to the community become involved in new crime, the human costs in terms of victimization and community destabilization—as well as the fiscal costs in terms of reincarceration—will be staggering" [Burke, 2001:12]. Therefore, a key issue is how best to achieve successful and safe re-entry for offenders. Thus, the question of prisoner re-entry is inextricably linked to concerns over present and future levels of community safety, as well as the financial and human costs of reoffending.

Getting prepared for release is essential if either parole or nonparole release is to be achieved with the most positive outcome. An important reason why prerelease effort is needed is indicated in the following observations:

> When supervision works well it provides some of the ballast people need during their first months in the community, but many newly released inmates find it hard to meet the broadly defined conditions of probation and parole. Accustomed to being told exactly what to do and how to do it, they often expect their supervision officers to forge a path for them—get them a job, find the right drug treatment program. Disappointed when their unrealistic expectations are not met, some people never form trusting relationships with those who supervise them. As for the officers, they begin the process with no information about how the people they have to supervise respond to authority figures and what they want to do with their lives. [Nelson and Trone, 2000:2]

Testing the water and getting used to forging one's own path are vital to offender resettlement in the community.

The public interest is served when prerelease and postrelease programs are put into place in ways that genuinely assist prisoners to adjust successfully to their after-prison lives. Public perceptions of leave and other forms of release may be negatively colored by poor execution of programs or by lack of clarity regarding program objectives and ends.

> People interested in improving or developing prerelease services first need to define what exactly they want to achieve. Many interventions have the potential to reduce recidivism while being worthy pursuits on their own. And these intermediate goals—such as providing job development services, guaranteeing that all physically and mentally ill inmates have medical insurance when they are released, and reuniting families before release—can be documented objectively and easily. [Nelson and Trone, 2000:6]

Thus, the positive benefits of prerelease services need to be recognized through widely circulated documentation of both underlying philosophy and outcomes.

17.2.3 Philosophy as a Driver of Intervention

How offenders are managed in the community as part of a release scheme is influenced as much as anything by the institutional structure and goals of community corrections in a given jurisdiction. The mission of community corrections as a specific form of justice intervention is informed by how punishment is viewed and what the intended outcomes of intervention are meant to be [Worrall, 1997]. The basic philosophies of community corrections generally involve either of two main orientations [White and Tomkins, 2003]:

Community incapacitation, in which the main emphasis is on the concepts of community safety and offender control. This involves intensive monitoring and supervision of offenders in community settings. The aim of community corrections, from this perspective, is to keep offenders under close surveillance and to thereby deter them from reoffending.

Community-level rehabilitation, in which efforts are made to change offender behavior in positive ways, as well as improving community relationships by use of supportive, participatory measures. The aim of community corrections, from this point of view, is to prevent recidivism through behavior modification via some type of therapeutic or skills-based intervention. The emphasis is on personal development and enhanced capabilities.

There may be a tension between "control and contain" strategies and "rehabilitative" strategies. So too, there may be differences between interventions designed as prison alternatives and those related to postprison transitions. Nevertheless, how community corrections workers actually carry out their task will largely be dictated by the dominant service philosophy. A third, and emergent, service philosophy is also evident. This is one that focuses on building stronger communal relationships through positive and constructive offender activities.

Restorative justice involves the offender in activities intended to repair the harm to victims and the wider community. The aim of community corrections, based on restorative assumptions, is to restore harmony through the offender doing something for and by themselves to make things better in the community. The emphasis is on improving the well-being of offender, victim, and community. [White and Tomkins, 2003]

The challenge, for supporters of the latter perspective, in particular, is to defend the importance of community corrections generally, rather than reliance on imprisonment, and further, to construe "good practice" within community corrections in the light of the theoretical and practical impetus of restorative principles.

There are numerous ambiguities and contradictions in the area of community corrections, and, if anything, these have intensified in recent years. Changes to the overarching political environment, in which "law and order" has come to the fore in many jurisdictions, have placed greater emphasis on punitive rather than rehabilitative or restorative principles. And yet the latter has become the guiding diversionary philosophy in areas such as juvenile justice [Cunneen and White, 2007; Mawby, 2007]. Meanwhile, government concerns with fiscal matters have frequently translated into more work, but fewer resources, being allocated to the corrections area, a problem not uncommon over the range of human services.

As the American experience seems to indicate, very often there are changes at the level of professional ideology and practice as well, and these too are making community corrections ever more complicated. For example, the heightened concern about victim involvement and perspectives in dealing with offenders, new procedures, and instruments in risk assessment as well as the slowly permeating influence of restorative justice ideals are currently being reworked into the professional lexicon and toolkits of parole and probation officers [Burke, 2001]. Where and how community corrections fit into the overall scheme of things is an issue of ongoing concern.

In the United Kingdom, similar issues are also apparent. The National Probation Service has been handed the task of tailoring services to fit victims, as well as to undertake the usual postrelease work with offenders. In fact, probation officers have long been involved with and have played a key role in the development of victim services in England and Wales [Goodey, 2005; Mawby, 2007]. Initiatives related to the introduction of restorative justice have intensified the engagement of parole and probation staff with victims. Further service obligations have recently been added with respect to the postrelease involvement of victims of serious crimes, specifically, contact, consultation, and support for victims whose offenders are about to re-enter the community. Victim support has now been adopted as a fundamental priority for the National Probation Service.

However, inadequate funding and resources for community corrections very much impede progress toward a successful multifunctional service. In jurisdictions such as Australia, the United States, and the United Kingdom, much more needs to be spent on the human infrastructure of corrections (rather than bricks and mortar), given the central importance of programs in opening the door for offenders to achieve futures in which offending becomes less of an option. When security costs outweigh service and program outlays, then prisons and community corrections become places of (temporary) containment and offender management, rather than opportunities for rehabilitation or restorative justice. Money is not spent for the purposes of change (of individual offenders, or with respect to community environment). The result inevitably is "more of the same": the failure of prison and corrections generally, as reflected in high recidivism rates [White, 2004].

It must be emphasized that if resources are not forthcoming to ensure an effective community corrections sector, and if intensive supervision and support are not provided in the prisons to those who most need them, then reoffending is guaranteed to stay the same or to increase. The net result of this is pressure to build more facilities—to expend capital on physical infrastructure, to house those who otherwise could be making a contribution to society, rather than being a drain on the public purse.

A restorative justice approach would appear to have great potential to effect change in an offender's behavior and attitudes in a positive direction. This is because it does not exclude people from the community (or, conversely, expose them to a school of crime, as in the case of prisons and detention centers), nor does it pathologize the offender (by placing most attention on their faults and weaknesses). The restorative perspective is driven by the idea that the offender deserves respect and dignity (they are persons) and that they already have basic competencies and capacities that need to be developed further (if they are not to reoffend). In this framework, the emphasis is on what the offender could do rather than should do [see also Ward and Maruna, 2007, on the "good lives" model of rehabilitation]. What is important is that offenders achieve at a concrete level, for themselves and for making reparation to their victim.

In the end, the point of dealing with offenders in particular ways is to reinforce the notion that they have done something wrong, to repair the damage done as much as possible, and to open the door for their reintegration into the mainstream of society. However, for any of this to be successfully implemented, certain preconditions to good practice are required. For a start, we need to be aware that different classes of prisoners may fit into release schemes in different ways.

For example, different objectives may be involved in selecting who is going to be eligible for prerelease programs. Factors to take into account include, for example:

- Universal programs designed so that every prisoner gets the opportunity for some type of prerelease experience (such as transition classes held outside the prison)
- Concentration of resources on certain inmates (e.g., by identifying only those inmates who would most likely benefit from job training)
- Limiting service provision to people more likely to reoffend (such as high-risk groups identified based on crime of conviction, criminal history, time served, age, and employment history)

From the standpoint of recidivism, it is important that some type of prerelease transition be put in place, that postrelease assistance systems be available to former prisoners, and that community corrections be resourced adequately to be of practical assistance.

Moreover, it is essential that the high-risk groups be an integral part of this process. Eventually, we have to live with those we punish, and this includes people with particularly bad records.

In many jurisdictions, high-risk offenders include people serving time for violent crimes or with a history of such convictions. Serving them involves taking some political risk but makes sense from a public safety perspective. [Nelson and Trone, 2000:6]

If no transitional pathway is provided for, then there is much greater likelihood that such offenders will reoffend—and thereby create even more victims than otherwise may be the case.

17.3 Victims' Rights: Supporting Those Who Have Been Harmed

The services available to victims vary greatly, as do the service providers [White and Perrone, 2005]. A range of initiatives to assist victims have developed worldwide over time. Some of these are outlined in Figure 17.2. They vary in nature, depending on the state and country of jurisdiction.

The main orientations of victim support programs and procedures include:

- A focus on *prosecution processes*, which center on the court case itself and the offender. Thus, the use of victim impact statements (VIS) is to assign penalty and to assist in the prosecution of offenders. It is

---

Victim notification—Victims are kept informed in about case developments and the hearing date.

Victim impact statements (VIS)—These include written statements, subdivided into either those that are formally structured and formatted and others that are unstructured and open ended. In some cases, there is an opportunity for victims to present their experiences orally in court.

Court orientation—Victims are introduced to the court system, so that they are able to identify the main players and feel comfortable with the court organization.

Transportation—Services are provided victims, enabling them to commute to and from court.

Escorting—This is basically a support service or "hand-holding" exercise, so that the victim is not left alone in the court and has someone to talk to throughout the proceedings.

Compensation—Some forms of physical and emotional injury may be compensated via state agencies such as a crimes compensation tribunal. Alternatively, victims may receive compensation either through civil proceedings (e.g., under the law of torts) or criminal proceedings, where a court orders that compensation be paid.

Victim–offender mediation—These are programs that are aimed at involving the victim in direct contact with the offender, who can then see the harm they have caused. This also enables victims and offenders to jointly be involved in attempts to resolve the harm done.

Restorative justice—This is an approach based on the idea of repairing the harm by involving offenders, victims, and communities as participants in the criminal justice process. It is widely used in the juvenile justice area and takes the form of juvenile conferences, circle sentencing, and community reparation schemes.

General support services—These include such programs as counseling services, youth and women's refuges, and alcohol and drug services. They are meant to center on victims' needs, both immediate and long term.

Figure 17.2 Victim services and participation.

not necessarily victim-centered per se, even though the victim may possibly gain some sense of satisfaction.

- A focus on *conflict resolution processes*, which involve some form of mediation and restorative justice. The intention here is on restoring dominion or personal liberty, both for the offender and the victim. Rather than focusing exclusively on the prosecution process, there is promotion of more active victim participation and attempts to "make good the harm" in a way that rectifies or improves relationships and resources for all concerned.

- A focus on *compensation*, so that the victim gains some type of financial recompense for harms suffered. The victim may be actively involved in determination of the level and nature of compensation. However, payment organization and administration are largely under the control of the courts and state compensation agencies.

- A focus on the *provision of support services*, which refers to areas such as counseling, funding of safe and secure refuges, the provision of information to victims so that they are better able to understand their victimization in a wider context, and so on. Central to this orientation is the idea of meeting victims' needs directly rather than by dealing with the offender.

Our concern in this section is not with victim services and support in general, but rather with those that specifically revolve around the offender. To appreciate and understand the nature of victim–offender issues in a transitional context, it is essential to consider the debates over victims' needs and victims' rights.

17.3.1 Victims' Rights and Needs

It is often clear that appeals to "victims' rights" are really code words for harsher penalties and reduced rights for offenders and suspects rather than means for addressing the practical concerns of victims, like compensation, counseling, assistance, and information. The rights and needs of crime victims should be taken extremely seriously. This, however, is not possible when they are viewed only in contrast or opposition to the rights of offenders. [Beyond Bars, 2002]

It is useful to distinguish between varying kinds of victims' "rights" and victims' "needs." The latter, generally speaking, do not involve civil liberty issues, in the sense that they refer to the provision of services and support structures that address the emotional and practical issues faced by victims. Victims' needs may also include such things as compensation and the right to be treated with dignity and respect by criminal justice officials. Other types of rights, however, have a direct impact on offender rights that are frequently seen in competition with victims' rights [Garkawe, 2002; Goodey, 2005]. Moreover, it is often the case that there is a perceived competition for community service funding, especially between victim and offender services, and this likewise can impinge on how "rights" issues are dealt with politically and administratively [Anderson, 1995].

Issues of access to justice and fair treatment on the part of victims have been addressed in provisions such as the following in the United Nations Declaration of Basic Principles of Justice for Victims of Crime and Abuse of Power.

The responsiveness of judicial and administrative processes to the needs of victims should be facilitated by:

1. Informing victims of their role and scope, timing and progress of the proceedings and of the disposition of their cases, especially where serious crimes are involved and where they have requested such information;
2. Allowing the views and concerns of victims to be presented and considered at appropriate stages of the proceedings where their personal interests are affected, without prejudice to the accused and consistent with the relevant national criminal justice system;
3. Providing proper assistance to victims throughout the legal process;
4. Taking measures to minimize inconvenience to victims, protect their privacy, when necessary, and ensure their safety, as well as that of their families and witnesses on their behalf, from intimidation and retaliation; and
5. Avoiding unnecessary delay in the disposition of cases and the execution of orders or decrees granting awards to victims.

Rights within criminal justice systems can broadly be distinguished in terms of "rights to information" and "participation rights." How these are interpreted and acted on in practice depends in part on how certain needs, such as the need for security and safety, are evaluated in relation to the balance of rights between (1) the victim, (2) the offender, and (3) the state. Three categories of victims' rights have been identified [Karmen, 1996; Garkawe, 2002]:

- *Those gained only at the expense of offenders* (e.g., where a victim's consent or willingness to participate can influence the rights of prisoners, as in the case of a parole process that negatively evaluates applications in which some kind of restorative justice program has not taken place)
- *Those gained only at the expense of the state*—that is, the criminal justice system and associated human services (e.g., the right to certain information and notification, as well as services and support workers)
- *Those gained at the expense of both offenders and the state* (e.g., the right to have input into system decision-making processes, such as bail or parole)

With regard specifically to issues of impending release, it is notable that in New South Wales, the victim has two kinds of rights [Garkawe, 2002:261]:

1. The right to be kept informed of the offender's impending release (or his or her escape) from custody, or of any change in security classification that results in the offender being eligible for unescorted absence from custody (i.e., *right to information*). This right has implications for system management but does not present any civil liberties concerns as such in relation to the inmate.
2. The right to make submissions with respect to decisions on whether "serious offenders" are eligible for unescorted leave of absence (i.e., *right to participation*). This right can have an impact on prisoner rights, in that victim submissions may influence the relevant authority (e.g., parole board, prison officials) either to disallow, defer, or place more stringent conditions on any external leave granted to the prisoner.

Given the impact that the exercise of different rights may have, it is essential to explore the rationale behind how such rights ought to be implemented in practice. For example, Garkawe [2002] discusses the specific contexts within which different rights ought to be exercised. It is acknowledged by most commentators that the "right to information" concerning criminal justice decision-making processes and outcomes is desirable and should be encouraged. However, the use of the "right to participate" does require certain qualifications. For example, the right of victims to present a submission to a parole hearing needs to be based on the requirement that any evidence so presented must be legally relevant and factually verifiable. In other words, participation by victims should be bounded by consideration of whether the evidence is "legally relevant" to the decision-making task at hand (e.g., documented threats or negative behavior directed toward the victim on the part of the prisoner).

Somewhat more contentiously, there are a range of subjective matters that also need to be evaluated. For example, it may well be that victims are fearful of an offender, that they perceive the offender to be untrustworthy, and that they may not have forgiven. Therefore, the question arises as to how, or if, the criminal justice system ought to respond to the emotional responses of victims. Here it is argued by Garkawe [2002:271] that victims' views may be of some relevance in a small minority of cases, where the conditions of parole (or day release) are involved. In other words, conditions relating to contact with victims or members of a victim's family or proximity to a victim's residence or commuting route might be subject to imposed special conditions, pursuant to victim submissions.

How victims feel about prisoner release ought to be fully integrated into any analysis of such programs. As demonstrated in Table 17.1, victims have

Table 17.1 What Victims Indicate They Are Most Concerned about or in Need of When Their Offenders Re-enter the Community

Need or Concern	Percentage
Information about whom to contact if victim has concerns	75
Notification of offender location	75
Notification of offender status	65
Protective or "no contact" orders	64
Input into conditions of release (victim impact statement)	33
Financial or legal obligations	29
Information about referrals	22
Offender programming that creates awareness	19
Input into interstate compact	16
Input into conditions of community service	15
Victim–offender programming (mediation)	12

Source: Seymour, 2001. *The victim's role in offender reentry: A community response manual.* Washington, DC: Office for Victims of Crime, U.S. Department of Justice.

a range of concerns relating to the re-entry of offenders back into the mainstream of society.

The emotional toll for victims anticipating the release of "their" offender ought not to be underestimated. From a community corrections point of view, this implies a number of challenges. For example, Seymour [2001:8] discusses the situation of victims of violent crime:

> For many violent [crime] victims, the thought of living in the same community as the person who caused them such terrible harm and deep psychological trauma is foreboding. Reentry partnership professionals and volunteers must accept this factor and find ways, to the degree possible, to honor the victim's wishes. This may mean establishing a geographic "safe zone" perimeter around the victim (for example, in California it is 30 miles from the victim's place of residence), and developing strict conditions of supervision that center on the victim's need for safety.

As suggested here, there are things that can be done to reassure the victim in regard to early and final release of offenders. To some extent, especially if the case involves parole, the decision regarding offender conditions of release are made well before the offender actually leaves the prison.

17.3.2 Victim Impact Assessment and Prerelease: Parole

The use of VIS in proceedings within court has engendered considerable debate in recent times [Erez and Rogers, 1999; Herman and Wasserman, 2001;

Seymour, 2001]. Many of the arguments revolve around the use of VIS as an objective rational account of the harm done by the offender to the victim or the emphasis on the harm and fear felt by the victim. Traditionally, the courts have held that the subjective accounts of the harm and suffering by the victim should not be the only consideration when passing sentence [Erez and Rogers, 1999]. The whole notion of a "victim perspective" has also raised questions about procedural fairness and justice as a concept, as illustrated in Figure 17.3.

The use of VIS in the parole process poses additional potential problems. For example, there is the possibility that VIS employment will involve de facto passage of second sentences on offenders, in effect extending the period of imprisonment beyond that intended by the sentencing court. This would constitute a form of double jeopardy for the inmate.

The inclusion of victims does not have to impinge on offender rights or freedoms. However, when victim testimony at parole hearings is given substantial weight, in some cases prisoner rights may well be eroded [Goodey, 2005]. A study of parole hearings in Alabama in the United States, for

---

Proposition:

There is no such thing as a "victim" perspective as such. Rather, different individuals respond differently to the event and effects of victimization. This has major consequences for how they encounter the criminal justice system and perceive their relationship with offenders. Consider the following scenarios. In each case the victim has suffered a physical assault at the hands of an assailant.

Victim 1

Retribution and punishment are all that this person can think about. The assault had a devastating impact on the life of the victim, who is angry and hostile. This victim wants a punitive response and to make the offender to suffer pain in some way. A VIS provides one mechanism to vent such emotions and to make the offender pay for the harm caused.

Victim 2

Forgiveness and understanding are the ultimate goals of this person. This person has been raised in a religious tradition that emphasizes peacekeeping, forgiveness, and love of one's enemies. The victim wants to understand why the offender did what he or she did. The victim also wants to assist with ways in which the offender can somehow find redemption for his or her deeds. A VIS is less important than the need to work with offenders to change their ways.

Victim 3

Forgetting and submerging the event, and not wanting to know any more about the offender, is what this person wants. The victim was traumatized by the assault and just wants to forget that it ever happened. The victim does not want to be bothered with confronting the offender, to forgiving the offender, or to contributing to a VIS. The victim simply does not want to relive the event in any way, shape, or form. It is time to move on and look to the future.

The orientation and role of victims within systems will vary according to the aims of the system as a whole: retribution, rehabilitation, or restoration. This, too, impacts the possible emotional state and contribution of each victim. Thus, for example, a retributive system will tend to generate vengeful punitive responses; in a restorative system, shame might be a key emotion for offender and victim alike.

Figure 17.3 A victim perspective: Three views.

example, found that victim and offender participation was significantly related to parole hearing outcomes. The study found that victim influences, in particular, were a highly predictive factor in the decision to grant or deny parole, even more so than the offender's behavior in prison or participation in rehabilitative programs. The more vocal and active the victim, the more likely a negative outcome for the offender [Morgan and Smith, 2005]. This places considerable power in the hands of articulate and proactive victims, while simultaneously undermining potential rehabilitation avenues and transitional pathways for offenders.

In many cases, the potential contribution of victims to parole board decisions does not relate so much to whether parole is granted but rather to the sort of conditions imposed on a parole order [Black, 2003]. What may be more important in the use and debate about VIS is that it may create classes of victims. This may well affect the parole selection criteria and parole conditions for inmates [John Howard Society, 1997]. If this were so, some prisoners would be disadvantaged in applying for parole depending on the social status, educational level, and ability to articulate the consequences of the offense on the victim's life because victims vary greatly in their skills to express the harm done [John Howard Society, 1997; White and Perrone, 2005]. Other victim differences have been noted in Figure 17.3.

More generally, Black [2003:5] points to a range of procedural issues that also require further attention:

> What should be done with new allegations against an offender? How should inflammatory or prejudicial material be dealt with and how should the veracity of victim submissions be determined? Should an offender have a right of rebuttal? These questions have serious ramifications, particularly if victim submissions are influential in parole decision-making. [Black, 2003:5]

Similar kinds of questions can be raised in relation to victim input into day release and other types of release from prison.

17.3.3 Victims' Rights in the Re-entry Process

The view of Victim Support Australasia, a victims' rights and support organization, is that corrective services should:

- Provide or facilitate restorative justice programs.
- Create a Victims Register, so that crime victims are kept informed of developments in the management and release of "their" offender.
- Provide victim awareness programs for prisoners and staff.
- Ensure the effective rehabilitation of offenders with the aim of preventing reoffending [Cook, David, and Grant, 1999:63].

When it comes to the re-entry process of offenders, victims have an interest across several domains [Seymour, 2001]. These include:

- **Victim notification**: Information about rights, processes, resources, options, and services
- **Victim protection**: Personal safety and security concerns, feelings of safety, actual fear, and perceived fear
- **Victim impact**: Harms or hurt suffered by the victim physically, emotionally, and financially
- **Victim restitution**: Financial compensation from offender, government compensation, and dialogue with the offender

The following subsections deal with issues surrounding victim notification and protection in greater depth.

17.3.3.1 Notification of Offender Status
The ways in which information is provided to victims and their families vary. The National Probation Service in the United Kingdom, for example, will normally write to particular victims (e.g., those who have suffered a sexual or violent offense for which the offender has been sentenced to 1 year or more in prison) within 2 months of the offender being sentenced. They will offer to meet with the victim for the following purposes:

- To give information about prison sentences in general and how prisoners can proceed through the system
- To ask victims whether they want to be contacted at key stages in the criminal justice process, as well as told when the prisoner is considered for final release
- To check whether victims have any concerns they feel should be taken into account when prisoners are considered for final release
- To give the name of someone the victim can contact at the probation office in the victim's area
- To explain how they will use any information the victim provides
- To tell the victim about any other services that may be able to help

The official position of the Probation and Community Corrections Officers Association of Australia (PACCOA) is that notification of victims is important and needs to be formally recognized [2003]. However, it is also acknowledged that any notification system has to balance several competing interests.

A primary victim's right to information about the status of an offender's progress through the criminal justice process should be balanced with that of an offender's right to privacy of personal information. In general, on victim request, offers of status and other information should be made proactively to the primary victim.

The sort of information that should be made available to a victim includes:

- General information about the role and meaning of court orders, and conditional release orders from prison or custody, and the victim programs within these settings
- Information about reparative, restorative, and restitution programs involving victims and offenders
- Notifications of postsentencing release decisions or outcomes, including work release, parole, pardon, community supervision orders, security classification and changes, placements, transfers and milestones, commitment to a mental health facility, or escape
- Notifications of relevant dates, such as review dates, release dates, and expiry or cancellation and suspension dates, and the implications (if any) of those dates

Unless legislation stipulates otherwise, PACCOA will only support the release of information on the proviso that:

- It will not be publicly disseminated in any way, including through the media, the Internet, or in any other form.
- It will not be used for any unlawful purpose that could cause harm or detriment to any person.
- Such information will not enable unwanted contact between offender or victim.
- Information divulged by victims to third parties must be restricted to the purposes of:
  - Self-protective measures to minimize risk of harm to themselves or immediate family.
  - Enhancing their healing within the confidentiality of treatment environments.
  - Disclosure to statutory authorities for legitimate business.

In general, PACCOA does not support the concept of issuing release notifications to communities, only to primary victims or their personal representatives (or statutory authorities where there is perceived risk to any individual in the community). PACCOA believes that victim services and probation–community corrections share the responsibility of both protecting their clients and assisting them in dealing with the fear and mistrust that each may hold for the other.

Garkawe [2002] points out that information about things such as the prisoner's place of detention, where the prisoner will reside after being released, and details of their treatment or participation in prison programs may breach the prisoner's privacy and may be used by some victims or their families to harass the prisoner or the prisoner's family. In the light of this, it is suggested that the privacy rights of prisoners should prevail in the absence of victims' genuine security needs.

These concerns are also obliquely reflected in the Victim's Register used in Tasmania at present. The Registration Form includes the following section:

> I understand and accept that the information supplied through the Victim's Register is confidential. I agree not to release this information for the purpose of public dissemination without approval from the Department. I agree not to use this information for any unlawful purpose which could cause harm or detriment to any person.

One question raised by the inclusion of this proviso is whether, and how, it might be enforced. Aside from moral pressure not to engage in a breach of "good faith," there appear to be two other options: to charge those who do not abide by these rules with an administrative offense (e.g., perhaps resulting in a fine) and/or to exclude victims from further notification and participation rights because of their infringement of the guidelines. Enforcement and compliance concerns, however, also beg the issues of how such breaches are to be investigated, what degree of proof and evidence are needed before a penalty is imposed, and whether mitigating circumstances can and ought to be taken into account.

17.3.3.2 Victim Protection

The PACCOA Statement on Victims [2003] also makes several comments relevant to the issue of victim safety, security, and protection. In the matter of victim protection, including from intimidation and harassment, PACCOA states:

> One of the most effective ways to encourage victim participation in the entire criminal justice process is to ensure their safety from intimidation or harm by offenders or those associated with offenders. Correctional agencies have an important obligation to protect victims from intimidation and harassment and/or harm from offenders under their supervision. A combination of sound policies, supervision procedures and modern technology may offer many innovative approaches to increasing and enforcing victim protection measures.

Concerning consideration of victim concerns and involvement in subsequent decision making, PACCOA states:

> In addition to providing information, it is important that all opportunities are provided by community corrections to enable victims to make representations to releasing bodies that are timely, and as far as is possible, informed.

Similarly, probation–community corrections should maintain accurate information on offender files about restrictions to the offender–victim relationship, for example, whether a protection or other court or releasing authority order is in existence and the conditions to it.

It is important that victims' needs be fully considered when assessing offender risk. Various detailed question-based systems have been developed in the United States that provide simple but effective ways to assess risk [Seymour, 2001]. Sample questions include such queries as: *Did the offender know the victim? Does the offender know where the victim lives? Was the offense committed at the victim's home or place of business? Did the offense involve personal violence or threats of violence?*

However, more discussion is needed on the nature of risk assessment and on how certain classes of offender are represented in risk discourse, in ways that lead to their control and confinement after release [Hughes and Edwards, 2002; Brown, 2008]. This is particularly the case with sex offenders, but easily accessible "criminal register" web sites open the door to surveillance and vigilante action across many different categories of offender. Thus, specific victim concerns may be transposed onto a notion of the universal victim, one that is premised on general risk and predictive models rather than personalized events and situations. This is an issue worthy of extensive discussion in its own right.

17.4 Impact of Crime on Victims: Offender Focus

One of the great misfortunes accompanying victimization is that all too often the emotional needs of the victim are forgotten in the criminal justice process. To some extent this is a matter of providing adequate counseling and other support services to guide victims through the difficult stages of transition and victim recovery. It is also vital that offenders be given the opportunity to be exposed to the victims' plight.

> No one can fully understand the victim's feelings or experience. Thus, one must allow victims to speak from the heart and let them know that we are listening with the heart as well. They have things to say that we might not understand; they often need answers to irresolvable questions; they have expectations that might not be met. We have to assume that what they say is important for us to hear and that we learn from our hearing it. Sometimes victims prove remarkably frank, blunt, or direct. It is important to respect these exchanges and the victim who shares them. [Nicholl, 2001:27]

There are two key issues here. One is how best to give victims a forum in which they can best and most positively voice their feelings. The second is how to arrange for offenders to "hear" the victim's voice without compromising their own safety, future opportunities, and rehabilitation processes. Options can range from face-to-face meetings between individual victims and individual offenders (in the community or in the prison), to family or juvenile group conferences that involve family members and support people, to "surrogate victims," in the form of panels of victims telling their stories to offenders [Nicholl, 2001].

The PACCOA Statement on Victims [2003] highlights the importance of offenders realizing the extent, nature, and pain of the harm experienced by victims. Support is given to the development and implementation of "victim awareness programs" for offenders to enable them to understand the impact that their criminal behavior has on victims, their families, and their communities.

PACCOA supports components that address offending behavior for prisoners and offenders that enable them to gain insight into and acknowledge the impact of crime on victims. PACCOA also recognizes that many offenders have themselves been victims and that in some cases this experience is directly linked to their offending behavior.

Raising consciousness among prisoners of the harms that they have caused can be achieved in different ways: for example, classes designed for adult and juvenile offenders, both nonviolent and violent, in diversion programs, probation, incarceration, detention, parole, and offender re-entry settings [Seymour, 2001].

17.4.1 Course Description

The objectives of this kind of class are for students to:

- Explore how they view the rights of other people.
- Raise their awareness of the long-term impact of their actions.
- Recognize their own possible victimization as children and how that abuse might impact them today.
- Provide opportunities to help them become nonabusive parents and good spouses or partners.
- Discuss their tendency to depersonalize the people they injure.
- Consider how they are accountable for the crimes they have committed.

Victim impact panels (VIP) involve a small panel of volunteer victims addressing a group of offenders in different settings [Fulkerson, 2001].

17.4.2 VIP Description

- Victims and offenders are provided an opportunity to meet in groups to discuss the nature of the harm.
- Victims are not allowed to speak on any panel in which the offender in their case is present.
- Subjects meet with a panel moderator for an orientation before the panel session.
- A security officer is present to ensure the safety of all victims.
- Victims get the chance to express their hurt and the effects of the harm on them.
- Offenders have an opportunity to learn from victims directly about the effects of their behavior.
- Offenders may see things in a different light because they are not directly threatened by their own victims but are still forced to deal with victim issues.

Community-based discussion groups involve a structured program in which convicted perpetrators of a particular offense (such as burglary) are subjected to a probation order that brings them into contact with burglary victims [Mawby, 2007]. This is similar in approach to the VIP described above. It has been commented that such processes were beneficial for offenders in that allowing victims to confront them about the nature of the harms perpetrated meant that the normal techniques of neutralization (e.g., the victim can afford it) were challenged. The result was that offenders had to acknowledge how their actions had impacted "real" victims.

Discussion of the preparation of prisoners for release, including in prerelease leave programs, requires that offenders at least begin to understand the impact of their actions on victims. Moreover, many jurisdictions also now demand some kind of involvement in restitution, reparations, or restorative justice activities, both while an offender is in prison and while they are on leave from prison or on parole. The importance of "restorative justice" in particular is emphasized by PACCOA [2003] and other organizations. Where appropriate, and where suitable human and material resources have been put into place, restorative justice mechanisms can be usefully applied in relation to prerelease programs and strategies.

Practical examples of how community corrections can be imbued with a restorative ethic at a concrete level are still relatively few and far between, although this is changing in some jurisdictions. The usual emphasis in community corrections work is what can be done to better supervise the offender, or what can be done to assist them to make the transition toward being a law-abiding citizen [e.g., Nelson and Trone, 2000]. Restorative justice inverts this relationship by making the offender an active contributor and participant. Thus, in the United Kingdom, "Offenders in some programmes carry out work for their own communities, which can help give the offenders a sense of social responsibility and an experience of social acceptance and recognition" [Marshall, 1999:14]. Seymour [2001] cites examples in the United States where the concept of "restorative community service" has taken hold. Relevant community work has included such things as youthful offenders escorting Alzheimer's patients from a local retirement center and their families for a day at a state fair, through to a licensed pharmacist who was convicted of forging drug documents performing 500 hours of community service at the free clinic in the neighborhood in which he had sold drugs.

Importantly, community service, as such, should not to be equated with restorative justice. Walgrave [1999] discusses how in some judicial settings, authorities use community service as a punishment (i.e., intended to inflict pain), whereas in other settings it is informed by a rehabilitative objective (as manifest in various forms of re-education and treatment). In contrast to these approaches, he argues that community service can also be used in a restorative sense, if it is meant to compensate for harm, restore peace in the community, and contribute to safety feelings in society.... Attention will now be turned to the harm and the restoration of it, including the reintegration of the offender, because this is an important item for restoring peace in the community [Walgrave, 1999:140].

This type of community service demands a clear appreciation of the philosophical foundations of restorative justice and how community corrections workers can achieve the potentials such a philosophy appears to offer.

17.5 Conclusion

Analysis of the relationship between victims and offenders during the transition from prison to community suggests a range of issues specific to each group, as well as matters that imply overlapping concerns and interests. Therefore, we conclude by considering the implications of this analysis for each group.

17.5.1 Victims and Offender Re-entry

If victims and offenders understand that people in their communities are paying attention—that the community has a vested interest in making sure that the re-entry process goes smoothly—it would change the whole dynamic. Victims would be less vulnerable; offenders would be more responsible; and the community would be looking out for its own people, actively engaging in maintaining a safer and healthier culture. [Melissa Hook, victim advocate, in Seymour, 2001:9]

Victims deserve and have a right to be engaged with the criminal justice system in many different ways and in relation to diverse rights and needs. However, how victims are involved specifically in relation to release matters needs to take into account, and be bounded by, several considerations:

- That any participation by victims be subject to the proviso that what they submit be "legally relevant" and based on objective evidence, when it comes to considerations of release
- That victim participation based on subjective fears and misgivings about offenders be directed at the conditions of release, rather than release itself
- That the exercise of victims' rights explicitly acknowledge certain responsibilities as part of this, as in the case of "confidentiality" considerations in relation to information about offenders
- That victim satisfaction cannot be guaranteed by the operation of the criminal justice system; only that victims' needs and rights be respected within an overall climate of rights-respecting institutions and human rights considerations
- That victims' rights do not automatically mean the diminishment of offender rights; rather, that rights are always constituted in relation to other rights, in relation to the intrinsic needs of specific categories of people, and in relation to universal standards (such as human rights)
- That an important role of the state is to safeguard citizens, including prisoners, from community prejudices and abuse of authority, and to protect victims from becoming offenders themselves (e.g., by taking the law into their own hands and engaging in violence against prisoners)

17.5.2 Offenders and Victim Interests

Almost all the people in Risdon will eventually live in my society. I want to live in a safe society, so I want rehabilitation for people in prison. I am less safe whenever these programmes are placed at risk. So I resent attempts to curtail them. I want good people coming out of prison, not angry resentful people. [Peter Flint, letter to the *Mercury* newspaper, Saturday, May 10, 2003]

Offenders, too, deserve and have a right to be engaged with the criminal justice system in many different ways and in relation to diverse rights and needs. How offenders are involved, specifically in relation to release matters, likewise needs to be taken into account, and be bounded by, several considerations:

- That offenders be sensitized to the real impact of their crimes on victims and appreciate the actual and ongoing damage and harm their actions have caused
- That offenders acknowledge that subjective fears and material harms to victims may well be ongoing, regardless of what has happened in their lives or what measures they may take to rehabilitate or change themselves
- That offenders have some obligation to repair the harm, and that this can take many different forms, including various kinds of community-based contributions
- That victim safety and perceptions of safety are paramount in relation to the conditions of their release and any subsequent activities on the part of the prisoner within certain communities
- That prison release programs are directed at transitional processes that are meant to bridge prison-community life and thereby to enhance the prospects of prisoners not reoffending, and as part of this, respect for the feelings of victims and other community members is essential

17.5.3 Institutional Requirements

This chapter opened with the observation that "justice" has to take into account the fact that most prisoners will eventually return to the community, that victims need to be supported, and that victims and offenders have particular interests in the criminal justice process.

One can only agree with the view of probation officers that offenders have the right to peaceful reintegration into the community at the earliest time that their sentence allows, and that the offender's reintegration ought to enable victims to continue their lives free from further risk from that individual [PACCOA, 2003]. For this to be achieved, there are a series of institutional measures that need to be borne in mind. These are outlined in Figure 17.4. The key message here is that fostering prisoner transition in ways that make sense and that are to the benefit of victims demands institutional commitment, resources, programs, and staffing.

In the end, the best way to support and enhance victims' needs, interests, and rights is not to juxtapose them with those of the offender. Rather, as this chapter has demonstrated, complex issues require sensitivity and close consideration of many different concerns. Victim–offender relationships are always going to be complex, and they are always going to be accompanied by intense emotional and moral debate. The concept of transitions implies

- That victims be fully briefed about the issues and dynamics of prison leave programs, and that they be cautioned about the importance of confidentiality in such processes
- That the relevant department develop explicit rules and guidelines to ensure compliance with confidentiality concerns involving victims, as well as mechanisms to resolve disputes emerging from victim–offender relations
- That victims be assured that their pain and stories are heard by prison authorities and are reflected in administrative processes (either through VIS or via victim advocates), and that mechanisms exist for offenders to learn about the harms experienced by victims
- That VIP be established and used in regard to prisoners, insofar as such panels enable victims to express their hurt and pain, and offenders to learn about the consequences of their actions, in a manner that depersonalizes the confrontation, but which allows greatest positive impact
- That all correctional staff undertake training and ongoing staff development in the area of victim services and victimology, so that offender programs and offender management are intrinsically linked to victim concerns, needs, and rights issues
- That the philosophical and practical rationale and justification for offender release programs be conveyed fully to all correctional staff, as well as to relevant victim of crime services agencies and victim advocacy groups
- That selection procedures for prison leave be administered by a formally constituted prison leave board (or its equivalent), that the criteria for granting leave be explicitly identified for each individual case, and that each individual case be assessed on its own merits, without fear or favor (particularly in relation to potential media reaction)
- That the conditions of leave be assessed in the light of victims' rights, needs, and responsibilities, as well as in the light of the offenders' experiences, rehabilitation needs, and institutional history, and that any conditions be specified in terms of present, rather than past, developments
- That the administration of release be subject to periodic review by the parole board to ensure consistency, transparency, and appropriate consideration of victim–offender issues
- That the relevant department explores fully the ways in which restorative justice principles and practices can be integrated into the prison leave program (and parole program), particularly as this would open the way for greater victim participation and satisfaction with criminal justice processes
- That victims and offenders be periodically surveyed regarding the processes and outcomes relating to victim notification, prisoner leave arrangements, and victim–offender relationships generally

Figure 17.4 Victim–offender relations in a transitional context: Institutional requirements.

movement and change. The challenge is to do this in ways that bring maximum benefit to victims, to offenders, and to the community as a whole.

References

Anderson, T. 1995. Victims' rights or human rights? *Current Issues in Criminal Justice* 6(3):335–45.
Begg, C. 1991. The halfway house—A program for currently serving prisoners. In *Keeping people out of prisons*, proceedings of conference held March 27–29, 1990, at Australian Institute of Criminology.

Beyond bars: Alternatives to custody. 2002. *Victims of crime*. Fact Sheet 3. Sydney: Beyond Bars coalition.

Black, M. 2003. Victim submissions to parole boards: The agenda for research. *Trends and issues in criminal justice* No. 251. Canberra: Australian Institute of Criminology.

Brown, M. 2008. Risk, punishment and liberty. In *The critical criminology companion*, ed. T. Anthony and C. Cunneen. Sydney: Hawkins.

Burke, P. 2001. Collaboration for successful prisoner reentry: The role of parole and the courts. *Corrections Management Quarterly* 5(3):11–22.

Cook, B., F. David, and A. Grant. 1999. *Victims' needs, victims' rights: Policies and programmes for victims of crime in Australia*. Research and Public Policy Series No. 19. Canberra: Australian Institute of Criminology.

Cunneen, C. and R. White. 2007. *Juvenile justice: Youth and crime in Australia*. Melbourne: Oxford University Press.

Ellis, T. and P. Marshall. 2000. Does parole work? A post-release comparison of reconviction rates for paroled and non-paroled prisoners. *Australian and New Zealand Journal of Criminology* 33(3):300–17.

Erez, E. and L. Rogers. 1999. Victim impact statements and sentencing outcomes and processes: The perspectives of legal professionals. *British Journal of Criminology* 39(2):216–39.

Garkawe, S. 2002. Crime victims and prisoners' rights. In *Prisoners as citizens: Human rights in Australian prisons*, eds. D. Brown and M. Wilkie. Sydney: The Federation Press.

Goodey, J. 2005. *Victims and victimology: Research, policy and practice*. Harlow: Pearson Education.

Grant, B. and C. Gillis. 1998. *Day parole outcome, criminal history and other predictors of successful sentence completion*, Report No. R-59. Research Branch, Correctional Services of Canada.

Herman, S. and C. Wasserman. 2001. A role for the victim in offender reentry. *Crime and Delinquency* 47(3):428–45.

Hughes, G. and A. Edwards. 2002. *Crime control and community: The new politics of public safety*. Cullompton, UK: Willan.

John Howard Society of Alberta. 1997. *Victim impact statements*.

Karmen, A. 1996. *Crime victims: An introduction to victimology*. Pacific Grove, CA: Brooks Cole.

Leggat, R. and K. Baohm. 1999. *Review of administration of prisoner leave programmes in Tasmania*. Hobart: Attorney-General's Office.

Mawby, R. 2007. Public sector services and the victim of crime. In *Handbook of victims and victimology*, ed. S. Walklate. Cullompton, UK: Willan.

Morgan, K. and B. Smith. 2005. Victims, punishment, and parole: The effect of victim participation on parole hearings. *Criminology and Public Policy* 4(2):333–60.

Neasey, F. 1993. *Report of an inquiry into the system of classification of prisoners in Tasmania and other related matters*. Hobart: Attorney General's Office.

Nelson, M. and J. Trone. 2000. *Why planning for release matters*. New York: State Sentencing and Corrections Program, Vera Institute of Justice.

Nicholl, C. 2001. *Implementing restorative justice: A toolbox for the implementation of restorative justice and the advancement of community policing*. Washington, DC: Office of Community Oriented Policing Services, U.S. Department of Justice.

Petersillia, J. 2001a. When prisoners return to the community: Political, economic, and social consequences. *Correctional Management Quarterly* 5(3):1–10.

____. 2001b. Prison reentry: Public safety and reintegration challenges. *The Prison Journal* 81(3):360–75.

Probation and Community Corrections Officers' Association. 2003. The foundations of corrections based services for victims of crime: A PACCOA position paper. *PACCOA Papers* 1(1):1–8.

Seymour, A. 2001. *The victim's role in offender reentry: A community response manual.* Washington, DC: Office for Victims of Crime, U.S. Department of Justice.

Walgrave, L. 1999. Community service as a cornerstone of a systemic restorative response to (juvenile) crime. In *Restorative juvenile justice: Repairing the harm of youth crime*, eds. G. Bazemore and L. Walgrave. Monsey, NY: Criminal Justice Press.

Walmsley, R. 2007. *World prison population list*, 7th ed. London: International Centre for Prison Studies, King's College.

Ward, T. and S. Maruna. 2007. *Rehabilitation: Beyond the risk paradigm.* London: Routledge.

White, R. 2004. Community corrections and restorative justice. *Current Issues in Criminal Justice* 16(1):42–56.

White, R. and S. Perrone. 2005. *Crime and social control.* Melbourne: Oxford University Press.

White, R. and K. Tomkins. 2003. *Issues in community corrections.* Briefing Paper No. 2, Criminology Research Unit, School of Sociology and Social Work. Hobart: University of Tasmania Press.

Worrall, A. 1997. *Punishment in the community: The future of criminal justice.* London: Longman.

Death of a Metaphor? Healing Victims and Restorative Justice

18

TOM DAEMS

Contents

18.1 Introduction

It might be illuminating to start this chapter with two small illustrations. The first is derived from the notorious Bobbitt case that received worldwide attention because of the specific details of the events. In June 1993, Lorena Bobbitt chopped off almost half of her husband's penis with an 8-inch kitchen knife while he was asleep. She then drove off and threw the severed piece out of the window of her vehicle. It was later found by police officers and reattached after more than 9 hours of surgery. Lorena was charged with "malicious wounding" but eventually was acquitted because she was deemed temporarily insane by the jury. Her defense lawyer welcomed the verdict with the following words: "This is a giant step forward for Lorena in the healing process."

Closer to my home and somewhat less notorious were the statements of the Flemish Minister of Mobility Renaat Landuyt in June 2005 following the release of a drunken driver who had killed an 18-year-old girl in a car accident. The Minister argued that the man had been freed too quickly from prison. The public prosecutor should have kept him behind bars "at least until after the funeral." The public prosecutor's office of the city of Antwerp was not happy with these public statements. The man was in remand custody, and, according to Belgian criminal law, this is only possible when there is a suspicion that the offender might commit new crimes, that he might try to escape, or that he might make evidence disappear. None of these three justifications for continuing remand custody were present.

What do these two illustrations have in common? In a reflection on the Bobbitt case, the American sociologist James Nolan Jr. drew attention to the somewhat strange reaction of the lawyer: Why did this person welcome the verdict as a giant step forward for Lorena in the healing process? Nolan suggested that, at first sight, a statement like "We are all glad that the law was upheld and justice prevailed" would have been more obvious [Nolan, 1998:77]. The reference to Lorena's healing process, however, becomes better understandable if we place it in a broader context, that is, the growing therapeutic influence on criminal law: Therapeutic language and concerns about mental health, as well as concomitant assumptions about trauma and emotional harm, have entered into the heart of the American criminal justice system [Nolan, 1998, 2001]. The wish of the Flemish Minister to keep the drunk driver in prison longer seemed to be inspired by a similar set of motives. There was no punitive or preventive logic at work here, that is, neither the harsh treatment of the drunk driver nor the prevention of future road traffic victims seemed to be his main preoccupation in this specific case. Rather, he worried about the psychological welfare of the relatives of the victim. He reasoned that by keeping the drunk driver behind bars "at least until after the funeral," the relatives would have the opportunity to mourn in silence and say farewell to their loved one [Daems, 2005].

Both the lawyer for Bobbitt and the Flemish Minister of Mobility hold law degrees, but, nevertheless, they surpassed a classical juridical way of reasoning: Bobbitt's defense lawyer reinterpreted the acquittal in terms of healing, and Minister Landuyt reimagined remand custody in the light of processes of mourning and recovery. In both cases, the needs of victims moved to the center of attention. However, one has to add that these needs entered the debate in a very specific manner and idiom: Victims' needs and appropriate remedies are formulated in terms of trauma, emotional harm, and recovery. It is this specific manner of speaking and acting about victims' needs that will be the subject of this chapter.

In the next section we explore how concerns about mental health problems have risen to prominence in recent times. In the third section, we discuss how a certain strand of evaluation research dealing with restorative justice programs focuses on the therapeutic effects of restorative interventions for victims of crime. In the penultimate section, we examine how the psychological restoration of victims as a goal and justification of penal interventions pervades other (non-)restorative parts of the criminal justice system. The fifth section offers a general discussion.

18.2 From 9/11 to Therapy Culture

We usually associate the aftermath of the tragic events of September 11, 2001, with a wave of law enforcement initiatives and surveillance measures: the USA PATRIOT Act, the stringent security regulations at airports and the targeting of "suspicious" individuals, the global-wide war against terrorism, the prison base at Guantánamo Bay, and the military invasions of Afghanistan and Iraq. It would be a mistake, however, to see 9/11 as the starting point of a new era of surveillance in Western societies. In his book *Surveillance after September 11*, David Lyon argued that the new surveillance measures were "just surface symptoms of deeper and longer-term shifts in political culture, governance and social control, not only in North America but throughout the world." Therefore, many of the "deeper shifts" "were already in process, and 9/11 served simply to accelerate their arrival in a more public way" [Lyon, 2003:3–4].

However, there was also another set of response to 9/11 that has received much less attention. In the introduction to their book *L'Empire du traumatisme: Enquête sur la condition de victime*, Didier Fassin and Richard Rechtman [2007] highlight the grand scale of interventions related to mental health care after the attacks on the Twin Towers in New York City. About 9,000 mental health specialists, including 700 psychiatrists, intervened to give psychological support to survivors, witnesses, and inhabitants. Numerous Internet web sites, surveys, and scholarly conferences were devoted to the traumatic impact of the events. These were concerned not only with survivors or witnesses but also with those who watched the images on television. The term *trauma* also came to be used in a more expanded sense, that is, America was a "traumatized nation." In view of the massive scale of violence of the attacks, this response, as well as its psychological framing, was perceived to be so self-evident and normal that nobody questioned it [Fassin and Rechtman, 2007:12]. However, so Fassin and Rechtman argue, this response was far from self-evident. Twenty-five years ago hardly anybody (with the exception of some closed circles of psychiatrists and psychologists) tended to speak in terms of traumatization, and also the large-scale crisis- and after-care interventions by mental health professionals were almost nonexistent. During the past 25 years these have become, slowly but surely, part of the standard response to many similar events. Like Lyon [2003], who insists on the continuities between pre- and post-9/11 developments related to surveillance, so Fassin and Rechtman [2007] argue against making the response to the "trauma" of 9/11 the starting point of a new era in mental health care: Its roots need to be situated in the early 1980s.

The book by Fassin and Rechtman is one of the most recent additions to the growing literature on how concerns with mental health have come to the fore in recent times. One of the decisive moments that scholars working in this field of research regularly point to is the inclusion of post-traumatic stress disorder (PTSD) in 1980 in the *Diagnostic and Statistical Manual of Mental Disorders*, third edition (DSM-III), after a successful campaign of traumatized Vietnam veterans and their supporters in the late 1970s [Scott, 1990]. PTSD quickly became a highly successful and closely studied diagnosis. A conservative count yielded more than 16,000 publications by 1999 [Summerfield, 2001:95]. An editor of the *American Journal of Psychiatry* observed in 1995, somewhat ironically, that PTSD is the only psychiatric diagnosis that patients want to have [Rechtman, 2004:914]. The attractiveness of PTSD is partly explainable by the fact that it uniquely supposes a single cause. As Summerfield [2001:97] notes: "What makes the disorder preferred to other potential diagnoses is the term 'post-traumatic' in its name, which seems to 'prove' a direct aetiological link between the present and an index event in the past that excludes other factors."

According to Rechtman, PTSD has to a large extent contributed to the recognition of the suffering of victims of all kinds of stressful events; however, so he adds, they have paid a price for this, that is, "a reconfiguration of this *condition of victim*, in which a *human condition*—being a victim—has come to be locked into a *clinical condition*—suffering from a *PTSD*" [Rechtman, 2002:778; present author's translation]. The price, then, is that human suffering comes to be captured in a specific language and framework of understanding: When there is a stressful event and the symptoms are identified, then suffering, according to the logic of PTSD, is equaled with traumatization. There is growing critical literature on how this way of reasoning has impacted on international interventions in war-affected countries. During the 1990s, the psychological effect of war on populations became a major preoccupation, and various psychosocial programs were promoted to facilitate psychological healing. This stands in sharp contrast with earlier humanitarian interventions that hardly took healing war trauma as a target and tends to override other—and, arguably, often more pressing—needs of people in postconflict situations, that is, rebuilding communities, schools, basic infrastructure, economic activity, and so forth. Pupavac speaks of an "international therapeutic governance" which "pathologizes war-affected populations as psychologically dysfunctional. As such, they are deemed to lack the capacity for self-government without extensive external management to break intergenerational cycles of psychosocial dysfunction" [Pupavac, 2004:378].

Pupavac's critique, as she stresses, is not meant to deny that people are marked by experiences but is directed at how current thinking presumes universal vulnerability and the necessity of intervention at the expense of resilience and survivorship. Moreover, this "therapeutic governance" often does not take into account how people in war-affected nations understand and experience their suffering and how they respond to it: The Western therapeutic model is supplanted to such regions without having regard to culture-specific coping strategies and positive capacities for self-government [Pupavac, 2002, 2004]. This is also why some have warned against using PTSD in non-Western war-affected countries: The category is built on Western-based assumptions of individuality that are often not shared in those countries; therefore, it tends to emphasize similarities in responses to trauma while underestimating the differences between cultural groups. As a result, also the assumption that individual treatment strategies developed in the West can be transferred to non-Western settings has been seriously questioned [e.g., Bracken et al., 1995; Summerfield, 1999].

Sociologists such as Nolan [1998] and Furedi [2004] have argued that preoccupations with mental health issues are not restricted to large-scale terrorist attacks or postwar zones but have pervaded Western cultures that tend to elevate emotional well-being to a most precious good. They speak of "therapeutic states" and "therapy cultures." Crucial thereby is that the cultural understanding of behaviors and experiences tends to change. As Furedi notes: "therapeutics does not simply reflect uncertainties it also cultivates a distinct orientation towards the world. It sensitises people to regard a growing range of their experiences as victimising and as trauma-tising" [Furedi, 2004:129]. Also for Furedi the response to the attacks of 9/11 exemplified the influence of the therapeutic: "The guidance offered to the public was underwritten by the conviction that most Americans required some form of therapeutic instruction to come to terms with the tragedy" [Furedi, 2004:13].

A culture becomes therapeutic, so Furedi argues, "when this form of thinking expands from informing the relationship between the individual and therapist to shaping public perceptions about a variety of issues" [Furedi, 2004:22; see also Fassin and Rechtman, 2007:18]. A therapy culture provides scripts through which people come to understand themselves and their relationships with others. They solve problems, and they face challenges through a therapeutic lens. Dramatic episodes in life then are made sense of in mental health terms, and coping with painful encounters is influenced by prevailing therapeutic frameworks. This does not imply that these authors see le trau-matisme or therapy culture as the sole cultural force impinging on people. Rather, they aim to highlight how a new language, new frameworks, and new forms of expertise have become available and impact on self-understanding and social organization.

In the next two sections, we will discuss how a similar therapeutic idiom has been used to speak about the needs of victims of crime and how this has come to inform formal responses to crime. In the third section, we have a closer look at how the psychological healing of victims has in recent years been addressed in a particular stream of restorative justice research. In the fourth section, we illustrate that such attention for victims of crime is not restricted to restorative justice but pervades different corners of the traditional criminal justice system.

18.3 Restorative Justice and Healing Victims

"Can Mediation Be Therapeutic for Crime Victims?" This is the title of a recent research article published by the *Canadian Journal of Criminology and Criminal Justice*. In the article, Wemmers and Cyr [2005] explore to what extent restorative justice may help the "healing process" of victims. They use "therapeutic jurisprudence" as a framework to study a group of crime victims who participated in a victim–offender mediation program in a large city in Quebec. The researchers explore themes such as victims' fear, whether participation in the program helped them to put the event behind them, whether they benefited from the meeting, whether they judged the process to be fair, and whether they were satisfied with the process followed in their case. The results discussed in the article led them, after considering the limitations of the study, to the conclusion that procedural justice facilitates "healing" and that mediation contributed to the victims' well-being.

This article is one recent example of how victims' needs start to enter the restorative justice research agenda in new—therapeutically imagined—ways. It inscribes itself in a new generation of empirical research on restorative justice where measuring positive effects on victims' well-being begins to occupy a central role. In early evaluation studies, the satisfaction rate ("To what extent are participants in a restorative program satisfied with the experience?") was already commonly used to measure the success of restorative interventions. But now we seem to be witnessing a qualitative shift: Notions such as "healing," "closure," "therapeutic effects," "emotional restoration," and "reducing the sense of alienation" point to something different, that is, restorative justice in these recent reformulations is no longer merely about making or keeping all participants satisfied (i.e., a consumer logic) but also, and increasingly, about making victims feel better (i.e., a therapeutic logic).

At his 2002 Presidential Address for the American Society of Criminology, Lawrence Sherman [2003], who plays a key role in these recent developments, pleaded for a new paradigm of emotionally intelligent justice. Modern criminology needs to reinvent justice around the emotions of victims, offenders, and society. The major part of his address was devoted to restorative justice and its potential contributions to such a new paradigm. However, he also suggested, *inter alia*, wider use of medical and nutritional programs for offenders to improve their emotional state. Sherman quoted research on the successful use of fluoxetine (Prozac) for reducing violence or aggressive incidents and referred to a study that found that a daily dose of supplementary vitamins and minerals had a substantial effect on reducing disciplinary mis-conduct in prison [Sherman, 2003:23]. "Is a world with more pharmacology and less prison better or worse than a world with more prison but less phar-macology?" he asks at the end of a section on medical and nutritional pro-grams [Sherman, 2003:25].

In her book *Repair or Revenge*, Heather Strang [2002a], a close collabora-tor of Sherman, presents the results of her study on victim-oriented expecta-tions and outcomes in relation to restorative justice conferencing. The study was conducted as part of a large empirical research program on restorative justice, the so-called RISE project.* The randomized design of RISE enabled Strang to compare the experiences of "court victims" (i.e., victims who were assigned to traditional court proceedings) with those of "conference victims" (i.e., victims who were assigned to a restorative justice conference). In gen-eral, victims who participated in the conferences seemed to have better expe-riences. Conferencing turned out to be especially successful with respect to "emotional restoration." Levels of anger and anxiety were reduced. The fear of revictimization was considerably lower than for court victims. Nearly four times as many conference victims received an apology [see also Strang, 2002b; Strang and Sherman, 2003].

At this moment Strang is codirector of the Jerry Lee Program on Randomized Controlled Experiments in Restorative Justice, a large research program based at the University of Pennsylvania.† The goal of the program is to further develop evidence-based theory and policy on restorative jus-tice. In a working paper, the aim of the project is formulated as "to learn whether a new kind of justice can change people's lives for the better, with long-term effects" [Sherman et al., 2004:2]. Interestingly, the program pays a lot of attention to victims and how participating in restorative initiatives may change their lives for the better. The first research question following the above quote goes as follows: "Can it cure the post-traumatic stress symptoms and improve the health of crime victims?" Somewhat further in the work-ing paper, in a section on "Victim Effects," the question is further specified:

---

* RISE stands for reintegrative shaming experiments, which started in 1995 in Canberra. It explicitly refers to the theory of reintegrative shaming of John Braithwaite [1989]. In his book, Braithwaite argued that shame is the missing element—the "glue"—that is able to connect different criminological theories (labeling, subcultural, control, oppor-tunity, and learning theories). In doing so, Braithwaite developed an ambitious general theory of crime with important policy implications: The key to tackle crime is shaming that reintegrates (as opposed to shaming that stigmatizes). Braithwaite was the strong man behind RISE and is a key figure in the international restorative justice movement.

† In a leaflet presenting the research program and emphasizing its scope, it is argued that "the Jerry Lee Program has initiated a total of 12 RCTs [RCTs are randomized controlled trials, my comment] in restorative justice, and has been funded to undertake a total of 16 RCTs, making it the largest coordinated program of controlled experiments in the history of criminology"; see http://www.sas.upenn.edu/jerrylee/research/rj_jlc_rct.pdf (accessed September 13, 2008).

"What are the long-term effects of restorative justice on crime victims' health, employment, happiness and lawfullness, and how long do these effects (if any) last?" [Sherman et al., 2004:2, 8].

It is not a coincidence that victims receive a great deal of attention in the program and that measuring victim effects is mentioned first in the "to do" list. The researchers conclude that benefits for victims are much more consistently demonstrated than those related to offenders: The evidence related to reducing reoffending is found to be much less clear-cut. In a recently published article they felt the need to respond to some scorning newspaper headlines. An Oxford University study that reported no crime-reducing effects of restorative justice (but neither crime increases) in the Thames Valley area provoked headlines such as "Saying Sorry Does Not Work" and "Thugs Who Say Sorry Reoffend." Interestingly, the response of the authors to these headlines was not to cite a long list of empirical studies that *do* find crime-reducing effects. Instead, they deplored that none of those newspaper articles asked whether victims derived any benefit from the restorative process [Strang et al., 2006:282]. This move makes sense not only from a scientific point of view (i.e., the benefits for victims are easier to measure and demonstrate) but also from a strategic point of view: A reform movement that aims to influence policymaking needs to be able to adapt itself to changing circumstances, new research findings, and external demands. From this perspective, it also becomes strategically more interesting to further explore potential benefits for victims of crime.

This exploration goes far. It has been suggested that the costs of crime should include emotional costs (victims' fear, anger, grievance, and loss of trust) and medical costs (post-traumatic stress symptoms [PTSS], which include reduced immune function, higher rates of disease, greater use of medical services, and higher mortality from cancer or cardiovascular disease) [Strang et al., 2006:281–82]. These newly added emotional and medical dimensions to the crime cost figure refer to changing emotional states of victims and furthering trauma recovery. One of the clearest illustrations of how this comes to be incorporated in research on restorative justice is the recent study by Angel [2005]. Angel investigated the impact of restorative justice conferencing on crime victims' PTSS. A sample of victims of burglary and robbery who participated in a London-based randomized controlled trial was divided in experimental and control groups. Both were phoned by Angel at two points: the first phone interview took place shortly after the restorative justice conference, and the second occurred 6 months after the first interview. These phone interviews lasted about 20 minutes: Roughly 10 minutes were allocated for the Parent Study (to which Angel's study was supplemented), and 10 minutes for the data collection of her study. The victim questionnaire included 12 questions on crime experience (e.g., Did you see the offender? Did you have any verbal interaction with the offender? Were you physically injured during the crime?), 16 attribution questions (e.g., With respect to the crime, have you thought "Why did this happen to me?" Do you blame yourself or place responsibility on yourself for the crime? Do you blame the offender for the crime?), and 22 questions probing for PTSS during the past 7 days before the interview took place (e.g., Any reminder brought back feelings about the crime? You had trouble staying asleep? Other things kept making you think about it?) [Angel, 2005:120–28].

Angel argued that her study yielded three major findings: "Conferences do not increase PTSS and thereby further psychologically harm victims; conferences, in fact, reduce the traumatic effects of crime and; conference participation is a predictor of lower PTSS six months following participation, while ruminating about 'why did this happen to me?' predicts greater PTSS" [Angel, 2005:vii]. In the discussion Angel suggested that there is "clinical therapeutic value to RJ conferences" [Angel, 2005:92]. And she continued: "given the range of psychological distress that victims will suffer as a result of their crime, conferences can provide them with a 'treatment' intervention without participants feeling the stigmatic associations of seeking counseling services" [Angel, 2005:93]. With these observations in mind and the expressed desire to shift toward Sherman's new paradigm of "emotionally intelligent justice"* she reimagined the criminal justice system as potentially the most widely available and accessible mental health service for crime victims: "The criminal justice system has a unique advantage over traditional clinically based treatment services since it encompasses such a wide net for catching victims" [Angel, 2005:93].

What is interesting for our discussion in this chapter is not that new victim needs are discovered (victimology has been mapping these for many years) but that arguments are put forward that formal reactions to crime should adequately respond to these needs. In other words, new *therapeutically imagined* elements are added to the discussion of penal reform to argue that victims are not properly taken care of in the classical criminal justice system. For example, to argue that restorative conferencing is better at reducing PTSS than the classical criminal justice system is not only an empirical statement but also a normative one: It assumes that formal responses to crime should have low PTSS scores as one of their objectives—an objective they never had. This goes further than arguing that criminal justice agencies, in their dealings with crime victims, should be vigilant for causing secondary victimization: The primary victimization itself (i.e., the harm caused by the crime) becomes the target for remedial interventions. Moreover, as we will elaborate further on in the fifth section, there is an assumption of the

---

* "The goal of this criminologist was to assist in re-inventing the current justice system as an 'emotionally intelligent' system, requiring justice authorities to take into account the emotional state of citizen participants throughout the process [Sherman, 2003]." [Angel 2005:81].

universality of victims' trauma embedded in this new wave of research: A set of normal reactions of victims to their victimization is reformulated as "symptoms" following a "traumatic" experience. Indeed, they all become classified in clinical terms as PTSS. This has deep implications not only for how we tend to perceive victims of crime (i.e., their experiences become pathologized and therefore tend to be judged as in need of treatment) but also for offenders and the criminal justice system at large.

18.4 Psychological Restoration and Broader Criminal Justice

Attention for victims' needs is not restricted to restorative justice interventions. The question: "How to offer an appropriate response to the needs, wishes, and desires of victims of crime?" is increasingly at the center of public debate, and it has become a standard ingredient of criminal justice reform proposals. Cesoni and Rechtman [2005] argue that criminal justice procedures and sanctions are given a function of reconstruction—which they refer to as "psychological reparation" (*réparation psychologique*); that is, it becomes imperative to assist victims to recover from the psychological consequences of the crime. According to the French philosopher Frédéric Gros [2001, 2006], we have witnessed the birth and rise of a new way of thinking about punishment. The three classical models—punishment as reaffirming the law (Kant), punishment as defending society (Hobbes), and punishment as educating an individual (Plato)—have been joined by a fourth: punishment as enabling victims to mourn, to recover, to cure. A similar transformation has been observed by scholars writing on transitional justice, truth and reconciliation commissions and other mechanisms to deal with postconflict situations: Truth-telling and reconciliation are perceived to fulfill a healing function [Moon, 2007, 2008; Brounéus, 2008]. They all point at how criminal (or transitional) justice procedures and sentencing should actively contribute to victims' well-being, how penal and other responses are claimed to produce positive therapeutic effects for victims of crime [see also Digneffe, 2004; Salas, 2004, 2005; Arènes, 2005].

More controversially, the most punitive of sanctions, that is, the death penalty, has been justified by having recourse to a similar kind of therapeutic language and a promise to "heal victims" and bring "closure" for the relatives. It is important to note from the outset that such claims, unlike the ones discussed in the previous section, are not built on scientific research. Indeed, in his book on capital punishment in the United States, Franklin Zimring argues that the term *closure* has been "a public relations godsend," and that it defies empirical studies because it is a "belief system," "a justification built on a foundation of faith" [Zimring, 2003:58, 63; see also Peterson Armour, and Umbreit, 2007]. The American experience with the death penalty demonstrates how a "folk wisdom" about victimization, a set of common sense assumptions about what victims need and how we should respond to those needs, informs penal practices and justifications. This folk wisdom needs to be differentiated from a victimological understanding, but it is interesting and important to observe that it tends to be couched in a similar-sounding therapeutic idiom; therefore, it serves as an additional indicator of how firmly the idea of "healing victims" as a goal or justification for criminal justice interventions has been settled in the minds of people and institutions.

At the beginning of his book *When the State Kills*, Austin Sarat refers to a decision by U.S. Attorney General Ashcroft to broadcast the execution of Timothy McVeigh, who was found guilty of the 1995 Oklahoma City bombing that killed 168 people, by means of a CCTV network.* Ashcroft argued that victims and their relatives had a unique and compelling claim to witness the execution: Watching McVeigh die came to be represented as a prerequisite for closure, a necessary condition for putting the victims' tragedy behind [Sarat, 2002:xii]. In fact, this way of reasoning runs against an age-old belief that decent citizens should not be exposed to the "spectacle of suffering," a belief that led to a gradual removal of the execution of punishment (whether by death or imprisonment) out of public view and behind high walls [e.g., see Banner, 2002; Pratt, 2002]. The therapeutic imagination, however, makes it possible to invent new alleged benefits for victims to get closely involved with the ceremony of execution.

Zimring argues that a kind of "personal service symbolism" is at work in the American imagery of capital punishment: "The death penalty ... is regarded as a policy intended to serve the interests of the victims of crime and those who love them, a personal rather than a political concern, an undertaking of government to serve the needs of individual citizens for justice and psychological healing" [Zimring, 2003:49]. This emphasis on harm and victim psychology is a fairly recent phenomenon but has come to play a profound role in how capital punishment is nowadays pictured in the United States. Especially the term *closure* has made impressive inroads in capital punishment talk: Before 1989 it did not appear in death penalty stories; however, in 2001 more than 500 stories combined "capital punishment" with "closure" [Zimring, 2003:60]. According to Furedi [2004:2] the terms *healing* and *closure* were the two most often-used words in reporting after the McVeigh case. And it did not remain restricted to reporting: The political "therapeutic" style of former U.S. President Bill Clinton—I know what you

---

* Around 2,000 victims were invited to witness the execution. In the end only 232 (or less than 12%) accepted the invitation. A journalist of the *Miami Herald* connected an interesting question to this observation: What does it say about the death penalty if more than 88% of those directly involved did not wish to witness an execution justified in their name? [Castro, 2001].

feel—also was welcomed after the fatal bombing. William Schnieder from the *Washington Post* wrote the following about this: "Remember all those jokes about how Clinton 'feels your pain'? Well, we were all feeling pain after the Oklahoma City bombing. The president expressed the country's pain eloquently at the memorial service. Clinton showed empathy and compassion— exactly what he does best" [Schnieder, cited in Nolan, 1998:288].

However, victims and suffering not only appear at the end of the whole process (i.e., the execution of the culprit), but also have come to the fore during trial. In fact, victims' suffering can be presented in different ways: Experts may testify in court; victims' experiences may be written down in reports that subsequently are presented in court; or victims themselves can testify orally in court about their suffering. The two latter forms are known as victim impact statements (VIS) and have a place in a range of Anglo-Saxon countries, and have recently also been introduced in the Netherlands [De Keijser and Malsch, 2002; Kelk, 2003; Kool and Moerings, 2004]. Advocates of VIS argue that it can perform two main functions: an instrumental (i.e., to influence decision making and affect sentencing) and an expressive (i.e., it provides an opportunity for victims to express themselves regarding the impact of the crime) function. It is especially the latter that is interesting here. It is argued that VIS has various "therapeutic" benefits and helps victims' "psychological healing" and "reduce their trauma" [Erez, 2000].

It is interesting to note that Erez, a long-time advocate of VIS, explicitly refused to touch on the link between VIS and capital punishment in a recent chapter where she discusses the advantages of VIS.* That link is a sensitive topic and probably makes VIS advocates feel somewhat uncomfortable: At the penalty stage, the available options are limited to death or life imprisonment, and an emotional testimony of how relatives of victims have suffered might tip the balance in favor of the first option. Legal scholars who are wary of a too grand role for victims in capital cases have expressed deep worries about the implications of VIS in the wake of the U.S. Supreme Court decision in *Payne v. Tennessee* in 1991. The case involved the killings of a young mother, Charisse Christopher, and her 2-year-old daughter, Lacie. Her little son, Nicholas, was stabbed. His grandmother would testify in court about the devastating emotional impact this experience had on the little boy. In its ruling, the Supreme Court allowed the admission of VIS in capital trials,

---

* The reason she gave for not addressing the use of VIS in capital cases sounds a little too easy: "This article does not address the use of VIS in capital cases, which has attracted much of the opposition to the VIS in the United States. Most Western countries do not use death sentences as a penalty option" [Erez, 2004:81, note 1]. The fact that the death penalty is not an option in most Western societies outside the United States should not prevent us from engaging seriously with the reasons why so many scholars are skeptical of VIS *because of* its use in capital cases.

thereby reversing its earlier case law.* In critical commentary that decision has variously been described as a "legitimation of revenge" [Sarat, 1997:165] and an "undifferentiated endorsement of harm as a sentencing factor" [Dubber, 1993:124; see also Simon, 2004].

18.5 Discussion

The research that we discussed in the third section seems to be built on the assumption that such a more pronounced orientation toward healing victims is also a highly desirable development. Moreover, the fact that conferencing and mediation yield better results in this respect can easily be transformed into a new and powerful argument to advance the cause of further implementing restorative justice approaches in the wider criminal justice system: Those who still doubt or those who oppose may be willing to abandon their reservations when they learn that victims benefit most of all parties involved. Victims service organizations, for example, which in the past have been critical about the instrumentalization of victims within restorative justice interventions that focused too much on rehabilitating offenders, may now look differently at restorative justice. The same holds for those who oppose restorative interventions because these are judged to be too soft for offenders: Suddenly the victim becomes the main benefactor, and the confrontation with the victim's suffering is, moreover, not all that pleasant. In sum, from a strategic point of view this focus on measuring victim effects may have a number of advantages because it may increase the social and political appeal of restorative justice in a victim-sensitive context, and, in addition, it may lead to a higher number of victims willing to participate in restorative programs. However, in the long run, this particular focus on victim effects may have deep implications for the future of restorative and criminal justice. In this section we explore some themes that, so it seems to us, are in need of further examination.

When criminal justice interventions are aimed at healing victims then this also impacts on the expectations being raised toward the offender as victimizer, that is, offenders are called on to contribute to the healing process of the victim. Consider, for example, the following reasons that Wemmers and Cyr [2005] presented for why victims felt less positive about their participation in a mediation program: One victim reported that she felt more fearful

---

* Four years earlier in *Booth v. Maryland* [1987] the majority of the Supreme Court found victim impact evidence to be unconstitutional under the Eighth Amendment's ban on "cruel and unusual punishment." Four reasons were given: (1) VIS creates a substantial risk of prejudice; (2) the focus should be on the wrong, not the harm; (3) use of VIS would turn the trial into a test of the rhetorical skills of the victim's relatives; and (4) VIS introduces passion and emotion and therefore would threaten the rational decision-making process [see Sarat, 1997:174].

because the offender did not regret his or her behavior; two victims felt worse after meeting with the offender because of his or her refusal to take responsibility for his or her actions; and for the same reason some victims suffered revictimization.

The conclusion that might be drawn from this (i.e., if such a therapeutic orientation toward victims is perceived to be desirable—which seems to be a settled question for both researchers) is that, to enhance the well-being of victims, offenders should regret their behavior and take responsibility for their actions. The same holds true for the importance that has been attributed to the role of apology. In *Repair or Revenge*, Strang [2002a:18–23] emphasized the "victims' need for apology," and in one of the studies coming out of the Jerry Lee Program it was used as a criterion to measure the success of restorative conferencing: "The criterion here is whether RJ conferences result in more apologies" [Sherman et al., 2005:373].

Such an emphasis on excuses, regret, apologies, and responsibility implies that victims' well-being comes, at least in part, to depend on action taken by the offender. Indeed, such research suggests that without an apology there is less chance of recovery. There is a danger for a different kind of instrumentalization here: not the victim who is being used to facilitate the rehabilitation of the offender, but the offender as the person who is assumed to hold the key to help the victim cure. This raises a number of questions that restorative justice advocates will need to address in the future: What are the implications of such expectations for the emotional dynamics of a restorative intervention? Does this facilitate a form of emotional conformity whereby only the "proper" emotions will be given space? What if an offender refuses to cooperate with the emotional restoration of the victim? [see also Acorn, 2004; Richards, 2005; Daems and Robert, 2006].

To argue that criminal justice systems should heal victims, that they should strive toward certain predefined mental health effects, is to assume that there is "something" to heal, that is, that victims are all damaged or traumatized in one way or another. After her review of some victimological research, Strang concluded the following: "All these research findings indicate the *universality of the trauma of victimization* and the high levels of dissatisfaction regarding the usual treatment victims receive at the hands of the criminal justice system" [Strang, 2002a:19, my italics]. After citing data from the British Crime Survey on fear of crime, various pieces of research that document victims' need for emotional support, evidence that victimization leads to "adverse mental health outcomes," and studies that have found that victims of property and violent crimes suffer problems that include "severe and persistent psychosomatic symptoms and impairment in social functioning," Angel concludes, on the very first page of her study, that "there is a large body of international research that illustrates *the enormity of the problem*" [Angel, 2005:1, my italics]. This conclusion then forms the starting point for her study whether restorative justice can contribute to solving this "enormous problem." For Angel, victims of crime, by definition, suffer from emotional problems and seem to be in need of professional help. Seen from this perspective, those who refused to participate in the experiment then are likely to be in denial and probably are even more in need of help than the others: "Roughly 45% of victims approached to participate in the Parent Study refused to do so, despite having a willing offender. By the nature of avoidant responses inherent to PTSD, it is quite possible that those most affected by PTSS and PTSD would decline to participate" [Angel, 2005:87].

The possibilities that these victims did not feel the need to participate in the program, that in the meantime things may have happened to them that gave their lives a positive turn, that their victimization was only a minor event in their life course, that PTSS did not dominate the victims' accounts of their suffering, that the natural healing process had made them recover, and/or that they received sufficient nonprofessional support from their social network are not mentioned as potential explanations. In particular, the latter is strikingly absent throughout the whole research: Somewhat paradoxically, the only event "social" in nature included in the study is the "treatment," that is, the restorative justice conference where victims are expected to be supported by figures from their social network. Family, relatives, friends, neighbors, and so forth only come into the picture for a couple of hours, that is, when they play their role in the experiment, but they then magically disappear during the many months that pass between the victimization and the follow-up interview.

Like with those earlier pathologizing assumptions about offenders, it is important to interrogate such images of victims. Indeed, such a general assumption of victims being "emotionally damaged" may be neither true nor very appealing for the persons labeled in that way. Sebba argues that "many—indeed, apparently most—victimizations are overcome within a relatively short period" [Sebba, 2000:60]. Fattah emphasizes the need for profound knowledge about the differential impact of victimization and the differential needs of crime victims: "The indisputable fact that crime victims constitute a highly diverse and heterogeneous group means that the impact of victimization and the consequences of the victimizing event will be extremely different from one victim group to another, and from one individual victim to the other" [Fattah, 1999:193; see also Fattah, 2006:93–95, 97–99]. Moreover, Fattah highlights how the "amplification of the negative effects of victimization" and the "pathologising of the normal reactions it evokes" lead to the creation of "a specific pattern of suffering that almost forces them to feel and behave in a certain manner. Victims feel compelled to conform to this pattern of suffering because otherwise they might not be, or be seen as, normal or typical victims" [Fattah, 1999:196].

Three years after his keynote address at the Ninth International Symposium on Victimology, where Fattah raised the above-mentioned worries, he predicted the "demise of victim therapy" in the "not too distant future." Fattah added that the "natural healing powers of the human psyche that are being interfered with, and hindered by, professional therapies, are bound to reaffirm themselves" [Fattah, 2000:41–42]. In light of our discussion in this chapter, this prediction may have turned out to be too premature. Moreover, the focus on "victim therapy" in the strict sense obfuscates how also traditional criminal justice responses may get "therapeutised" and, in their wake, lead to the implicit adoption and promotion of assumptions about victims being emotionally damaged. In this sense it is, for example, remarkable how the restorative justice literature in recent years has become oriented toward researching "victim effects" and advocating restorative programs as an attractive option for victim recovery. Indeed, such victim-oriented "therapeutisation" of restorative justice seems to be highly incompatible with some of its core values, such as active participation and reciprocal communication [Daems, 2007].

It should be clear that the ways in which we depict victims of crime and their needs have an impact on how we respond to criminal victimization. Indeed, even though, as we argued earlier in this section, the assumption overgeneralizes the impact of victimization and fails to differentiate between individual victims and groups of victims, it is, nevertheless, a powerful one that resonates with more wide-ranging preoccupations of mental health issues (see second section). One particular implication is that the image of the traumatized victim engenders new expectations toward their victimizers: The kind of person we expect offenders to be or become is not merely a law-abiding, industrious human but also a person who has the ability to empathize with the suffering of others and who is emotionally adequate him- or herself. Indeed, what Wemmers and Cyr perceived to be particularly problematic in view of the therapeutic value of mediation was that offenders were not taking responsibility for their actions or did not regret what they had done to the victim. When Strang and others highlight the need for an apology from the offender to further recovery, then it is, again, the emotional skills of offenders that are being problematized. Whether such offenders will reoffend is here (at least as long as there is no risk for revictimization of "their" victim), to a certain extent, beside the point: Offenders rather "fail" when they lack the vocabulary and skills to move themselves into the position of their victims, which, as such, may hamper their recovery [Daems and Robert, 2006:268]. When such expectations are prevalent, then also here (like in the case of Fattah's normal or typical victims who need to conform to a "specific pattern of suffering," see above) there is a risk that a specific pattern of behaving and feeling is established: The normal or typical victimizers then are those who produce the right set of emotions and make the expected gestures and moves. In a society preoccupied with emotional well-being, offenders may need to display not only conformity to the law but also an emotional conformity toward the victim.

18.6 Conclusion

The concern for the plight of victims of crime is often formulated by means of metaphorical language. One of the most common metaphors used by victimologists and reformers is the metaphor of "healing victims." Victims, in one way or another, need to be "healed": Their suffering needs to be alleviated; they need to be dealt with in such a way that their painful experiences soften and wither away, they become whole again, and they are enabled to recover from trauma or transform. Metaphors often can (and do) fulfill a critical function because they challenge the *status quo*; in this case, the *status quo* of a (perceived) offender-oriented criminal justice system that is insensitive to victims' needs. Metaphors can stimulate the imagination and offer an appealing and recognizable language that helps to increase public awareness of the perceived problem and that highlights the ways in which the problem needs to be solved.

However, metaphors involve the application of a word or phrase to something that it does not apply to literally. Recent developments in victimology and restorative justice research suggest, however, that we are no longer dealing with a metaphor: "Healing victims" has turned out to become something "real," to be applied "literally," and therefore stops being a metaphor. Healing victims tends to become a real objective, an emerging justification for penal interventions, a new way of looking at punishment and of evaluating criminal justice responses. If "healing victims" as a metaphor is in the process of dying, then this has deep implications for the ways in which we respond to crime and victimization, as well as for the ways in which we picture offenders and victims. Such topics then should move to the center of scholarly reflection in this area of research.

References

Acorn, A. 2004. *Compulsory compassion: A critique of restorative justice.* Vancouver: University of British Columbia Press.
Angel, C. M. 2005. Crime victims meet their offenders: Testing the impact of restorative justice conferences on victims' post-traumatic stress symptoms. Ph.D. diss., University of Pennsylvania.
Arènes, J. 2005. Tous victimes? *Études: Revue de culture contemporaine* 403(1/2):43–52.
Banner, S. 2002. *The death penalty: An American history.* Cambridge, MA: Harvard University Press.

Bracken, P. J., J. E. Giller, and D. Summerfield. 1995. Psychological responses to war and atrocity: The limitations of current concepts. *Social Science & Medicine* 40(8):1073–82.

Braithwaite, J. 1989. *Crime, shame and reintegration*. Cambridge: Cambridge University Press.

Brounéus, K. 2008. Truth telling as talking cure? Insecurity and retraumatization in the Rwandan Gacaca courts. *Security Dialogue* 39(1):55–76.

Castro, M. J. 2001. We kill for vengeance, not closure and justice. *Miami Herald* June 19. http://www.commondreams.org/views01/0619-05.htm (accessed September 13, 2008).

Cesoni, M. L. and R. Rechtman. 2005. La 'réparation psychologique' de la victime: Une nouvelle fonction de la peine? *Revue de droit pénal et de criminologie* 85(2):158–78.

Daems, T. 2005. Straf en therapie (andermaal). Van Kubrick naar Landuyt (en verder). *FATIK: Tijdschrift voor Strafbeleid en Gevangeniswezen* 107:16–18.

_____. 2007. De slachtofferdimensie van herstelrechtelijke interventies. Een sluimer-ende therapeutisering? *Tijdschrift voor Herstelrecht* 7(1):7–21.

Daems, T. and L. Robert. 2006. Victims, knowledge(s) and prisons: Victims enter-ing the Belgian prison system. *European Journal of Crime, Criminal Law and Criminal Justice* 14(3):256–70.

De Keijser, J. W. and M. Malsch. 2002. Is spreken zilver en zwijgen goud? Spreekrecht en het ontstemde slachtoffer. *Delikt & Delinkwent* 32(1):5–20.

Digneffe, F. 2004. Juger en démocratie. Les enjeux du procès pénal. In *Procès Dutroux. Penser l'émotion*, ed. V. Magos, 89–96. Brussels: Ministère de la Communauté française.

Dubber, M. D. 1993. Regulating the tender heart when the axe is ready to strike. *Buffalo Law Review* 41:85–156.

Erez, E. 2000. Integrating a victim perspective in criminal justice through victim impact statements. In *Integrating a victim perspective within criminal justice. International debates*, ed. A. Crawford and J. Goodey, 165–84. Aldershot: Ashgate.

_____. 2004. Integrating restorative justice principles in adversarial proceedings through victim impact statements. In *Reconcilable rights? Analyzing the tension between victims and defendants*, ed. E. Cape, 81–96. London: Legal Action Group Education and Service Trust Limited.

Fassin, D. and R. Rechtman. 2007. *L'Empire du traumatisme: Enquête sur la condition de victime*. Paris: Éditions Flammarion.

Fattah, E. A. 1999. From a handful of dollars to tea and sympathy: The sad history of victim assistance. In *Caring for crime victims. Selected proceedings of the 9th International Symposium on Victimology. Amsterdam, August 25–29, 1997*, ed. J. J. M. van Dijk, R. G. H. Kaam, and J. A. M. Wemmers, 187–206. Monsey, NY: Criminal Justice Press.

_____. 2000. Victimology: Past, present and future. *Criminologie* 33(1):17–46.

_____. 2006. Le sentiment d'insécurité et la victimisation criminelle dans une perspec-tive de victimologie comparée. In *Une criminologie de la tradition à l'innovation. En hommage à Georges Kellens*, ed. M. Born, F. Kéfer, and A. Lemaître, 89–106. Brussels: De Boeck & Larcier.

Furedi, F. 2004. *Therapy culture: Cultivating vulnerability in an uncertain age*. London: Routledge.

Gros, F. 2001. Les quatre foyers de sens de la peine. In *Et ce sera justice. Punir en démocratie*, ed. A. Garapon, F. Gros, and T. Pech, 11–138. Paris: Éditions Odile Jacob.

———. 2006. La victime, sujet de droit ou objet politique?. In *Le sexe et ses juges*, ed. E. Alt, 23–27. Paris: Éditions Syllepse.

Kelk, C. 2003. Slachtofferverklaringen in woord en geschrift. *Delikt & Delinkwent* 33(2):93–101.

Kool, R. and M. Moerings. 2004. The victim has the floor. The victim's right to be heard in writing or orally in the Dutch courtroom. *European Journal of Crime, Criminal Law and Criminal Justice* 12(1):46–60.

Lyon, D. 2003. *Surveillance after September 11*. Cambridge: Polity.

Moon, C. 2007. Reconciliation as therapy and compensation: A critical analysis. In *Law and the politics of reconciliation*, ed. S. Veitch, 163–84. Aldershot: Ashgate.

———. 2008. *Narrating political reconciliation. South Africa's truth and reconciliation commission*. Plymouth: Lexington Books.

Nolan, J. L., Jr. 1998. *The therapeutic state: Justifying government at century's end*. New York: New York University Press.

———. 2001. *Reinventing justice: The American drug court movement*. Princeton, NJ: Princeton University Press.

Peterson Armour, M. and M. S. Umbreit. 2007. The ultimate penal sanction and "closure" for survivors of homicide victims. *Marquette Law Review* 91:380–424.

Pratt, J. 2002. *Punishment and civilization*. London: Sage.

Pupavac, V. 2002. Pathologizing populations and colonizing minds: International psychosocial programs in Kosovo. *Alternatives* 27(4):489–511.

———. 2004. International therapeutic peace in Bosnia. *Social and Legal Studies* 13(3):377–401.

Rechtman, R. 2002. Être victime: Généalogie d'une condition clinique. *L'Évolution Psychiatrique* 67:775–95.

———. 2004. The rebirth of PTSD: The rise of a new paradigm in psychiatry. *Social Psychiatry and Psychiatric Epidemiology* 39:913–15.

Richards, K. M. 2005. Unlikely friends? Oprah Winfrey and restorative justice. *Australian and New Zealand Journal of Criminology* 38(3):381–99.

Salas, D. 2004. La nouvelle victime ou la dette sans réponse. In *Procès Dutroux. Penser l'émotion*, ed. V. Magos, 233–39. Brussels: Ministère de la Communauté française.

———. 2005. *La volonté de punir. Essai sur le populisme pénal*. Paris: Hachette Littératures.

Sarat, A. 1997. Vengeance, victims and the identities of law. *Social and Legal Studies* 6(2):163–89.

———. 2002. *When the state kills: Capital punishment and the American condition*. Princeton, NJ: Princeton University Press.

Scott, W. J. 1990. PTSD in DSM-III: A case in the politics of diagnosis and disease. *Social Problems* 37(3):294–310.

Sebba, L. 2000. The individualization of the victim: From positivism to postmodernism. In *Integrating a victim perspective within criminal justice*, ed. A. Crawford and J. Goodey, 55–76. Aldershot: Ashgate.

Sherman, L. W. 2003. Reason for emotion: Reinventing justice with theories, innovations, and research—The American Society of Criminology 2002 Presidential Address. *Criminology* 41(1):1–38.

Sherman, L. W., H. Strang, C. Angel, et al. 2005. Effects of face-to-face restorative justice on victims of crime in four randomized, controlled trials. *Journal of Experimental Criminology* 1(4):367–95.

Sherman, L. W., H. Strang, D. J. Woods, et al. 2004. *Restorative justice: What we know and how we know it*. http://www.sas.upenn.edu/jerrylee/research/rj_WorkingPaper. pdf (accessed September 13, 2008).

Simon, J. 2004. Fearless speech in the killing state: The power of capital crime victim speech. *North Carolina Law Review* 82:1377–413.

Strang, H. 2002a. *Repair or revenge: Victims and restorative justice*. Oxford: Oxford University Press.

_____. 2002b. Justice for victims of young offenders: The centrality of emotional harm and restoration. In *Restorative justice for juveniles. Conferencing, mediation and circles*, ed. A. Morris and G. Maxwell, 183–93. Oxford: Hart.

Strang, H. and L. W. Sherman. 2003. Repairing the harm: Victims and restorative justice. *Utah Law Review* 2003(1):15–42.

Strang, H., L. Sherman, C. M. Angel, et al. 2006. Victim evaluations of face-to-face restorative justice conferences: A quasi-experimental analysis. *Journal of Social Issues* 62(2):281–306.

Summerfield, D. 1999. A critique of seven assumptions behind psychological trauma programmes in war-affected areas. *Social Science & Medicine* 48:1449–62.

_____. 2001. The invention of post-traumatic stress disorder and the social usefulness of a psychiatric category. *British Medical Journal* 322:95–98.

Wemmers, J.-A. and K. Cyr. 2005. Can mediation be therapeutic for crime victims? An evaluation of victims' experiences in mediation with young offenders. *Canadian Journal of Criminology and Criminal Justice* 47:527–44.

Zimring, F. E. 2003. *The contradictions of American capital punishment*. New York: Oxford University Press.

The Healing Nature of Apology and Its Contribution toward Emotional Reparation and Closure in Restorative Justice Encounters

19

EYAL BROOK* AND SHARON
WARSHWSKI-BROOK

Contents

* An earlier draft of this essay was written while Eyal Brook was a student at the Institute of Criminology, University of Cambridge, UK.

To err is human; to forgive is divine.
—**Alexander Pope**

Learning to forgive is much more useful than merely picking up a stone and throwing it at the object of one's anger, the more so when the provocation is extreme. For it is under the greatest adversity that there exists the greatest potential for doing good, both for oneself and for others.
—**Dalai Lama**

19.1 Introduction

In the 1949 western *She Wore a Yellow Ribbon*, John Wayne plays the aging Captain Nathan Brittles, who advises his young successor: "Never apologize. It's a sign of weakness." This advice is ignored, and apologies are exchanged, which create stronger relationships between the younger officers [Young, 2001].

To a large extent, this advice still reflects a prevalent value, predominantly in the criminal justice prevailing in the Western legal society, according to which an apology is often perceived as an admission of guilt and therefore frequently ignored, albeit being an important tool and a powerful ritual that is necessary for emotional restoration.

However, despite the notable absence of apology in almost all areas of law, apology does have a limited legal history in Western culture. Martin Wright [1991] points out that in eighteenth-century England, criminal law was essentially carried out by crime victims, who decided whether to initiate prosecutions and what the charges would be. With the advent of professional prosecutors and the disappearance of the victim from the process, the role of apology in English criminal law came to an end.

The right to punish in most current criminal justice systems belongs to the state and not the victims, and many courts exclude testimony by victims or their relatives concerning the proper punishment. Wagatsuma and Rosett [1986] argue that apology survives today in many criminal law systems primarily to the extent that it could be viewed by a judge as a mitigating factor at a sentencing hearing. Such a situation, however, conflicts with many people's moral intuition because crime has a human face, which should have a say in the matter [Bibas, 2007]. Nevertheless, most victims say they do not want to be the arbiter of punishment for their offenders and have other priorities instead [Strang, 2002].

Victim studies during the past 2 decades show that what victims want the most is not material reparation but rather symbolic reparation, primarily an apology and a sincere expression of remorse* [Marshall and Merry, 1990; Dignan, 1992; Strang, 2002, 2004].

---

* When victims are asked what they want, the following replies were frequently encountered: a less formal process where their views count; participation in their case; more information about both the processing and outcome of their case; respectful and fair treatment, material restoration; and most importantly, emotional restoration, including an apology [Strang, 2004].

However, in general, victimology literature makes little mention of victims' desire for apologies from their offender [Strang and Sherman, 2003]. In many ways, apology has been neglected because victims have traditionally been removed from the criminal proceedings. Christie [1977] argued that conflicts have been taken away from victims. He claimed that victims have lost the chance to participate in their own case, and that offenders have lost the opportunity to deal with the consequences of their misdeeds.

Only in the past 20 years has there been a rise of the victim movement. Hence it is relatively recently that apology has come to be seen as central to the process of restoration. In restorative justice communications, apologies are one of the most common features [Braithwaite, 1999] and are usually seen as central to the process of emotional restoration. Almost all accounts of restorative justice emphasize the desirability of an apology as a prelude to meaningful reparation and reconciliation [Bottoms, 2003].

In this chapter, we discuss the importance of apology and its healing nature, as well as its contribution toward emotional restoration. In the next section, we present various definitions of apology and discuss its healing nature. We consider the benefits of apology to both offender and victim and discuss the requirements for an effective apology. We then discuss how apology can lead to forgiveness and free the victim from the desire for revenge. In the third section, we evaluate various reasons for the absence of apology in criminal justice, emphasizing the effects of the adversarial culture and legal education. In the fourth section, we discuss the importance of apology in restorative justice encounters, arguing that restorative justice conferences are more encouraging of apology compared with conventional justice. We also highlight the importance of the interpersonal element and face-to-face encounters, which are crucial if a true emotional restoration is to be achieved. Finally, we discuss Japan as an example of a society that attaches importance to apology and demonstrates a restorative nature, which, it has been suggested, may be associated with a low crime rate [Braithwaite, 1989].

We argue that the absence of apology in Western society and criminal justice constitutes a failure and will suggest its increased use.

19.2 The Importance of Apology and Its Healing Nature

We may not have to live in the past, but the past lives in us.
—**Samuel Pisar**
Of Blood and Hope

19.2.1 Definitions

Apologies are extremely complex forms of communication. According to Tavuchis [1991], an apology is an act of speech that fully acknowledges responsibility for wrongdoing. It is a form of ritual exchange in which words are spoken that may enable conclusion, or closure, of the criminal event. The efficacy of an apology can be attributed to its status as an act of speech. The offender must not only be sorry but also say so. Speech makes all the difference and is most effective because of its revelatory character. Tavuchis argued that apology should be viewed as a corrective ritual that restores a moral power imbalance between two parties. It is a diplomatic act in which the offender places him- or herself in an inferior position to the offended party and asks for forgiveness.

Words of apology are necessary to maintain interaction between the parties, following an injury of one by the other, be it physical, psychological, or financial. Apologetic words can be used to express sympathy, understanding, and regret; an apology, offered and accepted, has tremendous power to restore relationships. Apology can heal psychic wounds, teach lessons, and reconcile damaged relationships. It helps to subtract the insult from the injury, thereby minimizing the injured party's anger toward the offender [Cohen, 1999].

Various definitions of apology have been offered, many stressing an acknowledgment of the harm suffered by the victim. Cohen [1999] mentions that the word *apology* derives from the Greek root *logos*, meaning "speech" or "word." Although originally associated with a formal justification, defense, or explanation [as in Plato's *apologia*; see West, 1979], apology also refers to remarks made following an injury, whether intentional or not. In this latter usage, an apology is defined as, "an acknowledgement intended as an atonement for some improper or injurious remark or an act. An admission to another of a wrong or discourtesy done him accompanied by an expression of regret" [*Webster's Third New International Dictionary*, 1961] or "[a]n explanation offered to a person affected by one's action that no offense was intended, coupled with the expression of regret for any that may have been given; or, a frank acknowledgment of the offense with expression of regret for it, by way of reparation" [*Oxford English Dictionary*, 2nd ed., 1989]. The modern usage of the word refers to "an expression of error or discourtesy accompanied by an expression of regret" [see *Webster's Collegiate Dictionary*, 10th ed., 1998:55].

In accord with current restorative justice understandings, Goffman [1971:113] suggested that "an apology is a gesture through which an individual splits himself into two parts, the part that is guilty of an offence and the part that dissociates itself from the dereliction and affirms a belief in the offended rule." According to this view, the offender has a "blameworthy" self and a "sympathizing" self. Thus, the harm doer can be seen to have some portion of him- or herself that is worth forgiving.

Goffman described apology as a form of remedial work, the purpose of which is to alter the meaning of an act from harmful to acceptable.

He identified three ways in which to do this: "accounts," in which the harm doer provides an explanation but generally does not accept responsibility for the act; "apologies," in which a harm doer does accept responsibility for the act; and "requests," in which a person requests permission from another before committing an act that may be viewed as harmful [Goffman, 1971; Petrucci, 2002]. Goffman suggested [1971] that in its fullest form, an apology has several elements: expression of embarrassment; clarification that one knows better conduct had been expected and sympathizes with the application of negative sanction; verbal rejection, repudiation, and disavowal of wrongful behavior and vilification of one's self for wrongdoing; and espousal of the right way and an avowal henceforth to pursue that course.

Goffman's view is frequently cited, although some disagreement exists as to an apology's function, specifically relating to the presence of responsibility. Wagatsuma and Rosett [1986] have argued that a true apology must contain five elements: (1) an acknowledgment that an injurious act occurred and was wrong, (2) an acknowledgment of fault, (3) willingness to compensate the injured party, (4) a promise that the injurious act will not happen again, and (5) intention to work for good relations in the future. Concerning compensation, they argue that "apology without reparation is a hollow form, at least when the injured person has suffered a clear economic loss and when the actor has the capacity to make compensation" [ibid.:487]. Scheff [1998] added a further core element, "the expression of emotion by the offender, including feeling of sorrow, sadness, and visible shame," whereas Tavuchis [1991:3] suggests that an apology must minimally entail "acknowledgment of the legitimacy of the violated rule, admission of fault and responsibility for its violation, and the expression of genuine regret and remorse for the harm done."

Thus, some scholars perceive apology as an acknowledgment, a recognition, of a past injury that damages the bonds between the offending and offended parties, whereas others expand this notion to be not only past oriented but also future oriented (restitution and refraining from such future conduct).

19.2.2 The Healing Nature of Apology

> A man's very highest moment is, I have no doubt at all, when he kneels in the dust, and beats his breast, and tells all the sins of his life.
> —Oscar Wilde

Apology is a form of symbolic reparation, a ritual, acknowledging the harm done and reinstating the victim as someone to whom respect and reparation are due. Scheff [1998] identifies two types of reparation: material and symbolic. *Material reparation* is the result of a negotiated agreement between the victim and offender. *Symbolic reparation*, the more important of the two, occurs as a result of the direct communication between the victim and offender and hinges on social rituals of respect, courtesy, apology, and forgiveness. The concept of symbolic reparation has been widely emphasized, and it is considered essential if true reconciliation is to be achieved [Scheff and Retzinger, 1996]. It offers a way to heal the emotional damage caused by the offense.

At the heart of apology lies a genuine display of appeal to sorrow, as opposed to an appeal to reason. The key components of apology—an expression of remorse or regret, acceptance of responsibility, compensation, and a promise to avoid such behavior in the future—if performed in an authentic and emotional face-to-face interaction—and accepted by victims through forgiveness—could provide what Scheff and Retzinger[1996:316] refer to as the *core sequence*, the mechanism by which symbolic reparation occurs, allowing the victim to heal and the offender to take responsibility for the harmful act, be accepted back into society, and therefore have less reason to commit future offenses: "The core sequence generates repair and restoration of the bond between victim and offender.... It is the key to reconciliation, victim satisfaction, and decreasing recidivism." Moore [1993] suggests three factors that are important in this respect. First, victims are relieved to see and feel how other people share their anger, their humiliation as caused by the offense. Second, victim and offender achieve a sort of empathy, which in a sense makes the offender more normal. Third, concluding the reconciliation conference between the parties, the image of the offender no longer corresponds with a monster, and malice and hatred toward the offender are lightened.

Apology, although it might only be a brief moment in time, may often be the magic turning point that permits the conflicting parties to reconcile. An apology, if acknowledged, can restore trust. As Kastor [1998] puts it, "the past is not erased, but the present is changed." Tavuchis [1991:13] explains the social structural context of the apology, claiming that it "speaks to an act that cannot be undone, but that cannot go unnoticed without compromising the current and future relationship of the parties, the legitimacy of the violated rule and the wider social web in which the participants are enmeshed."

Apology is central to the process of restoration. Lazare [1995:40] suggests that "a genuine apology offered and accepted is one of the most profound interactions of civilized people. It has the power to restore damaged relationships between two people." He argues that apology offers a powerful exchange formula of shame and power:

> What makes an apology work is the exchange of shame and power between the offender and offended. By apologizing, you take the shame of your offence and redirect it to yourself. You admit to hurting or diminishing someone and, in effect, say that you are really the one who is diminished—I'm the one who was wrong, mistaken, insensitive, or stupid. In acknowledging your shame

you give the offended the power to forgive. The exchange is at the heart of the healing process. [ibid.:42]

Thus, apology also involves role reversal: The person apologizing relinquishes power and puts him- or herself at the mercy of the offended party, who may or may not accept the apology. This exchange, which is a dramatically powerful encounter, providing the victim with a moral supremacy, is at the heart of the healing process and contributes toward a change in the dynamics between the parties.

It seems that the spiritual and psychological functions of apology are frequently neglected. It is known that the basic human interaction process has significance for the victims in healing the psychological harm caused by crime. As Takahashi [2005] observes, "an apology cannot undo what has been done, but a sincere apology with remorse might increase the victim's empathy for the wrongdoer and open the door to forgiveness."

19.2.3 The Effective Apology

The effectiveness of an apology is related to various elements and has been defined by scholars in various terms: the genuine apology [Scheff, 1998], the meaningful apology [Wagatsuma and Rosett, 1986], the full-blown apology [Holtgraves, 1989], and the authentic apology [Tavuchis, 1991]. Three concepts surface as central to effective apologies: communicating emotions (such as remorse or sadness), a face-to-face interaction, and the timing of the apology [Petrucci, 2002]. The severity of the offense is another element that influences how these components should be executed. If it is successful, an apology can sometimes even work to place a relationship between two individuals on a higher level than it occupied before the injury.

One of the most important elements of the process is the degree of sincerity, meaning internal coherence and wholeheartedness. For an apology to comfort the injured party, it must be perceived to be sincere. It has been claimed that for an apology to work, the injured party must be convinced that the offender believes that he or she was at least partially responsible for an act that harmed the offended party and feels regret for the act [Levi, 1997]. For a genuine apology, the offender must drop all defenses. If the apology is perceived as insincere, there is a substantial risk of further alienation of the injured party.

Apology also has to demonstrate understanding of the nature of the wrongdoing and its effect on the person. Richard Nixon's famous resignation speech is a good example for what should *not* have been said. In his speech he said: "I regret deeply any injuries that may have been done in the course of the events that led to this decision [to resign]. I would say only that if some of my judgments were wrong, they were made in what I believed at the time to be in the best interest of the nation." This statement is far from a true apology. His expression of regret is linked both to the conditional and unspecified wrongs; neither meets the requirements of apology. The statement as a whole is an effort to justify and excuse deeds [Griswold, 2007]. To succeed, the apology has to be specific. The person who apologizes has to show that he or she understands the nature of the wrongdoing and the impact it had on the victim.

Furthermore, for the sincerity of the apology to be believed by the offended party, the intensity of the apology should reflect the intensity of the harm. A brief "I'm sorry" is unlikely to suffice in a case of a severe injury. A more serious and detailed apology is required to assuage the victim's feelings. Conversely, a brief apology may be sufficient in a case of a less severe impact [Ohbuchi et al., 1989]. However, such categorization can be problematic because the degree of severity is often a matter of subjective judgment.

The manner in which an apology is offered may also play a role in its perceived sincerity. Despite the fact that many lawyers may instinctively wish to speak for their clients, and many clients may wish to use their attorneys as spokespersons, there is no doubt that an apology offered directly by the offending party is much more effective [Bolstad, 2000]. The main issue is sincerity. Because an apology is meant to demonstrate the offender's sympathy and remorse, a direct apology from the offender should have greater impact. Echoing Buber's [1923] dialogical philosophy, which highlights the interpersonal nature of human existence,* it seems that the two parties are the central players, and no one can displace them in that role if the apologetic discourse is to be really meaningful [Bottoms, 2003].

The timing of an apology is also of importance in the valuation of its sincerity. An apology that is offered too quickly may be dismissed as inauthentic. However, in most cases, the longer one waits to apologize, the more harm may be done as a result, and the less chance the apology will be accepted [Tavuchis, 1991]. It is claimed that it is best to enable the victim to recount his or her story before the offering of an apology, thus reflecting a full comprehension of the injured party's loss [Goldberg et al., 1987].

Moreover, for an apology to be effective, it should also be voluntary—made of a party's own free will. And finally, the effectiveness of an apology is dependent not only on the speaker but also on the injured party. It is through acknowledging the apology and possibly forgiving that its recipient closes the circle, restoring the moral equilibrium between the two parties [Bolstad, 2000].

---

* Martin Buber [1923] in his dialogical philosophy emphasized the importance of the interpersonal dialogue, distinguishing between the "I-Thou," a relationship of mutuality and reciprocity necessary for authentic existence, and the "I-It," a relationship of separateness and detachment.

19.2.4 The Benefits of Apology for Victim and Offender

There is psychological evidence to the effect that an apology benefits both the offender and victim [e.g., see Ohbuchi et al., 1989; Lazare, 1995; Cohen, 1999]. An offender who fails to apologize may suffer feelings of guilt, and the victim who does not receive an apology may suffer the corrosive effect of accumulated anger. However, although the psychological benefits for the victim are widely recognized, those for the offender are often overlooked, especially by lawyers. As Gerald Williams [1996] writes:

> [W]e usually think the lawyers' role, when representing defendants, is to protect their clients from having to admit wrongdoing or having to make legal compensation for harms they cause. But … as there are negative psychological consequences to people who are harmed, there are psychological consequences to those who do the harming.

For the offender, an apology is important in various aspects. The emotional exchange postulated in an apology may help the offender to realize the harm he or she has caused. For the offender to confess and apologize with no neutralization techniques can be a powerful and shocking experience, which may lead to a real change. By directly addressing the harmful act, apologies may help offenders to more immediately realize the harm they have caused. Through apology, the offender may feel less negative about him- or herself, and it may help the offender separate the harmful act from his or her permanent identity [Petrucci, 2002]. By apologizing, the offender acknowledges his or her diminished moral stature and asks for restorative forgiveness.

It further appears that the expression of remorse and a genuine desire for reconciliation on the part of the offender is a significant predictor of offender's desistance from future offending [Zehr, 1984]. Morris et al. [1996] indicates that offenders who fail to apologize were three times as likely to reoffend as those who apologize.

Other matters worth mentioning include the spiritual and other psychological values of an apology. Within many religious and ethical systems, offering an apology for one's wrongdoing is an important part of moral behavior. Responsibility and respect, rather than denial and avoidance, lie at the core of apology. By apologizing for, rather than denying or avoiding, the damage one has inflicted, the offender becomes a better person. This constitutes an important aspect in a person's moral development, enabling him or her to feel empathy for others [Cohen, 1999].

For victims, clearly, apologies are also extremely important. Strang [2004] points out that the profound need for emotional restoration has partly to do with the need for vindication, an acknowledgment of the injustice they have suffered, and partly because of a desire to forgive, for their own sake, and to release and alleviate the burden of revenge, anger, and shame.

Murphy [1988] has observed the psychological process of victims in overcoming their anger to forgive wrongdoers. He suggests that we believe and expect other members of society to treat us in accordance with our own moral values and refers to "moral injury," a key to understanding the emotional impact on victims. Hence when wrongdoers cause harm, victims feel indignation toward the wrongdoers because their behavior conveys a message that victims are not valuable enough to be treated respectfully. The wrongdoer puts the victims in a lower status, undermining their value system and damaging their self-esteem [Takahashi, 2005].

Having been victimized, many victims often feel grief and anger. Although it naturally seems that victims immediately want vengeance, empirical evidence suggests that victims are far less vengeful that one might think [Mattinson and Mirrlees-Black, 2000; Strang, 2002]. What victims often really want is to understand the meaning of the event, the reasons that have led the offender to commit the crime, and go on a casual search to understand "why this happened to me." Ideally, victims would like to receive apologies, which often help to restore their sense of self-esteem and control; those who receive apologies generally find it easier to heal and forgive [Bibas, 2007]. They also would like to try to ensure that such an event will not recur. Many victims want to confront offenders face to face and present their stories.

It has been claimed that attribution theory [Weiner, 1992] has potentially valuable applications for understanding the process and benefits for victims [Petrucci, 2002]. As mentioned, crime victims are often likely to search for an explanation for the event. Attribution theory attempts to explain why an event has occurred and to link the cause (or attributes) to one's later expectations of behavior. The heart of the theory lies in its three causal dimensions: locus (internal or external), stability, and controllability, and their relationship to expectancy of success and to emotions and actions.

Thus, the theory provides a possible explanation of the cognitive and emotional processes that ensue for victims as a result of the process of apology, moving them from negative to positive self-attributions. Initially, victims may want to blame themselves and feel responsible for the crime. A face-to-face apology by the offender could potentially alter such self-attributions toward a more positive and neutral stance, by clearly explaining why the event occurred, and often placing the responsibility for the act on the shoulders of the offender.

19.2.5 Forgiveness

There is a link between apology, gratitude, and forgiveness—the healing of social hostility. Forgiveness is the natural goal of an apology because it completes the circle of interaction and enables the restoration of a normally functioning relationship, which can exist only where an emotional bond exists between offender and victim [Bolstad, 2000; Strang, 2002].

Forgiveness means letting go and acknowledging that the crime is past and that the time for healing is at hand. As Bibas [2007] mentioned, victims have a psychological need not only to express their feelings but also to feel that they are being heard. The power to forgive and dispense mercy changes the balance between the offender and the victim, placing the victim above the offender, thus empowering the victim.

Forgiveness and mercy are deeply ingrained within Judeo-Christian religious traditions. The most holy day in Judaism is the Day of Atonement, Yom Kippur. Before this day, Jews will ask forgiveness of those they have wronged during the previous year, and during the day itself they fast and pray for God's forgiveness for the transgressions that they have made against God himself. In fact, the *Talmud* declares that God created repentance before he created the universe. In Christian theology, forgiveness is an absolute value. In his sacrifice on the cross, Jesus personified the Christian belief that no act, however terrible, excludes a human from the possibility of God's grace, redemption, and forgiveness [Jacoby, 1985]. In Buddhism, in contemplating the law of Karma, we realize that what is important for a wronged party is not seeking revenge, but rather practicing *metta* (loving kindness) and forgiveness, for the victimizer is, truly, the most unfortunate of all [Sumedho, 1997]. Many writings, from ancient religious texts to modern psychology, argue that forgiveness is invariably good for mental (and spiritual) health and that vindictiveness is bad. Forgiveness involves overcoming one's resentment of an offender for having inflicted an injury. It involves an internal emotional change but also expresses itself in action [Murphy, 1998].

Forgiveness is important for both offenders and victims. *For offenders,* forgiveness may counteract the negative publicity and bad reputation frequently associated with a crime, making it easier for the offender to reintegrate into society.

Another important cluster of benefits to the offender is psychic. Many offenders often feel guilt for their misdeeds. Forgiveness may lighten such burden, making it easier for them to move on with their lives. As Arendt [1998:237] puts it:

> Without being forgiven, released from the consequences of what we have done, our capacity to act would, as it were, be confined to one single deed from which we could never recover; we would remain the victims of its consequences forever, not unlike the sorcerer's apprentice who lacked the magic formula to break the spell.

Forgiveness benefits *victims* as well. Until victims forgive, they are likely to feel anger, shame, fear, incomprehension, and even hatred and rage [Murphy and Hampton, 1988]. Apology begins as a process that enables the victim to transform the injury suffered to a new energy that enables him or her to move forward. This act of compassion enables the victim to look beyond fear, pain, and blame.

However, it seems that in modern American criminal justice in particular, there is little room for forgiveness. Bibas [2007] argues that it has become a plea-bargaining factory that speeds up cases and reduces costs by sacrificing the offender's and victim's day in court. Police and lawyers take control of the process from the moment the crime report is submitted, and they forbid or discourage offenders and victims from having any contact or discussing the case. The logic of adversarial legal combat leads each side to adopt an antagonistic posture, instead of engaging in dialogue and trying to understand each other's point of view. As Bibas [2007] claims, criminal justice need not be cold, abstract, and impersonal, as it currently is. Bibas also suggests that a more personalized criminal justice system could give much greater weight to the interests and desires of offenders, victims, and the community members. Apology and forgiveness are respected ways to restore offenders and victims and to enable them to move on with their lives.

19.2.6 Forgiveness as Freeing from the Desire for Revenge

Forgiveness, which flows from an internal transformation, provides a basis for mercy, an external remission of punishment [Bibas, 2007]. Thus, it involves a catharsis, a cleansing, of hatred. Forgiveness seems to have the power to release the victims from the desire for punishment and revenge, ultimately leading to closure, a conclusion of the criminal event.

Forgiveness helps victims to cleanse themselves of anger and vengeance, promoting emotional healing. Arendt [1958:240–41], in providing an analysis of the consequences of forgiveness in resolving a moral impasse, describes vengeance as a re-enactment of a wrong that leaves everyone bound to it. She describes forgiveness, the antithesis of vengeance, as "freeing from (the wrong's) consequences, both the one who forgives and the one who is forgiven":

> Forgiveness is the exact opposite of vengeance, which acts in the form of re-enacting against an original trespassing, whereby far from putting an end to the consequences of the first misdeed, everybody remains bound to the process, permitting the chain reaction contained in every action to take its unhindered course. In contrast to revenge, which is natural, automatic reaction to transgression and which because of its irreversibility of the action process can be expected and even calculated, the act of forgiving can never be predicted; it is the only reaction that acts in an unexpected way and thus retains, though being a reaction, something of the original character of action. Forgiving, in other words, is the only reaction which does not merely re-act but acts anew and unexpectedly, unconditioned by the act which provoked it and therefore freeing from its consequences both the one who forgives and the one who is forgiven.

A sanction imposed on a defendant that is intended to provide the victim with an emotional resolution of the crime experience, but that is based on revenge, will not provide true resolution but rather suppress it. Vengeance will not likely allow a victim to recover psychologically; its opposite, forgiveness, will enable the victim to be restored emotionally [Starkweather, 1992].

We will now address various reasons for the absence of apology, in particular in Western criminal justice, focusing on the nature of the adversarial system, the perceived role of lawyers, and on legal education.

19.3 The Absence of Apology in Conventional Justice

The heart has reasons that reason cannot comprehend.
—**Blaise Pascal**

19.3.1 The Absence of Apology in Conventional Justice and the Reasons Lawyers Neglect Apology

Despite the fact that apology and forgiveness play a pivotal role in social life, they play a fairly small role in the criminal process. Traditionally, the criminal law has focused on deterrence, incapacitation, rehabilitation, and retribution on individual offenders; it has neglected the power of remorse and apology [Bibas and Bierschbach, 2004]. Thus, despite clear indications of victim willingness to receive apologies from the offenders, and despite its clear advantages, apology is not a prevalent concept in law. It cannot, for example, serve the defense after an assault.

The biggest block to apologizing is normally the belief that it may be perceived as a sign of weakness and admission of guilt. This liability, or the fear thereof, is the main barrier to apology in most disputes. It is often the case that people are afraid that their apology will be used against them as an admission in court. Thus, lawyers tend to avoid any expression that might be construed as an admission of guilt.

The legal term *without prejudice* has been developed in many countries to preclude using an apology against a person in court. This is exemplified in Charles Dickens's *Bleak House*, with Mr. Guppy's proposal of marriage "without prejudice" to Esther Summerson. Under the common law, statements made during settlement negotiations were admissible in court, unless posed as hypothetical. Use of the words *without prejudice* preceding a statement helped ensure that it would be deemed hypothetical [Cohen, 1999].

The purpose of Rule 408 of the U.S. Federal Rules of Evidence (Fed. R. Evid. 408) was to expand the confidentiality of private statements made during settlement negotiations and to promote settlements by getting rid of the common law reliance on legal formalism [Bolstad, 2000]. Federal Rule of

Evidence 408 includes within its protection statements made during voluntary and court-ordered mediations. However, the rule does not require the exclusion of evidence when offered for another purpose, such as proving the bias or prejudice of a witness or contradicting an allegation of undue delay. It is perhaps the influence of the *adversarial system*, which precludes apology out of fear of establishing blame and admitting culpability. The adversarial system is structured as a contest, with a winner and a loser, rather than a win–win situation. It tends to view conflicts dichotomously and is essentially based on rationalization rather than emotions; it breeds defensiveness because apology involves legal vulnerability. Thus, it may in fact lead to disempowerment and a perception that justice has not been done. Delving into the emotional layers may lead to a more creative and beneficial solution for both parties. By contrast, restorative justice is now poised for reinventing justice around the emotions of victims, offenders, and society. Sherman [2003] argues that the justice system should become emotionally intelligent. It is based on the theory that "manners and emotional overtones of justice officials affect future offending rates as much or more than the formal decisions and severity of punishments" [Tyler and Huo, 2002], and that talking (and listening) can have major effects on future behavior matters.

Lawyers engaged in representing a party are unlikely to think of the possibility of apologizing, let alone to encourage it. In contrast to parents, for example, who normally teach their child to take responsibility when they have wronged someone and to apologize, lawyers typically advise their clients to do precisely the opposite. Most lawyers focus on how to deny responsibility. Such a difference perhaps can be attributed to the fact that parents generally care for the moral development of their child far more than lawyers do about that of their clients [Cohen, 1999].

Various reasons have been suggested as to why lawyers do not regularly discuss apology with clients [Cohen, 1999]. First, the legal system focuses on adjudicating rights rather than on repairing relationships. Second, the attitude of legal education focuses predominantly on individual rights and adversarial relationships, rarely on apology. Thus, most lawyers are unaware that the possibility of apologizing even exists. Many lawyers do not realize that there are legally "safe" ways to apologize. Cohen has advocated the use of safe apologies, namely, accompanying an apology with a statement that the speaker does not want the apology to be used against him or her to create liability. Although such an apology might lack the strength of one offered without any attempt at insulation from liability, it may still have some positive impact on the other party. Third, lawyers may fear that if they raise the issue of apology with their client-offender, the client will think the lawyer disloyal, too sympathetic to the other party's case.

Moreover, recommending an apology may run counter to the role expectations that both the lawyer and client bring to the relationship: that lawyers should be combative, not apologetic. Lawyers generally see their roles in adversarial terms and are reluctant to suggest apologizing for fear of being viewed by clients as disloyal or just insufficiently aggressive. Also, lawyer and client do not have identical interests. Lawyers derive much income from creating and escalating litigation, which apologies help to terminate.

The relative absence of apology in many Western legal systems may also be connected to the historic preoccupation of those legal systems with reducing all losses to economic terms, which can be awarded in a money judgment. Such absence may also be connected to the related tendency, in cases involving injury not easily reducible to quantifiable financial terms, either to not compensate at all or else to award extravagant damages [Wagatsuma and Rosett, 1986].

The focus of the criminal justice system is on achieving as just an outcome as possible with maximum efficiency. However, as Bibas and Bierschbach [2004] argue, the emphasis on efficiency exemplifies a larger trend. Criminal procedure has come to focus on serving procedural values such as fairness, efficiency, and accuracy to the exclusion of substantive values. Indeed, a major complaint of victims is that they are not encouraged to feel part of justice proceedings [Sebba, 1996].

In the courtroom setting, the opportunity for offenders to offer an apology directly to their victims is nearly zero, and even if apology is forthcoming, it only fulfills its aim to a limited extent because the victim is not normally present in court, and the apology is presented to the judge, who represents the society. Thus, there is no direct apology to the victim, often rendering the apology ineffectual because of the lack of an interpersonal and intimate, face-to-face dimension, a key element in communicating emotions. Sincere expression of remorse is something that victims almost never have the chance to hear in the courtroom [Sherman and Strang, 2003]. As a result, frustration, pain, guilt, and alienation frequently replace the potential for closure, reconciliation, and healing.

Furthermore, the failure to apologize may create a vicious circle. An offender who wants to apologize, but fears being sued, may refrain from doing so—and the absence of an apology is precisely what could trigger the suit.

In sum, it seems that criminal justice should be more oriented to encouraging defendants to pave the way for forgiveness by admitting guilt and expressing remorse. Apology feeds a deep human need that is essentially at the "heart" of a conflict, but that is often widely neglected in the mechanistic, lawyerized adversarial process. Incorporating apology into the legal repertoire would be a small change for most lawyers but could produce a dramatic change in how we settle disputes because an apology is a key element in resolving a dispute.

We now turn to evaluate the importance of apology in restorative justice encounters, as well as the contribution of such encounters to the process of emotional restoration, emphasizing the importance of interpersonal dialogue and the face-to-face elements as encouraging apology. We will end with a reference to Japanese society, which serves as an example of a society demonstrating restorative nature, *inter alia*, by attaching significant importance to apology.

19.4 Apology in Restorative Justice Encounters

19.4.1 The Nature of Restorative Justice

Although restorative justice is an umbrella concept, there is a general sense of what it means. It is commonly understood as a theory of criminal justice that focuses on crime as an act by an offender against another individual or community, rather than against the state. It is based on the belief that parties to a conflict ought to be involved in resolving it and mitigating its negative consequences. Restorative justice refers to a process for resolving crime by focusing on redressing the harm done to the victims and for holding offenders accountable for their action [Von Hirsch et al., 2003].

Restorative justice is not easily defined because it includes a variety of practices. One of the more accepted definitions described restorative justice as: "a process whereby parties with a stake in a specific offence collectively resolve how to deal with the aftermath of the offence and its implications for the future" [Marshall, 1999]. Restorative justice emphasizes the repair of the harm and ruptured social bonds resulting from crime. It is mainly concerned with restoration: restoration of victims, of offenders, and of the damage caused by crime to the community.

A fundamental element of restorative justice is that the parties themselves consider and decide what should happen. The core elements include an emphasis on the role and experience of victims in the criminal process and involvement of all the relevant parties (including the victim, offender, and their supporters) in discussing the offense, its impact, and what should be done to "repair the harm" [Daly, 2002].

One of the important aims of restorative justice is reintegration into society. Braithwaite [1989] introduced the notion of reintegrative shaming in restorative justice conferences, arguing for an integrative rather than stigmatizing response to crime. During this process, offenders are confronted with the misery they caused and with the reality that they have breached the moral norms of the community. They are encouraged to apologize and take responsibility for their misbehavior, with victims thus receiving recognition. Reintegrative shaming communicates shame to the offender in a way that encourages him or her to desist from like conduct in the future. He is treated as a good person who has done a bad act.

According to Braithwaite, apology is a critical element in the shaming process. Shaming the harmful act while respecting the individual will foster reintegration and avoid stigmatization. With reintegration, offenders have the opportunity to take responsibility for their behavior, express their shame in the presence of the victim, often in the form of apology, and have social support present while doing so [Braithwaite, 1989; Petrucci, 2002]. The importance of shame is also espoused by other scholars. According to Scheff and Retzinger [2001; Scheff, 1988], shame is a "master emotion." Most other emotions, from aggression to compassion, derive from it. Shame forces people to observe, empathize, and get involved.

One of the leading arguments for restorative justice involves the abandonment of victims' interests through the jurisprudence of retribution. Victims are recognized to be the neglected party in the criminal justice process. Neither their needs nor their preferences are usually taken into account in the prosecution and sentencing of offenders [Strang and Sherman, 2003]. In contrast to criminal justice, restorative justice theories attach paramount importance to apology, considered a key element and a main goal, alongside communications, healing, reparation and restoration, talking about the future, reintegration, and transformation [Shapland et al., 2006]. Shapland argues that in a sense, the whole restorative justice process, if it functions as intended, could be seen as symbolic reparation, in that "the offender has acknowledged responsibility for the offence, has agreed to come to a meeting, has stated they have done the offence, and has acknowledged that at least some harm has been done to the victim."

The informal procedures of restorative justice are often praised, compared with the formality of criminal justice. Compared with criminal proceedings, it seems that the restorative justice conference atmosphere is much more encouraging of rapprochement [Strang, 2002].

19.4.2 The Interpersonal Element in Restorative Justice as Encouraging Apology

Apology includes an interaction, a negotiation process. A restorative justice encounter seems more effective in encouraging apology than court proceedings because it is more personal and intimate, where body language and the relatively small distance play a role in creating a more personal setting.

The interpersonal relationship seems to be a key factor, if a true emotional restoration is to be achieved. An apology that occurs in a face-to-face interaction provides the most expedient means to communicate emotion, permitting an effective apology to be offered, and is considered a key ingredient to the communication of emotion in effective apology [Petrucci, 2002]. The face-to-face interaction has two purposes: The offender expresses shame and remorse for the act, thereby accepting responsibility; this then allows the victim to no longer feel shame because the victim sees that the offender accepts responsibility for the harmful act [Scheff, 1998]. Tavuchis [1991] also sees such "interpersonal orientation," found in restorative justice to a much greater extent than in conventional justice settings, as a key ingredient. The communication of sorrow, so central to the apology acceptance, can only occur in a face-to-face interaction in the presence of the harmed person.

Many claim that among humans, the face is perhaps the most expressive area of emotional embodiment. In a mutual gaze, we experience another person more intensively and intimately than most other animals are capable of doing [Cole, 2001]. Cole argues that one may not be able to feel the other's pain, but one can share his or her suffering. It is through behavior that this is possible. In this process of interpersonal relatedness, face does play an important role. Indeed, much communication remains nonverbal. In discussing how one person can know the mind of another, Pinker [1997] writes:

> The body is the ultimate barrier to empathy. Your toothache does not hurt me the same way as it hurts you. But genes are not imprisoned.... Love, compassions and empathy are invisible fibres that connect genes in different bodies.

In court, there is no victim–offender dialogue, no opportunity for face-to-face apology or expression of contrition. Restorative justice encounters, by contrast, provide various advantages compared with criminal proceedings. A restorative justice encounter inevitably entails a high degree of participation by both victims and offenders. Consequently, victims emphasize the personal nature of the process and the chance they have to play an active role in the delivery of justice as benefits that they value and that are not available in court [Strang and Sherman, 2003].

Evidence suggests that victims are more likely to feel better as a result of conferences [Daly, 1996; Strang and Sherman, 1997]. Conference victims had a beneficial effect on feelings of dignity, self-respect, and self confidence, which contributed toward greater emotional restoration than court victims [Strang, 2002].

Generally, such findings confirm that conferences have been more successful in providing the restoration sought by the victims, as well as forums for apology. Because of their intimate nature, restorative justice conferences tend to constitute an "emotional high point," producing more genuine and authentic apologies and generally leading victims participating in conference to believe that apologies are more sincere than victims feel in a court setting. Also, apologies offered at conferences seem to be more spontaneous than those offered in court, which generally seem coerced. Thus, restorative justice, focusing more on the needs of the participants, may lead to a better healing process and reconciliation, enabling the injured to get on with their lives.

19.4.3 Emotional Restoration

Restorative justice offers ample opportunity for emotional restoration. When offenders are able to apologize and express remorse effectively, and victims are able to accept the apologies, emotional restoration and repair are more likely to be achieved [Strang, 2002; Strang and Sherman, 2003]. The admission of guilt, explanation, or regret is meant, at least partially, to repair the damage to the victim's self-concept. Thus, as Tavuchis claimed, apology seems to possess almost miraculous qualities, and its magic in restoring the antecedent moral order is that, although it cannot undo the past, nevertheless "in a mysterious way and according to its own logic, this is precisely what it manages to do" [1991:5]. The "magical quality" is demonstrated, as in a sense nothing has happened, but from the exchange of a few words, everything has changed. A further important element of emotional restoration for victims is the regaining of a sense of safety and security and a reduced feeling of fear.

In a series of randomized controlled trials conducted in Canberra, Australia, known as the Reintegrative Shaming Experiments (www.aic. gov.au.rjustice.rise.index/html), Strang [2002] found that apology was of great importance in achieving emotional restoration. Thus, 90% of all victims, whether assigned to court or conference, felt they should receive an apology. However, one of the most significant differences between restorative justice and conventional justice was found in the prevalence of apology in conferences as opposed to courts. For victims assigned to conferences, 72% said their offender had apologized (86% of those who were in a conference) compared with only 19% of those assigned to court. Moreover, conference-assigned victims more often felt that the apologies were sincere (77% vs. 41%). These differences are striking and perhaps can partly be attributed to the unique and intimate atmosphere of a restorative justice conference that encourages apologies, as well as authentic behavior.

In addition, restorative justice conferences have also proved to alleviate the desire for revenge. When RISE victims were asked whether the conference had made them feel they could put the offense behind them, three times as many agreed as disagreed [Strang, 2002]. Overall, 20% of court victims said they would harm their offenders if they had the chance, compared with only 7% of conference victims [Strang, 2002]. In sum, it seems that restorative justice conferences produce more productive apologies, an important element of the restoration and closure processes.

A possible criticism is that the apology may not be sincere and can be offered for tactical reasons. If the apology is not sincere, the offender does not experience a moral catharsis; indeed, his engagement in flawed moral patterns could deepen. Moreover, if an apology is offered merely as a legal requirement (for instrumental means) and not as meaningful interaction (for moral purposes), it is of no value [Tavuchis, 1991]. Furthermore, if apology is not conducted properly, it can actually aggravate the dispute.

Moreover, in certain cases of extreme misdeeds or because of the personality of the victim or offender, either side may lack interest in apology or forgiveness. However, such cases are certainly not common and reflect a small portion of offender–victim interactions. Researchers have shown that most victims are equally likely to desire, or demand, apologies, whether for real or imagined transgressions, and that apologies are common to all levels and sectors of society [Tavuchis, 1991].

19.4.4 Learning from Japan: The Increased Use of Apologies

The contribution of restorative justice principles toward social cohesiveness, emotional restoration, and a reduced crime rate can be learned from Japan. Japanese society, in contrast to many in the West, does not perceive an apology as a sign of weakness but rather as a show of strength, honesty for admitting wrongdoing, and generosity for restoring the self-concept of those who were offended. Rather than apologies increasing the number of lawsuits in Japan, the opposite has occurred, namely, few lawsuits are filed.

In Japan, apologies occupy a prominent place in the resolution of conflicts and play a major role as a social restorative mechanism and a ritual role in the conservation of social harmony. Japan is a developed society that has perhaps the heaviest reliance on reintegrative shaming as an alternative to humiliation or outcasting criminals. Many scholars have remarked on the restorative nature of Japanese society, which attaches particular importance to apology. Braithwaite [1989] cited Japan as an example of a communitarian society with a strong cultural commitment to reintegrative shaming. He argued that reintegrative shaming is most likely to be found in societies that are characterized by communitarianism and a high level of interdependency among its members.

The use of apology in Japan is different from that in the United States and elsewhere in the West, where the emphasis is on individualism and freedom. In Japan, a society that stresses group cohesiveness, apology is far more prevalent than in the United States, which emphasizes individualism and hence individual responsibility. For the Japanese, maintaining a harmonious relationship among members of society is more important [Takahashi, 2005].

Japanese society consists of innumerable groups, not individuals. Each member represents these groups to the outside. Membership within a group is an important part of one's social identity; thus, apology plays a major role in maintaining harmonious relationships when social norms are infringed [Yoshida, 2003]. The fact that a member of a group may have committed a crime and has been apprehended could publicly shame not only the wrong-doer but also other members of the group. Being "under arrest," for example, is widely regarded as an admission of guilt by the neighbors, the media, and the public. The suspect loses the respect of others for breaking the social norm that one should have nothing to do with the police. Such involvement will lead other members of the group to be ashamed of being in the same group.

Because of strong interdependency within a group, the Japanese tend to be nervous about whether their behavior conforms to the rules of the group. The feeling of finding oneself different in conduct, and therefore exposed to the gaze of others, is the Japanese idea of shame. Thus, the Japanese intragroup formation provides both a sense of security and strong informal social control, and the Japanese, who are brought up with a strong sense of self-control and group orientation, are willing to apologize to avoid exclusion from one's group [Takahashi, 2005]. In this respect, an apology constitutes a statement that the harmony of the group is supreme to the interests of the individual.

It has been argued that the Japanese seem to focus more on the symbolic act and ritual of apology itself [Ikeda, 1993]. In Japan, apologizing is a sign of an individual's desire to restore or maintain a positive relationship with the other party, despite the temporarily disruptive and harmful act. Americans, in contrast, are more concerned with pragmatic solutions for the offense, such as restitution [Wagatsuma and Rosett, 1986].

Such cultural differences can sometimes be problematic. Japanese are inclined to apologize even for matters for which they are not really responsible, simply because they caused trouble to other members of their group. Thus, for example, in the case of a car accident, Western drivers are often instructed by their insurance companies to avoid admitting fault. Consequently, Japanese executives who move to the United States for business reasons are generally instructed by their corporate employers not to apologize if they are involved in a car accident. The advice is considered necessary because in a similar situation in Japan, the natural inclination would be to apologize, whether or not the driver is at fault [Wagatsuma and Rosett, 1986; Tannen, 1996].

Thus, the application of restorative justice principles in Japan seems to contribute toward a more cohesive social bond and reduced crime rate. Haley [1998], who conducted a comparative review of crimes rate in Japan and the United States, argues that it is the importance of apology and pardon that differentiates the two criminal justice systems. Whereas the crime rates per 100,000 persons tripled in the United States between 1960 and 1988, Japan's crime rate decreased, as has the number of actual offenders. Despite some increase in Japan's crime rate since the mid-1990s, its homicide rates are the lowest in the world, and lower than at any time since World War II, and theft rates (except for bicycle theft) are the lowest in the industrialized world, as well as lower than they were 15 years ago [Yoshida, 2003; Johnson, 2007].

19.5 Conclusion

Apology constitutes an important and powerful tool in everyday life. It significantly contributes toward closure and emotional reparation, and it is beneficial to both offender and victim. Recent evidence suggests that victims see reconciliation to be far more important than material reparation. Victims themselves say that emotional harm is healed, as opposed to compensated for, by an act of emotional repair. Apology seems to possess some "magical quality" because an exchange of a few words can often dramatically alter a situation.

However, notwithstanding its advantages, apology does not constitute an integral part of the criminal justice system. Yet beyond the material harm that crime victims may endure, there are emotional and psychological dimensions that are frequently neglected. It seems that the relative dearth of scope for apology in Western legal systems does not stem from a real human difficulty but more from cultural, social, and institutional values, emphasizing detachment and rivalry. The absence of apology in Western society seems to constitute a failure, given the importance of apology and forgiveness in Judeo-Christian culture. It seems that there is room for increased use of apology, as can be learned from the Japanese experience. A shift in judicial and legal discourse may be necessary. Surely apology merits higher priority than has been historically accorded by the criminal justice system and the academy.

Restorative justice, in which apology is a central feature, may provide a supportive framework for neutralizing this failure and for cultivating values of dialogue, empowerment, and reintegration. Restorative justice encounters, because of their personal nature, provide a good opportunity for the offender to offer an apology and for the victim to accept it, thus offering an emotional and spiritual transformative dimension: Victims recover from the injury, the conflict is addressed through dialogue, and the harmful act is shamed while the offender is not stigmatized. Recent evidence suggests that victims receive far more apologies in restorative justice encounters than they do in courts.

Apology seems to be a necessary cornerstone if emotional restoration is to be realized and a genuine healing process is to occur. It can often constitute a bridge and the route toward a more just result and a broader solution, while benefiting both the offender and the victim. Eventually, this may accomplish Braithwaite's [1999:2] inspirational words about the potential of restorative justice: "Crime is an opportunity to prevent greater evils, to confront crime with a grace that transforms human lives to paths of love and giving."

Acknowledgments

We are very grateful to Dr. Heather Strang and Professor Lawrence Sherman for their insightful comments on draft versions of this chapter.

References

Arendt, H. 1958. *The human condition.* Chicago: University of Chicago Press.

Arendt, H. 1998. *The human condition,* 2nd ed. Chicago: University of Chicago Press.

Bibas, S. 2007. Forgiveness in criminal procedure. *Ohio State Journal of Criminal Law* 4:329–48.

Bibas, S. and R. A. Bierschbach. 2004. Integrating remorse and apology into criminal procedure. *The Yale Law Journal* 114:85.

Bolstad, M. 2000. Learning from Japan: The case for increased use of apology in mediation. *Cleveland State Law Review* 48:545.

Bottoms, A. E. 2003. Some sociological reflections on restorative justice. In *Restorative justice and criminal justice: Competing or reconcilable paradigms?* ed. A. Von Hirsch, J. Roberts, A. E. Bottoms, K. Roach, and M. Schiff, 79–113. Oxford: Hart.

Braithwaite, J. 1989. *Crime, shame and reintegration.* Cambridge: Cambridge University Press.

_____. 1999. Restorative justice: Assessing optimistic and pessimistic accounts. *Crime and Justice: A Review of Research* 25:1–127.

Buber, M. 1923. *I and Thou,* trans. R. G. Smith (1958). New York: Charles Scribner's Sons.

Christie, N. 1977. Conflict as property. *British Journal of Criminology* 17(1):1–14.

Cohen, J. R. 1999. Advising clients to apologize. *Southern California Law Review* 72:1009–69.

Cole, J. 2001. Empathy needs a face. *Journal of Consciousness Studies* 8(5–7):51–68.

Daly, K. 1996. Diversionary conferences in Australia: A reply to the optimists and skeptics. Paper prepared for Presentation at the American Society of Criminology Annual Meeting, November 20–23.

Daly, K. 2002. Restorative justice: The real story. *Punishment and Society* 4(1):55–79.

Dignan, J. 1992. Repairing the damage: Can reparation work in the service of diversion? *British Journal of Criminology* 32(4):453–72.

Goffman, E. 1971. *Relations in public: Microstudies of the public order.* New York: Basic.

Goldberg, S. B., E. D. Green, and F. E. A. Sander. 1987. Saying you're sorry. *Negotiations Journal* 3:221.

Griswold, C. S. 2007. *Forgiveness: A philosophical exploration.* Cambridge: Cambridge University Press.

Haley, J. O. 1998. Apology and pardon, learning from Japan. *American Behavioral Scientist* 41:842–67.

Hayes, H. 2006. Apologies and accounts in youth justice conferencing: Reinterpreting research outcomes. *Contemporary Justice Review* 9(4):369–85.

Holtgraves, T. 1989. The function and form of remedial moves: Reported use, psychological reality, and perceived effectiveness. *Journal of Language and Social Psychology* 14:363–78.

Ikeda, R. 1993. A comparative study of apology: Japanese and Americans. *Nihongo Gaku* 12:12–21.

Jacoby, S. 1985. *Wild justice: The evolution of revenge.* London: Collins.

Johnson, D. T. 2007. Crime and punishment in contemporary Japan. *Crime & Justice* 36:371.

Kastor, E. 1998. The repentance consensus: A simple apology just doesn't cut it. *Washington Post,* 19 Aug.:D5.

Lazare, A. 1995. Go ahead, say you're sorry. *Psychology Today* January–February:40–76.

Levi, D. L. 1997. The role of apology in mediation. *N.Y.U. Law Review* 72:1166.

Marshall T. 1999. Restorative justice: An overview. Occasional paper. London: Home Office.

Marshall T. and S. Merry. 1990. *Crime and accountability: Victim–offender mediation in practice.* London: HMSO.

Mattinson, J. and C. Mirrlees-Black. 2000. Attitudes to crime and criminal justice: Findings from the 1998 British Crime Survey, 34–44. Home Office Research Study 200. London: Home Office.

Moore, D. 1993. Shame, forgiveness and juvenile justice. *Criminal Justice Ethics* 12(1):3–25.

Morris, A., G. Maxwell, J. Hudson, and B. Galaway. 1996. Concluding thoughts. In *Family group conference: Perspectives on policy and practice,* ed. J. Hudson, A. Morris, G. Maxwell, and B. Galaway. Sydney: Federation.

Murphy, J. and J. Hampton. 1988. *Forgiveness and mercy.* Cambridge: Cambridge University Press.

Ohbuchi, K. I., M. Kameda, and N. Agarie. 1989. Apology as aggression control: Its role in mediating appraisal of and response to harm. *Journal of Personality and Social Psychology* 56:219–27.

Petrucci, C. J. 2002. Apology in the criminal justice setting: Evidence for including apology as an additional component in the legal system. *Behavioral Sciences and the Law* 20:337–60.

Pinker, S. 1998/1997. *How the mind works.* London: Allen Lane, 1998 (first published New York: W.W. Norton, 1997).

Scheff, T. J. 1988. Shame and conformity: The deference-emotion system. *American Sociological Review* 53:395–406.

Scheff, T. J. 1998. Therapeutic jurisprudence forum: Community conferences: Shame and anger in therapeutic jurisprudence. *Revista Juridica Universidad de Puerto Rico* 67:97–119.

Scheff, T. J. and S. M. Retzinger. 1996. Strategy for community conferences: Emotions and social bonds. In *Restorative justice: International perspectives,* ed. B. Galaway and J. Hudson, 315–36. Monsey, NY: Criminal Justice Press.

Scheff, T. J. and S. M. Retzinger. 2001. *Emotions and violence: Shame and rage in destructive conflicts.* Lincoln: iUniverse.

Sebba, L. 1996. *Third parties: Victims and the criminal justice system.* Columbus: Ohio State University Press.

Shapland J., A. Atkinson, H. Atkinson, et al. 2006. Situating restorative justice within criminal justice. *Theoretical Criminology* 10(4):505–32.

Sherman, L. W. 2003. Reason for emotion: Reinventing justice with theories, innovations, and research—the American Society of Criminology 2002 Presidential Address. *Criminology* 41(1):1–38.

Sherman, L. W. and H. Strang, 2003. Repairing the harm: Victims and restorative justice. *Utah Law Review* 15:15–42.

Starkweather, D. A. 1992. The retributive theory of "just deserts" and victim participation in plea bargaining. *Indiana Law Journal* 67:853.

Strang, H. 2002. *Repair or revenge: Victims and restorative justice.* Oxford: Clarendon.

Strang, H. 2004. Is restorative justice imposing its agenda on victims? In *Critical issues in restorative justice,* ed. H. Zehr, and B. Toews. Monsey, NY: Criminal Justice Press.

Strang, H. and L. W. Sherman. 1997. The victim's perspective. RISE Working Papers No. 2. Canberra: Australian National University, Research School of Social Sciences. (www. aic.gov.au/rjustice/rise/index.html).

Sumedho, A. 1997. Universal loving kindness. *Forest Sangha Newsletter,* October, Number 42.

Takahashi, Y. 2005. Towards a balancing approach: The use of apology in Japanese society. *International Review of Victimology* 12:23–45.

Tannen, D. 1996. I'm sorry, I won't apologize. *New York Times Magazine.* Sunday, July 21:34–35.

Tavuchis, N. 1991. *Mea culpa: A sociology of apology and reconciliation.* Stanford, CA: Stanford University Press.

Tyler, T. and Y. J. Huo. 2002. *Trust in the law: Encouraging public cooperation with the police and courts.* New York: Russell Sage Foundation.

Von Hirsch, A., J. Roberts, A. E. Bottoms, K. Roach, and M. Schiff. 2003. *Restorative justice and criminal justice: Competing or reconcilable paradigms?* Oxford: Hart.

Wagatsume, H. and A. Rosett. 1986. The implications of apology: Law and culture in Japan and the United States. *Law and Society Review* 20(4):461–98.

Weiner, B. 1992. Attributional theories of motivation: persons as scientists. In *Human motivation: Metaphors, theories and research,* ed. B. Weiner, 221–89. Newbury Park, CA: Sage.

West, T. G. 1979. *Plato's apology of Socrates: An interpretation,* with a new translation. Ithaca, NY: Cornell University Press.

Williams, G. R. 1996. Negotiation as a healing process. *Journal of Dispute Resolution* 1:1–66.

Wright, M. 1991. *Justice for victims and offenders: A restorative response to crime.* Philadelphia: Open University Press.

Yoshida, T. 2003. Confession, apology, repentance and settlement out-of-court in the Japanese criminal justice system—Is Japan a model of 'restorative justice'? In *Restorative justice in context, international practice and directions,* ed. Elmar G. M. Weitekamp and H. J. Kerner, 173–96. Cullompton, UK: Willan.

Young, P. 2001. Mediation and the power of an apology: The case of the missing snowman. *Missouri Lawyers Weekly* 7 (April 9), reprinted at http:/www.mediate.com/articles/young3.cfm (2001) and at *The Communicator,* Vol. 3, No. 2 newsletter of the Association of Missouri Mediators (Summer 2001).

Zehr, H. 1984. Retributive justice, restorative justice. *New Perspectives on Crime and Justice* (No. 4, September). Akron, PA: Mennonite Central Committee Office of Criminal Justice.

Exploring the Effects of Restorative Justice on Crime Victims for Victims of Conflict in Transitional Societies

20

HEATHER STRANG

Contents

20.1 Introduction

Over the past 20 years the claims of restorative justice advocates have been considerable. They include the reduction and prevention of reoffending, greater social cohesion through joint problem solving by neighborhoods and communities, and more harmony in schools and other institutions. Research has addressed many of these claims, and much is now known about the effects of restorative justice on all these dimensions. However, the only claim for which unequivocal evidence now stands is the greater benefit that restorative justice offers victims of crime who are willing to meet their admitted offenders. This evidence emerges from a large number of observational and comparative studies conducted in recent years [e.g., Umbreit and Coates, 1992, 1993; Umbreit, 1994, 1995, 2001; Miers et al., 2001; Nugent et al., 2003] and from a meta-analysis of 35 restorative justice programs carried out by Latimer et al. [2001]. Perhaps the most compelling evidence, however, is offered by findings from randomized controlled trials comparing the benefits available to victims from restorative justice with that from courts and other formal justice procedures [Sherman and Strang, 2007].

In this chapter I will discuss the meaning of restorative justice for crime victims, review the most rigorous evidence for victim benefits of restorative justice in the criminal justice setting, and examine the ways in which restorative justice appears to be superior to formal justice in providing crime victims with the benefits they seek. I will then examine the issues most salient to victims in societies struggling with the aftermath of violent conflict, taking as a framework five areas of concern in transitional justice—truth-telling, prosecution and accountability, reparations, institutional reform, and reconciliation—and discuss findings from our research with crime victims that are relevant to each of these areas. Finally, I will broach the relationship between justice and peace and discuss some of the ways in which restorative justice may help achieve both in devastated communities.

20.2 Restorative Justice and Victims of Crime

There are almost as many definitions of restorative justice as there are practitioners, researchers, and policymakers. There are also considerable variation in the practices embraced by the term. Nevertheless, there is general agreement that restorative justice proceeds by bringing together all stakeholders affected by a harm—victims, offenders, their families and friends, and affected communities—who discuss in the presence of a trained facilitator what happened, how they have each been affected, and what should be done to right any wrongs suffered [Braithwaite and Strang, 2001].

However, it is the values attached to restorative justice that make the process unique and distinguish it from conventional court-based justice. These values are also contested [Braithwaite, 2002], but there is general accord that restorative justice entails undominated deliberation by all participants with opportunities for apology and forgiveness; furthermore, the objective is to repair the harm admitted by the offender and prevent it from happening again.

Although restorative justice processes may have existed for thousands of years and remain crucial mechanisms for traditional conflict resolution remedies in many parts of the world [Braithwaite, 2002], it is only during the past 2 or 3 decades that serious attempts have been made to (re)introduce restorative justice into Western criminal justice arrangements. As enthusiasm grew for an innovation that many claimed had the potential to improve on the perceived failings of the conventional justice system, so did calls for rigorous research that would demonstrate whether this potential was achievable and whether it represented a viable alternative paradigm to court-based justice.

Research initially focused inevitably on the effects of restorative justice on the behavior of offenders. Large claims were made based on dramatic experiences about the possibilities of truly altering offenders' lives by allowing them the opportunity to hear directly from their victims the full consequences of their actions. Findings to date show that restorative justice can indeed be effective in reducing reoffending for all kinds of offenders. The independent evaluation of seven experiments conducted by our research team in the United Kingdom found that this highly emotional process resulted in 27% fewer reconvictions for new crimes during a 2-year follow-up period by offenders who had experienced restorative justice compared with an equivalent group of offenders who had not done so but had only been dealt with by conventional justice in the usual way [Shapland et al., 2008]. Effects, however, seem to vary across different kinds of offenses and offenders, although available evidence points to restorative justice working better with more serious offenses. This may be related to the emotional basis for restorative justice: that offenders' remorse for having harmed a victim, especially when there is little social distance in terms of class, race, or ethnicity between them, is linked to the generation of empathy between them, a subject that I will return to later in this chapter. Still, work remains to be done on determining for whom and under what conditions restorative justice most effectively prevents future offending.

At the same time, the effects on victims of crime appear to be very consistently beneficial, and the evidence for this emerges strongly from the program of rigorous research undertaken by our team during the past 15 years [Strang, 2002; Strang and Sherman, 2003; Sherman et al., 2005; Strang et al., 2006].

All our field trials comparing face-to-face restorative justice conferences with conventional court-based criminal justice have randomly assigned eligible cases either to the usual conventional justice treatment alone or to a restorative justice meeting. The advantage of this methodology is that, for a sufficient number of cases, the differences between the two groups—the control and the experimental—in their social and demographic characteristics, their criminal histories, and life experiences will "wash out," so that we can be confident that any differences in outcomes—offender recidivism or victim satisfaction, for example—can be confidently attributed to the treatment each received rather than to any inherent differences between the groups.

These trials included four experiments in which we were able to seek detailed interviews with all the crime victims. Two of these came from a series conducted in Canberra, Australia, in 1995–2000, and two came from a second series conducted in the United Kingdom in 2002–2005.

These Canberra studies dealt with property crimes committed by juvenile offenders and with violent crimes committed by offenders aged less than 30 years. All these cases were of sufficient seriousness that they would normally have been dealt with in court. In all of them the offenders had admitted responsibility for the crime and said they would be willing to accept the restorative justice option if offered. Eligible cases were referred to the research team by arresting police officers for random assignment either to prosecution through the court in the usual way or diverted away from court to a face-to-face restorative justice meeting. Victims of the restorative justice group were then contacted by the case facilitator who explained the process and invited them to attend the meeting, together with anyone they wished to bring to support them.

The two United Kingdom studies in which victims were interviewed were carried out in London. These cases involved much more serious offenses than the earlier tests in Canberra: robbery and burglary prosecuted in the Crown Courts. The offenders were all aged more than 18 years, most had extensive criminal histories, and all had pleaded guilty in court to the offense that had brought them into our study. Because of the seriousness of the offense, they were all dealt with in court in the usual way: half of the eligible, consenting group was randomly assigned to attend a restorative justice conference as well. Most of these offenders had been remanded in prison before sentence, and most of them were given custodial sentences. Eligibility in these tests was based on both offender and victim consent [Shapland et al., 2005, 2006, 2007]. Around 80% of offenders approached agreed to meet their victims in this process, a surprisingly high figure given that it was made clear to them that participation was unlikely to affect their sentence. Victims of the consenting offenders were then contacted by facilitators who spent considerable effort in explaining the process, answering questions, offering reassurance about safety and security, and arranging events as far as possible around the victims' convenience.

Previous experience in the United Kingdom had led many to believe that victims were unwilling to take part in restorative justice, even in less serious cases where sometimes fewer than 10% of victims of juvenile crime agreed to meet their offenders [e.g., see Miers et al., 2001; Newburn et al., 2001]. Thus, we were pleased that around 45% of these victims of robbery and burglary, some of them seriously traumatized by their experiences, were willing to meet their offenders. We concluded that victim agreement to participate depended greatly on the degree of effort put into encouraging them to do so; we also suggest, based on what victims have told us [Strang, 2002], that they may be more likely to agree when the offense is a serious one because of the opportunity to ask questions directly of their offenders, to express their anger and outrage directly to those responsible for the suffering they have endured, and to seek reparations they themselves feel are appropriate.

It is the findings from this program of research conducted by my colleagues and me over the past 15 years that I will draw from in exploring what restorative justice may be able to offer victims of harms experienced in the course of armed conflict and civil strife. This is in some ways a daunting undertaking. Many of the restorative justice meetings we have observed have been extraordinarily powerful encounters following grievous crimes; some have even been shocking in their character and their consequences. Indeed, it is because this research has revealed such extraordinary benefits for so many different kinds of crime victims that I want to explore what may be beneficial also to victims of horrific events that occur in large-scale violent conflicts. Nevertheless, it is with some caution and humility that I will look for lessons to be learned from our research program for this wider context. My hope is that the experience of restorative justice in the criminal arena may give some indication of how best to help victims in transitional societies. However, before turning to specific applications of our research findings, I would like to make two preliminary comments.

First, we have learned in criminal justice that we must not promise too much to victims, or at least we must not promise what we cannot always deliver. Victims whose cases were randomly assigned to restorative justice in our Canberra experiments and who experienced a restorative justice meeting were significantly more satisfied about the way they were treated than those victims whose cases went to court in the usual way. However, the angriest and most frustrated victims in these studies were those who, for reasons beyond their control, did not have their promised restorative justice meeting—they were much angrier, as it turned out, than those victims to whom no promises of restorative justice had been made and whose cases were dealt with in court. We know that this can be a huge risk in the transitional justice arena, too: For example, a hard lesson was learned after the Sun City Accord of 2002 that resulted in the temporary cessation of the worst of the hostilities in the Congo's civil war and led to the establishment, among other entities, of a Truth and Reconciliation Commission. The perhaps unrealistically ambitious goals of the Accord seem to have left victims feeling frustrated and angry because the promise of a chance finally to tell of their suffering has not been fulfilled [Vanspauwen and Savage, 2008].

Second, the wisest course seems to be to allow restorative justice to work with the prevailing culture and not impose any particular view of the best way for parties in conflict to come together. Building on traditional conflict resolution processes appears to be desirable where they exist and where they conform with restorative principles of democratic dialogue. The primary example of success with this approach is the adoption and adaptation of Maori traditional practices in New Zealand's family group conferencing legislation. However, we must not assume that such practices always conform to restorative justice principles: A primary example of failure may be the attempt to use a New Zealand model of restorative justice with Australian Aboriginal youth. Our Canberra program backfired with Aboriginal youth at least in part, we surmise, for cultural reasons. For example, Aboriginal people are often taught that it is disrespectful to look people who are in authority in the eye; they may even have traditional relationships with family members (such as mothers-in-law) that forbid any direct contact or communication. They may be impervious to the might of the criminal justice system but highly susceptible to the authority of elders in their communities. We learned a great deal in our research about how *not* to conduct restorative justice with Aboriginal people and to make recommendations based on those findings about how better to use restorative justice techniques.

20.3 Justice in Transitional Societies

Kofi Annan [2006] observed that "roughly half of all countries that emerge from war lapse back into violence within five years" and that the United Nations (UN) system in the past has not effectively addressed the challenges of helping countries in the transition from war to lasting peace. It is clear that peace-keeping troops, resources for reconstruction, and even international courts have not always succeeded in overcoming the grievances, the sense of injustice and bitterness, and the breakdown in trust that provide the fuel for the next round of hostilities.

Restorative justice typically focuses on individual harm, on what each affected person requires to repair that harm, and on engendering empathy between victims and offenders. Some observers suggest that the sheer scale of atrocities following war renders this focus unworkable. We may be daunted by so much tragedy, but the reality is that formal justice can only be applied to a small number of those responsible and that inevitably it becomes the task of every town and village to engage in the process of repair. In Kosovo, for example, restorative interventions have been aimed at establishing contact and dialogue between ethnic groups who have had similar experiences, whether as victims or war veterans [Nikolic-Risanovic, 2008; Valinas and Arsovska, 2008]. These initiatives focus on the rebuilding of trust between those who fought each other. Bougainville, after a conflict lasting 9 years in which perhaps 10% of the population died, trained 10,000 people to conduct restorative justice at the grassroots level [Howley, 2003]. Again, the focus was on the acknowledgment of harm and the construction of opportunity for apology and even forgiveness. With that kind of commitment it seems entirely feasible to foster the aims of transitional justice from the bottom up and to multiply its effects through the sheer number of individual restorative justice encounters.

In the context of Northern Ireland, McEvoy and Eriksson [2006] have argued strongly that restorative justice principles are uniquely suited for societies in transition: that especially when state-based justice has been suborned by the conflict or where the state itself is guilty of human rights abuses, it makes sense for damaged communities to take primary ownership in justice reconstruction because of the greater legitimacy derived from their contributing to decisions about the kind of intervention that best suits them.

To address legacies of turmoil, reconciliation processes with principles of restorative justice at their heart have been used with varying degrees of success in a growing list of countries, from Northern Ireland to South Africa and from Kosovo to Bougainville, which have emerged from conflicts and are transitioning into a sometimes uncertain peace. As Karstedt [forthcoming] has documented, this is a relative recent response to the suffering of the victims of hostilities: Victims as individuals were invisible in the national and international tribunals that followed the Second World War and in most of the conflicts since that time. Despite the emergence of a human rights framework in international justice following the Universal Declaration of Human Rights in 1948, it was not until the late 1980s that victims of abuse and injustice perpetrated by the state or in the course of armed conflict began to be heard. Much has been accomplished in formal justice arenas in the past 2 decades in acknowledging the suffering of victims, but I will argue that international courts and even national tribunals and commissions can rarely cope with the sheer numbers of victims in the aftermath of violent conflict. The scale of the calamity of armed conflict creates an impossible burden for formal prosecution authorities, even those set up specifically to include the voices of victims, such as the International Criminal Tribunal for the former Yugoslavia and the South African Truth and Reconciliation Commission. When this leads to impunity through wide-scale amnesties or, worse, no prosecutorial action at all, the prospects for the recovery of relationships and the restoration of civil society diminish accordingly.

The issues facing postconflict societies are formidable, but lessons have been learned about what is required by societies in transition if justice is to be established. The former Deputy Chair of the South African Truth and Reconciliation Commission, Alex Boraine, has suggested that transitional justice requires attention to five principal areas:

- Truth recovery
- Prosecution and accountability
- Institutional reform
- Reparations
- Reconciliation

I will examine each of these dimensions of transitional justice to see what restorative justice may be able to offer these victims, based on what we know from our empirical research about the consequences of each for victims of crime.

20.3.1 Truth Recovery

Much as we might wish for truth to be self-evident to all who honestly seek it, our everyday experience tells us it is not so. Especially in encounters that engage our emotions, memories can be unreliable, and participants to the events may have good reason to bend their recollections to their own advantage. John Braithwaite [2005:291] has observed that "truth" in postconflict societies, as in ordinary crime, may be a "misleading shorthand [because] … what matters is not so much revealing an objective truth as a process that all stakeholders in an injustice see as a high-integrity process for revealing what may end up being multiple truths." He goes on to say that "this kind of truth-seeking must be deliberative, attentive to multiple sources of evidence, open to public scrutiny and critique."

We have found often in meetings of crime victims and perpetrators that a discussion of the "facts" of the case almost always runs into a stone wall of disputation, even when responsibility for the incident as a whole has been admitted. This seems to be replicated on the larger canvas of postconflict situations where we so often hear about truth "going missing"—that there have been very few successes in establishing the whole truth about atrocities when legal standards of evidence are required and victims have few opportunities to tell their side of the story in their own words.

Rather than rehearse the details of the offense, our facilitators learned to turn the discussion to the incontrovertible harm that the victim had suffered. The offender may be able to justify his or her actions in terms of provocation or self-defense but cannot deny the consequences of those actions as the victim describes them. Our experience showed that an emphasis on the harm rather than the objective facts, or "truth," is more productive in getting to questions about what should be done to repair it. A restorative encounter permits all the truths to be expressed by all parties, all the consequences explained, and all the harms heard.

Moreover, our research confirms the observation of Stan Cohen [1995] that for victims there is a burning need for something more than truth. What more often is sought and needed is acknowledgment, which Cohen describes [1995:18] as "what happens to knowledge when it becomes officially sanctioned and enters the public realm." It is here that truth-telling intersects with accountability. If there is no knowledge there can be no accountability, but I suggest that equally knowledge is of little use without a process of accountability.

20.3.2 Prosecution and Accountability

Often, in the context of international law, accountability is viewed as synonymous with prosecution. Formal justice after violent conflicts, with its focus on punishment, denunciation, and deterrence, leaves little opportunity for individual victims' voices to be heard. As Ivo Aertsen [2008] has observed, it is generally assumed, in a normative way, that "prosecution brings relief to victims by acknowledging the facts and recognising the harm and injustice done to victims" [p. 419], but there is little empirical evidence to support this view: Indeed, victims are rarely consulted on such questions.

In fact, when crime victims from different parts of the world have been asked about their views of the justice process generally, the findings have been astonishingly similar [e.g., Kitchling, 1991; Sebba, 1996; Shapland, 2000]. They resent their exclusion from a meaningful role in the prosecution process, other than the meager opportunity to act as witnesses in their own cases; they feel intimidated by the enormous social and even physical distance between themselves and the prosecutorial authorities and are perplexed by the rules of evidence. They are angered by the lack of information available to them from justice officials and by the disrespectful and unfair ways in which they are often treated. And whenever they are asked, they repeatedly call for less formal ways of dealing with their cases where their views would count.

The evidence we have from our restorative justice research confirms these findings [Strang, 2002]. When we compared the views of similar victims whose cases were randomly assigned either to court or to restorative justice, we found that those whose cases were dealt with by the formal justice system were often sorely dissatisfied with their treatment. We found that restorative justice was consistently superior in providing the opportunity to be as closely engaged with the processing and outcome of their case as they wished to be. One of the primary sources of victim dissatisfaction with the courts and the prosecution process was the difficulty of obtaining information about what was happening to their case. Those who experienced restorative justice were consistently much better informed and had an opportunity for direct input in the way their case was handled.

We found as well that victims believed restorative justice was better at giving them a participating role in their case. Victims whose cases went to court in the usual way had no formal role unless they were required as witnesses, but victims in restorative justice took an active part in the resolution of their cases; their views were central to the way in which it was handled. When the victims in our Canberra study were asked why they took part in restorative justice, we found that "having a say" and "expressing feelings directly to their offender" were major reasons. Although some commentators [e.g., see Brown, 1994] have suggested that the restorative justice forum may serve to suppress victims' feelings of outrage and loss and that they would be reluctant to express their anger directly to their offender, when we asked them they have almost never expressed any feelings of inhibition in the restorative justice setting, even when the crime itself was violent and traumatizing.

We found too that victims felt restorative justice is better than court at providing fair and respectful treatment. This may appear to be the minimum that could be expected by victims in the formal justice system, but research continues to find that is surprisingly rare. Even though most successful prosecutions rely on victims to provide witness testimony, victims often are treated with such discourtesy and disregard that the term *secondary victimization* by the criminal justice system is commonly used about their experience. Despite the lip service paid to the importance of witnesses in the prosecution process, little attention is usually given to them: They remain paradoxically both needed and unvalued. Our research consistently finds that victims who have experienced restorative justice report much higher levels of procedural fairness that do victims whose cases are only dealt with in court; furthermore, because they are central to the process, they also report much higher levels of respect from criminal justice officials.

Of course, there are circumstances in which only the full majesty of the law appears equal to the scale of a tragedy inflicted. For those who lead in encouraging or permitting gross human rights abuses, the courtroom may be the appropriate forum. However, no formal judicial institution is capable of dealing with all the crimes perpetrated during a conflict. Nor is it designed to contribute to the hard job of rebuilding trust among citizens, especially when victims and perpetrators live among each other. Raveling up broken relationships cannot be done from afar by distant formal institutions. As I mentioned earlier, restorative justice offers the possibility of starting the work of community rebuilding from the bottom up: Examples abound, from Bougainville to Kosovo, so that truth can be not only told but also acknowledged by those responsible in face-to-face restorative justice encounters, who can then be held to account by those they have harmed.

20.3.3 Institutional Reform

Although this topic is broader than the realm of justice alone, there is good reason to suggest that where vigorous traditional conflict resolution mechanisms exist, to the extent that they have community legitimacy, comply with accepted standards of human rights, and are based on principles of reconciliation and restoration, they will have an important role in the revival of civil society. Criticism has sometimes been made of the capacity of village councils and similar grassroots entities to address severe crimes on the grounds that they lack legal competence and that the remedies available to them as grossly incommensurate with the crimes they address [Kamwimbi, 2008]. Nevertheless, in the Democratic Republic of Congo, for example, civil society groups are reported "to play a critical role in promoting peace and stability, monitoring human rights violations and other abuses against innocent civilian populations and in promoting inter-ethnic dialogue and reconciliation at the local and regional levels" [Franciscans International, 2006]. Such entities need to be acknowledged for the role they play and the legitimacy they possess in any remaking of institutions of civil society, especially in the absence of, or because of the distrust of, more formal judicial entities. On the other hand, failure to adhere to restorative justice principles may undermine programs based on traditional conflict resolution techniques; for example, in Rwanda, *gacaca* may not be achieving its aims of truth and reconciliation because of its coerciveness, its failure to prioritize the practical needs of victims, and for other reasons associated with a failure to comply with values central to restorative practices [Waldorf, 2006].

In addressing the issue of how to incorporate restorative justice programs into a reformed justice system, it may be useful to consider our research findings on how best to conduct them. First and most important is the framework for restorative justice within the formal parameters of the rule of law. Restorative justice must be subject to the processes of accountability, reviewability, and appeal that this framework provides. Second, monitoring arrangements are essential to ensure that programs are operationalized as they were intended and that they comply with basic restorative justice principles of democratic deliberation by all the affected parties. Third, what turns out to matter most with successful criminal justice programs is not the professional background of the people running the program, nor the bureaucratic arrangements. Far more important are the quality of training and the standing in the community of those entrusted with restorative justice facilitation: They must be respected, and they must be seen to be impartial and fair-minded by all participants.

20.3.4 Reparations

International law sets out clearly the right to reparations. In the context of gross violations of human rights, the UN's Van Boven/Bassiouni Principles [United Nations General Assembly, 2005], which are generally regarded as an international charter of victims' rights, outline five aspects to public reparation programs: restitution, compensation, rehabilitation, public acknowledgment of the wrong, and guarantees of future security. They are designed to govern tangible efforts of the state to repair the harm to victims and attempt to encompass both the material and emotional dimensions of harm and repair. However, our research has demonstrated that restorative justice with its individual focus can effectively render both material and emotional restoration, often more effectively than state justice.

Our findings on material reparations to victims show that although they can be awarded monetary or other reparation by both the courts and via an restorative justice meeting, neither route provides any guarantee that payments or any other kind of compensation will be reliably forthcoming. We found that more of our court-treated victims than our restorative justice victims said they wanted financial restitution, but fewer of them received any. Although material reparation is a legitimate and significant part of the restorative process, it was interesting to find that our restorative justice victims did not always see it to be of primary importance: Afterward, fewer than one-third of them rated it as a primary reason for meeting their offender, although it may have been an important motivator for agreeing to take part. There were several meetings in our study where the victim arrived with a handful of bills, clearly intending to ask the offender for money, but left without presenting the bills, saying that they no longer felt it was appropriate or necessary to be financially repaid. However, clearly material reparations can be essential to the business of postconflict recovery, and restorative justice meetings provide the opportunity both to specify what victims need and to put in place personal arrangements to ensure that it is delivered. The failure of courts to order the payment of reparations or compensation when victims believe they have a just claim, as well as their failure to ensure its delivery when they do even in such a smoothly running judicial system as Canberra's, reveals how difficult it is for institutions to achieve this.

20.3.5 Reconciliation

Even though material and financial reparations are often essential for victim recovery, especially in postconflict societies, they need to be linked to other elements of the transitional justice processes if they are to be interpreted as anything more than "blood money." It is here that reparation intersects with reconciliation and the acknowledgment of the emotional consequences of victimization. Reconciliation lies at the heart of the idea of restorative justice. It implies a forward-looking coming-together of parties formerly locked in conflict. Boraine and Valentine [2006] argue that reconciliation can begin when the other elements of transitional justice are seen by victims to be underway: that truth is being sought, that perpetrators are being held accountable, that institutional reforms are underway, and that the issue of reparations is being addressed.

Although material elements of restoration may be important to victim recovery, time after time research with crime victims has found that it is the dimension of emotional harm that requires redress if the experience of victimization is ever to be satisfactorily resolved. Crime victims tell us that emotional reparation is usually far more important to them than material or financial reparation [e.g., Marshall and Merry, 1990; Umbreit et al., 1994;

Strang, 2002], even though they may not have realized it until after they have met their offender and understood the extent of the emotional damage they had endured. In our research we have consistently found that victims' anger, fear, and anxiety have all been at much lower levels after a restorative justice encounter with their offender than they were beforehand, most notably for victims of violent crime. Furthermore, their sense of dignity, self-respect, and trust increased commensurately after restorative justice. These findings contrast markedly with the experience of victims whose cases went to court and who had no opportunity to ask questions directly of their offender, no chance to make their own assessment of their offender's character or propensity for future crime, and no way of making sense of the harm they had suffered [Strang, 2002].

It appears that the most powerful "engine" for achieving this repair is apology. When we asked the victims in our Canberra experiments if they felt they should have received an apology from their offender, around 90% said they should have done. When we asked whether they had received an apology, more than four times as many victims who had experienced restorative justice said they had done so, compared with those whose cases went to court. When we asked them about the quality of the apology they had received, the restorative justice victims much more often rated it as sincere, probably because of the emotionally charged circumstances in which the apology was offered. The few victims whose cases went to court who received an apology much more often felt it was instrumental or had been coerced, whereas apologies in an restorative justice meeting usually emerged spontaneously as the discussion evolved and feelings of empathy developed between victim and offender [Strang, 2002].

Some commentators believe that empathy is an essential precursor to reconciliation: It certainly is central to the practice of restorative justice. It is through this mechanism that anger, fear, and a desire for revenge may be replaced by a degree of mutual understanding. We have demonstrated this empirically through our research with crime victims and their offenders [Strang, 2002]. Interviews with restorative justice participants reveal that each party—victims and offenders—influences the other in experiencing emotions of empathy. We were able to show conclusively in our research that the more empathy one party felt, the more the other felt as well.

For some, reconciliation implies forgiveness and putting the past behind. Certainly, if forgiveness can be offered in answer to genuine remorse, victims may be relieved of the burden of anger, bitterness, and the desire for vengeance resulting from a sense that their emotional hurt is unacknowledged [Arendt, 1958]. Usually, however, we assume that an expression of sincere remorse is an essential element in reconciliation, but perhaps even this is not the case. Two stories demonstrate the different forms that reconciliation may take.

20.3.5.1 A Tale of Two Victims

Natalie, a young woman aged 21 years at the time she came into our London study, had had a deeply troubled life. After being sexually assaulted at the age of 8 years, she was raped when she was 19, and again just before the robbery she committed that brought her into the study. She had 25 previous arrests, four of them for robbery, and had served one previous term of imprisonment.

Carol, the victim of Natalie's most recent robbery, was a nurse aged 56 years who had never before been the victim of a crime. Natalie had hit her over the head when she tried to grab her handbag, resulting in 70 stitches and a stay in hospital. Carol was severely traumatized by this attack. She gave up her job because she was too afraid to leave her home.

Carol was fearful too about meeting Natalie, and in the course of the restorative justice conference, she said very little. Natalie was very distressed, partly because of what her grandmother said at the conference when she expressed her shock and shame that Natalie could do such a thing to someone of a similar age and circumstances as herself. Natalie begged for Carol's forgiveness, but she did not respond until the very end of the conference. At that point, she asked Natalie to kneel in front of her, and when she did so she prayed for her and told her that she forgave her for her crime.

Carol found the experience of meeting Natalie a life-changing one. She returned to work soon afterward, after 5 months of isolation since the crime, and was able to resume her normal life. Although it was not common in our London study for prayers to be said, the fact that Carol and Natalie shared an Afro-Caribbean culture made Carol's response to Natalie's expressions of remorse extraordinarily meaningful to her. This event seems to meet at least some of the definitions and understandings about the nature of reconciliation.

20.3.5.2 A Tale of Two Offenders

In Canberra, two young men were involved in a violent altercation. One of them, Phil, had just been released from prison and had come looking for the other, Sam. Phil had heard that while he was in prison Sam had raped his girlfriend. When he found Sam he beat him severely; Sam's front teeth were knocked out, and he lost nearly two liters of blood before he was found in the street and taken to the hospital. When Phil was arrested, police asked him and his victim whether they would be prepared to meet in a restorative justice conference instead of having the case dealt with in court. Both of them agreed, and the meeting took place together with friends of each of them and a pastor who knew both of them through his work with Canberra's drug-dependent community. Phil was still extremely angry about the alleged rape, which Sam denied, although he did not deny having sexual relations with Phil's girlfriend. Sam was extremely upset about the loss of his teeth and demanded $3,000 toward their repair. Phil said he had no money and did not in any case feel any obligation to help Sam. The discussion meandered for a considerable period, neither party feeling an obligation to accept full responsibility for what had happened and both continuing to feel aggrieved. Both recognized that problems were likely to arise because they had a common drug dealer and were likely to encounter one another often. Finally, the suggestion was made that the two parties should simply ensure that they did not in future come within 100 meters of each other. Each agreed to this suggestion as a fair outcome. In the 5 years following the restorative justice conference, no arrest was recorded for either Phil or Sam.

So what was the value of this meeting? It did not meet traditional criteria for reconciliation—it certainly did not restore friendship or even harmony—and yet by some measures it was a highly successful event. Perhaps both parties acceded to one of the less common understandings of reconciliation, however—each had an opportunity to check their understandings of events against the other, and both accepted something unpleasant about the situation in which they found themselves. Furthermore, from the wider community's perspective, there was a peaceful outcome when there might otherwise have been ongoing feuding and violence.

Our research, moreover, reveals an unexpected benefit of restorative justice along another dimension entirely—that of desire for revenge. Whether victims of crime and conflict have a hard-wired "instinct" for revenge, or whether it derives from moral outrage, there is growing evidence that vengefulness itself can be ameliorated by restorative justice. In our early research in Canberra we inadvertently discovered large restorative justice effects in reducing victims' desire for violent revenge—inadvertently because we had no theoretical basis for testing restorative justice effects in this way. As part of a series of questions designed to test the feelings of victims toward their offenders after their cases had been concluded, we asked them whether they would now harm their offender if they had the chance. Among victims of violence, we found that almost half of those whose cases had gone to court said that they would do so compared with only 9% of those who had met their offender in a restorative justice encounter.

In our subsequent work in London involving much more serious crime—robbery and serious burglary—we measured the amelioration of revenge more systematically. In two-thirds of such incidents, victims had confronted the perpetrators in the course of the crime, had been threatened with a weapon (in one-third of cases), or sustained an injury (a further one-third). In eight of eight tests of the hypothesis, we found substantially fewer victims expressing a desire for physically violent revenge in the restorative justice group than in the control group [Sherman et al., 2005]. Overall, we found that for these crimes the desire for physical retaliation was up to nine times higher for victims in the control group than for those who had met their offenders.

We also measured the incidence of post-traumatic stress among these London victims using the diagnostic criteria of the American Psychiatric Association [1994; see also Angel, 2005]. These criteria require exposure to a traumatic event in which both of the following have been present: The person experienced, witnessed, or was confronted with an event or events that involved actual or threatened death or serious injury, or a threat to the physical integrity of self or others; and the person's response involved intense fear, helplessness, or horror. Among our London victims, 25% exhibited symptoms of post-traumatic stress when scored against a standardized instrument (Impact of Events Scale—Revised). We found a significant reduction in these symptoms in the restorative justice group compared with those who had not experienced restorative justice; furthermore, the differences between the two groups were sustained at a second interview 6 months later [Angel, 2005]. It appears that restorative justice may be one of the few interventions that have been shown to have any positive effect on this much underrated consequence of victimization. This finding is clearly of great relevance to victims of conflict, most of whom have no opportunity to receive counseling or other interventions that might relieve their symptoms of post-traumatic stress.

20.4 Concluding Remarks

It is often said that there can be no lasting peace without justice. Justice requires truth and truth needs to be sought, but we need to acknowledge the complexity of truth, which is so much more than facts. But how much truth can a society bear when it begins to recover from these events? Should truth be told at the expense of peace? And how do we deal with situations in which perpetrators of the horror justify their actions on the grounds that similar atrocities have been visited on them? How do we begin to address these cycles of revenge, these infinite regressions of truth that so often are used to justify the violence? If there can be no peace without justice assuredly there can be no justice without peace, however delicate and provisional. It is in that transitional time of physical and emotional exhaustion that restorative justice may reveal its strength as a process that does not require the Manichean view of formal justice, that recognizes the complexity and multilayered nature of truth, that prioritizes the stories of individuals, both victims and perpetrators, for resolution within devastated communities and provides a chance for the knitting up of division, alienation, and resentment. I suggest that our research findings in restorative justice in the arena of ordinary crime and criminality demonstrate that it has the potential to provide those spaces to begin the process of renewal from the ground up.

References

Aertsen, I. 2008. Racak, Mahne Yehuda and Nyabyondo: Restorative justice between the formal and the informal. In *Restorative justice after large-scale violent conflict*, ed. I. Aertsen, J. Arsovska, H-C. Rohne, M. Valinas, and K. Vanspauwen, 444–61. Cullompton, UK: Willan.

Angel, C. 2005. Victims meet their offenders: Testing the impact of restorative justice conferences on victims' post-traumatic stress symptoms. PhD dissertation, University of Pennsylvania.

Annan, K. 2006. *In larger freedom.* New York: United Nations. http://www.un.org/largerfreedom/chap3.htm (accessed January 3, 2009).

Arendt, H. 1958. *The human condition*, Chicago: University of Chicago Press.

Boraine, A. 2004. Transitional justice as an emerging field. Paper presented at the "Repairing the past: Reparations and transitions to democracy" symposium, International Development Research Centre, Ottawa, Canada. http://www.idrc.ca/en/ev-58817-201-1-DO_TOPIC.html (accessed January 3, 2009).

Boraine, A. and S. Valentine. 2006. *Transitional justice and human security*. Cape Town: International Center for Transitional Justice.

Braithwaite, J. 2002. *Restorative justice and responsive regulation*. Oxford: Oxford University Press.

Braithwaite, J. 2005. Between proportionality and impunity: Confrontation, truth, prevention. *Criminology* 43(2):283–306.

Braithwaite, J. and H. Strang. 2001. Introduction: Restorative justice and civil society. In *Restorative justice and civil society*, ed. H. Strang and J. Braithwaite. Cambridge: Cambridge University Press.

Brown, J. 1994. The uses of mediation to solve criminal cases: A procedural critique. *Emory Law Journal* 43:1247–1309.

Cohen, S. 1995. State crimes of previous regimes. Knowledge, accountability and the policing of the past. *Law and Social Inquiry* 20(1):7–50.

Franciscans International. 2006. Position paper. Paper presented at the fourth ordinary session of the African Commission on human rights, Banjul. http://www.franciscansinternational.org/docs/statement.php?id=475 (accessed January 3, 2009).

Howley, P. 2003. Restorative justice in Bougainville. In *A kind of mending: Restorative justice in the Pacific Islands*, ed. S. Dinnen. Canberra: Pandamus Books.

Kamwimbi, T. 2008. Between peace and justice: Informal mechanisms in the DR Congo. In *Restorative justice after large-scale violent conflicts,* ed. I. Aertsen, J. Arsovska, H.-C. Rohne, M. Valinas, and K. Vanspauwen. Cullompton, UK: Willan.

Karstedt, S. Forthcoming. From absence to presence, from silence to voice: Victims in transitional justice since the Nuremberg Trials. *International Review of Victimology.*

Kiltchling, M. 1991. Interests of the victim and the public prosecution: First results of a national survey. In *Victims and criminal justice*, ed. G. Kaiser, H. Kury, and H.-J. Albrecht. Frieburg I Br, Germany: Max Planck Institute for Foreign and International Penal Law.

Latimer, J., C. Dowden, and D. Muise. 2001. *The effectiveness of restorative justice practices: A meta-analysis*. Ottawa: Canadian Department of Justice.

Marshall, T. and S. Merry. 1990. *Crime and accountability: Victim–offender mediation in practice*. London: HMSO.

McEvoy, K. and A. Eriksson. 2006. Restorative justice in transition: Ownership, leadership and "bottom-up" human rights. In *Handbook of restorative justice: A global perspective*, ed. D. Sullivan and L. Tifft. London and New York: Routledge.

Miers, D., M. Maguire, S. Goldie, et al. 2001. *An exploratory evaluation of restorative justice schemes*. Crime Reduction Series, paper 9. London: Home Office.

Newburn, T., A. Crawford, R. Earle, et al. 2001. *The introduction of referral orders into the youth justice system*. HORS 242. London: Home Office.

Nikolic-Risanovic, V. 2008. Truth and reconciliation in Serbia. In *Restorative justice after large-scale violent conflicts*, ed. I. Aertsen, J. Arsovska, H.-C. Rohne, M. Valinas, and K. Vanspauwen. Cullompton, UK: Willan.

Nugent, W., M. Williams, and M. Umbreit. 2003. Participation in victim–offender mediation and the prevalence and severity of subsequent delinquent behavior: A meta-analysis. *Utah Law Review* 2003(1):137–66.

Sebba, L. 1996. *Third parties: Victims and the criminal justice system*. Columbus: Ohio State University Press.

Shapland, J. 2000. Victims and criminal justice: Creating responsible criminal justice agencies. In *Integrating a victim perspective within criminal justice*, ed. A. Crawford and J. Goodey. Aldershot: Ashgate.

Shapland, J., A. Atkinson, H. Atkinson, et al. 2006. *Restorative justice in practice: The second report from the evaluation of three schemes*. Sheffield: Sheffield Centre for Criminological Research, University of Sheffield.

Shapland, J., A. Atkinson, H. Atkinson, et al. 2007. *Restorative justice: The views of victims and offenders. The third report from the evaluation of three schemes*. Ministry of Justice Research Series 3/07. London: Ministry of Justice.

Shapland, J., A. Atkinson, H. Atkinson, et al. 2008. *Does restorative justice affect reconviction? The fourth report from the evaluation of three schemes*. Ministry of Justice Research Series 10/08. London: Ministry of Justice.

Shapland, J., A. Atkinson, E. Colledge, et al. 2004. *Implementing restorative justice schemes (Crime Reduction Programme): A report on the first year*. Home Office online report 32/04. London: Home Office. http://www.homeoffice.gov.uk/rds/pdfs04/rdsoir3204.pdf (accessed January 3, 2009).

Sherman, L., and H. Strang. 2007. *Restorative justice: The evidence*. London: Smith Institute.

Sherman, L., H. Strang, C. Angel, et al. 2005. Effects of face-to-face restorative justice on victims of crime in four randomized controlled trials. *Journal of Experimental Criminology* 1(3):367–95.

Strang, H. 2002. *Repair or revenge: Victims and restorative justice*. Oxford: Oxford University Press.

Strang, H. and L. Sherman. 2003. Repairing the harm: Victims and restorative justice. *Utah Law Review* 1:15–42.

Strang, H., L. Sherman, C. Angel, et al. 2006. Victim evaluations of face-to-face restorative justice experiences: A quasi-experimental analysis. *Journal of Social Issues* 62(2):281–306.

Umbreit, M. 1994. Crime victims confront their offenders: The impact of a Minneapolis mediation program. *Research on Social Work Practice* 4(4):436–47.

Umbreit, M. 2001. *The handbook of victim–offender mediation*. San Francisco: Jossey-Bass.

Umbreit, M. and R. Coates. 1992. The impact of mediating victim–offender conflict: An analysis of programs in three states. *Juvenile and Family Court Journal*:21–28.

Umbreit, M. and R. Coates. 1993. Cross-site analysis of victim–offender mediation in four states. *Crime and Delinquency* 39:565–85.

United Nations General Assembly. 2005. *Basic principles and guidelines on the right to a remedy and reparation for victims of gross violations of international human rights law and serious violations of international humanitarian law*. Office of the United Nations High Commissioner for Human Rights. http://www2.ohchr.org/english/law/remedy.htm (accessed January 3, 2009).

Valinas, M. and J. Arsovska, J. 2008. A restorative approach for dealing with the aftermath of the Kosovo conflict: Opportunities and limits. In *Restorative justice after large-scale violent conflicts*, ed. I. Aertsen, J. Arsovska, H.-C. Rohne, M. Valinas, and K. Vanspauwen. Cullompton, UK: Willan.

Vanspauwen, K. and T. Savage. 2008. Restorative justice and truth-seeking in the DR Congo: Much closing for peace, little opening for justice. In *Restorative justice after large-scale violent conflicts*, ed. I. Aertsen, J. Arsovska, H.-C. Rohne, M. Valinas, and K. Vanspauwen. Cullompton, UK: Willan.

Waldorf, L. 2006. Rwanda's failing experiment in restorative justice. In *Handbook of restorative justice: A global perspective*, ed. D. Sullivan and L. Tifft. London and New York: Routledge.

Victims and Social Divisions

VI

The Hidden Violent Victimization of Women

21

WALTER S. DEKESEREDY

Contents

21.1 Introduction

In response to public comments made by U.S. researchers and practitioners at a 2008 conference about the intense competition for grant money needed to support various types of work on sexual assault, a colleague of mine based in Ohio sarcastically stated that, "We should all relax. There is enough violence in this world for everyone to share." Certainly, there is much support for her claim. For example, in Canada where I live, citizens repeatedly hear, see, or read media accounts of gang-related shootings, muggings, soldiers either dying or being injured in Afghanistan and Iraq, and a myriad of other forms of interpersonal violence (e.g., bank robberies). As Renzetti and Edleson [2008:xxxiii] correctly point out, such violence:

> invades both the public and private spheres of our lives, many times in unexpected and frightening ways. Interpersonal violence is a problem that individuals may experience at any point during the lifespan—indeed, even before birth. From the use of amniocentesis to identify the sex of a fetus with the intention of aborting it if it is a female to the withholding of food or medication from an elderly person to punish him or her for some perceived

infraction, interpersonal violence is found not only throughout the life course, but also throughout the world. It is a global problem that includes war, genocide, terrorism, and rape of women as a weapon of war.

However, not everyone is at equal risk of being the victim of violent crime, and some victims get more attention than do others [Currie, 2008]. For example, although stranger-to-stranger murders are relatively rare, they receive much attention for weeks and sometimes years in daily Canadian newspapers [Mennie, 2008]. Consider the case of Jane Creba. On December 26, 2005, a stranger shot and killed this 15-year-old girl in downtown Toronto, and this murder was still frequently described 3 years later in the widely read and cited newspaper *Toronto Star* [Contenta et al., 2008]. However, this is not to say that Ms. Creba's untimely, violent death should be trivialized. It is, to say the least, deeply disturbing, and the pain and suffering experienced by her family and friends are immeasurable. Still, how often do the media report sexual assaults that routinely occur in university/college dating relationships? How frequently are male-to-female beatings in marital/cohabiting relationships featured on the televised evening news? And, how often do the media and politicians address the plight of women killed by male ex-partners during or after the process of separation or divorce? These and other victims of what Stanko [1985] refers to as "intimate intrusions" greatly outnumber the victims of predatory violent crimes that occur on the streets and in other public places (e.g., taverns), but the media generally character-ize male-to-female assaults in intimate relationships as either "exceptional incidents" or as the "result of a man's suddenly having 'snapped'" [Myers, 1997:110].

The violent abuse of women by intimate male partners is not restricted to a handful of countries. Rather, it is a worldwide public health problem [Shoener, 2008]. For example, the World Health Organization conducted a multicountry study of the health effects of domestic violence. More than 24,000 women who resided in urban and rural parts of 10 countries were interviewed, and the research team discovered that the percentage of women who were ever physically or sexually assaulted, or both, by an intimate partner ranged from 15% to 71%, with most research sites ranging between 29% and 62% [Garcia-Moreno et al., 2005]. Consider, too, that in Australia, Canada, Israel, South Africa, and the United States, 40–70% of female homicide victims were murdered by their current or former partners [Krug et al., 2002]. Another frightening fact is that 14 girls and women are killed each day in Mexico [Mujica and Ayala, 2008]. Of course, male violence against female intimates takes many other shapes and forms, such as honor killings, dowry-related violence, and acid burning [Watts and Zimmerman, 2002; Sev'er, 2008; Silvestri and Crowther-Dowey, 2008]. Sadly, right now, women around the world are being brutalized by their current or former male partners "in numbers that would numb the mind of Einstein" [Lewis cited in Vallee, 2007:22].*

There is ample evidence of what Canadian journalist Brian Vallee [2007] refers to as "a war on women," one that is all around us. It is a global problem that damages our public health, with many commentators asserting that intimate relationships and institutions across the globe are experiencing an epidemic of woman abuse. Actually, the concept of epidemic is out of place here. To health officials, an epidemic is a disease that devastates a population before eventually subsiding. Male-to-female physical, sexual, psychological, and other forms of violence, however, seem to be deeply entrenched in the world's population. Thus, if male-to-female abuse is a disease, then it is in its endemic phase [DeKeseredy et al., 2000], possibly to be compared with hard drug use (e.g., smoking crack cocaine) among truly disadvantaged North American inner-city residents [Currie, 1993; DeKeseredy and Schwartz, 2009].

In a current global political economic climate characterized by massive government cuts to women's programs [DeKeseredy and Dragiewicz, 2007], a rabid antifeminist backlash [Stanko, 2006], and other major threats to women's health and well-being, many people would agree with Silvestri and Crowther-Dowey's [2008:106] prediction that "things are set to get worse." Ironically, at a time when crime discussion in many parts of the world is dominated by calls for more prisons, more executions, and "what about the victim?," a market remains for belittling crime victims when they are women [Schwartz and DeKeseredy, 1994; DeKeseredy, 2009a]. For example, growing numbers of conservative fathers' rights groups, academics, politicians, and others intent on rolling back the achievements of the women's movement fervently challenge research showing alarmingly high rates of male-to-female beatings, sexual assaults, and other highly injurious patriarchal practices that typically occur behind closed doors and in intimate relationships [Stanko, 2006; DeKeseredy and Dragiewicz, 2007]. Moreover, although many people, especially men, are quick to point out human rights violations in totalitarian countries, they simultaneously whitewash or ignore the victimization of women in their own so-called democratic societies [Kallen, 2004; Silvestri and Crowther-Dowey, 2008].

The purpose of this chapter, then, is to help give voice to groups of women who, for the most part, suffer in silence. The challenges of gathering data on male violence against adult female intimates are presented, and two widely read and competing theoretical perspectives are reviewed. Some progressive policies are also briefly discussed, but it is first necessary to define violence against women.

---

* Stephen Lewis is the Cofounder and the Codirector of AIDS-Free World, a new international AIDS advocacy organization, based in the United States. He was also Canada's Ambassador to the United Nations from 1984 to 1988.

21.2 What Is Violence against Women?

What is violence against women? For many people, the answer to this question is simple—an intentional physical act such as a punch, kick, bite, or forced sexual penetration that results in physical trauma. Consider what happened to four 13-year-old girls at a Toronto, Ontario, middle school on September 25, 2007. Eight male students were videotaped restraining and groping them on school property and were thus charged with sexual assault. What the boys did is a violation of the Canadian Criminal Code and was dealt with accordingly by the police, but large numbers of people, including some conservative university professors [e.g., Fekete, 1994; Gilbert, 1994], would regard labeling the perpetrators' behaviors *sexual assault* as "definitional stretching." For example, one boy's mother was quoted as saying, "It's kids playing basketball. People touch people. [T]hey were just playing around" [cited in Powell and Brown, 2007:A27]. Nevertheless, just because people like this woman do not define what happened to the victims as serious does not mean that their perspective coincides with the girls' real life feelings and experiences. The reality is that these young women were traumatized [DeKeseredy, 2009b].

Again, when most people think of violence, they think of physical brutality. Many workers in battered women's shelters cynically refer to this definition as the *stitch rule*. They assert that many justice system workers believe that if you do not need to have stitches, you are not hurt [DeKeseredy and Schwartz, 1996]. However, there is ample evidence showing that many women who have experienced violence often say that it is the psychological, verbal, and spiritual violence that hurts the most and longest [DeKeseredy, 2009a]. Some women, like the person quoted below, say that most physical wounds heal, but the damage to their self-respect and ability to relate to others caused by emotional, verbal, and spiritual violence affects every aspect of their lives:

> I was raped by my uncle when I was 12 and my husband has beaten me for years. For my whole life, when I have gone to a doctor, to my priest, or to a friend to have my wounds patched up, or for a shoulder to cry on, they dwell on my bruises, my cuts, my broken bones. My body has some scars … that's for sure … I don't look anything like I did 15 years ago, but it's not my body that I really wish could get fixed. The abuse in my life has taken away my trust in people and in life. It's taken away the laughter in my life. I still laugh, but not without any bitterness behind the laughter. It's taken away my faith in God, my faith in goodness winning out in the end, and maybe worst of all, it's taken away my trust in myself. I can live with my physical scars. It's these emotional scars that drive me near suicide sometimes. [DeKeseredy and MacLeod, 1997:5]

Note, too, that Fitzpatrick and Halliday's [1992:76] respondents would often tell them that "they would rather be hit than endure the constant

put-downs and mind games inflicted on them by their abusive partners."
Another woman interviewed by MacLeod [1987:12] said:

> The thing that's most hurting for me is the way he makes me feel so dirty, so
> filthy. He treats me like a dog, worse even. He tells me I'm ugly and worthless.
> He spits on me. It's not enough to hit me and kick me. He spits on me.
> Sometimes I think the hitting is better than being made to feel so low.

In sum, then, many nonviolent, highly injurious behaviors are just as
worthy of in-depth empirical, theoretical, and political attention as those that
cause physical harm. Furthermore, physical abuse, sexual abuse, and psychological abuse are not mutually exclusive. Indeed, psychological abuse always
accompanies physical and sexual assaults in intimate relationships [Gelles
and Straus, 1988; DeKeseredy and Joseph, 2006]. Joan is a rural Ohio woman
interviewed by DeKeseredy et al. [2006:237] who was harmed by various
types of abuse during the process of exiting her relationship:

> Well, what happened was that he got drunk and wanted sex from me and I told
> him no. I said, "Stay away from me. I can't stand you when you're drinking.
> Get away from me." He started grabbing my butt, and playing with my legs,
> and trying to grab my boobs. And everything, anything to get what he wanted.
> And I told him. I kicked him in the leg and I told him, "Get away from me."
> And then [we] got into a fight over it and then he started throwing stuff at my
> face and I went to the phone and I said, "I'm gonna call your probation officer."
> I says, "If you don't leave me alone and you've been drinking, you're acting like
> an ass. Leave me the hell alone." And he wouldn't. He unplugged the phone.
> I plugged it in, I plugged it, you know. It was back and forth. He unplugged,
> I plugged it in. He unplugged it, I plugged it in…. When he was trying to
> prevent me from getting the phone, he stepped on my foot, which fractured
> the top of my foot. I was on crutches for two weeks.

Sometimes women are not the only ones injured by their current or former male partners. For example, 19% of DeKeseredy et al.'s [2006] 43 rural
Ohio respondents stated that their partners abused their children, and one
woman believes that her ex-partner raped her as a means of killing her
unborn child. Below is what Trina's ex-husband did to her daughter:

> He came back October of the same year for a so-called emergency visitation,
> and he was able to take my daughter away from me for eight hours even though
> the DNA had never been proven. And, when my daughter finally came back,
> she had severe diaper rash, smelled like cigarettes and alcohol, and had bruises
> right, right on her thighs and on her wrists. [ibid.:237]

Again, nonphysical acts should be considered part of any definition of
violence against women. However, here I focus mainly on assaults on women's

bodies because most of the social scientific research focuses on these harms. Certainly, much more work on other nonphysical hurtful behaviors is necessary for the above reasons.

Most people around the world perceive family/household settings and intimate relationships as "havens in a hostile world" [Lasch, 1977]. Further, numerous citizens of advanced Western industrial societies like to brag that they live in "the freest country on Earth" [Katz, 2006]. Perhaps they would change their minds if they knew what really goes on behind closed doors in many homes across their countries and exactly how much of it occurs.

21.3 The Challenges of Gathering Data on Violence against Women

What U.S. sociologists Richard Gelles and Murray Straus stated 20 years ago still holds true for women today: "You are more likely to be physically assaulted, beaten, and killed in your own home at the hands of a loved one than anyplace else, or by anyone else in society" [1988:18]. However, we really do not know exactly how many women are raped, killed, hit, punched, and kicked by their current or former male partners. Although many estimates are made, every data set underestimates the true extent of male-to-female violence [DeKeseredy and Schwartz, 1996; Rosenbaum and Langhinrichsen-Rohling, 2006]. For example, most criminologists argue that data on homicide are among the most accurate crime data of all, primarily because unlike property crime or even intimate and nonintimate assaults, the majority of homicides are reported to or are discovered by the police [Fox and Piquero, 2003]. However, leading experts on femicide (also referred to as the killing of women by current or former male intimates) point out that official statistics on this harm vary greatly. According to Mahoney, Williams, and West [2001:153], in the United States:

> This variance is due in large part to the problem of reliance on police reports and/or federal statistics for information on the relationship between the victim and perpetrator. Such information is often missing for a large percentage of cases (from 30% to 50% in many reports), and even when it is provided it may be incorrect.

There are other problems with homicide data. Consider that in the United States, former intimate partners are often labeled by the police as "acquaintances" or "friends" [Campbell, 1992]. Sometimes, too, bodies are hidden or victims are deemed to be "missing persons" because they cannot be located. Then, of course, there are cases where medical officials declare women as dying from accidental or suicidal causes when in fact they were murdered by their estranged or current male partners. Certainly, there is what some criminologists refer to as the "dark figure of homicide" [Brookman, 2005].

Think about how you would go about finding out how much nonlethal woman abuse exists. What would you do? Would you look at the records of the police or other public officials? Would you go door to door and ask women if they have been beaten and/or raped? Clearly, any method has limitations. Many women do not reveal their experiences to researchers or public officials because they are embarrassed or because they are terrified of retaliation or reprisal if their abuser finds out they revealed their victimization [DeKeseredy, 2009a]. Amazingly enough, some people have suffered such severe blows to their self-image that they think their experiences are too trivial to mention, whereas others do not wish to discuss their problems with researchers because they do not want to recall painful memories [Straus et al., 1981; Kirkwood, 1993; Smith, 1994; DeKeseredy and Schwartz, 1998].

Getting violent men to accurately disclose the amount of abuse they commit is even more difficult, especially during times when substantial media attention is being given to issues surrounding lethal and nonlethal forms of violence against women. Even if these men are guaranteed confidentiality and anonymity, they may fear that they will be punished for victimizing their current or former partners, or they may worry about being publicly humiliated. Moreover, sharp discrepancies exist between the physical and sexual violence estimates generated from talking to men and from talking to women. Women are more likely to report victimization experiences than men are to disclose their injurious behaviors. What accounts for these discrepancies? It is unlikely that men and women report differently because large numbers of women are lying. A much more likely explanation is that social desirability plays a key role in shaping male responses [DeKeseredy and Schwartz, 1998].

However, even if it is impossible to obtain totally accurate data on nonlethal assaults, some methods are more reliable than others. The best procedures are representative sample self-report and victimization surveys specifically designed to collect data on male-to-female assaults. This is not to say that other methods cannot provide valuable insight; however, only random sample surveys of various populations can give us fairly reliable estimates of how much violence takes place in cities, towns, countries, states, provinces, and on university and college campuses. The basic idea of a random sample survey is that, although it is impossible to question everyone in the country or city, if everyone has an equal chance of being selected as an interviewee, then, we would only need to question a smaller number of them.

For example, to interview everyone in Toronto, Canada, would require an extraordinary number of interviewers. Worse, by the time you tracked down everyone, the answers from the first people interviewed would be so old that they could not be properly compared with the responses from the most recent interviews. Thus, researchers would choose a representative sample of all the people in Toronto. If this is done correctly, experience has shown many times that their answers will adequately represent what we would have found if we had interviewed everyone. Of course, as a cautionary note, some surveys are more methodologically sound than others.

How violence against women is measured is another key issue that warrants careful attention. A research team can develop an excellent sampling plan but still underestimate the extent of male-to-female violence. For example, surveys that use questions derived from narrow, legal definitions of physical and sexual violence typically elicit rates that are markedly lower than studies that use operational definitions of intimate male-to-female violence that extend beyond the limited realm of criminal law [DeKeseredy, 2000]. Again, many women argue that psychological abuse is more painful than physical violence. Nevertheless, to this day, many people claim that "real battering" results in bruises and stitches, "not words that wound deeply or the terroristic household that frightens horribly" [Schwartz, 2000:819]. Thus, what happened to this woman and her children on Christmas Eve some years ago would not be counted because the perpetrator never touched her:

> Her husband arrived home late, drunk and angry, and upon entering the house and seeing the little tree, all fixed up, he became so angry that he took the tree and tore it up to pieces, took all the little gifts and presents off the tree and mutilated and destroyed them…. Not being satisfied with this, and while cursing and defaming the plaintiff, he took all of the table linens and mattresses and sheets and quilts off the bed, took them to the kitchen and dumped them on the floor, gathered up all the food there was in the house and spilled these on the floor, put the cooking utensils on the floor and then took the stove pipe and dumped soot over the bed linen and food and everything he had put on the floor and then turned water all over this mess, then broke and tore up all the furniture. [Peterson del Mar, 1966:124]

A major problem still remains even when researchers use broad definitions of violence. For example, we still see variance in incidence and prevalence rates across studies, even when they use similar measures. This problem is caused by sampling differences, different data-gathering techniques (telephone vs. computer surveys), and other methodological factors. Obviously, definitional consensus does not necessarily translate into scientific consistency. Still, definitional consistency, standard measures, and similar samples will not make much of a difference if respondents cannot understand the survey. Many immigrants and refugees do not read or speak English; thus, it is pointless to ask them to complete a survey unless it is translated into their native language. This approach is expensive, albeit empirically fruitful, because it results in improved response rates [Smith, 1987]. Additionally, administering surveys to ethnic minority booster samples can generate a sufficient number of minorities to allow for complex multivariate analyses of patterns of violence against women [DeKeseredy, 2000; Jones, MacLean, and Young, 2006]. Nevertheless, as DeKeseredy et al. [2003] discovered in their study of woman abuse in a Canadian public housing community, many recent refugees or immigrants not only have difficulties speaking English but also came from war-torn countries, dictatorships, or police states. Thus, it is possible that large numbers of minority women may not believe a research team's assurances of confidentiality [Schwartz, 2000].

Empirical attempts to "unsilence the voices of marginalized and oppressed women who are battered" must also address the plight of rural women [Sokoloff and Dupont, 2005:3]. However, as DeKeseredy and Schwartz [2009] remind us about doing such work in the United States, regardless of what theoretical or political position one takes or what methods are used, studying woman abuse in the "heartland" presents many challenges, especially in rural communities characterized by geographic and social isolation [Websdale and Johnson, 2005; Logan et al., 2006], inadequate (if any) public transportation [Lewis, 2003], the existence of a powerful "ole" boys network consisting of patriarchal criminal justice officials and some abusive men, and relatively low telephone subscription rates [Websdale, 1998].

Like other rural criminologists [e.g., Logan et al., 2004], DeKeseredy and Schwartz [2009] found that many abused women live far away from neighbors, other agents of informal social control, social service providers, and criminal justice officials. It should also be noted that Websdale's [1998] rural Kentucky female interviewees said that their abusers' assaults "feed off of" their partners' isolation. They often use such tactics such as destroying their current or ex-wives' cars, which are necessities in rural communities. One woman told Websdale that her ex-husband did not want her to have a car so that she would have to stay with him. In an attempt to get her back, he set her car on fire.

Similarly, a rural Ohio woman interviewed by DeKeseredy and Schwartz [2009] told them that, "I didn't have a car. I wasn't allowed to go anywhere." Her husband, however, had "plenty of cars" and would do the following to stop her from seeking freedom and independence:

> He would even take the brain off the car, because I figured out how to fix the distributor, so the brain started coming off. Because if you don't have the brain, your car don't start. It was plain and simple. He taught me a lot about cars and I knew what parts I need. And there would be no spare. So, I couldn't leave.

In rural parts of Ohio and elsewhere, there is also widespread acceptance of woman abuse, as well as community norms prohibiting survivors from publicly talking about their experiences and from seeking social support [DeKeseredy et al., 2007]. As an Appalachian Ohio woman interviewed by DeKeseredy and Joseph [2006:303] put it:

I don't sit around and share. I keep it to myself. Um, I, I believe that's part of my mental illness. I believe it takes a lot of it. But, I'm not one to sit around and talk about what's happened.

Then, of course, like a sizeable portion of their urban counterparts, many rural women are physically forced by their current or former male partners to keep their abuse a secret from friends, relatives, neighbors, and other people. Poverty also keeps many rural women from coming into contact with those who can help them or who will listen to their voices. Unable to afford telephones, cars, or to take taxis, they suffer alone [DeKeseredy and Schwartz, 2009]. In numerous cases, being economically disadvantaged is not simply the result of the inability to find work in a community plagued by joblessness. It is also a function of separation and divorce [Logan and Walker, 2004].

An even longer list of obstacles researchers encounter while conducting rural studies of male-to-female violence and other crimes could easily be provided. However, some of these problems can be overcome or minimized using methods similar to those used by DeKeseredy and his colleagues to gather data on rural separation/divorce sexual assault. For example, the advertisement presented in Box 21.1 was placed once a week during two different 6-week periods in a free newspaper available throughout parts of Athens County, Ohio. Also, posters about the study were hung in public places and were given to social service providers who come into contact with abused women.

Several other sample selection and recruitment strategies were used, including radio station advertisements and local support services "spreading the word" about the project.* Further, from early March 2003 until early

BOX 21.1   NEWSPAPER ADVERTISEMENT

Call for interested women of Athens, Hocking, and Vinton Counties for participation in an Ohio University research project

Have you ever had unwanted sexual experiences while trying to leave your husband or male live-in partner?

Or, have you ever had unwanted sexual experiences after you left your husband or male live-in partner?

We would greatly appreciate your participation in a confidential interview. Your name will not be given to anyone.

We will pay you $25.00 for your time and transportation costs. Also, we will talk to you at a time and location of your choosing.

---

* See DeKeseredy and Schwartz [2009] and DeKeseredy et al. [2006] for more in-depth information about the sample selection and recruitment strategies.

April 2004, two female research assistants carried cellular phones 24 hours a day to receive calls from women interested in participating in the study. Callers were told the purpose of the research and were then asked a series of screening questions to determine their eligibility to be interviewed. If they met the selection criteria, the women were invited to a semistructured face-to-face interview at a time and place of their choosing.

At the start of the interview, women were again told the purpose of the study and asked to sign a consent form. They were also reminded that the interview would be highly confidential, that they could end the interview at any time, and that they did not have to answer any of the interview questions. After the interview, the women were paid US$25.00 for their time and given $US7.75 for travel expenses and an index card listing the locations and phone numbers of local support services for survivors. Moreover, interviewees were invited to contact the research team at a later time if they had questions or concerns. Although the research team was deeply committed to generating rich qualitative data, it was more concerned with ensuring respondents' safety in communities where most residents know each other.

In sum, similar to what other criminologists found [e.g., Websdale, 1998], many rural women in the United States strongly adhere to privacy norms and have little, if any, faith that a promise of confidentiality will be guaranteed by survey researchers, especially those who are "outsiders" (e.g., people who are not from the community) [Lewis, 2003].* For these and other reasons noted by DeKeseredy and Schwartz [2009], feminist means of gathering data on rural woman abuse are necessary. Still, the methods used by DeKeseredy and his colleagues are not unorthodox. For example, the sample selection techniques are akin to those used by Bowker [1983] to recruit Milwaukee women who have successfully "beaten wife-beating" and to procedures used by DeKeseredy et al. [2003] to recruit people to participate in their Canadian study of poverty and crime in public housing. These methods are also comparable with those used by Logan et al. [2006] to recruit female victims of stalking in both rural and urban communities.

Indeed, methodological improvements are needed in future rural studies. We also require better means of studying other types of male-to-female violence, such as hate-motivated sexual assaults on women. One positive step in this direction is a representative sample survey administered by DeKeseredy et al. [2008] of students enrolled at two Canadian institutions of higher learning. To the best of my knowledge, before this project, not one North American survey was specifically designed to generate data on hate-motivated sexual assaults on campus. DeKeseredy and his colleagues found that slightly less than 11% (10.2%; $n = 39$) of the women in the sample stated that they experienced one or more of five variants of hate-motivated sexual

* Pilot work for Logan et al.'s [2006] stalking study also revealed that rural communities are more distrustful of researchers and/or strangers than are urban areas.

assault. As expected, the overall rate for the same types of victimization experienced since the age of 16 was markedly higher (27.9%; $n = 107$). What makes these two rates especially alarming is that they are underestimates. As is the case with surveys that focus on woman abuse in intimate relationships, there is a variety of reasons that hate crime victims do not disclose incidents, including embarrassment and fear of reprisal.

While the "multicultural women's movement has utterly transformed the cultural landscape" on Canadian university and college campuses [Katz, 2006:1], DeKeseredy et al. [2008] offer evidence that on top of having to worry about abusive acts committed by male intimates and acquaintances, as well as random acts of male "stranger danger" that "come out of the blue," many women live in fear of being attacked by their peers because of a perception that they have overstepped their boundaries. It is not surprising, then, that for many female students there is "no safe place" [Wolfe and Guberman, 1985]. It is probably the norm for Canadian female undergraduates to remain "hyper-vigilant—sometimes 24/7" about the likelihood of being sexually assaulted from many different directions [Katz, 2006].

21.4 Summary

More than 20 years ago, Fine [1985:397] argued that:

> [F]eminists have dealt inadequately with the question of whether some women are more vulnerable than others. Eager to repudiate class and race-biased analyses of abuse, we have promoted universal risk arguments, criticizing methodologies that define some women as more vulnerable than others. But this refutation of classism and racism obscures our ability to wrestle with this question of vulnerability and therefore eligibility criteria.

Of course, the neglect to examine variations in violence against women across many different socioeconomic status categories can just as easily be said about social science in general throughout the twentieth century. However, only a few social scientific areas of inquiry have moved as far and as fast as the study of male-to-female physical, sexual, and psychological abuse. For example, only 37 years ago, a comprehensive bibliography of North American sources on wife-beating would fit on an index card. Today, hundreds of journal articles, scores of books, and several important journals specifically address a variety of forms of woman abuse across the world. We now have rich empirical information and a wide variety of theories on woman abuse in a variety of relationships and social settings, making it clear that living in conditions of tyranny is a dangerous attack on a woman's psychological and physical health [Mattley and Schwartz, 1990; DeKeseredy and Schwartz,

2002]. Nevertheless, reading the extant literature makes it clear that we still have a long way to go to create effective means of getting large numbers of women to "speak to the unspeakable" to the research community.

As Abraham [2002:xi] correctly points out, "[W]hen we assume there is one overarching problem and one way to address it, we limit both our vision and our ability to individually and collectively contribute to the struggle to end domestic violence." More researchers need to recognize that their empirical techniques must be tailored to fit different groups of women's unique backgrounds and that there is considerable "domestic violence at the margins" [Sokoloff, 2005].

21.5 "Why Does He Do That?" Two Competing Theoretical Perspectives on Violence against Women

Included in the above heading is the title of Lundy Bancroft's [2002] book on angry and controlling men. It is also a variation of a question often asked by students, journalists, and others not immersed in the woman abuse literature. Perhaps the most common answer people give is that men who beat, kill, or sexually assault female intimates must be "sick" or mentally disturbed. How could a "normal" person punch, kick, stab, or shoot someone he deeply loves and depends on? Certainly, the media help to build that myth [Adams, 2007]. Violence against women is also generally portrayed in fiction, television, and films as involving a drunken, foreign, or criminal assailant [Gelles and Straus, 1988].

Psychological perspectives on woman abuse are not as popular among criminologists as they were in the 1970s. Nevertheless, several prominent researchers still claim that the majority of men who beat, kill, or sexually assault their current or estranged female intimate partners do so because they are mentally ill or suffer from personality disorders [e.g., Dutton and Bodnarchuk, 2005; Dutton, 2006].* Much of the popular British sensibility on battered women was formed on the parallel theory, popularized by J. J. Gayford [1975] that the women themselves can be seen as deviant or mentally ill, thus bringing the violence on themselves.†

It is difficult for many people to view men who assault women as anything other than sick. However, this "commonsense perspective" lacks empirical support for several reasons [Loseke et al., 2005]. Certainly, woman abuse is occasionally a function of psychopathology; however, a large body of research shows that most abusive men are "less pathological than expected"

---

* Some researchers [e.g., Dutton, 2006] who make this claim also call for marginalizing the consideration of gender in the etiology of violence against women. See DeKeseredy and Dragiewicz's [2007] feminist response to this call.
† There is a propensity for many male psychiatrists to blame female victims for their male partners' abusive behavior [Stark, 2007].

[Gondolf, 1999]. Further, large- and small-scale North American surveys show that woman abuse in a wide variety of intimate relationships "happens with alarming regularity" [Lloyd, 1991]. For example, at least 11% of the women in marital/cohabiting relationships are physically abused by their male partners on an annual basis in Canada and the United States, and approximately 25% of North American female undergraduate students experience some variation of sexual assault on an annual basis [DeKeseredy and Flack, 2007; DeKeseredy, 2009b].

If only a handful of men abused their current or former partners, it would be very easy to accept nonsociological accounts of their behaviors. They must be disturbed individuals. Unfortunately, as feminist theorists point out, in Canada and in other advanced industrial nations (e.g., the United States), a substantial number of injurious male actions, values, and beliefs are microsocial expressions of broader patriarchal forces [Smith, 1990; Stanko 1997; DeKeseredy and Schwartz, 2009]. This means that the problem is not one in which individual men simply all happen to suffer from the same psychopathology, or weak ego, or whatever. Rather, they all live in the same society, and the single individual man is partially a reflection of the values and beliefs that are expressed by the broader society. As Jackson Katz [2006:28] notes in his analysis of men who abuse women:

> Most men who assault women are not so much disturbed as they are disturbingly *normal*. Like all of us, they are products of familial and social systems. They are our sons, brothers, friends, and coworkers. As such, they are influenced not only by individual factors, but also by broader cultural attitudes and beliefs about manhood that shape their psyches and identities. And *ours*. (Emphasis in original)

A large body of literature shows that gang rapes and other similar crimes are frequently committed by "homegrown products of contemporary American society" [Katz, 2006:28].* An even larger mass of scientific literature shows that sexual, physical, and psychological abuse is common in North American heterosexual relationships.† Again, men who abuse women are not acting in a deviant manner completely opposite to everything they have ever learned about the way to treat women. Of course, some abusive men have clinical pathologies [O'Leary, 1993], but most do not [Pagelow, 1992, 1993; DeKeseredy and Schwartz, 2009]. Some researchers claim that fewer than 10% of all incidents of intimate violence are caused by mental disorders and that psychological perspectives cannot explain the other 90% [Gelles and Straus, 1988].

---

* See Schwartz and DeKeseredy [1997] for an in-depth review of sociological research on gang rapes committed by college students.
† See Bachar and Koss [2001], DeKeseredy [2009b], and Mahoney, Williams, and West [2001] for reviews of studies of the incidence and prevalence of woman abuse.

Although the majority of men perhaps never sexually or physically assault women, certainly all North American men, including those who live in rural communities, live in a society that can accurately be termed a "rape culture" [Buchwald et al., 1993], where no man can avoid exposure to patriarchal and pro-rape attitudes. For example, rare is a man who is not been exposed to pornographic media, to mainstream television shows or movies depicting women as inferior to men, and to rap videos and songs referring to women as "bitches" and "hoes" [Schwartz and DeKeseredy, 1997; Katz, 2006]. In fact, pornography plays a major role in woman abuse [DeKeseredy and Schwartz, 1998; Bergen and Bogle, 2000; DeKeseredy et al., 2006].

From the standpoint of many feminist scholars [e.g., Dworkin, 1994], pornography is also a variant of hate-motivated violence against women, and it, too, has become "normalized" or "mainstreamed" in North America and elsewhere [Jensen and Dines, 1998], despite becoming increasingly more violent and racist. Jensen [2007:17] observes:

> There is no paradox in the steady mainstreaming of an intensely cruel pornography. This is a culture with a well-developed legal regime that generally protects individuals' rights and freedoms, and yet it also is a strikingly cruel culture in the way it accepts brutality and inequality. The pornographers are not a deviation from the norm. Their presence in the mainstream shouldn't be surprising because they represent mainstream values: the logic of domination and subordination that is central to patriarchy, hyper-erotic nationalism, white supremacy, and a predatory corporate capitalism.

Returning to the issue of rap songs, some journalists assert that rap artist Eminem and others who write and sing songs like his are creative. On the other hand, many feminists refer to these "musicians" as promoters of "hate humor" [Katz, 2006]. It is hard to disagree with this after hearing Eminem sing, "Put anthrax on your Tampax and slap you till you can't stand" [cited in Katz, 2006:159]. Nevertheless, despite recognizing the pain caused by such lyrics, a few feminists, such as popular singer and recording artist Tori Amos, oppose the censorship of violent, misogynist rap because they view it as functional for women. According to Amos:

> If you're singing songs that are about cutting women up, usually these guys are tapping into an unconscious male rage that is real, that's existing and they're just able to harness it. So to shut them up isn't the answer. They're a gauge; they're showing you what's really happening in the psyche of a lot of people. [cited in MTV.com, 2001:1]

Similarly, other feminists, such as Gronau [1985], contend that feminists should oppose the censorship of pornography, even its most violent forms. She claims that pornography serves to remind women of the rampant sexism that victimizes and exploits them. If pornography is censored, then the evidence of sexism is hidden. Gronau further argues that it is more difficult to mobilize women to fight hidden sexism than it is to fight the obvious and extreme form of sexism manifested in pornography. However, this functional conception of pornography as benefiting women represents a minority view among feminists who have written on the topic [Alvi, DeKeseredy, and Ellis, 2000].*

Most people would never dare to praise or support musicians, filmmakers, or actors who say hateful things about people's ethnic/cultural backgrounds or spirituality. However, it seems that our media and society in general do not view hateful songs about women as problematic. Consider Katz's [2006:169] commentary on the marketing of Eminem as a legitimate "rebel" to youth, especially to young white males:

> [I]f you focus on contents of his lyrics, the "rebellion" is empty. If you are a "rebel," it matters who you are and what you are rebelling against. The KKK are rebels, too. They boast about it all the time. They fly the Confederate (rebel) flag. But most cultural commentators would never dream of speaking positively about the KKK as models of adolescent rebellion for American youth because the content of what they advocate is so repugnant. Likewise, Eminem would be dropped from MTV playlists and lose his record contract immediately if he turned his lyrical aggression away from women and gays and started trashing people of color, Jews, Catholics, etc. In that sense, Eminem's continued success makes a statement about how this culture regards women and gays. Sadly, it is a statement that many progressive, feminist, egalitarian, and non-violent people in this era of white male backlash find quite deflating.

If pornography and sexist rap songs contribute to male violence against women, the same can be said about men's adherence to the ideology of familial patriarchy, which is a discourse that supports the abuse of women who violate the ideals of male power and control over women in intimate relationships [Smith, 1990; DeKeseredy and Schwartz, 1993]. Relevant themes of this ideology are an insistence on women's obedience, respect, loyalty, dependency, sexual access, and sexual fidelity [Dobash and Dobash, 1979; Barrett and McIntosh, 1982; Pateman, 1988; DeKeseredy and Schwartz, 1998].

Familial patriarchy is a subsystem of societal patriarchy. These two components really cannot be pulled too far apart, and one variant cannot be fully understood without reference to the other [Smith, 1990]. Although the definition of societal patriarchy is subject to much debate, here it refers to the type of male domination at the societal level. Moreover, following Dobash and Dobash [1979], societal patriarchy is made up of two elements: a structure

---

* See Vance [1984] for a nonfunctional, anticensorship, and feminist approach to pornography.

and an ideology. Structurally, the patriarchy is a hierarchical social organization in which males have more power and privilege. Certainly, North America is known for being a continent characterized by gross gender inequity. For example, in 30 U.S. states, under law, a man can be awarded conditional exemptions if he raped his wife [Bergen, 2006].* Moreover, despite decades of ongoing struggle and activism around the issue of pay equity, women continue to earn about 73% of what men do in the United States [Lips, 2005]. Note, too, that on October 3, 2006, Bev Oda, then federal Minister for the Status of Women Canada (SWC), announced that women's organizations would no longer be eligible for funding for advocacy, government lobbying, or research projects. Further, SWC was required to delete the word "equality" from its list of goals [Carastathis, 2006]. This seriously challenges Donald Dutton's [2006:ix] claim that, "Women rights have finally been acknowledged after centuries of religion-based political oppression."

Of course, in many parts of the world, every major social institution, such as the family, the workplace, and the military, has been affected by some laws and other means of eliminating sexism [Renzetti and Curran, 2002; DeKeseredy, Ellis, and Alvi, 2005]. Nevertheless, as Stanko [1997:630] observes, "Despite the advantages for some women who have achieved educational and employment recognition, our concern about physical and sexual integrity remains one of our main worries." And, "there is little evidence that the general patterns of men's abuse have been interrupted" [1997:630].

Many more examples of patriarchal discourses and practices can easily be provided. Still, examples such as the above do not answer a number of questions. Why do men maintain this power? Why don't they, in the spirit of fair play, simply give up enough power to equalize the power between men and women? Why don't more women rebel against the patriarchy? The answer is the other part of patriarchy: the ideology. The ideology of patriarchy provides a political and social rationale for itself. Both men and women come to believe that it is "natural" and "right" that women be in inferior positions. Men feel completely supported in excluding women, and up to a point women feel that exclusion is correct [DeKeseredy and Schwartz, 1993; Katz, 2006]. To someone (male or female) who believes completely in the ideology of patriarchy, the entire concept of equal rights or women's liberation is a controversial topic, sounding not only wrong but also unnatural [Bacchetta and Power, 2002].

Obviously, there are other factors that contribute to violence against women, including life-events stress [Hardesty, 2002], social class [DeKeseredy and Schwartz, 2002], membership in male patriarchal subcultures of violence [Bowker, 1983; Schwartz and DeKeseredy, 1997], and poverty [Sokoloff, 2005]. However, all attempts to explain any form of woman abuse should

---

* A husband is exempt in these states if his wife is mentally or physically impaired, unconscious, asleep, or unable to consent [Bergen, 2006].

always be "grounded in women's lived experiences" [Hardesty, 2002:618]. As Stanko [2006:546] notes based on her experiences as Director of the Economic and Social Research Council Violence Research Program in the United Kingdom:

> We had to learn to hear ordinary women about ordinary violence. Now we sometimes listen to what they say. But all too often, in so many areas around the world, we still do not listen enough or effectively. If we did, perhaps we would challenge violence against women—and all violence—more effectively.

Regardless of which current or new theory best explains the causes of the pain and suffering described throughout this chapter, for women at risk of experiencing violence or who are subjected to it, the creation of effective policies should be the top priority. Moreover, as Logan et al. [2004:58] put it, "Creative solutions must be developed in order to serve women with victimization histories within the context of the specific communities where these women live."

21.6 What Is to Be Done about Male-to-Female Violence?

Violence against women is not a relatively new problem. For example, wife-beating has existed for close to 3,000 years [Dobash and Dobash, 1979]. However, before the 1970s, it was ignored by social scientists.[*] Consider that the prestigious *Journal of Marriage and Family*, from its beginning in 1939 through 1969, did not contain any articles on wife abuse [O'Brien, 1971]. As stated earlier, since the early 1970s, however, the number of studies on violence against women has increased dramatically. Nevertheless, research alone does little, if anything, to prevent the problems addressed in this chapter. Hence practitioners and activists assert that we should devote most of our time, energy, and other resources to the development of prevention and control strategies. This point is especially well taken, given that the rates of various types of violence against women have not decreased during the past several decades [Stanko, 1997; DeKeseredy, 2008]. Moreover, in millions of North American intimate relationships men use a myriad of nonviolent means of coercive control that reflect what Evan Stark [2007:5] refers to as the "deprivation of rights and resources that are critical to personhood and citizenship."

There are also numerous examples of government cuts to progressive efforts aimed at interrupting the patterns of male-to-female violence. One of the most popular pieces of U.S. legislation is the Violence Against Women Act, but most American programs dealing with the results of woman abuse

---

[*] Feminist activists—not social scientists—are responsible for the "discovery" of woman abuse [Breines and Gordon, 1983].

operate on shoestring budgets. Worse, for a long and complicated set of reasons, those who try to provide services for abused women find that to maintain funded facilities they must conform to strict governmental requirements. To get funds from county mental health budgets, their clients often must have diagnoses and prognoses. Services must be aimed at the individual problems of the client [Schwartz and DeKeseredy, 2008]. Also in the United States, Child Protection Services often are required in the first instance to try to maintain the family, even if one member is a batterer or child sexual abuser. Services, money, and programs do not deal with broader social forces in North America. As Miller and Iovanni [2007:294] put it, "These concessions have shifted the discourse and action away from challenging the root causes of battering—including issues related to power and privilege—and away from prevention efforts."

Some of the responses to National Football League player Michael Vick constitute another highly problematic example of how contemporary North American society responds to violence against women. He was sent to prison for operating an illegal dog-fighting ring, and there was a broad national sense of outrage about his crime. Why do people get so upset by the death of animals but not by the murder of women? In Pittsburgh, a sports radio personality pointed out that Michael Vick would have never gotten into as much trouble if he had limited himself to raping women. He was removed from the air, but the fact remains that he was right. Why, in North America, do most athletes accused of battering or rape end up with the charges dismissed and the woman complainant vilified [Bennedict, 1997; Katz, 2006]? The outrage and economic pressure (e.g., losing lucrative endorsements) just are not there in North America for people who harm women, just dogs [Schwartz and DeKeseredy, 2008].

Historically, many governments opposed and actively resisted women's efforts to improve their quality of life. For example, in the 1970s, Canada, a country consistently ranked by the United Nations as one of the best countries in the world to live in, was led by a government that viewed the feminist movement as a major potential threat to its political, economic, and social order. In fact, Royal Canadian Mounted Police infiltrated the women's movement at that time and "amassed thousands of pages worth of surveillance records" on groups like the now defunct Toronto Women's Caucus [Bronskill, 2008:A2]. Twenty years later, the politicians guaranteed us that, "the barricades have fallen" and "women's fight for equality has largely been won" [Faludi, 1991:ix]. As vividly described by Hammer [2002] and many others who made progressive contributions to an interdisciplinary understanding of the enduring discrimination against women [e.g., Cross, 2007], most of us still live in a climate characterized by vitriolic attacks on feminist scholarship, practice, and activism intended to secure women's basic human rights [Stanko, 2006; DeKeseredy and Dragiewicz, 2007; Dragiewicz, 2008]. Note, too, as Vallee [2007:322] observes:

Those fighting to end gender inequality and its often lethal effects find themselves swimming in a sea of red herring—in the form of a conservative backlash determined to prove that women are just as violent as men, and that solutions to the problem of domestic violence must be gender neutral.

What, then, is to be done? Resistance to efforts to end violence against women and other symptoms of gender inequality are part and parcel of every-day life and will never disappear. However, this should not be interpreted as a call for sitting back and doing nothing. Moreover, we already know about many effective prevention and control strategies, and we could reduce much pain and suffering around the world if "existing policies and protocols were diligently executed and enforced" [Vallee, 2007:345]. Thus, here, I briefly sug-gest a few additional ways of mobilizing communities to work together to change the harmful *status quo*.

We live in a society riddled with factoids that challenge efforts to curb violence against women. The *Merriam-Webster Online Dictionary* [2005:1] defines a *factoid* as "an invented fact believed to be true because of its appear-ance in print." Researchers, activists, and practitioners struggling to end violence against women are all too familiar with factoids, which often become much more than what this dictionary refers to as "brief and usually trivial news items" [ibid.:1]. "But women do it too" is one factoid that is especially troubling and is frequently used by fathers' rights groups, right-wing politicians, and others intent on blocking programs designed to save women's lives.

As pointed out in my earlier work [see DeKeseredy, 2007], there are many ways of challenging factoids in a highly intelligible fashion and in public are-nas. One strategy is to organize inexpensive conferences open to practitioners, researchers, journalists, and the general public. This approach is vital, given that right-wing men's and fathers' rights groups are organizing such events to further support the above factoid and the erroneous claim that violence against women is a statistically insignificant harm committed by a handful of pathological men.

Organized by the Sheila Wellstone Institute, Camp Sheila Wellstone is a prime U.S. example of an effective initiative that, among other things, provides practitioners and advocates guidance on how to develop effective messages to send out to the community. Camp Sheila Wellstone also teaches people how to influence decision makers and how to build coalitions. More information on the Sheila Wellstone Institute can be found at http://well-stone.org. People around the world can also turn to it for innovative ideas aimed at challenging factoids.

Proactive steps need to be taken to disseminate well-crafted research and critiques of factoids to the media. Volunteering to appear on talk shows and holding press conferences are some examples of the ongoing efforts to "get the word out." That people who are advocates for survivors of abuse have been called on by the media [e.g., Cross, 2007] reveals that journalists do not totally disregard the research and views of people who challenge danger-ous factoids and erroneous interpretations of data and policies [Caringella-MacDonald and Humphries, 1998; DeKeseredy, 2007].

In 2006, Nancy Neylon, Director of the Ohio Domestic Violence Network, suggested to me that daily conversations with community groups, neighbors, friends, service providers, and others about violence against women should always include statements that challenge factoids. This is an important point because advocates spend much more time in the community, police departments, hospi-tals, shelters, and courts than they do at conferences or on television shows.

As one of my Swedish friends repeatedly states, "communication is the key." If more people become aware of the true extent of various types of violence against women and of the problematic nature of factoids such as "women are as violent as men," more people may voice their discontent with apathetic government responses to one of the world's most compelling social problems. They may also elect politicians who are committed to enhancing the health and safety of women who continue to suffer in silence.

Will the above and other progressive strategies make a difference? This is a question that can only be answered by evaluating their effects. Regardless of what strategy is pursued, we must remember that there are people who will develop initiatives to support factoids and thus our work will be ongoing and ever changing. Another point to keep in mind is that ending violence against women in intimate relationships and in other social settings also requires schol-ars moving beyond trying to "win a point" in the "name of science" [Renzetti, 1997:vi]. Additionally, we must remember that no matter how we study or try to explain violence against women, the perspectives we offer are often irrel-evant to those who are hurt by it [DeKeseredy and Dragiewicz, 2007]. After all, who knows more about violence than the people who are targets of it?

Acknowledgments

I would like to thank Drs. Knepper and Shoham for their guidance and comments. Some of the research reported here was supported by National Institute of Justice Grant 2002-WG-BX-004, financial assistance provided by Ohio University, and by a federal Canadian grant from the Social Sciences and Humanities Research Council to Walter DeKeseredy and Barbara Perry.

References

Abraham, M. 2002. *Speaking the unspeakable: Marital violence among south Asian immigrants in the United States.* New Brunswick, NJ: Rutgers University Press.
Adams, D. 2007. *Why do they kill? Men who murder their intimate partners.* Nashville, TN: Vanderbilt University Press.

Bacchetta, P. and M. Power. 2002. Introduction. In *Right wing women: From conservatives to extremists around the world*, ed. P. Bacchetta and M. Power, 1–15. New York: Routledge.

Bachar, K. and M. P. Koss. 2001. From prevalence to prevention: Closing the gap between what we know about rape and what we do. In *Sourcebook on violence against women*, ed. C. M. Renzetti, J. L. Edleson, and R. K. Bergen, 117–42. Thousand Oaks, CA: Sage.

Bancroft, L. 2002. *Why does he do that? Inside the minds of angry and controlling men.* New York: Berkley.

Barrett, M. and M. McIntosh. 1982. *The anti-social family.* London: Verso.

Benedict, J. 1997. *Public heroes, private felons: Athletes and crimes against women.* Boston: Northeastern University Press.

Bergen, R. K. 2006. Marital rape: New research and directions. *VAWnet* February 14:1–13.

Bergen, R. K. and K. A. Bogle. 2000. Exploring the connection between pornography and sexual violence. *Violence and Victims* 15:227–34.

Bookman, F. 2005. *Understanding homicide.* London: Sage.

Bowker, L. H. 1983. *Beating wife-beating.* Lexington, MA: Lexington Books.

Breines, W. and L. Gordon. 1983. The new scholarship on family violence. *Signs: Journal of Women in Culture and Society* 8:491–531.

Bronskill, J. 2008. RCMP spied on Rita MacNeil: Feminist singer of "women's lib songs," among dozens under scrutiny in early '70s. *Toronto Star* August 5:A2.

Buchwald, E., P. R. Fletcher, and M. Roth (eds.). 1993. *Transforming a rape culture.* Minneapolis, MN: Milkweed Edition.

Campbell, J. C. 1992. If I can't have you, no one can: Power and control in homicide of female partners. In *Femicide: The politics of women killing*, ed. J. Radford and D. Russell, 99–113. New York: Twayne.

Carastathis, A. 2006. New cuts and conditions for Status of Women Canada. *Toronto Star* October 11. www.dominionpaper.ca/canadian_news/2006/10/11 new_cuts_a.html (accessed October 11, 2006).

Caringella-MacDonald, S. and D. Humphries. 1998. Guest editors' introduction. *Violence Against Women* 4:3–9.

Contenta, S., J. Rankin, B. Powell, and P. Winsa. 2008. Why getting tough on crime is toughest on the taxpayer. *Toronto Star* July 19:A1, A14–A15.

Cross, P. 2007. Femicide: Violent partners create war zone for women. *Toronto Star* July 6, AA8.

Currie, E. 1993. *Reckoning: Drugs, the cities and the American future.* New York: Hill and Wang.

____. 2008. Pulling apart: Notes on the widening gap in the risks of violence. *Criminal Justice Matters* 70:37–38.

DeKeseredy, W. S. 2000. Current controversies on defining non-lethal violence against women in intimate heterosexual relationships: Empirical implications. *Violence Against Women* 6:32–50.

____. 2007. Factoids that challenge efforts to curb violence against women. *Domestic Violence Report* 12:81–82, 93–95.

____. 2008. *Thoughts on day one.* Paper presented at the National Institute of Justice Sexual Violence Research Workshop, Arlington, VA.

_____. 2009a. Patterns of violence in the family. In *Families: Changing trends in Canada*, ed. M. Baker, 6th ed, 179–205. Whitby, Ontario: McGraw-Hill Ryerson.

_____. 2009b. Girls and women as victims of crime. In *Women and the criminal justice system: A Canadian perspective*, ed. J. Barker, 313–45. Toronto: Emond Montgomery.

DeKeseredy, W. S., S. Alvi, M. D. Schwartz, and E. A. Tomaszewski. 2003. *Under siege: Poverty and crime in a public housing community*. Lanham, MD: Lexington Books.

DeKeseredy, W. S., J. F. Donnermeyer, M. D. Schwartz, K. D. Tunnell, and M. Hall. 2007. Thinking critically about rural gender relations: Toward a rural masculinity crisis/male peer support model of separation/divorce sexual assault. *Critical Criminology* 15:295–311.

DeKeseredy, W. S. and M. Dragiewicz. 2007. Understanding the complexities of feminist perspectives on woman abuse: A commentary on Donald G. Dutton's rethinking domestic violence. *Violence Against Women* 13:874–84.

DeKeseredy, W. S., D. Ellis, and S. Alvi. 2005. *Deviance and crime: Theory, research and policy*. Cincinnati, OH: LexisNexis.

DeKeseredy, W. S. and W. F. Flack, Jr. 2007. Sexual assault in colleges and universities. In *Battleground criminal justice*, ed. G. Barak, 693–96. Westport, CT: Greenwood.

DeKeseredy, W. S. and C. Joseph. 2006. Separation/divorce sexual assault in rural Ohio: Preliminary results of an exploratory study. *Violence Against Women* 12:301–11.

DeKeseredy, W. S. and L. MacLeod. 1997. *Woman abuse: A sociological story*. Toronto: Harcourt Brace.

DeKeseredy, W. S., B. Perry, B. Pearson-Nelson, and M. D. Schwartz. 2008. *Campus sexual assault as hate crime: Results from a Canadian representative sample survey*. Oshawa, Ontario: University of Ontario Institute of Technology.

DeKeseredy, W. S. and M. D. Schwartz. 1993. Male peer support and woman abuse: An expansion of DeKeseredy's model. *Sociological Spectrum* 13:394–414.

_____. 1996. *Contemporary criminology*. Belmont, CA: Wadsworth.

_____. 1998. *Woman abuse on campus: Results from the Canadian national survey*. Thousand Oaks, CA: Sage.

_____. 2001. Definitional issues. In *Sourcebook on violence against women*, ed. C. M. Renzetti, J. L. Edleson, and R. K. Bergen, 23–34. Thousand Oaks, CA: Sage.

_____. 2002. Theorizing public housing woman abuse as a function of economic exclusion and male peer support. *Women's Health and Urban Life* 1:26–45.

_____. 2009. *Dangerous exits: Escaping abusive relationships in rural America*. New Brunswick, NJ: Rutgers University Press.

DeKeseredy, W. S., M. D. Schwartz, and S. Alvi. 2000. The role of profeminist men in dealing with woman abuse on the Canadian college campus. *Violence Against Women* 6:918–35.

DeKeseredy, W. S., M. D. Schwartz, D. Fagen, and M. Hall. 2006. Separation/divorce sexual assault: The contribution of male peer support. *Feminist Criminology* 1:228–50.

Dobash, R. E., and R. Dobash. 1979. *Violence against wives: A case against the patriarchy*. New York: Free Press.

Dragiewicz, M. 2008. Patriarchy reasserted: Fathers' rights and anti-VAWA activism. *Feminist Criminology* 3:121–44.

Dutton, D. G. 2006. *Rethinking domestic violence*. Vancouver: University of British Columbia Press.

Dutton, D. G. and M. Bodnarchuk. 2005. Through a psychological lens: Personality disorder and spousal assault. In *Current controversies on family violence*, ed. D. R. Loseke, R. J. Gelles, and M. M. Cavanaugh, 5–18. Thousand Oaks, CA: Sage.

Dworkin, A. 1994. *Pornography happens to women*. http://www.nostatusquo.com/ACLU/dworkin/PornHappens.html (accessed July 15, 2008).

Faludi, S. 1991. *Backlash: The undeclared war against American women*. New York: Crown.

Fekete, J. 1994. *Moral panic: Biopolitics rising*. Montreal: Robert Davies.

Fitzpatrick, D. and C. Halliday. 1992. *Not the way to love*. Amherst, NS: Cumberland County Transition House Association.

Fox, J. A. and A. R. Piquero. 2003. Deadly demographics: Population characteristics and forecasting homicide trends. *Crime and Delinquency* 49:339–59.

Garcia-Moreno, C., A. F. M. H. Jansen, M. Ellsberg, L. Heise, and C. Watts. 2005. *WHO multi-country study on women's health and domestic violence against women: Initial results on prevalence, health outcomes, and women's responses*. Geneva: World Health Organization.

Gayford, J. J. 1975. Wife-battering: A preliminary survey of 100 cases. *British Medical Journal* 1:194–97.

Gelles, R. J. and M. A. Straus. 1988. *Intimate violence: The causes and consequences of abuse in the American family*. New York: Simon and Schuster.

Gilbert, N. 1994. Miscounting social ills. *Society* 31:18–26.

Gondolf, E. W. 1999. MCMI-III results for batterer program participation in four cities: Less "pathological" than expected. *Journal of Family Violence* 14:1–17.

Gronau, A. 1985. Women and images: Feminist analysis of pornography. In *Women against censorship*, ed. C. Vance and V. Burstyn, 127–55. Toronto: Douglas and McIntyre.

Hammer, R. 2002. *Antifeminism and family terrorism: A critical feminist perspective*. Lanham, MD: Roman and Littlefield.

Hardesty, J. L. 2002. Separation assault in the context of postdivorce parenting: An integrative review of the literature. *Violence Against Women* 8:597–621.

Jensen, R. 2007. *Getting off: Pornography and the end of masculinity*. Cambridge, MA: South End.

Jensen, R. and G. Dines. 1998. The content of mass-marketed pornography. In *Pornography: The production and consumption of inequality*, ed. G. Dines, R. Jensen, and A. Russo, 65–100. New York: Routledge.

Jones, T., B. D. MacLean, and J. Young. 1986. *The Islington crime survey*. London: Gower.

Kallen, E. 2004. *Social inequality and social injustice: A human rights perspective*. Basingstoke, UK: Palgrave Macmillan.

Katz, J. 2006. *The macho paradox: Why some men hurt women and how all men can help*. Naperville, IL: Sourcebooks.

Kirkwood, C. 1993. *Leaving abusive partners*. Newbury Park, CA: Sage.

Krug, E., L. Dahlberg, J. Mercy, et al. 2002. *World report on violence and health*. Geneva: World Health Organization.

Lash, C. 1977. *Haven in a heartless world: The family besieged*. New York: Basic Books.

Lewis, S. H. 2003. *Unspoken crimes: Sexual assault in rural America*. Enola, PA: National Sexual Violence Resource Center.

Lips, H. M. 2005. *Sex and gender: An introduction.* New York: McGraw-Hill.

Lloyd, S. 1991. The dark side of courtship: Violence and sexual exploitation. *Family Relations* 40:14–20.

Logan, T. K., J. Cole, L. Shannon, and R. Walker. 2006. *Partner stalking: How women respond, cope, and survive.* New York: Springer.

Logan, T. K., L. Evans, E. Stevenson, and C. Leukefeld. 2004. Rural and urban women's perceptions to barriers to health, mental health, and criminal justice services: Implications for victim services. *Violence and Victims* 19:37–62.

Loseke, D. R., R. J. Gelles, and M. M. Cavanaugh. 2005. Controversies in conceptualization. In *Current controversies on family violence*, ed. D. R. Loseke, R. J. Gelles, and M. M. Cavanaugh, 1–4. Thousand Oaks, CA: Sage.

MacLeod, L. 1987. *Battered but not beaten: Preventing wife battering in Canada.* Ottawa: Advisory Council on the Status of Women.

Mahoney, P., L. Williams, and C. M. West. 2001. Violence against women by intimate relationship partners. In *Sourcebook on violence against women*, ed. C. M. Renzetti, J. L. Edleson, and R. K. Bergen, 143–78. Thousand Oaks, CA: Sage.

Mattley, C. and M. D. Schwartz. 1990. Living under tyranny: Gender identities and battered women. *Symbolic Interaction* 13:281–89.

Mennie, J. 2008. Statistics no comfort: Police want to heighten public's sense of security. *Montreal Gazette* July 18:A3.

Merriam-Webster Online. 2005. *Factoid.* http://www.m-w.com//cgi-bin/dictionary?book=Dictionaryandva=factoid (accessed June 11, 2007).

Miller, S., and L. Iovanni. 2007. Domestic violence policy in the United States. In *Gender violence: Interdisciplinary perspectives*, ed. L. L. O'Toole, H. R. Schiffman, and M. L. Kiter Edwards, 287–96. New York: New York University Press.

MTV.com. 2001, September 28. *Tori Amos says Eminem's fictional dead wife spoke to her.* http://www.thedent.com/mtvart0901.html (accessed July 18, 2008).

Mujica, A. and A. I. U. Ayala. 2008. *Femicide in Morelos: An issue on public health.* Paper presented at the World Health Organization's 9th World Conference on Injury Prevention and Safety Promotion, Yucatan, Mexico.

Myers, M. 1997. *News coverage of violence against women: Engendering blame.* Thousand Oaks, CA: Sage.

O'Brien, J. E. 1971. Violence in divorce-prone families. *Journal of Marriage and the Family* 33:692–98.

Pagelow, M. D. 1992. Adult victims of domestic violence: Battered women. *Journal of Interpersonal Violence* 7:87–120.

———. 1993. Response to Hamberger's comments. *Journal of Interpersonal Violence* 8:137–39.

Pateman, C. 1988. *The sexual contract.* London: Polity.

Powell, B. and L. Brown. 2007. 8 boys charged with sex assault on school grounds: 12- and 13-year-old students accused of restraining and groping girls; parents fear charges overblown. *Toronto Star* October 5:A1, A27.

Renzetti, C. M. 1997. Foreword. In *Woman abuse: A sociological story*, ed. W. S. DeKeseredy and L. MacLeod, 5–7. Toronto: Harcourt Brace.

Renzetti, C. M. and D. J. Curran. 2002. *Women, men, and society.* Boston: Allyn and Bacon.

Renzetti, C. M. and J. L. Edleson. 2008. Introduction. In *Encyclopedia of interpersonal violence*, vol. 1, ed. C. M. Renzetti and J. L. Edleson, 33–4. Thousand Oaks, CA: Sage.

Rosenbaum, A. and J. Langhinrichsen-Rohling. 2006. Meta-research on violence and victims: The impact of data collection methods on findings and participants. *Violence and Victims* 21:404–09.

Schwartz, M. D. 2000. Methodological issues in the use of survey data for measuring and characterizing violence against women. *Violence Against Women* 6:815–38.

Schwartz, M. D. and W. S. DeKeseredy. 1994. People without data attacking rape: The Gilbertizing of Mary Koss. *Violence Update* 5:5, 8, 11.

———. 1997. *Sexual assault on the college campus: The role of male peer support.* Thousand Oaks, CA: Sage.

———. 2008. Interpersonal violence against women: The role of men. *Journal of Contemporary Criminal Justice* 24:178–85.

Sev'er, A. 2008. Discarded daughters: The patriarchal grip, dowry deaths, sex ratio imbalances and foeticide in India. *Women's Health and Urban Life* 7:56–75.

Shoener, S. J. 2008. Health consequences of intimate partner violence. In *Encyclopedia of interpersonal violence*, vol. 1, ed. C. M. Renzetti and J. L. Edleson, 326–27. Thousand Oaks, CA: Sage.

Silvestri, M. and C. Crowther-Dowey. 2008. *Gender and crime.* London: Sage.

Smith, M. D. 1987. The incidence and prevalence of woman abuse in Toronto. *Violence and Victims* 2:173–87.

———. 1990. Patriarchal ideology and wife beating: A test of a feminist hypothesis. *Violence and Victims* 5:257–73.

———. 1994. Enhancing the quality of survey data on violence against women: A feminist approach. *Gender and Society* 8:109–27.

Sokoloff, N. J. (ed.). 2005. *Domestic violence at the margins: Readings on race, class, gender, and culture.* New Brunswick, NJ: Rutgers University Press.

Sokoloff, N. J. and I. Dupont. 2005. Domestic violence: Examining the intersections of race, class, and gender—An introduction. In *Domestic violence at the margins: Readings on race, class, gender, and culture*, ed. N. Sokoloff, 1–14. New Brunswick, NJ: Rutgers University Press.

Stanko, E. A. 1985. *Intimate intrusions: Women's experiences of male violence.* London: Routledge and Kegan Paul.

———. 1997. Should I stay or should I go? Some thoughts on variants of intimate violence. *Violence Against Women* 3:629–35.

———. 2006. Theorizing about violence: Observations from the Economic and Social Research Council's Violence Research Program. *Violence Against Women* 12:543–55.

Stark, E. 2007. *Coercive control: How men entrap women in personal life.* New York: Oxford University Press.

Straus, M. A., R. J. Gelles, and S. K. Steinmetz. 1981. *Behind closed doors: Violence in the American family.* New York: Anchor.

Vallee, B. 2007. *The war on women.* Toronto: Key Porter.

Vance, C. 1984. *Pleasure and danger: Exploring female sexuality.* London: Routledge and Kegan Paul.

Watts, C. and C. Zimmerman. 2002. Violence against women: Global scope and magnitude. *The Lancet* April 6:359.

Websdale, N. 1988. *Rural woman battering and the justice system: An ethnography.* Thousand Oaks, CA: Sage.

Images of Criminality, Victimization, and Disability

22

MANUEL MADRIAGA AND
REBECCA MALLETT

Contents

The loose association between what we would now call disability and criminal activity, mental incompetence, sexual license, and so on established a legacy that people with disabilities are still having trouble living down. [Davis, 1995:37]

22.1 Introduction

This chapter aims to open up discussion about the relationship between disability and notions of criminality and victimhood. This discussion is underpinned with a radical-critical victimological stance [Mawby and Walklate, 1994] that sees the victimization of disabled people beyond the narrow confines of criminal law [van Dijk, 1999; Zednar, 2002; Goodey, 2005]. The rationale for this chapter is that the discipline of disability studies has inadequately addressed this relationship, whereas in the areas of criminology and victimology there has been a lack of engagement with the relatively recent debates around what it means to be disabled. This chapter hopes to unearth these inadequacies to advance the idea that broadening and combining relatively new understandings of disability with developing concepts of criminology and victimology could benefit future work in both areas.

The following chapter outlines recent debates within disability studies around understanding and conceptualizing disability. It is here where we will also highlight the failure of disability studies to address the criminalization and victimization of disabled people. This is followed by an exploration of the concomitant failure of criminology and victimology to take into account the changing conceptions of impairment and disability. Our motivation for pursuing this aim is to propel the idea that, rather than a biological circumstance, disability is a social process that is constructed from everyday notions of "normalcy," or "everyday eugenics," that both disabled and nondisabled people take for granted [Davis, 1995; Snyder and Mitchell, 2006]. Reflecting on the works of Davis [1995] and Snyder and Mitchell [2006], in the final section we explore how an everyday eugenics plays its part in creating and perpetuating cultural images of disabled people. We maintain a dual focus on criminals and victims as we argue that the conflation between disabled people and criminals amounts to a different yet nonetheless significant sort of victimization deriving from, what we are calling, everyday eugenics. We conclude that the cultural representation of disabled people as either villains or victims can tell us much about disabled people's present position as an oppressed minority.

22.2 Disability Studies: The Criminalization and Victimization of Disabled People?

Twenty years ago there was no such thing as disability studies [Barton and Oliver, 1997:ix].

Although the study of "disability" is currently a burgeoning domain of academic inquiry [Swain et al., 2003], such was not always the case. Following a considered investigation of the available literature, Abberley [1987:5] concluded that the state of "the sociology of disability" in the mid-1980s was "both theoretically backward and a hindrance rather than a help to disabled people." It has been argued that this inadequacy was connected to a failure to realize the significance of disability and disabled people to the wider sociological project, and this has been mirrored in relation to other disciplines with history [Kudlick, 2003], anthropology [Oliver, 1996], geography [Chouinard, 1994], and psychology [Shakespeare and Watson, 1997] cited, along with sociology, as historically failing to take the socially orientated study of disability seriously.

Although this generalized picture of academia in the mid-1980s is bleak, there were movements afoot that sought a greater profile for disability in social and political contexts. By this time, Paul Hunt [1966] had offered essays on disability in his collected volume *Stigma: The Experience of Disability*, the Union of the Physically Impaired Against Segregation (UPIAS) [1976] had published their pioneering *Fundamental Principles of Disability*, and Vic Finkelstein [1980], in association with the World Rehabilitation Fund, had published *Attitudes and Disabled People: Issues for Discussion*. Slowly, an alternative explanation of disability gained momentum, and with it, the beginnings of a legitimacy for both a new wave of political activism and a new area of academic study.

The birth, development, and allied associations of an academic discipline named *disability studies* have been narrated in a number of ways; however, it is the Open University that most widely receives the foundational credit. In response to the increasing politicization of disabled people, in 1975 the Open University produced a new undergraduate course entitled "The Handicapped Person in the Community" [Finkelstein, 1998]. Shortly afterward, the University of Kent followed suit with a master's degree program [Barton and Oliver, 1997], and in 1981 the Open University produced its first disability reader entitled *Handicap in a Social World* [Barnes, 1999]. In the years that followed "the steady and evergrowing stream of writings emerging from disabled people themselves" [Barton and Oliver, 1997:ix] enabled the study of disability to find its way onto the curriculum, with some of the earliest writers to become canonical within the resulting discipline being initially activists in the Disabled People's Movement [e.g., Hunt, 1966; Finkelstein, 1980, 1993, 1998; Barnes, 1991a&b, 1992, 1997, 1998].

Although links with the political movement are more dispersed today, debate between the Disabled People's Movement and the discipline it spawned is vibrant when compared with the debate between it and disability studies' "source" disciplines [Shakespeare and Watson, 1997]. Indeed, with regard to geography, in 1998 Park et al. noted that "the disability rights movement has scarcely begun to make a significant impact on the literature" [Park et al., 1998:226]; the situation has changed little in the decade since. Given the focus of this chapter, we would also add criminology and victimology to the list of disciplines that continue to pay little attention to socially orientated study of disability.

Although disability studies is a relatively new area of academic inquiry [Gleeson, 1997], in its broadest sense, it is distinguishable by its commitment to a shift in focus "away from a prevention/treatment/remediation paradigm to a social/cultural/political paradigm" [Pfeiffer and Yoshida, 1995:480]. It is also discernible by its vibrant interdisciplinarity: "drawing on sociology, linguistics, economics, anthropology, politics, history, psychology and media studies" [Swain et al., 2003:33].

Given this focus on the social/cultural/political aspect and its inter-disciplinarity it seems odd that the criminalization and victimization of disabled people have not been more fully explored within disability studies itself. The relationship between crime and disability has been explored and examined in other areas such as law [Williams, 1995; Peay, 2002; Littlechild and Fearns, 2005], criminology [Chappell, 1994; Petersilia, 2001; Peay, 2002], and psychiatry [e.g., Holland et al., 2002; Lindsay, 2002; Lindsay et al., 2002], but as yet disability studies has not adequately engaged with the topic. This seems even more surprising when we consider the presence of a passing but nonetheless heartfelt recognition that, throughout history, disabled people have been the victims of violence. For example, Barnes [1992:20] discusses how the "ancient Greeks and Romans were enthusiastic advocates of infanticide for disabled children," as well as how the nineteenth century saw the rise of a scientific legitimacy for eugenics resulting in forced sterilization and, ultimately, led to the Holocaust. In total, an estimated 275,000 disabled people were killed [Disability Rights Advocates, 2001; Kudlick, 2003].

Paradoxically, the reason for this neglect may stem from an adherence to the social model of disability within disability studies in the United Kingdom. Despite it being, for many, the essence of the contemporary study of disability, it has marginalized people labeled with certain impairments (especially those labeled with learning difficulties), as well as marginalizing discussion of impairment itself:

> The social model has become the conceptualisation of disability with the most resonance and support in the British disabled people's movement, and, as such, is the reference point for those both within and outside that movement and Disability Studies who want to take a social understanding of disability further, or in different directions. [Thomas, 1999:13]

The social model, which has been described as the Disabled People's Movement(s) "big-idea" [Hasler, 1993], understands disability as the product of a disabling society that "is geared to, built for and by, and controlled by non-disabled people" [Swain et al., 2003:2]. As Thomas suggests above, it has become *the* reference point for this new field of political activism and academic inquiry. Oliver [1990] credits the UPIAS [1976] for conjuring a sociological understanding of disability. According to UPIAS [1976:3–4]:

> In our view, it is society which disables physically impaired people. Disability is something imposed on top of our impairments, by the way we are unnecessarily isolated and excluded from full participation in society. Disabled people are therefore an oppressed group in society. It follows from this analysis that having low incomes, for example, is only one aspect of our oppression. It is a consequence of our isolation and segregation, in every area of life, such as education, work, mobility, housing, etc.

In describing the social model of disability, Oliver juxtaposes it with traditional conceptions of disability, which he termed the individualization and medicalization of disability. Instead of viewing disability as an indicator of individual failing or one's own (medical) "problem," the social model of disability comprehends disability as purely social phenomena. This means that disabled people are *disabled* by society, not by their impairments. Distinguishing disability and impairment is essential in grasping the social model of disability. Citing UPIAS [1976:14] again:

> Disability is something imposed on top of our impairments by the way we are unnecessarily isolated and excluded from full participation in society. Disabled people are therefore an oppressed group in society. To understand this it is necessary to grasp the distinction between the physical impairment and the social situation, called "disability," of people with such impairment. Thus we define *impairment* as lacking part of or all of a limb, or having a defective limb, organ or mechanism of the body; and *disability* as the disadvantage or restriction of activity caused by a contemporary social organisation which takes no or little account of people who have physical impairments and thus excludes them from participation in the mainstream of social activities. Physical disability is therefore a particular form of social oppression. (Italics added)

Thus, although a person may have a physical impairment that may require wheelchair use, he or she may only be disabled if presented with flights of stairs. Having the option of an elevator or lift would eliminate the disabling barrier of the stairs.

Although the social model of disability has become symbolic of the political mobilization among disabled people in the United Kingdom, it has been contended that people labeled with certain impairments have been marginalized from the mainstream disability movement and therefore also marginalized within disability studies. As Goodley [2001:211] pointed out:

> Whereas people with physical impairment are rightfully afforded a socio-historical position in the social model ... people with "learning difficulties" are consistently underwritten. Thrown into the category of naturalised, irrational "other." Closed in, isolated and confined by a "mental impairment" devoid of meaning and history, pre-social, inert and physical. People with "learning difficulties" are personal tragedies of their unchangeable "organic impairments." That these assumptions are so strongly held is particularly worrying in light of the concerted attempts by disability theorists and activists to expose the *social character of humanity* in relation to disablement. (Emphasis in the original)

This marginalization of people with so-called "learning difficulties" and "mental impairments" in the political disability movement has been reflected within the realm of disability studies [Chappell, 1998; Goodley, 2001]. With (some) people labeled with learning difficulties appearing to have an "organic impairment," their "place in the context of the social model of disability" has been "decidedly shaky" [Goodley, 2001:213]. This is the result of the social model's theoretical distinction between disability and impairment, where the former is understood as being socially constructed and the latter is consigned "to the domain of medical discourse and authority" [Molloy and Vasil, 2002:663]. It is this thinking that perpetuates the perception that the social model of disability is reserved for people with physical impairments rather than people with learning difficulties [Goodley, 2001:212]. Thus, in response to the limited discussion on impairment, disability studies writers, like Goodley [2001], have called for a shift of emphases from the social processes of disability toward the social construction of impairment [e.g., Molloy and Vasil, 2002]. We will return to the importance of considering the social construction of impairment in a later section, but for now we will explore the impact of marginalizing people labeled with learning difficulties.

The consequences of an emphasis of disability over impairment in regard to exploring the criminalization and victimization of disabled people can be seen most clearly in the case of people labeled with learning difficulties. Instead of disability studies being at the forefront of this exploration, the disciplines of criminology, law, and psychiatry are relied on. This is a cause of concern because the latter disciplines have streams of Lombrosian thinking within them [Garland, 2002], where people with learning difficulties, for example, remain *fixed objects* of inquiry in regard to criminal and deviant acts [Chappell, 1994]. In the next section, we consider what a rethinking of how to constitute "disabled people" would mean for criminology and victimology.

22.3 Criminology and Victimology: Reconsidering the Constitution of Disabled People

Since its inception, criminology has had a key interest in impaired people. For example, phrenology, the practice of measuring dimensions of peoples' skulls, was used as a criminological method in the nineteenth century to determine one's personal qualities and distinguish the "normal" from the "deviant" [Davis, 1995:45]. It was from this practice of phrenology where notions of normalcy were congruent with notions of white supremacy [Eze, 1997] and "ableism" [Davis, 1995]. One's intelligence and tendency to commit crimes was supposedly determined by variance away from a normal cranium measurement. Because cognitive impairments are often *hidden* (not as visible as physical impairments), examining external physical features, such as one's cranium size, was perceived as offering valuable insight into one's mind. This practice is part of the legacy of criminology. It is attributed to the work of early criminologists in the nineteenth century like Cesare Lombroso, who was part of a "positivist criminology" that "claimed to have discovered evidence of the existence of 'criminal types' whose behaviour was [biologically] determined rather than chosen and for whom treatment rather than punishment was appropriate" [Garland, 2002:11]. This notion of criminal types being *determined* justified early eugenicist thinking, as Holland et al. [2002:7] explained:

> The "eugenics" movement of the past century provided some important lessons about the distorting effects of the political agenda, "scientific" theories, prejudice and preconceptions, and loose and tautological definitions. Once the assumption was made that feeble-mindedness and criminality were linked, it was not difficult to find apparent supportive evidence.

A consequence of this has been fear of the "mentally disordered" [Peay, 2002; Littlechild and Fearns, 2005], which is a criminal justice ill-defined, all-encompassing category of people that includes people labeled with schizophrenia and learning difficulties [Holland et al., 2002:7]. This fear is paralleled with criminological interest in this particular group of disabled people [Glaser and Deane, 1999; Jahoda, 2002; Peay, 2002; Gendley and Woodhams, 2005; Littlechild and Fearns, 2005; Hayes, 2007]. Acknowledging this sense of anxiety, or even possibilities of risk and uncertainty [Goodey, 2005] of the so-called mentally disordered, we are reminded that people so-labeled as having learning difficulties or mental health difficulties are not to be distinguished from other disabled people covered under current UK disability discrimination legislation, the Disability Discrimination Act of 2005. With this in mind, *disabled people* have been portrayed in criminological studies as dangerous, menacing, violent sexual predators [Chappell, 1994; Jahoda, 2002; van den Bergh and Hoekman, 2006], which is largely unwarranted and highly stereotypical [Hiday, 1995]. It is such fear that informed the passage of UK legislation such as the Mental Deficiency Act of 1913, the first systematic legal attempt to remove disabled people from wider society [Chappell, 1994; Holland et al., 2002]. The legacy of this legislation and its subsequent consequences of segregation practices are still apparent as disabled people, particularly people labeled with cognitive impairments, are overly represented in UK prisons [Riches et al., 2005; Hayes, 2007; Hayes et al., 2007]. It is in prisons where they often receive treatment to be "normalized." The paradox of this is that the responsibility for change "has been laid at the feet of the disabled [sic], not the community" at-large [Glaser and Deane, 1999:353].

Because disabled people are over-represented in prisons [Riches et al., 2006; Hayes, 2007; Hayes et al., 2007] and disproportionately vulnerable to being victims of crime [Chappell, 1994; Sobsey, 1994; Williams, 1995;

McCarthy and Thompson, 1996; Read and Baker, 1996; Kelly and McKenna, 1997; Keilty and Connelly, 2001; Petersilia, 2001; Berzins et al., 2003; Disability Rights Commission/Capability and Scotland, 2004; Wood and Edwards, 2005; Radford et al., 2006; van den Bergh and Hoekman, 2006; Hunter et al., 2007], there is a need for a disability studies perspective to critically address the processes of criminalization and victimization of disabled people. The latter requires particular emphasis as disabled people are considered "life-long victims" of crime [Williams, 1995:17]:

> Most victim studies base their conclusions on an analysis of isolated incidents. Whilst studies may discover the incidence of specific crimes, the criminogenicity of various settings, or the propensity of certain groups to offend, they rarely reveal the cumulative nature of victimization in the lives of individuals. It is the stories of cumulative, individual victimization that most distinguishes the experience of people with learning disabilities; they are often lifelong victims. *Events which may seem trivial* in themselves, take on much greater significance when they happen to the same person. (Italics added)

These "trivial events" are everyday criminal acts made against disabled people that go unnoticed and unreported, such as experiencing daily harassment in the local neighborhood [Hunter et al. 2007] or crimes of assault and battery [Williams, 1995]. Of course, more attention needs to be drawn to the victimization of disabled people; however, persistent cultural images of disabled people as criminals or "villains" act as barriers toward having constructive discussion. As Williams [1995:102] recognized, "Government committees produce copious reports about the 'mentally disordered' offenders, and nothing about the victims." The lack of discussion of crime from a disability perspective has left legal experts, medical practitioners, and media outlets unaccountable in perpetuating a link between disabled people and crime.

In the next, section, we return to the idea of considering the social construction of impairment before exploring further the role of cultural images of disabled people.

22.4 Constructing Impairment: An Everyday Eugenics

As the social model of disability has been symbolic of the political mobilization of disabled people in the United Kingdom, it has also been critically challenged from those within disability studies, as touched on above and from others overseas. Snyder and Mitchell [2006], for example, in the United States have taken the above criticisms of the social model of disability into account to introduce their concept of the cultural model of disability. In the cultural model, there is a split *within* the term *impairment* as opposed to the social model where impairment is split *from* disability and considered a "neutral bodily difference":

> The cultural model has an understanding that impairment is both human variation encountering environmental obstacles *and* socially mediated difference that lends group identity and phenomenological perspective…. In recognising this split in the conceptualization of impairment, the cultural model of disability does not jettison embodiment but views it as a potentially meaningful materiality. An embodied experience can be embraced while also resulting in social discrimination and material effects (such as pain, discomfort, or incapacity)… this divided understanding of impairment is encompassed by the larger, politicised term *disability*… disability is once removed from impairment in that the concept depends upon both conditions of impairment being met—namely embodied difference that precipitates social discrimination…. The formulation of a cultural model allows us to theorize a political act of renaming that designates disability as a site of resistance and a source of cultural agency previously suppressed—at least to the extent that groups can successfully rewrite their own definition in view of a damaging material and linguistic heritage. (Italics in original) [Snyder and Mitchell 2006:10]

In critiquing the social model's take on impairment, Snyder and Mitchell offer another epistemological perspective in understanding disability where impairment is emphasized and explored rather than pushed to the side. They take into account impairments as social constructions, while also accounting for the meanings and experiences attached to impairments as being significant in marking the ill effects of a disablist world (or "ableist" world as termed in the United States). More importantly, their cultural model highlights the agency of disabled people. The social model with its emphasis on social boundaries and discrimination does not take into account how these processes of discrimination inform identities of disabled people. Snyder and Mitchell's explanation of this process is reminiscent of social anthropological models of social identity.

For example, the work of Jenkins [2008a&b] on social identity is relevant in explaining the significance of agency of disabled people in having and "rewriting their own definition" of their group identity [Snyder and Mitchell, 2006:10]. Jenkins introduces the dialectical process of group identification (social groups) and social categorization (social categories). In describing this process and the distinction between social groups and social categories, Jenkins uses Marx's famous contrast of "class in itself" (group) and "class for itself" (category):

> In this understanding of the development of class consciousness, the working class(es)—a *social category* that was initially defined, with reference to their immiseration and alienation from the means of production, and to their threat

> to the established order, by others such as capitalists, agencies of the state,
> socialist activists, etc.—becomes a *social group*, the members of which identify
> with each other in their collective misfortune, thus creating the possibility of
> organised collective action on the basis of that identification. (Italics added)
> [Jenkins, 2008b:56]

In relation to identity politics and disability, government officials and
medical practitioners may categorize and subsequently segregate people
labeled with physical impairments into institutions. This experience may
inform a shared experience among those who are segregated because of
their impairment. This collective experience informs the making of a *social
group*. It creates that sense of "us" from "them." This, in turn, can create the
possibility of organized collective action or what Snyder and Mitchell refer
to as groups *rewriting their definitions*.

The formation of UPIAS may best be representative of this kind of *rewriting*
when it first conceptualized the social model of disability. Members of
this group shared a collective experience of living in segregated institutions.
This experience formed a sense of collectivity, a sense of "us" against a "them"
whoever "them" might be, such as medical practitioners or care professionals.
It can also be everyday people who perpetuate disabling barriers, discount-
ing structural access issues that people labeled with physical impairments
confront. In response to "them," (some) people with physical impairments
organized themselves collectively, *redefined* themselves as UPIAS, and drew
up the tenet that became known as the social model of disability.

In the examples given of class consciousness and UPIAS above, group
identity is initially formed through being categorized *by* a powerful Other.
For Marx, this powerful Other was the established order and capitalists.
In the case of UPIAS, this powerful "them" would be the combination of
the medical profession and the nondisabled world. Jenkins [2008a] understands power to be the capacity to intervene in one's life. The ability for
medics to categorize a group of people as being "physically impaired"
requires a sense of power. The ability to distinguish and label children as
having autism or having learning difficulties requires one to have power,
or specialist knowledge in the Foucauldian sense [Molloy and Vasil, 2002].
For Davis [1995] and Snyder and Mitchell [2006], this sense of power that
medical professionals and practitioners use in categorizing disabled people
stems from historical remnants of eugenics that is continually perpetuated
in our everyday lives.

This idea of power has been touched on by Davis [1995] in explaining
the extent of "normalcy"—the social construction of being "normal" as a nondisabled person—in taken-for-granted notions of citizenship and nationality. Davis [1995:31] traces this normalcy to the eugenics movement of the
past century where eugenicists "became obsessed with the elimination of

'defectives,' a category which included the 'feebleminded,' the deaf, the blind, the physically defective, and so on." For this to occur, eugenicists adopted theories in statistics in defining notions of the ideal norm, looking at particular desirable traits such as a person's height or intelligence. This was problematic for disabled people as "eugenicists tended to group together all allegedly 'undesirable traits.' So, for example, criminals, the poor, and people with disabilities might be mentioned in the same breath" [Davis, 1995:35]. Snyder and Mitchell [2006] also highlight the historical significance of the eugenics movement and how its legacy continues to be unmarked in contemporary understandings of disability. Their reflection on eugenics cannot be separated from previous discussions of race theorists [e.g., Hall, 1997] and the role of scientific racism in rationalizing an ideology of white supremacy [Eze, 1997]. The pervasiveness of white supremacy, or "whiteness," is taken for granted to the extent that it is invisible [Frankenberg, 1993, 1997; Madriaga, 2005, 2007]. It is the presence of *different*, dark-skinned Others that an axiomatic relationship between "whiteness" and "normality" become apparent. Similar thinking is conveyed by Davis [1995] and Snyder and Mitchell [2006] as they suggest an axiomatic relationship exist between nondisability and normal. Thus, instead of focusing on social barriers and the social construction of disability, Davis argues for examining the construction of normalcy. He stated, the problem "is not the person with disabilities; the problem is the way that normalcy is constructed to create the 'problem' of the disabled person" [Davis, 1995:24]. In calling for a deconstruction of normalcy, Davis comprehends that a sense of power is implicit in being normal. It is the (re)production of normalcy that marks out and categorizes disabled people as different, even deviant. This process is two-way, informing conceptions of normalcy versus deviancy, distinguishing "us" from "them" [Jenkins, 2008a]. Thus, marking deviancy informs everyday conceptions of normalcy, of who "we" are from "them." It divides and homogenizes. It distinguishes disabled people from nondisabled people. While dividing, it provides senses of "us" for both sides of the dichotomy. However, this dichotomy is unbalanced as an everyday eugenics heralds the nondisabled person without "defects" [Davis, 1995]. Disabled people are not absent in this (re)production of normalcy or what is being termed here as an "everyday eugenics." Both nondisabled and disabled people participate and perpetuate in this oppressive process, blurring the boundaries between "us" and "them." This has been evidenced in Deal's [2006] findings of a hierarchy of impairments where disabled people, like nondisabled people, ranked people with certain impairments as being more acceptable than others.

Having said this, our aim in this chapter is not to reaffirm divisions within the Disabled People's Movement [Humphrey, 1999] but rather to convey how the (re)process of an everyday eugenics is represented through the criminalization and victimization of disabled people. A cultural model of disability is a welcome contribution to disability studies and is the theoretical backbone of this chapter. It also provides ways of challenging the power, or specialist knowledge, of medical professionals and practitioners who are traditionally relied on in criminology to constitute disabled people. It offers an understanding that *everyone, everyday* may be active, unwitting agents in eugenics. Disability is much more than barriers and incidents of discrimination (as suggested in the social model of disability). As students and teachers of disability studies, our role is to mark the pervasiveness of eugenics that we take for granted in our everyday lives. Considering the work of critical white scholars like Frankenberg [1997] in uncovering everyday whiteness, we see identifying everyday eugenics as marking the *invisible* in the *visible*. This has been observed by Davis [1995:43] in his reading of English literature where he argues for a disability studies consciousness that alters "the way we see not just novels that have main characters who are disabled but any novel." It is through these lenses that the next section reflects on cultural texts and how they perpetuate an everyday eugenics that criminalizes and victimizes disabled people. As Chappell [1994:29] has argued in reference to stereotypes of people with learning difficulties:

> Eugenicist beliefs have created a legacy of stereotypes which have rendered [disabled people] vulnerable to wrongful conviction. On the one hand, they may be viewed as child-like, passive, malleable and objects of ridicule. On the other, they can be stereotyped as sexually dangerous, menacing, cunning and prone to violence.

22.5 Deformed, Unfinished: Cultural Images of Criminality, Victimhood, and Disability

> I, that am curtailed of this fair proportion,
> Cheated of feature by dissembling Nature,
> *Deformed, unfinished*, sent before my time
> Into this breathing world, scarce half made up,
> And that so lamely and unfashionable
> That dogs bark at me as I halt by them.
> (*Richard III*—Shakespeare [2005] [c.1592–93]: I.i.18–23—emphasis added)

One area where disability studies has, to some extent, considered the criminalization and victimization of disabled people is in cultural representations. For example, Longmore [1987:65] discusses how disabled characters occupy a range of positions citing "crippled criminals," blind detectives, and "disabled victims or villains." Moreover, Barnes' [1992] 11 stereotypes of disabled people include "The Disabled Person as Sinister and Evil" and "The Disabled Person as an Object of Violence." In this section we want to explore how the representation of disabled people in cultural texts is, in part, contingent on the notions of everyday eugenics discussed earlier and feeds into the ongoing social construction of impairment and disability. Although we would argue that a disability consciousness [Davis, 1995] demands readings of texts beyond those which include central characters that are explicitly impaired, we will focus here on some of the more obvious examples in literature and on film. We could have equally considered the print media, television, theater, or advertising, and although some small examples from those forms may be referred to it will be literature and film that demand our closest attention. We will look at the what (content) and offer some suggestions for why these images persist. Our ultimate aim, as noted in the introduction, is to demonstrate how many representations of disabled people in relation to crime and violence rely on notions of everyday eugenics and are, therefore, like Shakespeare's Richard III, deformed, unfinished, and scarcely half-made up and amount to a different, yet nonetheless significant, sort of victimization. We consider representations that rely on notions of (1) malevolency, (2) monstrosity, and (3) violence and death before moving on to a brief consideration of (4) heroes and counternarratives.

22.5.1 Malevolency

> Disability has often been used as a melodramatic device.... Among the most persistent is the association of disability with malevolence. Deformity of body symbolizes deformity of soul. [Longmore, 1987:66]

Examples of impairment acting as a cause, and thereafter an emblem, of malevolence are many. Both Kreigel [1987] and Barnes [1992] discuss Captain Ahab in Melville's Moby Dick and Shakespeare's Richard III. Kreigel [1987:34] says of both of them, they "are what they are because they have been crippled." For Kreigel [1987:35], from such a circumstance comes frustration, which results in resistance of the values of "normals" and thus, such a characterization frightens the normals with the threat of "a rage so powerful that it will bring everything down in its wake." Barnes [1992:22] argues that the sound of "Ahab's false leg tapping back and forth across the deck in the middle of the night" signals the use of impairment to heighten the sinister atmosphere of the book. He also discusses how disabled characters are even added to a storyline for the sole purpose of intensifying a sinister and menacing atmosphere. For example, although absent in Mary Shelley's book, in the 1931 film version of Frankenstein staring Boris Karloff, Fritz, a character with a "hunchback," was added as Baron Frankenstein's only assistant. His addition is significant because he is portrayed as the true creator of the monster as, when asked to fetch the brain, he retrieves one of a known criminal rather than the one requested by the Baron [Barnes, 1992].

Barnes [1992] goes on to discuss the presence of such villainous characterizations in films such as *Dirty Harry* (1971), *The Sting* (1973), and numerous James Bond films. We would also add here the eponymous *Hook* (in the 1991 film version of J. M. Barrie's *Peter Pan*) or even the albino villain, Silas, in Dan Brown's *The Da Vinci Code* (2006).

Longmore [1987] also turns to films and discusses the first James Bond film, *Doctor No* (1962), and *Dr. Strangelove* (1964). Again the impairments of both seemingly result from misadventures in their experiments: "They are "crippled" as a consequence of their evil" [ibid.:67]. Longmore [1987:67] further suggests that such villains reflect and reinforce three common prejudices about disabled people: "disability is a punishment for evil; disabled people are embittered by their 'fate'; disabled people resent the nondisabled and would, if they could destroy them." As he goes on to point out, and as our earlier discussion noted, it has been the nondisabled world that would, and has tried, to destroy disabled people. As outlined in the introduction, our dual focus on criminals and victims allows us to examine the conflation between disabled people and criminals and to suggest that the popular representation of disabled people as villains can tell us much about how impairment is constructed in the social consciousness. Longmore [1987:67–68] likens the portrayal of disabled people to that of other minorities and suggests that the "unacknowledged hostile fantasies of the stigmatizers are transferred to the stigmatized." In other words, through such characterization the general social consciousness is allowed to disavow its fears by blaming the villains. By making them responsible for their own circumstances (remember Captain Ahab, Richard III, Doctor No, and Doctor Strangelove are blamed for their own impairments), a nondisability consciousness abdicates responsibility, distances itself from interaction, and, to maintain that distance, creates a threat so powerful it prohibits the divide being crossed.

One way that this divide between danger and safety is reinforced is an overemphasis on the sexual deviancy of such characters. Longmore [1987:72] discussed how criminal disabled characters are often portrayed as having a "kinky, leering lust for sex with gorgeous 'normal' women." He cites Dr. Loveless in the TV adventure series *Wild Wild West* (1965–1969), as well as the central character in the film *Dr. Strangelove* (1964).

Another, perhaps less pervasive, device uses the characterization of a disabled person to represent the dangers of the modern world. Kriegel [1987] discuss how D. H. Lawrence's Clifford Chatterley (*Lady Chatterley's Lover*) mirrors Richard III's bitterness but is bereft of his poetry. Instead Clifford Chatterley's demonism stems from a soullessness created by industrialization. Here the disabled person is simultaneously a villain and a victim of modern industrial society, further supporting our contention that villainous representations of disabled people amount to a different, yet nonetheless significant, sort of victimization.

22.5.2 Monstrosity

Closely related to such characterizations, the disabled person as a "monster" can be seen in horror classics such as *The Hunchback of Notre Dame* (1939) and *The Phantom of the Opera* (1962). Often involving some form of visible impairment, these characterizations forward the idea that impaired bodies are inhabited by impaired souls that cannot be trusted to remain in balance. Thus, the danger such characters present, as a result of the threat of a violent loss of self-control, results in their exclusion from society. As with criminal portrayals, portrayals of disabled people as monsters also draw on notions of sexual deviancy, particularly in relation to the menacing of "women who would ordinarily reject them" [Longmore, 1987:72]. For example, the Phantom (from *The Phantom of the Opera*) kidnaps a woman, whereas Quasimodo (from *The Hunchback of Notre Dame*) rescues and cares for the women he loves. With both, the sexual deviancy of the monster is compounded by the possibility of the divide between the impaired and the nonimpaired (or "normal") being involuntarily bridged (on the part of the nondeviant). The sexualization of the danger only serves to heighten the threat the monster/disabled person poses and reinforces the normalcy "truth" that some people are essentially different and should be segregated. We would also add here films where characters that have a "mental disorder" are portrayed as dangerous, menacing predators, such as Alfred Hitchcock's *Psycho* (1960), Billy Bob Thornton's *Slingblade* (1996), and James Mangold's *Identity* (2003).

Despite Zola [1987] suggesting that the "out-and-out monster" portrayals are on the wane, they remain incredibly informative about how disabled people are perceived. Longmore [1987] makes a significant point here when he argues that even though the audience is invited to be sympathetic to the "monster" and consider him or her a "victim of fate," characters such as Quasimodo (*The Hunchback of Notre Dame*) and Lennie (*Of Mice and Men*) are ultimately shown to be justifiably ostracized. Again, the dual presence of monster and victim means that the two cannot be meaningfully examined alone.

This duality is best demonstrated in the characters Norman Bates, the antagonist in Alfred Hitchcock's *Psycho*, and Karl Childers, the protagonist in Billy Bob Thornton's film *Slingblade*. With the former having the label of "split personality" and the latter labeled with learning difficulties, they both are portrayed as monstrous murderers. Toward the ending of each film, after both are discovered by authorities as having committed heinous crimes, there are images of both characters incarcerated in specialized institutions for the "mentally disordered." Before the climax, and in contrast to the monstrous images, both characters are also portrayed as having childlike qualities. For example, in *Psycho*, Alfred Hitchcock vividly reveals Norman Bates' childlike qualities by displaying images of his toys in his bedroom. There is also an image of his bed along with a stuffed animal. In *Slingblade*, Karl Childers' childlike qualities come in the form of his friendship with a child, Frank Wheatley. Their friendship becomes more cohesive as they experience harassment and abuse within Frank's household. Of course, this may stir sympathy for the "monsters" [Longmore, 1987] as their ties to childhood link them to being vulnerable victims [Williams, 1995]. At the same time, these images may also hint of the risk and uncertainty of childhood, or "the youth problem," where the behavior of the young maybe difficult to predict. In other words, being a child may represent a period of irrationality where cognitive skills of reason and rational thought are underdeveloped [France, 2000:322]. Therefore, instead of being dialectically opposed, this relationship between childlike and a monster maybe congruent. It is this underdevelopment of being rational, or "normal" in a eugenic sense, that not only perpetuates images of disabled people as being vulnerable victims but also, and paradoxically, maintains images of them being villains and monsters.

22.5.3 Violence and Death

For Longmore [1987:69], and crucially for our argument in this chapter, "the final and only possible solution" for malevolent or monstrous characters is death. For villainous characters death is presented as a justifiable punishment, whereas for monstrous characters death is tragic but an "inevitable, necessary, and merciful outcome" [ibid.].

Considering characters with impairments in general, research has shown that on television, when fictional dramas include a disabled character they are more than three times as likely to be dead at the end of the show than their nondisabled counterparts [Cumberbach and Negrine, 1992]. Of these deaths more than half were violent and one-fifth of those were suicides, all committed by "mentally ill" characters, supporting the belief that disabled people are also in need of protection from themselves. Barnes [1992:22] echoes Longmore's [1987] point above and states that such portrayals "reinforce, albeit implicitly, the eugenic conviction that the 'natural' solution to the problems associated with impairment is a violent one." This is supported by Zola's [1987] observation that the most common cause of impairment (where one can be identified) in the crime-mystery drama is trauma. Less represented are congenital conditions and even less present are disease-related impairments.

Another, and related, area of representation is what Barnes [1992] refers to as "The Disabled Person as an Object of Violence." We appreciate disabled people are not only often subject to abuse and violent attack but also find the justice system disabling, as Petersilia [2001:656–57] has stated:

> Not only are people with developmental disabilities at higher risk of victimization, but they also face innumerable barriers when reporting their

victimization, when having their cases investigated and prosecuted, and in receiving emotional support.

Nevertheless, the perpetuation of imagery that draws solely on such a weak characterization reinforces an equally damaging belief that disabled people are helpless, vulnerable, and in constant need of protection.

Related to this is the gendered use of visible impairments to symbolize villainy. Zola [1987:488] has commented that "from the earliest crime-fiction writing as well as in illustrations and silent films, one could easily recognize the villain by his/her features." When undertaking an analysis of the visibility of scars in terms of gender, Zola [1987:492] argues that "[m]en's scars are all over their bodies, almost randomly distributed. Women's scars are more likely to be facial or in their sexual organs and thus are more purposefully inflicted." In positioning men's scars as "badges" of their villainy and/or their heroism, whereas women's scars are often badges of dishonor, Zola [1987:493] expands his comments and concludes that "men are thus 'at risk' of disablement because of what they do, women, children and older people are 'at risk' because of who they are." Here a disability consciousness has been joined by one of gender and suggests that the perpetuation of "in need of protection" is a particular issue in relation to the feminized characters.

22.5.4 Heroes and Counternarratives

Of course, the above discussion has not incorporated all "types" of portrayals of disabled people. Indeed, during Zola's [1987] consideration of the portrayal of disability in the crime-mystery drama he admitted surprise at the concomitant history of disabled people being portrayed as the hero/protagonist. More recent examples of this can be seen on television and in literature with characters such as the wheelchair-using *Ironside* (1967–1975) and the obsessive-compulsive disorder (OCD)-labeled *Monk* (2002–present), along with Jonathan Letham's Lionel Essrog, a private detective labeled with Tourette's syndrome in his 1999 novel *Motherless Brooklyn*. Furthermore, in Andrew Niccol's science fiction film *Gattaca* (1997), the character Vincent Freeman, who was diagnosed with a heart condition and labeled with attention deficit disorder (ADD) as a child, is the protagonist against a eugenicist-dominated society. The futuristic society portrayed in the film practices "geno-ism," where discrimination is based on notions of genetically superiority and inferiority, not on notions of social class or race. The genetically inferior, like Vincent Freeman, are referred to in the film as "the invalids." Given a lack of opportunities because of his perceived impairments, Vincent Freeman commits fraud and passes himself off as being genetically superior. This means modifying his physique and other physical traits such as eye color and fingerprints. It also means him illegally purchasing blood and urine samples from another character, Jerome Eugene Morrow, who is genetically superior but suffered a serious injury and uses a wheelchair. The climax of the film is Vincent Freeman being able to realize his dream of flying into space, an opportunity only reserved for the genetically superior.

Although television shows such as *Monk* and films like *Gattaca* offer a useful counterpoint to malevolent and monstrous representations that rely on violence and death for their resolution, they do not offer a space for the sort of *rewriting* we discussed earlier [Snyder and Mitchell, 2006]—a rewriting of definitions where senses of power are deconstructed and challenged to form the basis for organized collective action. A collective action fashioned similarly along the lines of the black power movement in the United States during the 1960s and early 1970s where slogans such as "Black is beautiful" emerged challenging white supremacist ideology. For example, although *Gattaca* offers insights and a critique about everyday eugenics, it did not offer a rewriting that could empower disabled people. It still perpetuates stereotypical prejudices and assumptions, such as disabled people being embittered by their fate or resenting the nondisabled world [Longmore, 1987]. The character Jerome Eugene Morrow encapsulates these stereotypes as he is portrayed as a depressed, angry drunk, resentful of his status as a wheelchair user. Toward the end of the film, there is a scene where he commits suicide supposedly pleased that his friend, Vincent Freeman, has been able to achieve his dream. This scene reaffirms the portrayal of the violent solution to problems associated with impairments discussed above [Longmore, 1987; Barnes, 1992], as well as confirms the greater likelihood that disabled characters will be dead at end of fictional dramas compared with their nondisabled counterparts [Cumberbach and Negrine, 1992].

However, such rewriting can be seen in the work of Liz Crow, director and producer of "Roaring Girl" films, who is currently engaged in producing a moving-image installation about one of the most substantial crimes against disabled people, *Aktion T-4*, a program of systematic killing of 250,000 disabled children and adults during the Nazi's reign of Germany. There have also been some theatrical attempts to rewrite the social construction of impairment; some of them have been collected together in *Beyond Victims and Villains: Contemporary Plays by Disabled Playwrights* [2006], edited by Victoria Ann Lewis. Furthermore, an academic consideration that draws heavily on the work of performance artists, Petra Kuppers, *The Scar of Visibility: Medical Performances and Contemporary Art* [2007], takes the scar as a place of production, repetition, and difference. In exploring the significance of medical images in visual culture, the topics she covers include representations of the AIDS virus in the National Museum of Health and on *CSI: Crime Scene Investigations*.

Although we do not have room here to explore these counternarratives in any depth, their emergence and continuation strike a blow for, what could be called, the "mainstream" representation of disabled people as either victims in need of protection from themselves or criminals/villains who are victims the world is in need of protection from. The consistency with which death occurs as a resolution to these mainstream narratives signals a close link with an everyday eugenics that seeks to remove deviancy and maintain normalcy at all costs. It could be argued that the social construction of impairment is clearer to see in cultural representation, not least because literary, cultural, and film studies are now well-equipped to provide the tools with which to unpack them. However, it must be remembered that we have used cultural representations here as illustrative examples and would argue that such everyday eugenics is at work in other parts of society, such as courts of law, hospitals, domestic violence units, and police stations. The number of people labeled with learning difficulties such as autism currently with an ASBO (Anti-Social Behaviour Order in the United Kingdom and Republic of Ireland) tells us that social construction of impairment as deviant has very real effects [Hunter et al., 2007]. Part of our argument in this chapter has been that cultural representations can help us understand the workings of these constructions and what sort of everyday logics are being perpetuated.

22.6 Conclusion

Disabled people are victims of an everyday eugenics that continually marks them as deviant. The legacy of the eugenics movement from the nineteenth century continues to be reproduced in contemporary cultural representations of disabled people. This legacy cannot be unhinged from the early developments of criminology where phrenology was taken for granted as a detector of normalcy [Davis, 1995; Holland et al., 2002]. Whereas early criminology attempted to distinguish prospective criminals, it also provided "scientific" rationale for segregating disabled people from mainstream society for their own safety. By not fitting within parameters of normalcy, they were considered potential offenders on the one hand and vulnerable victims on the other [Chappell, 1994].

It is an everyday eugenics that places disabled people at risk of repeat victimization of criminal acts, such as harassment and hate crime, to the extent that Williams [1995] describes disabled people as being lifelong victims. However, discussion on the phenomena of repeat victimization of disabled people has gone relatively unnoticed compared with the disproportionate amount of attention drawn to the offending of disabled people [Williams, 1995]. With this in mind, recent legal policies that address this gap, such as UK policy for prosecuting cases of disability hate crime, are welcome:

> Safety and security, and the right to live free from fear and harassment, are fundamental human rights and the CPS recognises the wider community

impact of disability hate crime where it strikes at all disabled people by
undermining their sense of safety and security in the community. For this
reason we regard disability hate crime as particularly serious. Such crimes are
based on ignorance, prejudice, discrimination and hate and they have no place
in an open and democratic society. [Crown Prosecution Service, 2007:3]

Not just restricted to the arena of criminal justice, an everyday eugenics
perpetuates disturbing cultural representations of disabled people. As evidenced above, the simultaneous dualism of being villainous criminals and
vulnerable victims has been represented in cultural images of disabled people in literature and films. For example, this dualism was represented in the
characters of Norman Bates in *Psycho* and Karl Childers in *Slingblade*. Both
characters were simultaneously portrayed as monsters and childlike. These
images of monstrosity and childlike characterize disabled people as lacking
reason and rational thought. These images also demarcate notions of eugenicist normalcy from deviant Others [Davis, 1995].

With the pervasiveness of everyday eugenics, there is an assumed sense of
power in identifying and categorizing another as being normal from abnormal. Longmore [1987:67–68] touched on this when discussing stigmatizers
transferring their hostile fantasies to the stigmatized. In transferring hostile
fantasies, the stigmatizers draw on conceptions of normalcy in stigmatizing
disabled people. The pervasiveness of everyday eugenics relies on cultural
representations that negatively portray disabled people as monsters, villainous criminals, or vulnerable victims. In perpetuating these images, stigmatizers maintain the capacity to intervene in the lives of disabled people. The
(re)production of everyday eugenics is a two-way process that informs the
identities and boundaries of stigmatizers (perpetuators and beneficiaries of a
nondisabled world) from the stigmatized (disabled people) and vice versa. As
everyday eugenics assures stigmatizers of their sense of normalcy, it structures the way disabled people perceive themselves, particularly when having
to identify with stigmatized categories and labels.

Of course, politically charged collectives of disabled people, like UPIAS,
challenged everyday eugenics by rejecting labels imposed on them and then
by rewriting who they were as a group. Snyder and Mitchell [2006] have advocated for this type of organized collective action as it requires disabled people
to be agents of change. This means rejecting stigmatized, eugenicist labels of
the nondisabled world to rewrite their own definitions.

A possible way to progress toward this end of disabled people rewriting
their own definitions is to challenge and mark out processes of everyday
eugenics that perpetuate damaging representations of disabled people as
criminals and victims. This will require interdisciplinary work between
disability studies and areas of criminology and victimology. This call for
"joined up" work has been echoed by Goodey [2005:38–39] when she stated

that victimologists and criminal justice practitioners and those from other disciplines should consider the plight of victims who fall outside traditional criminal justice but who fall within models of social justice and welfare assistance. Possible outcomes of interdisciplinary work may spark a rethink about some of the taken-for-granted terms and definitions used to describe disabled people in the area of criminal justice. For example, much of the criminological and victimological work on disabled people focuses on offenders so-labeled mentally disordered. The latter is an ill-defined, umbrella term used to describe people labeled with learning difficulties and people with mental health difficulties. The use of the term attempts to distinguish a particular group of disabled people from other disabled people based on the appearance of "organic" [Goodley, 2001] rather than physical impairments. This distinction only reifies a hierarchy of impairments [Deal, 2006].

To address this issue, an instilling of a disability studies consciousness [Davis, 1995] within criminology and victimology will be a positive step forward in empowering disabled people to rewrite their own definitions. This may help to deconstruct its legacy and untie itself from a eugenicist past. At the same time, disability studies needs to account and draw closer attention to criminological and victimological work that revolves around issues pertinent to the lives of *all* disabled people. Thus far, it has inadequately done so. The lack of attention in this area from a disability studies perspective has been attributed to a hierarchy of impairments where the so-called mentally disordered and their interests are pushed to the periphery by both nondisabled and disabled people. Despite this, there is much to look forward to in the future of disability studies. New models in understanding disability have been introduced like the cultural model of disability [Snyder and Mitchell, 2006], where discussion has moved beyond talk of barriers toward critiquing the everyday processes of eugenics that all people, disabled or nondisabled, may be active, unwitting participants. It could possibly be from this premise that further work examining the criminalization and victimization of disabled people will be initiated.

References

Abberley, P. 1987. The concept of oppression and the development of a social theory of disability. *Disability, Handicap and Society* 21:5–19.

Barnes, C. 1991a. *Disabling comedy and anti-discrimination legislation.* www.leeds. ac.uk/disability-studies/archiveuk/archframe (accessed February 10, 2003).

_____. 1991b. Discrimination: Disabled people and the media. *Contac* 70(Winter): 45–48. www.leeds.ac.uk/disability-studies/archiveuk/archframe (accessed June 5, 2003).

_____. 1992. *Disabling imagery and the media: An exploration of the principles for media representations of disabled people.* Halifax: BCODP/Ryburn.

_____. 1997. Disability in the writing of Irvine Welsh: A discussion paper. Paper presented at the Disability Studies Conference, Glasgow, Scotland. www.leeds. ac.uk/disability-studies/archiveuk/archframe (accessed June 5, 2003).

_____. 1998. The social model of disability: A sociological phenomenon ignored by sociologists. In *The disability reader: Social science perspectives*, ed. T. Shakespeare, 65–78. London: Cassell.

_____. 1999. Disability studies: New or not so new directions? *Disability & Society* 14(4):577–80.

Barton, L. and M. Oliver. 1997. The birth of disability studies. In *Disability studies: Past, present and future*, ed. L. Barton and M. Oliver, 9–14. Leeds, UK: Disability Press.

Berzins, K., A. Petch, and J. M. Atkinson. 2003. Prevalence and experience of harassment of people with mental health problems living in the community. *British Journal of Psychiatry* 183:526–33.

Breckman, A. 2002–present. *Monk.* Television program. Burbank, CA: Mandeville Films.

Chappell, A. L. 1994. Disability, discrimination and the criminal justice system. *Critical Social Policy* 14:19–33.

_____. 1998. Still out in the cold: People with learning difficulties and the social model of disability. In *The disability reader: Social science perspectives*, ed. T. Shakespeare, 211–20. London: Cassell.

Chouinard, V. 1994. Reinventing radical geography: Is all that's left right? *Environment and Planning D: Society and Space* 12:2–6.

Crown Prosecution Service (CPS). 2007. *Disability hate crime: Policy for prosecuting cases of disability hate crime.* London: Crown Prosecution Service.

Cumberbach, G. and R. Negrine. 1992. *Images of disability on television.* London: Routledge.

Da Vinci Code. 2006. Directed by Ron Howard. Culver City, CA: Columbia Pictures.

Davis, L. 1995. *Enforcing normalcy: Disability, deafness and the body.* London: Verso.

Deal, M. 2006. Attitudes of disabled people toward other disabled people and impairment groups. PhD diss., City University, London.

Dirty Harry. 1971. Directed by Don Siegel. Los Angeles: Malpaso.

Disability Rights Advocates. 2001. *Forgotten crimes: The holocaust and people with disabilities.* Oakland, CA: Disability Rights Advocates. http://www.dralegal.org/publications/forgotten_crimes.php (accessed August 7, 2008).

Disability Rights Commission/Capability Scotland. 2004. *Hate crime against disabled people in Scotland: A survey report.* Stratford upon Avon, UK: Disability Rights Commission.

Doctor No. 1962. Directed by Terence Young. London: Eon Productions.

Dr. Strangelove or: How I Learned to Stop Worrying and Love the Bomb. 1964. Directed by Stanley Kubrick. UK: Hawk Films.

Eze, E. C. (ed.). 1997. *Race and the enlightenment: A reader.* Oxford: Blackwell.

Finkelstein, V. 1980. *Attitudes and disabled people: Issues for discussion.* New York: World Rehabilitation Fund.

_____. 1993. The commonality of disability. In *Disabling barriers—Enabling environments*, ed. J. Swain, V. Finkelstein, S. French, and M. Oliver, 9–16. London: Sage in association with the Open University Press.

_____. 1998. Emancipating disability studies. In *The disability reader: Social science perspectives*, ed. T. Shakespeare, 28–49. London: Cassell.

France, A. 2000 Towards a sociological understanding of youth and their risk taking. *Journal of Youth Studies* 3(3):317–31.

Frankenberg, R. 1993. *The social construction of whiteness: White women, race matters.* Minneapolis: University of Minnesota Press.

____. 1997. Introduction: Local whitenesses, localising whiteness. In *Displacing whiteness*, ed. R. Frankenberg, 1–33. Durham, NC: Duke University Press.

Frankenstein. 1931. Directed by James Whale. Universal City, CA: Universal Pictures.

Garland, D. 2002. Of crimes and criminals: The development of criminology in Britain. In *The Oxford handbook of criminology*, ed. M. Maguire, R. Morgan, and R. Reiner, 7–50. Oxford: Oxford University Press.

Garrison, M. 1965–1969. *Wild Wild West.* Television program. Los Angeles: Bruce Lansbury Productions.

Gattaca. 1997. Directed by Andrew Niccol. Culver City, CA: Columbia Pictures.

Gendley, K. and J. Woodhams. 2005. Suspects who have learning disability: Police perceptions toward the client group and their knowledge about learning disabilities. *Journal of Intellectual Disabilities* 9(1):70–81.

Glaser, W. and K. Deane. 1999. Normalisation in an abnormal world: A study of prisoners with an intellectual disability. *International Journal of Offender Therapy and Comparative Criminology* 43(3):338–56.

Gleeson, B. 1997. Disability studies: A historical materialist view. *Disability & Society* 12(2):179–202.

Goodey, J. 2005. *Victims and victimology: Research, policy and practice.* Harlow: Pearson Education Limited.

Goodley, D. 2001. "Learning difficulties," the social model of disability and impairment: Challenging epistemologies. *Disability and Society* 16(2):207–31.

Hall, S. 1997. The spectacle of the "Other." In *Representations: Cultural representations and signifying practices*, ed. S. Hall, 223–90. London: Sage.

Hasler, F. 1993. Developments in the disabled people's movement. In *Disabling barriers—Enabling environments*, ed. J. Swain, V. Finkelstein, S. French, and M. Oliver, 278–84. London: Sage in association with the Open University Press.

Hayes, S. C. 2007 Women with learning disabilities who offend: What do we know? *British Journal of Learning Disabilities* 35:187–91.

Hayes, S., P. Shackwell, P. Mottram, and R. Lancaster. 2007. The prevalence of intellectual disability in a major UK prison. *British Journal of Learning Disabilities* 35:162–67.

Hiday, V. 1995. The social context of mental illness and violence. *Journal of Health and Social Behavior* 36(2):122–37.

Holland, T., I. C. H. Clare, and T. Mukhopadhyay. 2002. Prevalence of criminal offending by men and women with intellectual disability and the characteristics of offenders: Implications for research and service development. *Journal of Intellectual Disability Research* 46(Supplement 1):6–20.

Hook. 1991. Directed by Steven Spielberg. Universal City, CA: Amblin Entertainment.

Humphrey, J. C. 1999. Disabled people and the politics of difference. *Disability & Society* 14(2):173–88.

The Hunchback of Notre Dame. 1939. Directed by William Dieterle. Los Angeles: RKO Radio Pictures.

Hunt, P. 1966. *Stigma: The experience of disability.* London: Geoffrey Chapman.

Hunter, C., N. Hodge, J. Nixon, S. Parr, and B. Willis. 2007. *Disabled people's experiences of anti-social behaviour and harassment in social housing: A critical review.* Sheffield: Centre for Education Research and Social Inclusion (CERSI) and Disability Rights Commission.

Identity. 2003. Directed by James Mangold. Culver City, CA: Columbia Pictures.

Jahoda, A. 2002. Offenders with a learning disability: The evidence for better services? *Journal of Applied Research in Intellectual Disabilities* 15:175–78.

Jenkins, R. 2008a. *Social identity*, 3rd ed. London: Routledge.

_____. 2008b. *Rethinking ethnicity: Arguments and explorations*, 2nd ed. London: Sage.

Keilty, J. and G. Connelly. 2001. Making a statement: An exploratory study of barriers facing women with an intellectual disability when making a statement about sexual abuse to police. *Disability & Society* 16(2):273–91.

Kelly, L. and H. P. McKenna. 1997. Victimization of people with enduring mental illness in the community. *Journal of Psychiatric and Mental Health Nursing* 4(3):185–91.

Kriegel, L. 1987. The cripple in literature. In *Images of disability, Disabling images*, ed. A. Gartner and T. Joe, 31–46. New York/London: Praeger.

Kudlick, C. J. 2003. Disability history: Why we need another "Other." *The American Historical Review* 108:103. www.historycoop.org/cgi-bin (accessed July 22, 2003).

Kuppers, P. 2007. *The scar of visibility: Medical performances and contemporary art.* Minneapolis: University of Minnesota Press.

Lawrence, D. H. 1928. *Lady Chatterley's lover.* London: Penguin Books.

Letham, J. 1999. *Motherless Brooklyn.* London: Vintage.

Lewis, V. A. (ed.). 2006. *Beyond victims and villains: Contemporary plays by disabled playwrights.* New York: Theatre Communications Group.

Lindsay, W. R. 2002. Research and literature on sex offenders with intellectual and developmental disabilities. *Journal of Intellectual Disability Research* 46(Supplement 1):74–85.

Lindsay, W. R. et al. 2002. A treatment service for sex offenders and abusers with intellectual disability: Characteristics of referrals and evaluation. *Journal of Applied Research in Intellectual Disabilities* 15:166–74.

Littlechild, B. and D. Fearns. (ed.). 2005. *Mental disorder and criminal justice: Policy, provision and practice.* Lyme Regis: Russell House.

Longmore, P. K. 1987. Screening stereotypes: Images of disabled people in television and motion pictures. In *Images of disability, disabling images*, ed. A. Gartner and T. Joe, 65–78. New York/London: Praeger.

Madriaga, M. 2005. Understanding the symbolic idea of the American dream and its relationship with the category of whiteness. *Sociological Research Online* 10(3): http://www.socresonline.org.uk/10/3/madriaga.html (accessed September 15, 2009).

_____. 2007. The star-spangled banner and whiteness in American national identity. In *Flag, nation and symbolism in Europe and America*, ed. T. H. Eriksen and R. Jenkins, 53–68. London: Routledge.

Mawby, R. I. and S. Walklate. 1994. *Critical victimology.* London: Sage.

McCarthy, M. and D. Thompson. 1996. Sexual abuse by design: An examination of the issues in learning disability services. *Disability & Society* 11(2):205–17.

Melville, H. 1988. [1851] *Moby Dick.* Edited with an introduction and notes by Tony Tanner. Oxford: Oxford University Press.

Molloy, H. and L. Vasil. 2002. The social construction of Asperger syndrome: The pathologising of difference? *Disability & Society* 17(6):659–69.

Oliver, M. 1990. *The politics of disablement*. London: Macmillan.

_____. 1996. A sociology of disability or a disablist sociology? In *Disability and society: Emerging issues and insights*, ed. L. Barton, 18–42. London: Longman.

Park, D. C., J. P. Radford, and M. H. Vickers. 1998. Disability studies in human geography. *Progress in Human Geography* 22(2):208–33.

Peay, J. 2002. Mentally disordered offenders, mental health, and crime. In *The Oxford handbook of criminology*, ed. M. Maguire, R. Morgan, and R. Reiner, 746–91. Oxford: Oxford University Press.

Petersilia, J. 2001. Crime victims with developmental disabilities: A review essay. *Criminal Justice and Behavior* 28(6):655–94.

Pfeiffer, D. and K. Yoshida. 1995. Teaching disability studies in Canada and the USA. *Disability & Society* 10(4):475–500.

Phantom of the Opera. 1962. Directed by Terence Fisher. Weybridge, UK: Hammer Film.

Psycho. 1960. Directed by Alfred Hitchcock. Universal City, CA: Shamley Productions.

Radford, J., L. Harne, and J. Trotter. 2006. Disabled women and domestic violence as violent crime. *Practice: Social Work in Action* 18(4):233–46.

Read, J. and S. Baker. 1996. *A survey of the stigma, taboos and discrimination experienced by people with mental health problems*. London: Mind.

Riches, V. C., T. R. Parmenter, M. Wiese, and R. J. Stancliffe. 2006. Intellectual disability and mental illness in the NSW criminal justice system. *International Journal of Law and Psychiatry* 29:386–96.

Shakespeare, T. and N. Watson. 1997. Defending the social model. In *Disability studies: Past, present and future*, ed. L. Barton and M. Oliver, 263–73. Leeds: Leeds Disability Press.

Shakespeare, W. 2005 [1592–3]. *Richard III*, ed. with a commentary by E. A. J. Honogmann. London: Penguin.

Slingblade. 1996. Directed by Billy Bob Thornton. New York: Miramax Films.

Sobsey, D. 1994. *Violence and abuse in the lives of people with disabilities: The end of silent acceptance?* Baltimore: Brooks.

Snyder, S. L. and D. T. Mitchell. 2006. *Cultural locations of disability*. Chicago: University of Chicago Press.

Steinbeck, J. 1937. *Of mice and men*. London: Penguin Red Classics.

The Sting. 1973. Directed by George Roy Hill. Los Angeles: Zanuck/Brown.

Swain, J., S. French, and C. Cameron. 2003. *Controversial issues in a disabling society*. Buckingham/Philadelphia: Open University Press.

Thomas, C. 1999. Female forms: Experiencing and understanding disability. London: Routledge.

UPIAS. 1976. *Fundamental principles of disability*. London: Union of the Physically Impaired Against Segregation.

Van den Bergh, P. M. and J. Hoekman. 2006. Sexual offences in police reports and court dossiers: A case-file study. *Journal of Applied Research in Intellectual Disabilities* 19:374–82.

Van Dijk, J. J. M. 1999. Introducing victimology. In *Caring for crime victims*, ed. J. J. M. van Dijk, R. G. H. van Kaam, and J. Wemmers, 1–12. New York: Criminal Justice Press.

Williams, C. 1995. *Invisible victims*. London: Jessica Kingsley.

Wood, J. and K. Edwards. 2005. Victimization of mentally ill patients living in the community: Is it a lifestyle issue? *Legal and Criminological Psychology* 10(2):279–90.

Young, C. 1967–1975. *Ironside*. Television program. Universal City, CA: Harbour Productions Limited.

Zednar, L. 2002. Victims. In *The Oxford handbook of criminology*, ed. M. Maguire, R. Morgan, and R. Reiner, 419–56. Oxford: Oxford University Press.

Zola, I. 1987. Any distinguishing features? The portrayal of disability in the crime-mystery genre. *Policy Studies Journal* 15(13):487–513.

The Psychological Impact of Victimization 23
Mental Health Outcomes and Psychological, Legal, and Restorative Interventions

SIMON N. VERDUN-JONES AND
KATHERINE R. ROSSITER

Contents

23.1 Introduction

The victims of crime are diverse, and their responses to criminal victimization vary widely as a result. Victimization, regardless of the form it takes, can lead to both short-term emotional difficulties and long-term psychological suffering for victims. Victims of crime may suffer deeply from a wide range of physical, psychological, and economic difficulties, and the degree of suffering may be determined by a number of factors, including the characteristics of the crime itself, the characteristics of the offender, the nature of the victim–offender relationship, and structural and individual-level factors characterizing the victim. This chapter addresses the mental health outcomes of criminal victimization for victims, highlighting several key factors, such as gender, age, and psychiatric disability, all of which render certain groups of individuals particularly vulnerable to victimization. Indeed, those who are most vulnerable to victimization are also those who may face the greatest barriers when attempting to access support in the criminal justice and mental health systems.

The victims' rights movement has been instrumental in advocating for the rights and needs of victims, including their needs for crisis intervention and counseling, information about their cases, participation at various stages of the criminal justice process, and opportunities for recovery and healing from the psychological impact of victimization [Roach, 1999]. Acknowledging that criminal victimization may profoundly affect the psychological and emotional well-being of victims, this chapter explores some of the psychological, legal, and restorative interventions that have been developed to reduce adverse mental health outcomes and improve the psychological health and well-being of victims. The chapter concludes with recommendations for policy and services that are designed to assist crime victims, and directions for future research on the psychological impact of crime and interventions that are calculated to reduce the impact of crime on victims.

23.2 Mental Health Outcomes of Criminal Victimization

The mental health outcomes of victimization and trauma exist along a continuum from relatively mild and short-lived distress to life-altering and debilitating psychiatric disorders [Weaver and Clum, 1995; New and Berliner, 2000]. The dynamic responses of victims to criminal victimization emerge from complex interactions among crime, offender, and victim characteristics. In the first part of this chapter, we identify the most common mental health outcomes of criminal victimization, as well as several key factors or characteristics that play a role in determining the nature and severity of psychological responses to victimization and trauma.

As noted above, at the far extreme of the continuum of psychological responses to criminal victimization are psychiatric disorders, where sets of symptoms reach clinically significant levels and begin to interfere with victims' daily functioning. Although there are many diagnoses that may be appropriate in the aftermath of criminal victimization, the most commonly described psychiatric disorder among victims is post-traumatic stress disorder (PTSD). This diagnostic category first emerged in the third edition of the American Psychiatric Association's [APA, 1980] *Diagnostic and Statistical Manual of Mental Disorders* (DSM-III) and represented a significant and controversial moment in the history of psychiatry [Lasiuk and Hegadoren, 2006]. The construct has been expanded to explain psychological responses to a broad range of traumatic experiences, including physical and sexual abuse or assault, violence experienced or witnessed in combat, and natural disasters [Lasiuk and Hegadoren, 2006]. Several psychological constructs, such as abused child syndrome, rape trauma syndrome [Burgess, 1995], and battered woman syndrome [Walker, 2000], have been more recently subsumed within the diagnostic category of PTSD [Lasiuk and Hegadoren, 2006].

According to the *Diagnostic and Statistical Manual of Mental Disorders*, fourth edition, text revision (DSM-IV-TR) [APA, 2000], the criteria for a diagnosis of PTSD include having experienced or witnessed a traumatic incident that involved actual or threatened death or serious bodily injury to the self or others, and having experienced significant fear, helplessness, or horror as a result. Post-traumatic stress symptoms fall into three categories: persistent re-experiencing of the traumatic incident (e.g., intrusive images, dreams, flashbacks), avoidance of stimuli associated with the trauma (e.g., thoughts, people, places, activities), and increased arousal (e.g., irritability, hypervigilance). Symptoms must be present for at least 1 month and result in impairment of social and occupational functioning [APA, 2000]. If symptoms last for fewer than 3 months, PTSD is considered to be acute, whereas symptoms that persist for longer than 3 months indicate chronic PTSD. In the case where symptoms manifest themselves shortly after the traumatic incident but last for less than 1 month, a diagnosis of acute stress disorder may be more appropriate.

Victims of crime may suffer from a host of other emotional and psychological problems, which fall along various points on the continuum of psychological responses to victimization, including depression, substance abuse, suicidal ideation, and suicide attempts [Kilpatrick and Acierno, 2003]. It is not uncommon for victims to suffer from depression following criminal victimization, and, in some cases, depression develops in association with PTSD. The likelihood of experiencing concurrent disorders, such as PTSD and depression, is particularly high for women who are assaulted by a stranger [Kilpatrick and Acierno, 2003]. Evidence also suggests that victims who suffer from PTSD are more likely to develop secondary substance abuse disorders [Kilpatrick and Acierno, 2003]. However, there is an ongoing debate as to whether substance use develops as a result of experiencing trauma or whether pre-existing substance use is responsible for increased vulnerability to trauma [Kilpatrick and Acierno, 2003]. The relationship between substance use and trauma is likely to be bidirectional, with substance abuse acting as both a cause and consequence of traumatic victimization [Kilpatrick and Acierno, 2003].

Some scholars have suggested that the existing diagnosis of PTSD inadequately reflects the broad range of complex psychological responses to chronic or repeated victimization. Based on the notion that symptoms of post-traumatic stress may be more appropriately classified as a spectrum of disorders, Herman [1997] advanced the concept of "complex post-traumatic stress disorder" to describe the psychological impact of prolonged victimization and trauma. Other emotional and mental health problems that commonly develop among victims with PTSD include dissociation, anxiety, and phobia [Bloom, 1997; Kilpatrick and Acierno, 2003; Briere and Scott, 2006].

The mental health consequences of crime do not always reach clinically significant levels or result in diagnoses of mental disorder, and it is clear that the majority of victims do not suffer such overwhelming effects. More common among victims of crime are changes in cognitive schemas, beliefs, expectations, and assumptions about themselves and others [McCann and Pearlman, 1990]. Victimization challenges victims' beliefs about their own invulnerability, their perceptions of the world as an inherently benign and meaningful place, and their trust in others [Yoder, 2005]. Victimization may cause victims to see themselves in a more negative light, and trauma may also impair both memory and decision-making functions [Bloom, 1997]. Victims of sexual and physical assault may be at risk of engaging in self-injurious behaviors and disordered eating practices, often as a coping mechanism for dealing with the symptoms of trauma.

We have now identified some of the most common psychological responses to victimization and emerging trends in the description and classification of the psychological sequelae of trauma. It is clear that the mental health outcomes of victimization vary widely both in terms of the type and severity of mental suffering. It is important, however, to consider the various factors that affect these mental health outcomes. We turn now to crime, offender, and victim characteristics that may play a role in determining the degree and duration of psychological suffering for victims of crime.

23.2.1 Crime Characteristics

The primary characteristics that determine the psychological impact of crime are characteristics of the crime itself. Crime characteristics can be classified as either objective or subjective and are responsible in part for determining the presence and severity of psychological distress following criminal victimization [Kilpatrick and Acierno, 2003]. Objective factors include type of offense, duration of victimization, degree of force exerted, use of a weapon, and physical injuries sustained [Weaver and Clum, 1995; Kilpatrick and Acierno, 2003]. Subjective factors, on the other hand, include perceived threat of death or bodily injury, the victim's perceived sense of control, and the victim's sense of responsibility or self-blame [Weaver and Clum, 1995; Kilpatrick and Acierno, 2003]. Although both objective and subjective crime characteristics play a role in determining victims' psychological responses to crime, subjective factors have been found to have a significantly greater influence than objective factors for victims of interpersonal violence [Kilpatrick and Acierno, 2003].

Crimes are ordinarily classified in three categories: violent crimes (e.g., robbery, physical assault, sexual assault, and homicide), property crimes (e.g., theft, fraud, and arson), and crimes against the public order (e.g., drug possession and trafficking, gambling, and prostitution) [Schmalleger and Volk, 2008]. Public order crimes are generally considered to be "victimless," but both violent and property offenses may have a significant impact on the mental health and well-being of victims. Violent crimes are typically thought to result in more severe and long-lasting psychological problems for victims; however, the psychological impact of victimization cannot be predicted with any degree of certainty based on the offense type alone. Indeed, victim and offender characteristics may play an important role in determining the impact of specific crimes, and, in some cases, the victims of nonviolent offenses may suffer more adverse outcomes than victims of violence, owing to the complex interaction of these factors.

Crimes can also be differentiated according to the number of victims and the group membership of those who are victimized. Mass victimization itself refers to a broad range of crimes, including school shootings (e.g., the Columbine, Virginia Tech, and Montreal massacres), terrorist attacks (e.g., the 9/11 World Trade Center attacks in New York), and genocide (e.g., the Holocaust in Nazi Germany, and Rwandan genocide). In the United States, Canada, and Australia, beginning in the late nineteenth century and continuing into the late twentieth century, Aboriginal children were removed from their families and placed in Indian residential/boarding schools or with white families, where many suffered extensive psychological, physical, and sexual abuse. The Canadian "60s scoop" and Australian "stolen generation" are considered by many to be examples of cultural genocide, and the lasting impact on future generations of Aboriginal people is reflected today in extraordinarily high rates of poverty, substance abuse, family violence, and suicide, as well as significant over-representation as offenders in the criminal justice system [York, 1989; La Prairie, 1990; Griffiths and Verdun-Jones, 1994; Roberts and Melchers, 2003]. The psychological impact of mass victimization is arguably greater than victimization at the individual level, if only because the experience of victimization is so widespread and, as in the case of the Holocaust and Indian residential schools, may lead to cultural and/or intergenerational trauma, impacting future generations [Sigal and Weinfeld, 1989; Raphael, Swan, and Martinek, 1998]. Many of the mass victimizations described above involve the targeting of victims who belong to various distinctive groups, whether based on gender, ethnicity, or religion. Hate crimes are offenses motivated by bias, whereby individuals are targeted based on their membership in a minority group that is defined by a common race, religion, ethnicity, gender, sexual orientation, or disability [McDevitt et al., 2007].

The impact of victimization also varies according to the nature of the victim's experience. The victim may have personally suffered the consequences of a crime (primary victimization) or may have witnessed a crime committed against another person or other persons (secondary victimization). The psychological impact of victimization often reaches beyond the primary victims to their families, friends, and communities. Witnessing violence at the individual level (e.g., domestic violence, homicide) and in the context of mass victimization (e.g., school shootings, combat in war) may leave people severely traumatized despite not having experienced the crime firsthand. Children who witness domestic violence between parents are especially likely to experience adverse mental health outcomes owing to their vulnerability and dependency on both victim and perpetrator [Osofsky, 1995; Finkelhor, 2007]. PTSD is also common among family and friends of homicide victims [Kilpatrick and Acierno, 2003], in which case trauma may be compounded by grief, a construct known as "traumatic grief" [Jacobs, 1999; Pfefferbaum et al., 2001]. Even professionals working with crime victims may experience significant distress and symptoms of trauma, a phenomenon that has been variously described as "vicarious traumatization" [McCann and Pearlman, 1990], "secondary traumatic stress" [Figley, 1995], and "traumatic countertransference" [Herman,1992].

Although broad differences between violent and nonviolent victimization, individual and mass victimization, and experienced or witnessed violence are clearly important in determining the psychological impact of victimization, details of individual offenses also affect the mental health outcomes of victimization. These factors include the duration of the incident, the amount of force used against the victim, the use of weapons in carrying out the offense, the extent to which victims suffer physical injuries, the perceived threat of grievous bodily injury or death, the degree of control victims felt they had during the victimization, and the degree to which they blame themselves for their own victimization [Kilpatrick and Acierno, 2003]. As noted above, although each of these factors may influence the likelihood that victims develop PTSD, there is evidence to suggest that subjective factors play a greater role than objective factors in determining the mental health outcomes of victimization [Kilpatrick and Acierno, 2003]. As the concept of victimization continues to expand and new types of crime and victimization continue to emerge (e.g., cyber-bullying, human trafficking), it will be important to continue to broaden our understanding of the psychological impact of crime and to develop interventions to minimize the negative effects of victimization [Finkelhor, 2007; Young et al., 2007].

23.2.2 Offender Characteristics

Offender characteristics are less frequently discussed than crime and victim characteristics in the literature concerning the mental health outcomes of victimization. However, several important factors, such as the role or position of the perpetrator and the victim–offender relationship, may also influence the psychological impact of victimization. The mental health consequences of criminal victimization may be particularly detrimental in cases where perpetrators are in (or purport to be in) positions of trust and authority. For example, offenders may be parents or guardians, religious leaders, police officers, legal representatives, caregivers, clinicians, or medical practitioners. Although a violation of trust may be damaging for victims of all ages, the psychological impact of victimization by someone in a position of trust may be especially profound for children [Dominelli, 1989; Feinauer, 1989]. Public perceptions of crime are created and reinforced by media accounts of criminal victimization, leading the public to fear crime committed by strangers disproportionately to the actual risk of victimization by strangers [Kidd-Hewitt, 2002]. On the contrary, there is significant evidence to suggest that crimes committed by persons known to the victim are considered to be more traumatic than those involving perpetrators who are strangers [Marley and Buila, 2001].

Violence occurring within families, such as child abuse, intimate partner abuse, and elder abuse, may be particularly traumatic and often occurs within a broader context of control. Victims may be less likely to report crimes committed by known perpetrators to the authorities for fear the perpetrator will retaliate or because they do not consider these events to be criminal. Victims of intimate partner violence are typically isolated and controlled by their abusive partners and thus may develop a psychological response known as learned helplessness [Walker, 1979]. This response is part of an overall cycle of violence that consists of three stages: a tension-building stage, an acute battering incident, and a stage of loving contrition, often referred to as the "honeymoon" stage [Walker, 2000]. When victims are dependent on those who victimize them, they may suffer from a loss of independence, a loss of trust, fear of revictimization, a sense of betrayal, and embarrassment [Heisler, 2007].

23.2.3 Victim Characteristics

Victim characteristics are likely to have the greatest impact on the psychological responses of victims to criminal victimization. Characteristics of individual victims that influence their psychological responses to crime include both structural factors, such as gender, age, race, ethnicity, and socioeconomic status, and individual-level factors, including previous experiences of victimization and trauma, pre-existing mental illness, and social support.

Gender is one of the most important structural factors affecting the psychological impact of crime and is closely linked to the types of crimes perpetrated against women and men. It is well-known that men are more likely to be both the perpetrators and victims of crime across the life span, but that women and girls are at significantly greater risk of being the victims of some particular types of offense, such as sexual assault [Finkelhor, 2007]. Furthermore, women experience more types of victimization across the life span and are more likely to be victimized repeatedly and to know the perpetrator of the crime [Marley and Buila, 2001]. Women are also more likely than men to develop PTSD [Brewin, Andrews, and Valentine, 2000; Kilpatrick and Acierno, 2003]. Gender differences in relation to PTSD are the greatest following physical assault (i.e., women are far more likely than men to develop PTSD after being physically attacked) but become comparable for both men and women following sexual assault (i.e., women and men are equally likely to develop PTSD following sexual assault). It is important to recognize, however, that sexual assault is more frequently committed against women [Kilpatrick and Acierno, 2003]. Men who develop PTSD following crimes that are of a nonsexual nature tend to have experienced or witnessed particularly overwhelming violence, a trend that is clearly reflected in combat stress among war veterans [Kilpatrick and Acierno, 2003]. Finally, there appear to be significant gender differences in relation to the coping mechanisms used by men and women who have been victimized. For example, Green and Diaz [2008] found that although victimized women experienced higher levels of depression, PTSD, anxiety, and anger, they were also more likely than men to make use of "emotion-focused" coping strategies and manifested higher levels of both mental and spiritual well-being.

Another important structural factor in determining the severity and impact of psychological distress on the victims of crime is age, or stage of the life course, at the time of the offense. Children and youth are particularly vulnerable to victimization, and, according to a developmental theory of victimization, early traumatic experiences shape the life course of victims in significant ways [Macmillan, 2001; Paolucci, Genuis, and Violato, 2001]. Developmental victimology is devoted to understanding the victimization of children, a phenomenon some have argued has been inadequately theorized and under-researched [Finkelhor, 2007]. Children who have experienced childhood sexual abuse are at significant risk of developing PTSD, substance abuse disorders, eating disorders, depression, and dissociation and may display suicidal ideation in adolescence and/or adulthood [Arboleda-Florez and

Wade, 2001; Lansford et al., 2002; O'Sullivan and Fry, 2007]. There is also a body of research that indicates that childhood sexual abuse is associated with the later emergence of sexually risky behavior in adulthood [Holmes, Foa, and Sammel, 2005; Roxburgh, Degenhardt, and Copeland, 2006], although it has been pointed out that this research is yet to establish a causal connection [Senn, Carey, and Vanable, 2008].

Emerging evidence also suggests that child abuse and maltreatment may result in permanent biological changes and brain dysfunction for young victims [Heide and Solomon, 2006]. The nature and scope of the negative consequences of early childhood abuse vary from one individual to another. Recent research suggests that some part of this variation may be explained by genetic predisposition. For example, Caspi et al. [2002] found that the impact of early childhood abuse may be moderated by specific genotypes, which may increase or decrease the likelihood that an abused child will subsequently engage in antisocial behavior. Despite the clearly devastating consequences of victimization for children, crimes committed against children do not often come to the attention of authorities owing to the stigma associated with certain types of victimization, such as incest, and the limited capacity of children to report crimes committed against them [Finkelhor, 2007; O'Sullivan and Fry, 2007].

Victimization among elderly persons is relatively uncommon, except where specific types of crimes, such as elder abuse, are considered. As noted earlier, this form of abuse is often perpetrated by caregivers, whether they are family members or paid workers in nursing homes. Despite their lower risk of victimization, elderly people have generally expressed high levels of fear of crime [Yin, 1982; Greve, 1998]. However, it appears that those who do become victims of crime are not particularly likely to develop psychiatric disorders, such as PTSD and depression, as a result of victimization [Kilpatrick and Acierno, 2003]. Scholars caution against overlooking the psychological impact of crime on older adults; however, they also suggest that it is possible that older adults manifest post-traumatic stress symptoms somatically [Averill and Beck, 2000]. It is clear that the psychological impact of victimization varies according to age; however, more research is needed to better understand differences in the severity and duration of symptoms throughout the life course, from childhood through adolescence and adulthood, and into older adulthood.

Like gender and age, the psychological impact of crime may not be uniform across racial and ethnic groups. Evidence is mixed concerning racial differences in the likelihood of being victimized and the likelihood of developing PTSD following victimization, with some studies reporting that African Americans experience more distress following trauma despite lower rates of victimization and others finding weak or no race-based differences [Brewin, Andrews, and Valentine, 2000; Kilpatrick and Acierno, 2003].

As noted above, race and ethnicity play a central role in some types of crime, such as hate crimes motivated by racial or ethnic bias, and in genocide. Some scholars have questioned the applicability of PTSD, as a clinical construct based on a medical model of mental illness, to other races and cultures [Marsella and Christopher, 2004; Lasiuk and Hegadoren, 2006], arguing that symptoms of psychological distress following victimization may not manifest themselves in common ways across diverse cultural groups [Briere and Scott, 2006].

A final structural factor in determining the psychological impact of victimization is socioeconomic status, which is a concept reflecting education level, employment status, and income [Brewin, Andrews, and Valentine, 2000]. Persons who have extremely low socioeconomic status may experience chronic or episodic poverty and homelessness, conditions that increase their vulnerability to victimization and the degree of psychological distress resulting from victimization. For example, research has found that socioeconomic inequality, as measured by unemployment status, increases both the risk of victimization and psychological distress following victimization [Wohlfarth et al., 2001]. Individuals who are homeless report very high levels of stress and fear, both on the streets and in shelters [Daiski, 2007], whereas homeless persons who suffer from mental illness and substance use disorders represent an even more vulnerable subgroup within this population [Lam and Rosenheck, 1998; Sullivan et al., 2000; Walsh et al., 2003]. Some scholars have concluded that violent victimization is so common in the lives of homeless women who are suffering from mental illness that it may be considered "normative" [Goodman, Dutton, and Harris, 1995]. Establishing safety may be the first stage of the trauma recovery process [Herman, 1992]; however, because of their limited social supports and diminished sense of safety and security in their daily lives [Simons, Whitbeck, and Bales, 1989], the recovery process may be impeded for persons who are homeless.

It is well-known that previous experience of victimization is the best predictor of future victimization [Lam and Rosenheck, 1998]. However, despite a substantial and growing body of knowledge about the experience and impact of victimization, relatively little is known about repeat victimization and even less is known about the cumulative impact of ongoing or chronic victimization [Follette et al., 1996]. Research has consistently found that a significant proportion of victims of violence, particularly women, have been victims of violence in the past, and that many female victims of childhood abuse go on to experience violence in adulthood [Herman, 1997]. Furthermore, research suggests that the impact of trauma is cumulative insofar as individuals who experience repeated or chronic victimization exhibit higher levels of post-traumatic distress following revictimization [Follette et al., 1996; Brewin, Andrews, and Valentine, 2000; Gearon et al., 2003; Kilpatrick and Acierno, 2003]. In addition to the negative effects of repeated victimization, revictimization may also impede the trauma recovery process [Follette et al., 1996]. Evidence that revictimization throughout the life course compounds the psychological impact of trauma has led scholars to propose alternative constructs, such as complex PTSD, that more adequately describe the symptoms of chronic revictimization [Herman, 1997].

Another individual-level factor that has a significant impact on the psychological impact of victimization is mental disability [Brewin, Andrews, and Valentine, 2000]. Persons with mental illness are at greater risk of victimization and trauma than those without mental illness [Hiday et al., 2001; Silver et al., 2005]. For example, Hiday et al. [1999] have found that the rate of violent criminal victimization for individuals with severe mental illness was 2.5 times greater than for the general population. Mentally disordered persons are more susceptible to violent victimization because they are more likely to be impoverished and homeless. They are also more likely to reside in socially disorganized areas, where victimization may be a common experience [Hiday, 1997, 2006; Hiday et al., 2001; Silver, 2006; White et al., 2006; Sirotich 2008]. In addition, residing in socially disorganized areas increases the probability that mentally disordered individuals will be exposed to—and engage in—illicit substance abuse, a factor which is independently associated with an elevated risk of violent victimization [Hiday, 1997, 2006; Silver, 2002; Sells et al., 2003; White et al., 2006]. Furthermore, owing to their clinical symptoms and occasionally bizarre conduct, mentally disordered individuals are also more likely to become involved in conflicted social relationships, which have the potential to result in violence [Hiday, 1997; Silver, 2002; Gearon et al., 2003]. Pre-existing mental health problems and mental illness may increase victims' risk of developing PTSD and other psychiatric symptoms [Goodman et al., 1999], but mental health professionals should be careful not to misdiagnose individuals who present with ambiguous symptoms. Post-traumatic stress symptoms may resemble—and overlap with—other psychiatric disorders, increasing the likelihood that the mental health problems experienced by victims of crime may be misdiagnosed and improperly treated [Gearon et al., 2003].

Evidence suggests that mentally ill persons, including those who themselves come into conflict with the law, constitute a severely traumatized population [Goodman et al., 1999; Spitzer et al., 2006; Mezey, 2007]; however, trauma and the symptoms of post-traumatic stress are often overlooked in clinical interviews with persons suffering from mental illness [Adshead, 1994; Mueser et al., 1998; Walsh et al., 2003]. Persons with mental illness who do become victims of crime may not report their experiences, particularly if they are homeless and victimization is a fact of their daily lives [Padgett and Struening, 1992]. Stereotypes about mentally ill persons and stigma toward those who suffer from psychiatric disorders may also lead service providers to make assumptions about the reliability of their reports [Marley and Buila, 2001]. Research has found, however, that the reports of mental health outpatients concerning their histories of victimization were reliable over time, with regard to the occurrence and severity of abuse, as well as the severity of PTSD symptoms [Goodman et al., 1999]. The validity of these patients' reports was not assessed, however, and thus it remains unclear whether patients' reports of abuse, although consistent over time, are accurate [Goodman et al., 1999]. Nevertheless, scholars note that PTSD is often underdiagnosed among women who have severe mental disorders and concurrent substance use disorders, and subsequently it often fails to receive treatment [Eilenberg et al., 1996; Mueser et al., 1998].

Previous victimization and pre-existing mental health problems may increase the risk of trauma and its sequelae, but various individual-level factors, such as social support, may serve to mitigate this risk and protect victims of crime from adverse mental health outcomes [Briere and Scott, 2006]. The role of informal social support will be discussed in the second part of this chapter, which explores psychological, legal, and restorative interventions for victims of crime.

23.3 Interventions for Victims of Crime

Victims have a broad range of needs, including the need to regain a sense of personal safety and control, the need to tell their stories, the need to have their experiences acknowledged or validated, and the need to reconnect with themselves and others [Herman, 1992, 2003; Bloom, 1997; Yoder, 2005]. In this section, we highlight various psychological, legal, and restorative interventions designed to mitigate the negative mental health outcomes of criminal victimization and improve the psychological well-being of crime victims. Before reviewing interventions for victims of crime, however, two important points must be made. First, trauma recovery is an ongoing process and "recovery is never complete" [Herman, 1997]. Thus, interventions may assist victims in the recovery process; however, this process is neither linear nor expected to reach the final stage, at which point survivors may claim full recovery status. Second, owing to the complex nature of the interaction between crime characteristics, offender characteristics, and victim characteristics in determining the psychological impact of victimization, no single intervention will be suitable or therapeutic for all victims. However, these three categories of characteristics may inform which interventions would be most appropriate and meaningful for individual victims of crime. We now turn to various psychological, legal, and restorative interventions that may offer hope to victims of crime for recovery and improved mental health.

23.3.1 Psychological Interventions

The focus in this section will be on the formal and informal supports, services, and mechanisms developed to reduce psychiatric symptoms, improve mental health, and promote trauma recovery. Victims differ widely with regard to the type, intensity, and duration of supports and services that are required to address their needs. Some victims will benefit little from formal services but may rely heavily on informal supports to receive emotional and practical assistance following a traumatic incident. Informal social supports provided by family, friends, and members of the community are both commonplace and valuable to crime victims. Support networks can provide immediate and long-term assistance to victims, addressing both practical and emotional needs [Davis, 2007]. Little research has been conducted on the impact of informal social support for victims' mental health; however, existing evidence suggests that this type of support has a greater impact on problems immediately following victimization than on the long-term effects of victimization. Undoubtedly, inappropriate and unsupportive responses from family and friends may serve only to exacerbate the negative psychological outcomes of victimization [Davis, 2007]. Ideally, informal support persons should connect with professionals to enhance their efforts to support victims of crime [Davis, 2007].

Victims of crime may benefit enormously from mental health and victims' services; however, research suggests that the majority of victims do not access such services [New and Berliner, 2000]. Among the factors influencing the likelihood that victims will seek treatment are the crime, offender, and victim characteristics identified above, such as the type and severity of the crime, frequency and duration of victimization, and the relationship between victim and offender. The nature and severity of psychological distress or psychiatric symptoms resulting from crime also play a role in determining whether victims decide to seek mental health treatment, insofar as those who access services are also those reporting greater distress following victimization [Follette et al., 1996; New and Berliner, 2000]. In some jurisdictions, victims may be able to access victim compensation funds to cover the costs of mental health treatment; however, research suggests that, despite financial support for mental health care, victims remain reluctant to seek treatment. Those who do seek treatment tend to be female victims of sexual assault or intimate partner violence, who suffer from post-traumatic stress symptoms [New and Berliner, 2000].

A wide array of psychological or clinical interventions have been developed to reduce the psychological costs of victimization, including psychoeducation (e.g., dispelling myths about victimization and trauma, assisting victims with safety planning), distress reduction and affect-regulation training (e.g., breathing techniques, trigger awareness), cognitive interventions (e.g., victim empowerment, narrative coherence), emotional processing (e.g., exposure, desensitization), and techniques to improve relational functioning [Briere and Scott, 2006]. Crisis intervention services focus on helping victims to re-establish a sense of safety, assisting victims with practical needs following victimization, and providing victims with a safe place to tell their stories [Young et al., 2007]. Given that the impact of trauma is cumulative, it is imperative that mental health professionals and victims' services workers inquire about victims' histories of trauma and abuse to better respond to their needs for recovery [Follette et al., 1996].

Victims of crime may seek services from mental health and criminal justice professionals in the immediate aftermath of victimization, and the sensitivity and care with which these professionals treat victims may play an important role in the recovery process [Mezey, 2007]. Indeed, trauma survivors may be inadvertently revictimized by mental health and criminal justice workers if these professionals are insensitive to their needs, engage in victim-blaming, or do not believe their reports of victimization [O'Sullivan and Fry, 2007]. For victims who are stigmatized based on mental health status, disability status, homelessness status, or legal status, negative interactions with helping professionals may be more common and more psychologically damaging.

23.3.2 Legal Interventions

Victims have traditionally played a very limited role in the criminal justice process and have typically served as witnesses in offender-centered courtroom proceedings. Until recently, the criminal justice system had neither formally established victims' rights nor adequately attended to their practical and psychological needs. During the past several decades, however, the role of victims has progressed from passive involvement as witnesses in criminal justice proceedings to more active involvement in the justice system [Erez and Roberts, 2007]. Indeed, the victims' rights movement is credited with numerous legal reforms that have resulted in increased recognition of the needs of crime victims and greater opportunities for victims to be active participants in the processing of their cases through the court system [Herman, 2003].

Victims' rights in relation to the criminal justice system include the right to general information about the criminal justice system, the right to be notified about the details and progress of their case (e.g., dates of hearings, release of the offender), the right to attend criminal justice proceedings, the right to consult with criminal justice officials, the right to have a voice in the criminal justice process, the right to protection by criminal justice officials (e.g., employment protection laws, no contact orders, victim/witness protection programs), the right to have their cases progress through the justice system without unreasonable delays, the right to restitution or reimbursement of financial costs resulting from the crime, and the right to privacy and confidentiality [Herman, 2003; Erez and Roberts, 2007; Howley and Dorris, 2007]. Victims also have the right to access services and supports within the criminal justice system, such as victims' services offered by the police and court advocacy programs [Erez and Roberts, 2007]. The 1960s also saw the development of programs providing financial compensation to victims of crime who have incurred financial and other significant costs as a result of their victimization [Howley and Dorris, 2007].

One of the most significant advancements concerning the victim's role in the criminal justice process was the development of victim impact statements (VIS), statements written by victims to convey to the court the financial costs of the crime and the impact of the crime on their physical and psychological well-being [Howley and Dorris, 2007]. VIS may offer victims a voice in the courtroom at pretrial, plea bargaining, sentencing, and/or parole hearings [Erez and Roberts, 2007]. However, there are important jurisdictional differences regarding the role of victims at various stages of the criminal justice process. For example, in Canada, victims are permitted to submit VIS at sentencing and parole hearings but, unlike in many U.S. states, cannot submit written or oral statements in pretrial or plea bargaining processes [Verdun-Jones and Tijerino, 2002, 2004]. VIS serve both instrumental and expressive functions, and may benefit crime victims by formally acknowledging the harm caused to them and by restoring their sense of dignity, power, and control [Erez and Rogers, 1999; Arrigo and Williams, 2003; Verdun-Jones and Tijerino, 2005].

Victims' rights advocates consider the development of VIS to be an important advancement in the victims' rights movement; however, VIS may not be suitable or therapeutic for all victims and, in some cases, may even be antitherapeutic. For victims who are not psychologically prepared to do so, for example, confronting the offender in legal proceedings may be psychologically damaging. Although VIS were developed to give victims a voice in criminal justice proceedings, some scholars have suggested that they have also silenced victims [Erez and Rogers, 1999]. To support the emotional well-being of victims and minimize the potential psychological harm for those who wish to have a voice in criminal justice proceedings, it is critical that processes designed to include victims in the criminal justice process remain flexible. Additionally, victims should be clearly informed about the role that VIS play in criminal justice proceedings. That is, VIS are intended to give victims a voice in court and to relay the impact of victimization in their daily lives, but they do not typically influence sentencing decisions [Erez and Roeger, 1995; Howley and Dorris, 2007]. If victims believe their statements will have an impact on sentencing decisions, the realization that their words have not been influential may cause further psychological distress. In the future, it may well be beneficial for victims if the courts were also to make use of VIS as a means of identifying the appropriate support services that individual victims may need and to exercise their authority to facilitate the timely provision of these services.

Some scholars and legal representatives question the role of emotion in criminal justice proceedings and argue that it is neither appropriate nor desirable for VIS to influence sentencing outcomes [Arrigo and Williams, 2003]. In a study of the use and effects of VIS in Australia, legal representatives (e.g., judges, Crown prosecutors, and defense lawyers) reported that VIS serve important symbolic, political, and therapeutic purposes, but that they have little impact on sentencing decisions [Erez and Rogers, 1999]. Based on evidence that VIS did influence the decision making of jurors in capital cases, however, Arrigo and Williams [2003] called for the abolition of VIS in such cases. Their central argument is that the emotional nature of these statements interferes with the right of the accused to a fair trial and thus that VIS seriously undermine the fundamental principles of justice.

It is possible that VIS may be inappropriate at some stages of the criminal justice process or for particular types of cases and criminal proceedings. Victims have typically had fewer rights in cases where the offender has been adjudicated "not criminally responsible on account of mental disorder" (NCR-MD in Canada) or "not guilty by reason of insanity" (NGRI in the United States). Limited emphasis on victims and their rights in these proceedings stems from the fact that, when processed in the forensic mental health system, the accused is not convicted of a crime and thus is treated as a mental health patient rather than as a convicted offender [Howley and Dorris, 2007]. Indeed, there is reason to believe that the inclusion of VIS in review board hearings may be antitherapeutic for both the victim and the accused. A victim's request to submit an oral VIS at the disposition hearing of an NCR-accused person should be considered on a case-by-case basis and take into account the potential psychological impact of such victim participation for both the NCR-accused person and the victim [Verdun-Jones and Tijerino, 2005].

The potential implications of participation in the criminal justice process are significant for victims; however, the majority of victims do not participate in the criminal justice process [Herman, 2003]. There are countless reasons for victims to avoid seeking justice, including legitimate fears of retaliation from the offender (e.g., in the case of intimate partner violence, where the offender may live with the victim and exert significant control over the victim's life), distrust of the criminal justice system and persons in positions of authority (e.g., in the case of refugees, where criminal justice processes in their home countries have been characterized by corruption and abuses of power), and skepticism about the capacity of an adversarial and offender-centered legal system to offer the victim any sense of justice [Herman, 2003].

Just as positive experiences of participation in the criminal justice system offer significant benefits to the mental health of victims, negative experiences with the justice system may exacerbate trauma symptoms and worsen victims' psychological well-being [Herman 2003]. Participation in the criminal justice system may be stressful and embarrassing for victims, and, in some cases, the justice system contributes to the retraumatization of victims [Herman, 2003]. When the victims of crime are children and they serve as witnesses in court, the criminal justice system must be particularly sensitive to their needs and vulnerabilities to minimize the stress and revictimization that may accompany their participation in criminal justice proceedings [Whitcomb, 2003]. Research suggests that child victims of sexual abuse may experience psychological stress when testifying in court but that the adverse effects of their participation in criminal justice proceedings do not appear to produce long-term psychological distress [Whitcomb, 2003]. Regardless of the victim's age, however, negative experiences and involvement in the criminal justice system may further exacerbate post-traumatic stress symptoms for both primary victims and their families and friends [Kilpatrick and Acierno, 2003].

There is an ongoing need to consider the rights and needs of victims in the criminal justice system, but opportunities for victim involvement in criminal justice proceedings should be carefully considered and evaluated to maximize the benefits and minimize the harms of victim participation. Therapeutic jurisprudence, or the potential of the law to act as a therapeutic agent [Wexler, 1990], offers an approach for reducing harm and improving the psychological well-being of those involved in the legal system, without overlooking the fundamental principles of justice [Goldberg, 2005; Wemmers, 2008]. Therapeutic jurisprudence provides the underlying theoretical framework for specialty or "problem-solving" courts, such as drug courts, domestic violence courts, and mental health courts and may contribute to the psychological well-being of both victims and offenders [Petrila, 2003].

Victims have a wide range of practical and psychological needs, and their experiences in the criminal justice system may have a significant impact on their mental health and well-being. Victims' needs include the need for information, compensation, support, respect, recognition, a sense of control, and a voice in the criminal justice process [Wemmers, 2008]. When these needs are not met, the criminal justice system may be considered antithera-peutic for victims and risks exacerbating the adverse mental health outcomes of victimization. Although the victims' rights movement has significantly improved the plight of victims, new developments and processes must be evaluated to ensure that they are in the best interests of victims, keeping in mind that victims' needs are diverse and cannot be adequately met with one-size-fits-all solutions.

23.3.3 Restorative Interventions

Restorative justice approaches offer an alternative to the traditional, retributive, and adversarial justice system, and have sought to address the limited capacity of the criminal justice system to address the needs of victims, offenders, and their communities. Restorative justice focuses on the harms done to victims and communities as a result of crime, addresses obligations and responsibilities, and emphasizes the needs of victims, including participation and empowerment [Zehr, 2002]. Specific restorative justice initiatives include victim–offender mediation, family group conferencing, community justice conferencing, and sentencing and peacemaking circles [Herman, 2003]. In contrast to formal inclusion of victims in criminal justice proceedings, restorative justice processes offer victims a chance to express their emotions, convey the psychological impact of victimization, and begin to heal from the emotional and psychological impact of victimization [Arrigo and Williams, 2003].

Like psychological and legal interventions, restorative interventions may not be appropriate in all cases, depending on crime, offender, and victim characteristics. For example, feminist debates continue about the suitability of restorative justice in cases of gendered violence, such as sexual assault and intimate partner violence [Curtis-Fawley and Daly, 2005; Herman, 2005; Cameron, 2006]. Despite the benefits of restorative justice processes, victims' advocates share concerns about the potential for these approaches to revictimize victims of crime, exacerbate power imbalances between victim and offender, appear to be "soft" on crime, and contribute to the privatization of gendered violence [Curtis-Fawley and Daly, 2005]. Feminist concerns about the use of restorative justice in cases of gendered violence do not necessarily mean these approaches are unsuitable for other types of crime. For example, a meta-analysis of restorative justice practices suggested that victim satisfaction with participation in restorative justice processes was significantly greater than victim satisfaction with participation in the traditional criminal justice system [Latimer, Dowden, and Muise, 2005].

Alongside local initiatives, restorative interventions have developed globally, on a much greater scale, to respond to the needs of victims of mass atrocities, where whole communities and cultures have been traumatized by mass victimization and human rights violations. Truth commissions are "official bodies set up to investigate a past period of human rights abuses or violations of international humanitarian law" [Hayner, 1994]. They may be governmental or nongovernmental, are established only temporarily, and are granted significant authority to document abuses and violations over a certain period in a country's past [Hayner, 1994]. Victims and witnesses of human rights violations may be invited to testify and tell their stories, thereby actively breaking the silence of the past, a process which may be therapeutic for both individuals who testify and whole nations or cultures [Chapman and Ball, 2001]. Truth commissions are distinguishable from war crime tribunals in that they seek "truth" and aim to prevent similar atrocities in the future rather than seeking "justice" and the prosecution of individuals charged with crimes against humanity [Hayner, 1994]. An important component of truth commissions is the acknowledgement of harm, which is critical for compensation and healing of victims and their families.

Truth commissions typically produce a report that acknowledges the widespread victimization and trauma experienced and, in some cases, includes recommendations for reform and reparations for victims [Hayner, 1994]. Truth commissions have been established in numerous countries to date, including Uganda, Bolivia, Argentina, Uruguay, Zimbabwe, the Philippines, Chile, Chad, South Africa, Germany, El Salvador, Rwanda, Ethiopia, Nepal, Sri Lanka, Haiti, Guatemala, Nigeria, Peru, Panama, Yugoslavia, Sierra Leone, and Ghana [Hayner, 1994; Chapman and Ball, 2001]. On June 1, 2008, Canada established the Indian Residential Schools Truth and Reconciliation Commission to acknowledge and document the experiences and consequences of the Indian Residential School legacy for Aboriginal peoples. In Australia, where similar abuses have been perpetrated against Aboriginal peoples, the government issued a formal apology on February 13, 2008, for the treatment of its indigenous peoples throughout history, but no truth commission has been established.

Research into the therapeutic value of the South African Truth and Reconciliation Commission (TRC) found that testifying offered victims an opportunity to express—and share—their experiences of physical suffering (e.g., bodily harm, death), mental suffering (e.g., shock, fear, anger), and collective suffering (e.g., mistrust, shared trauma). Healing was considered to be a private, public, individual, and collective process that was achieved through storytelling and remembrance, financial and symbolic reparation, and psychological and spiritual support systems [de la Rey and Owens, 1998]. Some scholars have argued that, despite claims of healing, the TRC process revealed widespread mental health problems that had been inadequately addressed, and that the process did not serve as a therapeutic agent, as envisioned in the therapeutic jurisprudence approach [Allan, 2000].

Continued evaluation of the suitability and value of restorative interventions, at both the individual and cultural levels, is clearly warranted. Although restorative justice initiatives may appear to be beneficial to victims, this is not always the case, and some scholars have argued that evaluation of existing restorative processes should precede the development of new initiatives [Cameron, 2006]. Evaluations of restorative initiatives may include an assessment of their impact on the psychological health and well-being of victims, and will hopefully shed light on various conditions under which restorative justice processes are therapeutic or, alternatively, antitherapeutic for victims. This knowledge and evidence will ultimately serve to inform restorative justice practice and support the recovery of victims.

23.4 Conclusions

The psychological impact and adverse mental health outcomes of crime and victimization are significant and may reach far beyond primary victims to their families, their communities, witnesses, and the public. Individuals, groups, and entire cultures may suffer tremendously from experiencing or witnessing violence, and the mental health outcomes of victimization, which range from relatively low levels of distress to life-altering and debilitating psychiatric disorders, depend on the complex interaction of crime, offender, and victim characteristics. Criminological theory suggests that victimization plays a role in future aggression and criminal behavior, and feminist criminologists, in particular, have acknowledged a cycle of violence in the lives of women victims and offenders. As a result, a "pathways to crime" approach has evolved in the field of feminist criminology that recognizes the histories of physical and sexual victimization and trauma in the lives of women, especially Aboriginal women, who come into conflict with the law [Comack, 1996].

Despite significant human suffering, many victims of crime have great resilience and are able to recover and heal from their experiences, abandoning their "victim" status and coming to see themselves as survivors. The positive psychology movement seeks to disrupt the illness ideology in clinical psychology and focus instead on notions of strength, resiliency, recovery, and growth for individuals who experience significant mental anguish. This paradigm has gained strength in recent years and, with the emergence of new concepts such as post-traumatic growth, is beginning to significantly shape the field of traumatic stress [Figley, 1988; Tedeschi and Calhoun, 2004; Ai and Park, 2005; Joseph and Linley, 2008].

The broad range of mental health outcomes and diverse needs of victims presents a significant challenge for criminal justice and mental health policy makers and service providers. Policies and practices designed to respond appropriately to individual victims' unique situations and needs must be flexible and avoid "one-size-fits-all" solutions for victims. Responses should be tailored to the unique needs of victims as much as possible and should not rely on assumptions about the psychological impact of crime based solely on characteristics of the crime, offender, or victim. Indeed, different people who experience the same crime may have vastly different psychological responses to their victimization, and individuals who experience different types of criminal victimization may respond in surprisingly similar ways [Weaver and Clum, 1995]. Victims' services and interventions must be attentive to the age, gender, race, ethnicity, and ability of the victim [Whitcomb, 2003]. Victims' participation in the criminal justice process must also be supported to ensure that victims are empowered rather than revictimized as a result of their participation [Herman, 2003].

Researchers should seek to better understand the way in which the various crime, offender, and victim characteristics interact and the implications of these interactions for mental health and victims' services. Of critical importance are the identification of vulnerable victim populations (e.g., the homeless; rural populations; ethnic, racial, and sexual minorities; persons with mental illness) and the barriers these victims face when seeking to access mental health and victims' services [Muscat and Walsh, 2007]. There is also a need for further research and theoretical development in the field of post-traumatic stress and post-traumatic growth to better understand the experiences of trauma, recovery, and growth for victims and witnesses, their families and friends, professionals working with victims, and the communities that are affected by criminal victimization [Calhoun and Tedeschi, 2008]. More evaluation research is clearly required to assess the success of existing psychological, legal, and restorative interventions for victims of crime, and to suggest reforms and alternatives that promise better outcomes for victims.

Researchers studying the mental health outcomes of crime and interventions for victims will continue to be challenged by new categories of crime, which produce new types of victims and an ever-expanding comprehension of the complexities of trauma. Globalization has resulted in new forms of international crime, and technological advancement has opened up new categories of Internet crime. Finally, it is critical to expand our perceptions of "victims" and to begin to appreciate that the boundaries between "victims" and "offenders" are often blurred and that it is frequently the case that perpetrators of crime have also been victims of crime themselves. Recognition of these blurring boundaries will have significant implications for theories of crime and victimization, victims' services, policy development, and future research on the psychological impact of victimization.

References

Adshead, G. 1994. Damage: Trauma and violence in a sample of women referred to a forensic service. *Behavioral Sciences and the Law* 12:235–49.

Ai, A. L. and C. L. Park. 2005. Possibilities of the positive following violence and trauma: Informing the coming decade of research. *Journal of Interpersonal Violence* 20(2):242–50.

Allan, A. 2000. Truth and reconciliation: A psycholegal perspective. *Ethnicity and Health* 5(3–4):191–204.

American Psychiatric Association. 1980. *Diagnostic and statistical manual of mental disorders*, 3rd ed. Washington, DC: American Psychiatric Association.

_____ 2000. *Diagnostic and statistical manual of mental disorders*, 4th ed. Washington, DC: American Psychiatric Association.

Arboleda-Florez, J. and T. J. Wade. 2001. Childhood and adult victimization as risk factor for major depression. *International Journal of Law and Psychiatry* 24:357–70.

Arrigo, B. A. and C. R. Williams. 2003. Victim vices, victim voices, and impact statements: On the place of emotion and the role of restorative justice in capital sentencing. *Crime & Delinquency* 49(4):603–26.

Averill, P. M. and J. G. Beck. 2000. Posttraumatic stress disorder in older adults: A conceptual review. *Journal of Anxiety Disorders* 14(2):133–56.

Bloom, S. 1997. *Creating sanctuary: Toward the evolution of sane societies*. New York: Routledge.

Brewin, C. R., B. Andrews, and J. D. Valentine. 2000. Meta-analysis of risk factors for posttraumatic stress disorder in trauma-exposed adults. *Journal of Consulting and Clinical Psychology* 68(5):748–66.

Briere, J. and C. L. Scott. 2006. *Principles of trauma therapy: A guide to symptoms, evaluation, and treatment*. Thousand Oaks, CA: Sage.

Burgess, A. W. 1995. Rape trauma syndrome. In *Rape and society: Readings on the problem of sexual assault*, ed. P. Searles and R. J. Berger, 239–45. Boulder, CO: Westview.

Calhoun, L. G. and R. G. Tedeschi. 2008. The paradox of struggling with trauma: Guidelines for practice and directions for research. In *Trauma, recovery, and growth: Positive psychological perspectives on posttraumatic stress*, ed. S. Joseph and P. A. Linley, 325–38. Hoboken, NJ: John Wiley.

Cameron, A. 2006. Stopping the violence: Canadian feminist debates on restorative justice and intimate violence. *Theoretical Criminology* 10(1):49–66.

Caspi, A., J. McClay, T. E. Moffitt, et al. 2002. Role of genotype in the cycle of violence in maltreated children. *Science* 297:851–54.

Chapman, A. R. and P. Ball. 2001. The truth of truth commissions: Comparative lessons from Haiti, South Africa, and Guatemala. *Human Rights Quarterly* 23:1–43.

Comack, E. 1996. *Women in trouble: Connecting women's law violations to their histories of abuse*. Halifax, NS: Fernwood.

Curtis-Fawley, S. and K. Daly. 2005. Gendered violence and restorative justice: The views of victim advocates. *Violence Against Women* 11:603–38.

Daiski, I. 2007. Perspectives of homeless people on their health and health needs priorities. *Journal of Advanced Nursing* 58(3):273–81.

Davis, R. C. 2007. The key contributions of family, friends, and neighbors. In *Victims of crime*, ed. R. C. Davis, A. J. Lurigio, and S. Herman, 267–76. Thousand Oaks, CA: Sage.

De la Rey, C. and I. Owens. 1998. Perceptions of psychosocial healing and the truth and reconciliation commission in South Africa. *Peace and Conflict: Journal of Peace Psychology* 4(3):257–70.

Dominelli, L. 1989. Betrayal of trust: A feminist analysis of power relationships in incest abuse and its relevance for social work practice. *British Journal of Social Work* 19(1):291–307.

Eilenberg, J., M. T. Fullilove, R. G. Goldman, and L. Mellman. 1996. Quality and use of trauma histories obtained from psychiatric outpatients through mandated inquiry. *Psychiatric Services* 47:165–69.

Erez, E. and J. Roberts. 2007. Victim participation in the criminal justice system. In *Victims of crime*, ed. R. C. Davis, A. J. Lurigio, and S. Herman, 277–98. Thousand Oaks, CA: Sage.

Erez, E. and L. Roeger. 1995. The effect of victim impact statements on sentencing patterns and outcomes: The Australian experience. *Journal of Criminal Justice* 23(4):363–75.

Erez, E. and L. Rogers. 1999. Victim impact statements and sentencing outcomes and processes: The perspectives of legal professionals. *The British Journal of Criminology* 39(2):216–39.

Feinauer, L. L. 1989. Comparison of long-term effects of child abuse by type of abuse and by relationship of the offender to the victim. *The American Journal of Family Therapy* 17(1):48–56.

Figley, C. R. 1988. Toward a field of traumatic stress. *Journal of Traumatic Stress* 1(1):3–16.

_____ 1995. *Compassion fatigue: Coping with secondary traumatic stress in those who treat the traumatized.* London: Routledge.

Finkelhor, D. 2007. Developmental victimology: The comprehensive study of childhood victimizations. In *Victims of crime*, ed. R. C. Davis, A. J. Lurigio, and S. Herman, 9–34. Thousand Oaks, CA: Sage.

Follette, V. M., M. A. Polusny, A. E. Bechtle, and A. E. Naugle. 1996. Cumulative trauma: The impact of child sexual abuse, adult sexual assault, and spouse abuse. *Journal of Traumatic Stress* 9(1):25–35.

Gearon, J. S., S. I. Kaltman, C. Brown, and A. S. Bellack. 2003. Traumatic life events and PTSD among women with substance use disorders and schizophrenia. *Psychiatric Services* 54:523–28.

Goldberg, S. 2005. *Judging for the 21st century: A problem-solving approach.* Ottawa: National Judicial Institute.

Goodman, L. A., M. A. Dutton, and M. Harris. 1995. Episodically homeless women with serious mental illness: Prevalence of physical and sexual assault. *American Journal of Orthopsychiatry* 65(4):468–78.

Goodman, L. A., K. M. Thompson, K. Weinfurt, et al. 1999. Reliability of reports of violent victimization and posttraumatic stress disorder among men and women with serious mental illness. *Journal of Traumatic Stress* 12(4):1573–98.

Green, D. L. and N. Diaz. 2008. Gender differences in coping with victimization. *Brief Treatment and Crisis Intervention* 8(2):195–203.

Greve, W. 1998. Fear of crime among the elderly: Foresight, not fright. *International Review of Victimology* 5(3/4):277–309.

Griffiths, C. and S. N. Verdun-Jones. 1994. *Canadian criminal justice.* Toronto: Harcourt Brace.

Hayner, P. B. 1994. Fifteen truth commissions—1974 to 1994: A comparative study. *Human Rights Quarterly* 16(4):597–655.

Heide, K. M. and E. P. Solomon. 2006. Biology, childhood trauma, and murder: Rethinking justice. *International Journal of Law and Psychiatry* 29:220–33.

Heisler, C. J. 2007. Elder abuse. In *Victims of crime*, ed. R. C. Davis, A. J. Lurigio, and S. Herman, 161–88. Thousand Oaks, CA: Sage.

Herman, J. L. 1992. *Trauma and recovery: The aftermath of violence—from domestic abuse to political terror*. New York: Basic Books.

———— 1997. *Trauma and recovery: The aftermath of violence—from domestic abuse to political terror*. New York: Basic Books.

———— 2003. The mental health of crime victims: Impact of legal intervention. *Journal of Traumatic Stress* 16(2):159–66.

———— 2005. Justice from the victim's perspective. *Violence against Women* 11:571–602.

Hiday, V. A. 1997. Understanding the connection between mental illness and violence. *International Journal of Law and Psychiatry* 20(4):399–417.

———— 2006. Putting community risk in perspective: A look at correlations causes and controls. *International Journal of Law and Psychiatry* 29(4):316–31.

Hiday, V. A., J. W. Swanson, M. S. Swartz, R. Borum, and H. R Wagner. 2001. Victimization: A link between mental illness and violence? *International Journal of Law and Psychiatry* 24(6):559–72.

Hiday, V. A., M. S. Swartz, J. W. Swanson, R. Borum, and H. R. Wagner. 1999. Criminal victimization of persons with severe mental illness. *Psychiatric Services* 50(1):62–68.

Holmes, W. C., E. B. Foa, and M. D. Sammel. 2005. Men's pathways to risky sexual behavior: Role of co-occurring childhood sexual abuse, posttraumatic stress disorder, and depression histories. *Journal of Urban Health* 82(1 Suppl 1):i89–i99.

Howley, S. and C. Dorris. 2007. Legal rights for crime victims in the criminal justice system. In *Victims of crime*, ed. R. C. Davis, A. J. Lurigio, and S. Herman, 299–314. Thousand Oaks, CA: Sage.

Jacobs, S. 1999. *Traumatic grief: Diagnosis, treatment, and prevention*. Philadelphia: Taylor & Francis.

Joseph, S. and P. A. Linley. 2008. Positive psychological perspectives on posttraumatic stress: An integrative psychosocial framework. In *Trauma, recovery, and growth: Positive psychological perspectives on posttraumatic stress*, ed. S. Joseph and P. A. Linley, 3–20. Hoboken, NJ: John Wiley.

Kidd-Hewitt, D. 2002. Crime and the media: A criminological perspective. In *Criminology: A reader*, ed. Y. Jewkes and G. Letherby, 116–29. Thousand Oaks, CA: Sage.

Kilpatrick, D. G. and R. Acierno. 2003. Mental health needs of crime victims: Epidemiology and outcomes. *Journal of Traumatic Stress* 16(2):119–32.

La Prairie, C. 1990. Role of sentencing in the over-representation of aboriginal people in correctional institutions. *Canadian Journal of Criminology* 32(3):429–40.

Lam, J. A. and R. A. Rosenheck. 1998. The effect of victimization on clinical outcomes of homeless persons with serious mental illness. *Psychiatric Services* 49:678–83.

Lansford, J. E., K. A. Dodge, G. S. Pettit, J. E. Batew, J. Crozier, and J. Kaplow. 2002. A 12-year prospective study of the long-term effects of early child physical maltreatment on psychological, behavioral, and academic problems in adolescence. *Archives of Pediatrics & Adolescent Medicine* 156(8):824–30.

Lasiuk, G. C. and K. M. Hegadoren. 2006. Posttraumatic stress disorder Part I: Historical development of the concept. *Perspectives in Psychiatric Care* 42(1):13–20.

———— 2006. Posttraumatic stress disorder Part II: Development of the construct within the North American psychiatric taxonomy. *Perspectives in Psychiatric Care* 42(2):72–81.

Latimer, J., C. Dowden, and D. Muise. 2005. The effectiveness of restorative justice practices: A meta-analysis. *The Prison Journal* 85:127–44.

Macmillan, R. 2001. Violence and the life course: The consequences of victimization for personal and social development. *Annual Review of Sociology* 27:1–22.

Marley, J. A. and S. Buila. 2001. Crimes against people with mental illness: Types, perpetrators, and influencing factors. *Social Work* 46(2):115–24.

Marsella, A. J. and M. A. Christopher. 2004. Ethnocultural considerations in disasters: An overview of research, issues, and directions. *Psychiatric Clinics of North America* 27:521–39.

McCann, I. L. and L. A. Pearlman. 1990. Vicarious traumatization: A framework for understanding the psychological effects of working with victims. *Journal of Traumatic Stress* 3(1):131–49.

McDevitt, J., A. Farrell, D. Rousseau, and R. Wolff. 2007. Hate crimes: Characteristics of incidents, victims, and offenders. In *Victims of crime*, ed. R. C. Davis, A. J. Lurigio, and S. Herman, 91–108. Thousand Oaks, CA: Sage.

Mezey, G. 2007. Victims and forensic psychiatry: Marginal or mainstream. *Criminal Behaviour and Mental Health* 17:131–36.

Mueser, K. T., L. A. Goodman, S. L. Trumbetta, et al. 1998. Trauma and post traumatic stress disorder in severe mental illness. *Journal of Consulting and Clinical Psychology* 66(3):493–99.

Muscat, B. T. and J. A. Walsh. 2007. *Reaching underserved victim populations: Special challenges relating to homeless victims, rural populations, ethnic/racial/sexual minorities, and victims with disabilities.* Thousand Oaks, CA: Sage.

New, M. and L. Berliner. 2000. Mental health service utilization by victims of crime. *Journal of Traumatic Stress* 13(4):693–707.

O'Sullivan, C. S. and D. Fry. 2007. Sexual assault victimization across the life span: Rates, consequences, and interventions for different populations. In *Victims of crime*, ed. R. C. Davis, A. J. Lurigio, and S. Herman, 35–54. Thousand Oaks, CA: Sage.

Osofsky, J. D. 1995. Children who witness domestic violence: The invisible victims. *Social Policy Report: Society for Research in Child Development* 9(3):1–16.

Padgett, D. K. and E. L. Struening. 1992. Victimization and traumatic injuries among the homeless: Associations with alcohol, drug, and mental problems. *American Journal of Orthopsychiatry* 62(4):525–34.

Paolucci, E. O., M. L. Genuis, and C. Violato. 2001. A meta-analysis of the published research on the effects of child sexual abuse. *Journal of Psychology* 135(1):17–36.

Petrila, J. 2003. An introduction to special jurisdiction courts. *International Journal of Law and Psychiatry* 26:3–12.

Pfefferbaum, B., J. A. Call, S. J. Lensgraf, et al. 2001. Traumatic grief in a convenience sample of victims seeking support services after a terrorist incident. *Annals of Clinical Psychiatry* 13(1):19–24.

Raphael, B., P. Swan, and N. Martinek. 1998. Intergenerational aspects of trauma for Australian aboriginal people. In *International handbook of multigenerational legacies of trauma*, ed. Y. Danieli, 327–40. New York: Plenum.

Roach, K. 1999. *Due process and victims' rights: The new law and politics of criminal justice.* Toronto: University of Toronto Press.

Roberts, J. V. and R. Melchers. 2003. The incarceration of Aboriginal offenders: Trends from 1978 to 2001. *Canadian Journal of Criminology and Criminal Justice* 45(2):211–42.

Roxburgh, A., L. Degenhardt, and J. Copeland. 2006. Posttraumatic stress disorder among female street-based sex workers in the greater Sydney area, Australia. *BMC Psychiatry* 6(1):24.

Schmalleger, F. and R. Volk. 2008. *Canadian criminology today: Theories and applications*, 3rd ed. Toronto: Pearson Education Canada.

Sells, D. J., M. Rowe, D. Fisk, and L. Davidson. 2003. Violent victimization of persons with co-occurring psychiatric and substance use disorders. *Psychiatric Services* 54(9):1253–57.

Senn, T. E., M. P. Carey, and P. A. Vanable. 2008. Childhood and adolescent sexual abuse and subsequent sexual risk behavior: Evidence from controlled studies, methodological critique, and suggestions for research. *Clinical Psychology Review* 28(5):711–35.

Sigal, J. J. and M. Weinfeld. 1989. *Trauma and rebirth: Intergenerational effects of the holocaust*. New York: Praeger.

Silver, E. 2002. Mental disorder and violent victimization: The mediating role of involvement in conflicted social relationships. *Criminology* 40:191–212.

_____ 2006. Understanding the relationship between mental disorder and violence: The need for a criminological perspective. *Law and Human Behavior* 30(6):685–706.

Silver, E., L. Arseneault, J. Langley, A. Caspi, and T. E. Moffitt. 2005. Mental disorder and violent victimization in a total birth cohort. *American Journal of Public Health* 95(11):2015–21.

Simons, R. L, L. B. Whitbeck, and A. Bales. 1989. Life on the streets: Victimization and psychological distress among the adult homeless. *Journal of Interpersonal Violence* 4(4):482–501.

Sirotich, F. 2008. Correlates of crime and violence among persons with mental disorder: An evidence-based review. *Brief Treatment and Crisis Intervention* 8(2):171–94.

Spitzer, C., C. Chevalier, M. Gillner, H. J. Freyberger, and S. Barnow. 2006. Complex posttraumatic stress disorder and child maltreatment in forensic inpatients. *Journal of Forensic Psychiatry & Psychology* 17(2):204–16.

Sullivan, G., A. Burnam, P. Koegel, and J. Hollenberg. 2000. Quality of life of homeless persons with mental illness: Results from the course-of-homelessness study. *Psychiatric Services* 51(9):1135–41.

Tedeschi, R. G. and L. G. Calhoun. 2004. Posttraumatic growth: Conceptual foundations and empirical evidence. *Psychological Inquiry* 15(1):1–18.

Verdun-Jones, S. N. and A. A. Tijerino. 2002. *Victim participation in the plea negotiation process in Canada: A review of the literature and four models for law reform*. Ottawa, ON: Policy Centre for Victim Issues, Department of Justice Canada.

_____ 2004. Four models of victim involvement during plea negotiations: Bridging the gap between legal reforms and current legal practice. *Canadian Journal of Criminology and Criminal Justice* 46(4):471–500.

_____ 2005. *Victim participation in disposition hearings involving accused persons who have been found not criminally responsible on account of mental disorder*. Report submitted to Research and Statistics Division, Department of Justice Canada.

Walker, L. E. 1979. *The battered woman*. New York: Harper and Row.

Walker, L. E. A. 2000. *The battered woman syndrome*, 2nd ed. New York: Springer.

Walsh, E., P. Moran, C. Scott, et al. 2003. Prevalence of violent victimisation in severe mental illness. *British Journal of Psychiatry* 183:233–38.

Weaver, T. L. and G. A. Clum. 1995. Psychological distress associated with interpersonal violence: A meta-analysis. *Clinical Psychology Review* 15(2):115–40.

Wemmers, J. 2008. Victim participation and therapeutic jurisprudence. *Victims & Offenders* 3(2/3):165–91.

Wexler, D. B. 1990. *Therapeutic jurisprudence: The law as a therapeutic agent*. Durham, NC: Carolina Academic.

Culture and Wife Abuse
An Overview of Theory, Research, and Practice

24

CARLA MACHADO, ANA RITA DIAS,
AND CLÁUDIA COELHO

Contents

24.1 Introduction

It is almost common sense to say that wife abuse is a cultural problem and that cultural change is needed to eradicate this form of violence. However, this does not translate into the way scientific research in the area has been conducted. In fact, wife abuse research has for many years been dominated by prevalence and impact studies in which cultural dimensions are, at best, superficially debated. At the theoretical level, although cultural factors are always mentioned when debating risk factors for violence, the focus has been on the family and individual factors that facilitate intimate violence.

The past few decades mark, however, a significant change in this regard. Prevalence and impact studies have extended to different regions of the globe and to various ethnic groups. Phenomena such as globalization and migrations have reinforced the difficulties of defining and identifying violence, and it is no longer possible to ignore the hyper-representation of minority and poor groups among those families submitted to some form of judicial intervention [Abney, 2002]. On the theoretical level, this has stimulated an awareness of the intersectionality [Crenshaw, 1994] of gender, class, and race in the experience of wife abuse and the concomitant need to rethink former explanations for this phenomenon. On the practical side, there is growing concern over the cultural competence of professionals and the unfair treatment of minorities by help professionals, police officers, and the courts.

This chapter will try to provide an overview of the current state of knowledge generated by this "new" concern over the cultural dimension of wife abuse, finishing with a discussion of the concept of culture, its potentialities, and risks.

24.2 Theoretical Perspectives on Culture and Wife Abuse

24.2.1 Attitudinal and (Sub)Cultural Theories

The relationship between violent behaviors and attitudes has received significant attention from criminological research, especially in the past few decades. According to this thesis, culturally transmitted attitudes and values are responsible for violence, and sociodemographic disparities in violence levels are the result of differences in attitudes, values, and norms between social groups. According to Markowitz [2001:207], several "studies have found that attitudes explain significant portions of age, gender, and SES (socioeconomic status) differences in violence against non-family targets."

A recent cross-cultural analysis [Archer, 2006] has, in fact, shown that sexist attitudes and approval of violence against women were related to variations in women victimization rates. A number of other studies reinforce the idea that violence legitimization attitudes are important predictors of intimate violence [e.g., O'Keefe, 1997] and found out that perpetrators of wife abuse tend to endorse more violence-prone attitudes [e.g., Sugarman and Frankel, 1996; Machado et al., 2007].

It must, however, be emphasized that these results are not consensual, with some authors finding evidence that attitudes, although important, do not explain demographic differences in wife abuse [e.g., Markowitz, 2001]. Others stress that low levels of violence legitimization do not automatically translate into the erosion of violent behaviors [e.g., Michalski, 2004]. A possible explanation for this paradox is the finding that, although people may disapprove of violence on a general level, they find it acceptable in some forms and situations [cf. Carlson and Worden, 2005]. This may signal the coexistence of "conflicting values and attitudes" [Parke and Lewis, 1981:173] toward intimate violence.

Cultural explanations for violence, such as those we have been examining, are frequently described as derived from the "subculture of violence" theory developed by Wolfgang and Ferracuti [1967]. This theory considers that violence is grounded on group cultural norms that differ from commonly shared beliefs and according to which violence is justifiable and even honorable. According to this theory, among certain social groups, especially lower-class males, violence is perceived as a common and legitimate means to address interpersonal conflicts and, moreover, as a source of power and status among peers [ibid.]. The transmission of these beliefs and values may be explained through social learning theory, according to which the group provides the context for the violence learning process, offering both the role models and the cultural norms that justify violence.

Applied to our theme, this would mean that wife abuse results from a violent male subculture that considers violence against women as acceptable or even as a proof of masculinity and dominance [Levinson, 1989]. This would explain the uneven distribution of violence among social classes, namely, the higher prevalence rates found in the more deprived families [cf. Michalski, 2004].

Since its conception, the subculture of violence theory has known many variations, one of them being its extension from the subcultural to the cultural level. According to some authors, differences in the frequency or severity of violence between countries or societies can be explained by their cultural norms regarding violence and its acceptability [cf. Levinson, 1989]. This means that "some societies have a basic set of values and beliefs that emphasize aggression and violence" [ibid.:40], and that in these societies violence constitutes a common pattern of behavior, observable in several spheres of life (e.g., family, sports, education). Authors such as Barash and Webel [2002] notice, for example, the widespread acceptance of violence in the United States, giving examples from television, films, and folklore.

The (sub)culture of violence theory has been tested by several researchers [e.g., Levinson, 1989; Counts, Brown, and Campbell, 1999], and some associations were found between wife beating and rates of other violent offenses or broader patterns of violent conflict management. However, there are studies that find no correlation between domestic violence and other violent offenses [e.g., Archer, 2006], and, even among those with some positive results, the findings are not consistent about the specific forms of interpersonal violence correlated with domestic abuse [cf. Levinson, 1989]. According to Counts et al. [1999], the very notion of a subculture of violence receives only marginal support from cross-cultural research.

On a theoretical level, the (sub)culture of violence theory has received many critiques, namely, the fact that it does not explain the origin of subcultural norms or the way they change over time [Gelles and Straus, 1979]. It also has been accused of neglecting the specific structural circumstances that make family violence different from common criminal violence, namely, the emotional bind between offenders and victims, the intimacy context, and the fact that female victims of violence frequently also engage in violent behaviors [Grandin and Lupri, 1997]. Finally, because of its particular application to the explanation of violence among minority groups, namely, African Americans, it has been accused of presenting a stereotypical and distorted view of that culture and its values [cf. Barnes, 1999].

(Sub)culture of violence theory has, however, in our opinion, made an interesting point when it stressed that wife abuse can be the product of cultural norms, rather than just a norm violation that derives from individual maladjustment. It also shed some light into the gendered nature of intimate aggression, relating it to conceptions of masculinity and peer status, topics that were later readdressed by feminist researchers.

24.2.2 Systemic and Ecological Approaches

The ecological approach is one of the most well-known and accepted theories in the field of family violence. Although it does not emphasize culture over other levels of influence, this theory conceives violence as the product of a complex web of influences that go from the microindividual to the macrocultural level. It is based on the early work on development conducted by Bronfenbrenner [1979], later applied to the etiology of child abuse [Belsky, 1993; Garbarino, 1993] and, to a lesser extent, to wife abuse [Dutton, 1995; Malley-Morrison, 2004; Stith et al., 2004; Brownridge, 2006].

According to Belsky [1993], family violence explanations should take into account the "developmental-psychological context" of individuals (onto-genetic level), the "immediate interactional context" between family members (microsystem), the formal and informal contexts that influence family life (exosystem), and the cultural context (macrosystem).

Although the relationship between these levels of influence has been conceptualized in different ways, Malley-Morrison's [2004] cognitive-ecological approach seems to us particularly relevant, given the emphasis it places on the cultural level. According to this framework, individuals act based on their individual implicit theories about the acceptability of violence, these implicit theories being developed in the broader cultural context. In this model, implicit theories are a part of the cultural heritage of the subject and translate into his or her way of thinking and judging specific situations and the way to respond to them. Reliance on these theories is especially likely to occur when subjects are confronted with ambiguous and stressful situations, such as interpersonal conflict. These theories may include assumptions about family and gender roles, the justifiability of aggression and its effects, as well as representations of the self and relationships (e.g., collectivist vs. individualist views of the self).

The ecological approach has some unique advantages over other theoretical models, namely, the ability to consider at the same time micro- and macrolevel variables, and taking into account the way socioeconomic and cultural structures influence family life [Garbarino, 1993]. The ecological approach also has the advantage of decentering the attention away from pathological characteristics and interactions to focus it on the way family violence is related to "normal" family interactions and wider cultural definitions of normative parental and couple roles.

However, in Gelles' [1997] opinion, the ecological approach has been lacking in empirical research; therefore, its premises have not been sufficiently tested. The complexity of the theory may be an important reason for these difficulties.

The complexity of relationships among several systems is also a central construct of the general systems theory. Straus [1973, cited in Michalski, 2004] was one of the first authors who applied the general systems theory to domestic violence, conceiving it as part of a pattern that involves the whole family and not only the dyadic relationship.

In the systemic approach, violence is seen as the result of family dysfunction, such as poor communication, indirect expression of feelings, inflexible rules, secrecy, problems in setting limits, and isolation from the outside world [cf. Margolin, Sibner, and Gleberman, 1988; Anderson and Schlossberg, 1999]. This dysfunction is translated into repetitive sequences of interaction, in which all family members participate, perpetuating the problem [McConaghy and Cottone, 1999].

According to this perspective, violence is, therefore, not the product of a lineal process of causality [cf. Dell, 1989] but rather an interactive pattern maintained by the whole relational system, victims and perpetrators participating in a reciprocal manner in the conflict [Greenspun, 2000].

It is precisely this notion of circular causality [Bateson, 1972, cited in Dell, 1989] that constitutes the main target of critiques to the systemic perspective. In fact, as Goldner [1999:2] points out, "to argue that partners mutually participate in an interactional process does not mean they are mutually responsible for it." This is a critique commonly addressed to general systems theory by feminist authors [e.g., Kurz, 1998], also considering that its focus on the family as a unit of analysis, its gender-blind language, and its conceptualization of violence as a symptom of family dysfunction, more than as a problem in itself, have lead to the minimization or neglect of wife abuse [Saraga, 1996].

On the empirical side, cross-cultural research has found mixed results for one of the main assumptions of the systemic perspective, the idea that all forms of family violence are interconnected. For example, Counts et al. [1999] found a pattern of only partial association between child and wife abuse, whereas Levinson's [1989] data suggest that wife beating is a distinct phenomenon from child abuse, requiring different theoretical explanations.

Finally, the general systems theory can also be criticized by focusing on the family level, noticing but rarely exploring the contributions of the wider cultural system to the violent interactions that occur within it. Gender asymmetries in the distribution of power, both in the family as in the macrosocial and cultural system, have also been paid little attention by family systems theory [Saraga, 1996; Goldner, 1999].

24.2.3 Feminism and Multiculturalism

Feminist perspectives[*] address precisely this gendered nature of wife abuse. According to these, violence is rooted in the unequal distribution of power between genders in the society, being used by men as a means to exert dominance and control over women, keeping them in subordinate positions [Foreman and Dallos, 1993; Marin and Russo, 1999; Yllo, 2005]. This means that violence can be used both as an expression of the male power in the relationship or when the man feels his power threatened, acting to re-establish dominance over his partner [Foreman and Dallos, 1993; Hearn, 1996].

According to this perspective, there is a continuum between normal family structure and interactions and wife abuse [Hearn, 1996]. This means that the patriarchal culture and social organization lead to an unequal distribution of power, resources, and roles within the "normative" family, in which the subordination of women is still perceived as the rule. Wife abuse corresponds to an extreme manifestation of this rule, being exerted especially when the man feels his power and privileges are endangered and

---

[*] Because there is not a unified feminist theory, we prefer the term *feminist perspectives*.

when other strategies to obtain subordination from the woman have failed. As Yllo [1983:277] points out, "The brutalization of an individual wife by an individual husband is not an individual or 'family' problem. It is simply one manifestation of male dominance which has existed historically and cross-culturally."

Although this hypothesis is probably too complex to be tested, a number of cross-cultural studies have reinforced some aspects of the feminist thesis. As an example, we can refer to Levinson's [1989] study of 90 preliterate and peasant societies around the world, in which he concluded that "the key inequality predictors of wife beating are male economic power in the family, male decision-making power in the family, and restrictions on the freedom of women to divorce their husbands" [ibid.:84]. Another case is the cross-cultural comparison of 52 developed countries conducted by Archer [2006], which has found that women's victimization was inversely correlated with gender equality.

As the former paragraphs make obvious, culture plays a fundamental role in feminist explanations for wife abuse. Among the cultural conditions that facilitate abuse are the belief that men are "naturally" entitled to obedience from their wives, the objectification of women, the persuasion of women to accept domination, and the cultural acceptance of wife battering, for which no meaningful sanction is provided [Crichton-Hill, 2001].

Therefore, violence has its core in the normative process of male socialization and in culturally transmitted patriarchal attitudes and beliefs about gender roles and relationships [Dobash and Dobash, 1980]. This also includes ideas about masculinity and femininity, namely, that it is the woman's role to care for the relationship and that her personal and social value depends on her capacity to build and maintain a marital relationship [Foreman and Dallos, 1993]. On the male side, cultural prescriptions for "hegemonic masculinity" [Connell, 1987] refer to physical, economical and/or intellectual dominance, emotional restraint, invulnerability, and self-sufficiency. These types of gender beliefs have become institutionalized and incorporated into the legal system and social structures [Marin and Russo, 1999] and are continually transmitted and reproduced (although not always without critique) in the family, by the media, and in the daily actions of individuals. Masculinity theorists have asserted that when men fail to live up to these prescriptions they can resort to violence to "do gender," drawing their sense of masculinity and control from the physical subordination of others [Jefferson, 1997].

Therefore, we can consider that feminist perspectives are, among those we examined, those that attribute a bigger role to cultural factors in the explanation of wife abuse. They can, however, be criticized for the fact of limiting their cultural approach to gender issues, neglecting other important cultural dimensions, such as class or race. Multiculturalist perspectives address precisely this critique to feminist researchers and concentrate on the intersection of gender, class, and race in the explanation and experience of wife abuse.

Multicultural feminists have, during the past decade, made an important contribution to wife abuse theory, noticing that "white feminism" has conceived power relations as structured only around gender, and assuming "a type of tunnel vision in which white experience is assumed to describe human experience" [Yllo, 2005:24]. The concept of "intersectionality," developed by Crenshaw [1994], addresses precisely the multiple structures of subordination that can co-occur in women's lives and that shape their experience of violence. As Sokoloff and Dupont [2006:2] explain, "the battered women's oppression is often multiplied by their location at the intersections at particular race, ethnic, class, gender, and sexual orientation systems of oppression and discrimination." This means, for example, that the very experience of intimate abuse and the responses to it are necessarily different for a white middle-class professional woman with no kids or for a black unemployed immigrant who is a mother of five. Economic constraints, religious values, group norms, race solidarity bonds, language barriers, fear of deportation, and mistrust of the police can play important roles in shaping individual responses to violence in a way that goes beyond gender [Kasturirangan, Krishnan, and Riger, 2004].

This means, for example, that a black woman can feel a stronger identification with the daily experience of her male abuser than with the white woman she works for as a domestic servant. This also relates to the fact that most lower-class women of color feel reluctant over reporting their victimization to the police or to the social services because of their experiences of intrusion, vigilance, and violence at the hands of these same institutions. They have frequently testified, when not directly experienced, having their children removed from home, their husbands and sons arrested, and their houses searched. Therefore, when they are battered, their responses are shaped by these previous experiences of humiliation and hostile treatment, an experience that is shared with their male partners. This certainly plays a part in explaining why it is that women from minority groups tend to be reluctant in calling the police even when they are badly hurt [Saraga, 1996]. The need to belong to a family or a community, the desire to present a positive image of that community to the eyes of the dominant society, and the fear of risking their children opportunities are other factors that may contribute to women immigrants' reluctance to report the abuse or divorce their husbands [Dasgupta, 1998].

This has important implications both in the theoretical and political arena. The idea of a unified gender experience must be deconstructed, and the multiplicity of women's experiences has to be recognized [Yllo, 2005], at the same time perceiving that there are women-on-women structures of domination (based on race, class, age, or sexual orientation). In fact, one of the critiques that can be addressed to "mainstream" feminism is the fact of assuming a unified gender identity for women, supposing the commonality of women's experiences. This is further compounded, sometimes, by the implicit assumption that women's identity is fundamentally based on their experiences of victimization [Pratt and Sokoloff, 2006]. This corresponds to a form of gender essentialism and hides the different experiences and histories of battered women, as well as the complex nature of power relations.

Multicultural theorists have claimed the need of a more complex understanding of the meaning of culture and its relation to wife abuse. Adopting a very critical stance over the hypothesis that women's victimization among ethnic minority groups is the result of their culture, they challenge the idea that other cultures are much more accepting of wife abuse than the occidental one and criticize the implicit assumption contained in this thesis, according to which wife abuse is mainly located in the lower classes and ethnic minorities [Dasgupta, 1998; Sokoloff and Dupont, 2006]. They also defy common representations of women from minority groups, such as "Asian women are passive," "Latina women are dependent," or "Black women are aggressive," pointing out that these stereotypes have prevented effective interventions to protect these women [Saraga, 1996; Sokoloff and Dupont, 2006]. Finally, multicultural feminists have appealed to a more complex understanding of the very notion of culture, its multiplicity and contradictions, as well as have deconstructed the linear and biased way in which some cultures are described. "What do we mean by culture?" and "Why beliefs and customs that oppress women gain recognition as 'culture'?" [Dasgupta, 1998:217], whereas other, more empowering, cultural traits remain in obscurity, are some of the important questions raised by multicultural feminists, questions we will come back to at the end of this chapter. Before that, we will take a look at the empirical research on the topic of culture and wife abuse.

24.3 A Typology of the Research on Culture and Wife Abuse

24.3.1 Anthropological and Ethnographic Studies

The anthropological tradition of research offers in-depth, dense, descriptions of the lives and traditions of communities. Some of these texts make only passing references to family violence, whereas others make rich and complex description of family life and patterns of intimate violence. A few of these studies have taken a comparative approach, providing information from different societies across the globe, trying to develop tests of the theories previously described. Whereas most authors discuss their comparative findings and their theoretical implications remaining within the qualitative tradition of anthropology, others, such as Levinson [1989], resort to quantitative methods to advance cultural research. In his seminal work, Levinson produced the first worldwide study of family violence among small-scale societies, quantifying the qualitative data previously collected by several ethnographic reports.

These comparative studies have shown that wife abuse is a widespread phenomenon. Family violence seems to be absent only in small-scale societies (wife abuse was absent or very rare in only 15.5% of the 90 societies studied by Levinson). Wife abuse seems, in fact, to be more common than child maltreatment, some authors even saying that it is a nearly universal variable [Counts et al., 1999].

Although common, wife abuse differs greatly in frequency and severity among cultural contexts. Counts et al. [1999], for example, differentiate societies characterized by patterns of *wife beating* (occasional acts of minor to moderate violence) from others where *wife battering* (severe and recurrent aggression, in a context of coercive control) is the norm. Levinson [1989] also makes reference to societies that tolerate wife aggression only in adultery situations, whereas others accept violence whenever it is perceived as deserved by the wife, and others, although rare, that have a more indiscriminate acceptance of violence against women. Counts et al.'s [1999] findings corroborate this idea, showing that most cultures have some kind of norms to regulate violence, establishing parameters within which it is acceptable to hit one's wife but accepting external interference if the aggression is perceived as excessive, undeserved, or dangerous.

Anthropological studies have also shown an association between wife abuse and the social status and value ascribed to women. The categories of women who "deserve" to be hit also seem to be culturally defined, namely, unfaithful wives and women who transgress other social and sexual gender norms. This is corroborated by recent revisions of studies conducted in several communities and tribes in Africa [Rotimi, 2007] and India [Segal, 1999], which enumerate a number of punishments women may receive if they do not comply with their attributed obligations (e.g., neglecting the children, disobeying or talking back to the husband).

Data also suggest an association between risk of violence and men's control of economic resources and social isolation of the woman [Levinson, 1989]. On the reverse, immediate external intervention in wife abuse episodes, clear social sanctions (legal, moral, or religious) against violence, and support structures for women who intend to leave home seem to be associated with lesser levels of wife abuse [Levinson, 1989; Counts et al., 1999].

An interesting result of these studies is the ambivalent role that women-to-women relationships seem to play concerning violence. On the one hand, female solidarity networks seem to be protective against violence [Levinson, 1989], whereas on the other they can also stimulate and legitimize it. When a hierarchical gender structure couples with an age hierarchy and with cultural norms that deeply value women chastity and submission, older women can approve violence against younger relatives, either to preserve their social value (e.g., genital mutilation) or to reinforce their own power or family interests (e.g., the dowry tradition) [Counts et al., 1999; Mehrotra, 1999; Levesque, 2001].

24.3.2 Prevalence Studies

24.3.2.1 National or Local Prevalence Studies

A recent review [Machado and Dias, 2008] of the articles that describe wife abuse prevalence rates published between 1985 and 2005 in several databases* found nearly 70 articles. For the purpose of this chapter, we had another look at the texts published since then, and the number has grown to 120 papers.

North America is undoubtedly the region of the globe where wife abuse has been examined for a longer period, both through large-scale surveys and with more specific samples. Compared with North America, European studies on the theme began later, especially in eastern and southern European countries. Although several prevalence surveys have been published since the 1980s, no consistent effort has been developed to provide a global view of the European situation [Hagemann-White, 2001]. Asian research on this subject is even more recent [cf. Machado and Dias, 2008], as well as African studies, which began in the mid-1990s [Bowman, 2003]. This is easily comprehensible if we take into account the economic, humanitarian, and political problems of the African continent, a context in which wife abuse could not acquire the status of a major social problem [Rotimi, 2007]. Studies in Latin America also seem to have begun late, with most publications dating from the past 10 years. Finally, the research seems to be just beginning in the Arab countries, where this is considered a highly sensitive theme [Almosaed, 2004].

These prevalence studies have been, at best, national in scope. In fact, very few cross-cultural studies have been published, and cross-cultural data are mostly accessible through literature reviews that try to gather information from studies realized in different cultural settings. This is the case of the World Report on Violence and Health [World Health Organization, 2002], which assembles information from 38 countries and suggests lifelong prevalence rates that oscillate between 10% and 67%.

More specific analysis of the situation found similar data in Africa (10–62%) [cf. Rotimi, 2007], as well as in Asian studies (5.6–77%) [cf. Machado and Dias, 2008]. Flake and Forste's [2006] study of five Latin America countries found lifelong prevalence rates a bit inferior to these (16–39%), although

---

* PsycARTICLES; PsycINFO1887; Sociology: A SAGE Full-Text Collection; EBSCO-HOST: Research Databases; and IBSS—International Bibliography of the Social Science.

Machado and Dias' [2008] review of the literature suggests much higher rates of wife abuse in some locations of that continent. European rates of lifelong victimization also seem to be high, varying between 10% and 50% in the studies analyzed by Machado and Dias [2008]. Finally, Malley-Morrison and Hines [2004], in their review of the self-report studies conducted in the United States, describe prevalence numbers of lifelong victimization that range from 17.4% to 25.5%.

However, these are numbers we must look at with some caution because studies widely vary in their types of samples (many are convenience samples), scope (relatively few national studies) and sample size, the types of violence considered (many studies include only physical violence, whereas others integrate emotional violence and coercion), time intervals considered (lifelong, past 5 years, past year, not specified), and data collection methods (questionnaires, interviews).

In an attempt to overcome some of these methodological problems, Garcia-Moreno et al. [2006] conducted a recent study of partner violence in 15 locations in 10 countries, with a sample of 24,097 women. According to this study, the lifelong prevalence of partner abuse ranged from 15% to 71% (two locations presenting rates less than 25%, seven between 25% and 50%, and six between 50% and 75%), and past year prevalence rates varied from 4% to 54%.

Taken together, and despite the methodological problems, all these results reinforce the idea that family violence is a very common problem around the globe. In all but one of the contexts studied by Garcia-Moreno et al. [2006], women's risk of aggression from their partners was higher than that from any other person.

Considering the sociodemographic correlates of wife abuse, aggression seems to be higher among traditional rural settings and less frequent in industrialized contexts [Garcia-Moreno et al., 2006]. The authors interpret these findings in relation with the options women have when trying to leave abusive relationships. Other authors stress that higher rates of violence are associated with lesser gender equality [e.g., Machado and Dias, 2008], a finding that reinforces feminist explanations for wife abuse. Finally, the role of lack of resources and poverty has also been emphasized by several studies [e.g., Flake and Forste, 2006; Rotimi, 2007].

24.3.2.2 Prevalence Studies with Specific Ethnic Groups

Although most national or regional prevalence studies present their findings as a whole, some researchers have recently tried to uncover wife abuse rates in specific ethnic groups, namely, blacks, Asians, and Hispanics. Most of these studies have been conducted in the United States or in Canada.

Malley-Morrison and Hines' [2004] review of the ethnic minority research conducted in the United States shows, once again, that wife abuse rates vary widely from study to study. On the whole, the literature suggests higher rates of abuse among African-American and Hispanic communities, but these differences in many cases diminish or disappear if sociodemographic variables, such as low income or poverty, are controlled [cf. Malley-Morrison and Hines, 2007]. The situation in the Asian community is less well known, with some authors considering that "empirical studies of domestic violence among Asian American communities are relatively uncommon" [Lee, 2007:142]. However, some studies with this population also found high prevalence rates [e.g., Kim and Sung, 2000; Lee, 2007].

Globally, large-scale surveys tend to report prevalence rates inferior to those found in smaller-scale studies. Language barriers, fear of revealing the abuse, distrust of the authorities, and cultural prescriptions about secrecy probably contribute to these findings and suggest the need for more culturally sensitive research. The expansion of studies with ethnic minorities to other contexts rather than North America is also essential.

Despite these problems, the existing findings reinforce the association between the structural disadvantages ethnic minorities face and their vulnerability to abuse. Poverty and racism contribute to higher levels of stress and violence, whereas at the same time they increase social control and visibility of abuse among minorities. Finally, specific cultural attitudes about wife abuse embraced by different ethnic groups can influence violence rates.

24.3.3 Cultural Values and Attitudes Studies

Despite the variability we just observed on prevalence numbers, most studies consider that available rates are underestimated because of a set of cultural factors that justify, obscure, or deny the problem of wife abuse around the world. Our revision of the literature on these cultural values and attitudes found four main types of research:

1. General descriptions of the values and beliefs of certain societies, regions, or ethnic groups
2. Empirical studies conducted with specific social or ethnic groups, most of them using qualitative methodologies and small samples
3. Comparative studies among different cultures, nationalities, or ethnic groups
4. Studies on the media representations of gender relationships and wife abuse

The first type of texts have addressed such different contexts as India [Segal, 1999], Africa [Rotimi, 2007], Japan [Kozu, 1999], China [Tang and Lay, 2008], and Russia [Horne, 1999]. Despite the specificities of each setting, all authors emphasize cultural norms that promote the acceptance of violence, its cultural perception as something normal in a marriage, and the idea that this is a private problem that should not be discussed outside the family. All authors also stress the connection between wife abuse and the patriarchal organization of the family and socialization into traditional gender roles.

Empirical studies seem to confirm this description. In such different cultural contexts as Jordan [Haj-Yahia, 2002], Saudi Arabia [Almosaed, 2004], India [Go et al., 2003], Poland [Kwiatkowska, 1998], and Haiti [CHREPROF, 1996, cited in Gage, 2005], violence seems to be perceived as an acceptable means to discipline a woman who fails to behave in accordance with traditional gender norms. Cultural definitions of "appropriate" femininity and masculinity and the belief that women who transgress those gender norms deserve to be punished are also pervasive in many cultural contexts and promote tolerance of wife abuse [Tang, Wong, and Cheung, 2002]. Cultural conceptions of love and romance also tend to endorse ideas that lead to the minimization of wife abuse, such as the notion that violence and control are expressions of love, or that "true love" will change an abusive partner [Romkens and Mastenbroek, 1998; Tang et al., 2002].

Despite these similarities, some of the few cross-cultural studies published suggest that differences may be found regarding the cultural sanctioning of wife abuse in different social groups. Vandello and Cohen [2003], for example, compared Brazilian and U.S. students and confirmed the idea that cultures that place a strong emphasis on women's fidelity (according to the authors, Brazil corresponds to a honor culture) tend to perceive violence as a means to restore male reputation. Therefore, violence is, although not approved, more easily excused in these cultures. Nayak et al.'s [2003] study with students from different cultural contexts also showed evidence that those from societies with a strong collectivist accent and more restrictive gender roles tend to be more tolerant of wife abuse. In a similar manner, Markowitz [2001] found higher levels of support for violence against women in the nonwhite population, although nonwhites actually reported lower levels of violence against their spouses.

However, Carlson and Worden's [2005] study with six New York communities seems to contradict these findings. In this study, participants' attitudes and estimates of prevalence did not differ according to their ethnic group. In fact, not only did African Americans' attitudes (contrary to what is frequently believed) not diverge from those of other groups as "when other factors (such as socioeconomic status and education) were controlled, they offered lower estimates of the prevalence of domestic violence in their communities" [ibid.:1214].

The sparse number of these cross-cultural attitudinal studies and their contradictory findings make evident the need for more research in this area, as well as the call for comparative studies that go beyond the usual comparisons of ethnic minorities with the white majority in the United States. We could also question the fact that researchers tend to focus almost exclusively on the cultures of minorities, as if the occidental culture was not accountable for the problem of wife abuse in North America and Europe.

An interesting exception to this rule is the case of media studies, mainly focused on the mainstream occidental representations of wife abuse. According to several authors, this is an especially important topic of research because media representations of family violence can be understood as a barometer of cultural attitudes and discourses [Schofield, 2004], at the same time that they constitute a main resource that people use to make sense of social life [Gamson, 1992].

However, there are few media studies that focus directly on the issue of wife abuse. Analyzing the discourse about it in political and men's magazines, Berns [2001] considers that it "degenders" male responsibility for the violence, whereas it places the burden of putting an end to it on the woman ("gendering the blame"). Female magazines also convey the idea that it is the woman's responsibility to solve the problem, usually recommending the woman to seek therapeutic help or to leave the relationship [Berns, 1999]. They tend to emphasize the victim's personality, self-esteem, and previous victimization history, therefore reinforcing an individual approach and hiding the cultural and social roots of the problem.

Another study, conducted by Carll [2003], analyzed media coverage of wife abuse in the United States. According to the author, although this is a theme frequently reported by the media, they convey the notion that violence against women is less common than other forms of aggression. According to Meyers [1994], the media present incidents of aggression against women as isolated events, reinforcing the notion of individual pathology and denying social responsibility. Whereas male aggression tends to be reported as a routine minor crime, marital aggression by women is treated as an exceptional and abhorrent event [Carll, 2003].

The few authors who analyzed media coverage in other cultural contexts seem to confirm these ideas. In Greece, Antonopoulou [no date, cited in Carll, 2003] says that media stories about male violence emphasize the justifications for those actions, frequently placing the aggressor in the role of victim or characterizing him as someone whose psychological problems explain violence. On the contrary, violent women are described as possessive, irrational, unfaithful, or immoral. "Passional" crimes by men are still described in terms of honor, whereas those by women are characterized as cruel and calculated. A study of this theme in Portugal [Dias and Machado, forthcoming] found similar results: (1) an emphasis on psychological or situational explanations for male violence, (2) the description of women aggressors as evil and cold, and (3) the search for media "novelty" (e.g., an emphasis on aggression by women, distracting the attention away from the much more common male violence against wives).

On the other hand, the media can also contribute to social change and to the growing awareness of wife abuse as a social and cultural problem. Cultural changes during the past few decades have redefined what are the appropriate themes for media coverage and led the media to pay more attention to wife abuse. According to Sacco [1995], the O. J. Simpson trial was, in the United States, the turning point after which the media began to explore the prevalence and causes of this problem, the inadequacy of the judicial responses, and the need for legislative changes. Carll [2003] also considers that the media have brought several other forms of violence against women to the public attention, such as "honor killings," dating violence, and stalking.

Therefore, the role of culture in the perpetration of wife abuse has begun to be widely recognized, even by cultural agents themselves. However, culture does not only play a role in the social acceptance of wife abuse and its perpetration. The role of culture in the explanation of the way wife abuse is experienced and coped with by its victims has also begun to be the object of research.

24.3.4 Impact Studies

As Carlson [2005:123] says, "Culture can be expected to moderate the effects of traumatic exposure and may influence the process of healing from the effects of trauma, violence, and abuse." The literature on this theme suggests to us at least five main ways through which culture influences the impact of wife abuse on victims: Culture seems to affect the length of time women endure violence, its psychological consequences, specific ways of coping with violence, received social support, and help-seeking behavior.

Cultural values and attitudes described in the latest section make it easy to understand the fact that immigrant and minority women tend to endure abuse for longer periods, some of them only seeking help in life-threatening situations [Hassouneh-Phillips, 2001; Shirwadkar, 2004]. In fact, besides the common difficulties battered women face when trying to leave the abusive relationship, cultural values about the importance of family, privacy, and gender roles make it more difficult for women to recognize the abuse and to escape from it. According to Yoshioka et al. [2003], *familism* (the perceived value of family ties and their preservation) and *collectivism* (the perceived importance of the community versus the self) are cultural values shared by South Asian, African, and Hispanic communities. *Machismo* (associated with male sexual prowess and aggression), *marianismo* (female submission and self-sacrifice), and *respect* (deference to older family members, especially men) have also been described as dominant traits of the Latino culture that pressure women to bear the abuse [Edelson, Hokoda, and Ramos-Lira, 2007]. Shame has also been pointed out as an important reason for women to endure violence. Cultures that value family honor and social image above individual freedom, such as Asian ones, may cause women to stay longer in abusive relationships [Chiu, 2004; Lee, Pomeroy, and Bohman, 2007].

In fact, several studies suggest that battered women from minority cultures frequently experience their victimization as a source of shame and disgrace and attribute violence to their own flaws as wives. This degradation of the self-image was noticed both in Asian [Chiu, 2004; Shirwadkar, 2004] and in Latina women [Edelson et al., 2007]. In accordance with this, in Edelson et al.'s [2007] study, battered Latina women showed significantly higher post-traumatic symptoms and depression than their non-Latino counterparts.

Culture also seems to influence the coping strategies women resort to for dealing with abuse. For example, Hyman et al. [2006] report that African-American women use prayer more frequently as a coping strategy when compared with whites. The importance of using coping strategies prescribed by the culture was documented by Yoshihama [2002], according to whom focusing on the positive and trying to engage in calming activities seem to reduce the psychological distress of battered Japanese women. Therefore, cultural beliefs and practices may simultaneously promote violence and provide some sort of relief from it. Religion, community festivities, traditional food, and shared beliefs can provide consolation to battered women and help them cope with violence [Kasturirangan et al., 2004].

Family also plays a central role in the way battered women cope with abuse, especially for immigrant women who are estranged from their other sources of support and face numerous obstacles that prevent them from seeking formal help. However, disclosure to the family is not without problems. In fact, according to Chiu [2004], in the Chinese culture, sharing one's problems, even with family members, is perceived as a breach of the cultural rule of privacy and self-reliance. Therefore, "far from being a source of support, the family came to be seen as a potential threat to the subject's self-image" [ibid.:158]. What is more, family does not always provide the support battered women need. In a study with Samoan women, Cribb and Barnett [1999] found that families usually advise women to stay home and maintain their marriages. A similar pattern was found by Yoshioka et al. [2003] with South Asian women. However, it must be noted that in this study almost half of the Asian women were told to leave their abusive marriage and that most Hispanic and African-American women were recommended by their families to do so.

Therefore, the family is sometimes a source of support and other times a source of pressure for battered women. In fact, minority battered women who abandon the relationship frequently face family and community disapproval and become isolated. These reactions have been documented especially in Arab Muslim [Hassouneh-Phillips, 2001] and South Asian communities [Shirwadkar, 2004]. When the family and the community reactions are so adverse, leaving the relationship is not only a difficult decision but also one that implies redefining both personal identity and the personal relationship to cultural values and expectations [Horsburgh, 2006], and even renegotiating their religious faith [Hassouneh-Phillips, 2001].

In this context of isolation and interpersonal strain, the access to professional help would be fundamental to wife abuse victims. However, most studies suggest that immigrant and minority women tend to refrain from seeking external help when they are battered, in particular from formal agencies such as the police. Some factors stressed by multicultural activists, such as lack of knowledge, language difficulties, fear of deportation, dependency on the husband, mistrust of the police, and economic problems, have been said to make it difficult to access formal services for Asian [Shirwadkar, 2004; Lee et al., 2007], Latina [Edelson et al., 2007], and African [Yoshioka et al., 2003] women. Cultural factors also play a role in this lack of resorting to the police or other formal sources of help. In fact, some studies suggest that stronger adherence to traditional beliefs, such as the importance of preserving family, of protecting it from shame, and of being a good wife, influence women's reluctance to report the abuse and ask for external help [Yoshioka et al., 2003]. Several studies also found that the degree of acculturation into Western culture increases the tendency for Latina [Garcia, Hurwitz, and Kraus, 2005] and Asian [Bui, 2003, cited in Hyman et al., 2006] women to report the abuse.

However, the estrangement minority women suffer from formal sources of help is not only imputable to their own difficulties. The type of response offered by professionals to these victims has also recently begun to be questioned, as well as the ways to improve this relationship.

24.4 Cultural Competency and Professional Responses to Victims

24.4.1 Culture and the Legal System Response to Victims

Police officers are frequently accused of inflicting secondary victimization on victims of wife abuse through behavior that reflects cultural myths concerning marital violence and conventional cultural attitudes about the role of women.

Research has shown that this is pervasive to multiple cultural contexts. For example, a Portuguese study aimed at evaluating police officers' beliefs and attitudes concluded that, despite the fact that most police officers generally disagree with wife abuse, a considerable number of them still believed the problem was concentrated in deprived and/or alcoholic families, and defended family privacy, therefore restricting their own action when facing wife abuse incidents [Machado et al., 2005]. Similar results were found by

Tam and Tang [2005] in Hong Kong, when comparing police officers' and social workers' perceptions on wife abuse. Their study concluded that police officers had more conservative attitudes toward gender, marital, parental, and social roles, endorsed more wife abuse myths, and had more restrictive definitions of wife abuse than social workers.

Narayanan [2005] went a bit further, exploring the organizational culture of the police in Singapore and its relations with the lack of police responsiveness to victims of wife abuse. According to this author, the police subculture expresses discomfort with the effect that the criminalization of wife abuse may have on the institution of family, considers it difficult to distinguish between offenders and victims in domestic disputes, believes that police intervention will prove pointless if victims withdraw their charges, and categorizes victims into those "deserving" or "undeserving" of protection, based on the woman's adhesion to gender stereotypes.

Therefore, patriarchal beliefs, the predominantly masculine composition of the police forces, and the organizational subculture can be important causes of police failure in addressing wife abuse victims' needs. This is especially aggravated, as we noticed before, in the case of immigrant victims, who sometimes have to face, in addition to the cultural difficulties previously discussed, negative attitudes and behaviors of police officers toward members of minorities [cf. Menjívar and Salcido, 2002].

Besides the interaction with police officers, other authors have studied the immigrant victim's contact with courts, namely, the widely discussed issue of the cultural defense in intimate violence incidents. The possibility of invoking culture as a justification for the actions of the abuser is an area of substantial controversy, evoking the "old" discussion between supporters of cultural relativism and those who defend the universality of human rights. Whereas the former defends that it is necessary to understand behaviors within the cultural frame of reference of the perpetrator and accuse the West of imposing its values on other cultures, the latter considers that the cultural defense allies with the offenders' system of self-justification and promotes the systematic abuse of women from minority groups. According to Hoeffel [2006], it also leads to the negative stereotyping of the defendant's entire culture to justify his actions, and it has the risk of promoting the generalization of this type of behavior.

24.4.2 Culture and the Support System Response to Victims

The incorporation of patriarchal beliefs toward gender relations and wife abuse, as well as its impact on the response to victims, has also been documented with helping professionals. Haj-Yahia and Uysal [2008], for example, concluded that a considerable number of Turkish medicine students embraced negative beliefs about women and patriarchal attitudes about marriage, supported victim blaming, and tolerated wife abuse. Despite the fact that the majority was willing to help the victim, only about half thought the husband was responsible for his abusive behavior and even less accepted divorce as a solution for violence or defended the punishment of the aggressor. These results were in part attributed by the authors to the assimilation of the Turkish collectivist and patriarchal ideology, which favors family cohesion and male dominance.

However, in more individualistic countries, such as the United States, victims of wife abuse may also face difficulties when seeking health professionals. Studies with nurses, for example, show that they often believe victims are manipulative and resistant to treatment as a result of their lack of trust, hostility, and impulsivity [Locsin and Purnell, 2002].

Once again, these problems are especially felt by ethnic minority women. For example, Ahmad et al. [2004] questioned South Asian women living in Canada and noticed that 29.8% believed domestic conflicts could not be discussed with doctors or nurses. This can reflect the aforementioned cultural tendency to keep domestic issues private, but also the idea that health care professionals do not promote dialogue about family violence. In a similar way, a study conducted by Yoshioka et al. [2003] showed that, when comparing disclosure patterns of battered South Asian, African-American, and Hispanic women, none of the members of the first two groups revealed the abuse to doctors, and only a small percentage of Hispanic women turned to these professionals for help. Reliance on counselors was higher, especially in the African-American and Hispanic samples.

These results probably reflect the previously discussed cultural prescriptions about (not) seeking external help, but also may be influenced by the way some professionals respond to these victims and their culture. According to some studies, therapists frequently experience difficulties when their own cultural values clash with those of their clients [Taylor et al., 2006], and sometimes culture is conceived simply as a new element to add to the case or even as a problem that needs to be addressed and solved in therapy [cf. Almeida and Dolan-Delvecchio, 1999].

24.4.3 Developing the Cultural Competence of Professionals

As a result from these findings and from multicultural theoretical approaches, there is a growing concern with the training of culturally competent professionals. According to Bent-Goodley [2005], cultural competences are useful in preventing and correcting the conceptual mistakes about cultures identified by Minnich [1991, cited in above source], such as faulty generalizations, circular reasoning, mystified concepts, and partial knowledge, which result from sparse information and lack of empirical evidence.

To respond to this demand, some professionals' curricula have included the topic of cultural competences, and there have been recommendations to integrate cultural diversity into the fabric of the professional organizations themselves, for example, through hiring policies [Sumter, 2006; Gillum, 2008].

However, there is the question of what does a culturally competent practice in fact mean. There are numerous suggestions in this regard, starting with the obvious need for professionals who are fluent in the victims' language and who belong to the same ethnic group. Others have emphasized the attention to the roles family, community, and religion play in victims' lives [e.g., Lee, Oh, and Mountcastie, 1992]. In a study with battered Latina women, they expressed precisely the desire for bicultural and/or bilingual counselors, who should understand the importance of family in their lives and work within a familiar approach, also recognizing that bearing suffering is a source of pride in their culture and that family and religion are important support systems for them [Kasturirangan and Williams, 2003].

The positive impact of delivering help in culture-specific settings, through the inclusion of pictures or artwork, has also been noticed, as well as the importance of providing holistic services to victims, given the multiplicity of problems they face [Gillum, 2008]. Outreach strategies also have been discussed, namely, the importance of divulging the message and services in community settings, such as churches, beauty salons, or grocery stores [Crichton-Hill, 2001; Kasturirangan et al., 2004; Gillum, 2008].

Besides the direct interaction with victims, other authors suggest alternative culturally competent approaches to work with minority communities. Most of these authors agree that individualistic approaches to deal with battered women do not fit the collectivist orientation of several minority cultures [Haj-Yahia, 2000, cited in Hassouneh-Phillips, 2001] and therefore seek to involve the victims' community in the response to the problem. Latta and Goodman [2005], for example, defend an educational approach toward key elements of these communities, such as religious leaders, who have the power to influence and orient other community members. The active support for reformist members of minority communities is also suggested by Shirwadkar [2004], whereas others propose more global efforts of community education [e.g., Hassouneh-Phillips, 2001]. These actions could use traditional myths and stories to pass along their message [Kasturirangan et al., 2004] and should be attentive to the importance of spirituality [Gillum, 2008] and oral communication in some cultures (not placing too much emphasis on written material) [Crichton-Hill, 2001]. Because minority victims tend to resort primarily to their families and those of the offenders, Yoshioka et al. [2003] emphasize the need to educate and mobilize this wide family network to provide victims the support they need and to reduce their shame and isolation.

Several authors stress that this involvement with the community should extend to the discussion of the problem at hand and the community's preferred way of dealing with it, as well as a dialogue about the type of help most needed to overcome it. This requires an open position of the technical staff, together with enough confidence to be able to disagree with interlocutors and "challenge those aspects of ... culture that might interfere with the safety or rights of the ... victim" [Crichton-Hill, 2001:210].

Finally, concerns over culturally competent research have also been raised. Yick [2007], for example, recommends that ethical principles for research should take into account cultural issues such as language and power dynamics, which might influence participants' autonomy, ability to provide informed consent, and understanding of confidentiality and its limits. Kasturirangan et al. [2004] go a bit further, offering detailed suggestions about how to incorporate cultural sensitivity in all phases of the research project. First, they stress the need to verify the applicability of the concepts derived from studies with white middle-class samples to different contexts or groups. Other suggestions are ethnic heterogeneity in sampling, seeking information with privileged informants from the community, prolonged contact with the community, formulation of questions in daily-life language, including open questions, and being careful not to interpret difference as deficit or pathology. Malley-Morrison and Hines [2007] add other suggestions, such as the need to "unpack" ethnic variables through detailed information on the respondents' cultural identification, country of origin, religion, and socioeconomic status, and the utility of oversampling ethnic minorities to have big enough samples to make within-group comparisons. Detailed proposals on how to conduct statistical analysis to analyze ethnicity both as an independent and as a moderator variable, as well as how to discuss findings in a culturally sensitive manner, are also offered by Malley-Morrison and Hines [2007].

24.5 Deconstructing "Culture": Critical Reflections on Theory and Research

This chapter has tried to summarize the available theory and research about the cultural aspects of wife abuse, reflecting, as a result, the main assumptions in the field. However, these assumptions are not to remain unquestioned. In fact, several authors have endorsed critiques to the way culture and cultural influences on wife abuse have been conceptualized. We will next discuss some of these assumptions and the critiques that can be addressed to them.

24.5.1 The Assumption of Culture as a Reified Entity

In a previous section, we invoked Dasgupta's [1998:217] question: "What do we mean by culture?" This is a very pertinent remark because very frequently cultural explanations and research tend to conceive culture as a coherent and static entity, composed by a given set of defined and homogeneous beliefs, values, and practices. This is the kind of perspective that allows explanations such as "people are violent because of their culture" or "culture makes women submissive." Culture is, in this sense, conceived as something similar to an internal trait people have (something that has been learned but that has become rigidly internalized) or as an external unit people are a part of [Levesque, 2001].

This assumption ignores three main facts. The first one is that culture changes with time [Crichton-Hill, 2001; Kasturirangan et al., 2004], being permanently transformed under the influence of factors such as contact with other cultures, migrations, media exposure, racism, and sociopolitical processes.

The second is that culture does not exist apart from each person's reconstruction of it. That is, each person interacts with culture; therefore, culture is constantly involved in a process of interpretation, negotiation, and redefinition [Levesque, 2001; Kasturirangan et al., 2004].

The third fact is that culture is not monolithic and that each culture has space for dissent, contradiction, and even resistance [Dasgupta, 1998; Volpp, 2006]. This is especially important because research has been focused on the majority's point of view, neglecting other perspectives inside the culture, some of them particularly relevant in the fight against wife abuse. According to Dasgupta [1998], this has contributed to the neglect of important dimensions of culture that are empowering to women. She proceeds into asking "why beliefs and customs that oppress women gain recognition as 'culture' ... and the aspects that enable women are doomed to obscurity" [p. 217]? According to Levesque [2001] this happens precisely because what we come to know as "culture" in fact represents the unstable outcome from a power confrontation between different groups inside that culture, in which the most powerful strive for their own values and interests being defined as "the culture."

24.5.2 The Assumption of Culture as a Phenomenon of the "Other"

Cultural explanations are usually invoked only to explain the violence perpetrated by ethnic minorities [Dasgupta, 1998; Pratt and Sokoloff, 2006], whereas the violence committed by members of the dominant culture tends to be explained through personality or family causes. This means that the deviance of minority members tends to be interpreted as an example of that group's usual behavior and culture, whereas the deviant behavior of dominant group members tends to be read as something exceptional, apart from the cultural rule, resulting from individual abnormality [Volpp, 2006].

This fact has contributed to a negative view of "Other" cultures and to their stigmatization as being violent, misogynistic, ignorant, and underdeveloped [Sokoloff and Dupont, 2006]. The superficial understanding of "Other" cultures also contributes to these stereotypes [Kasturirangan et al., 2004], reinforcing labeling processes that influence, as we have seen before, even the professionals who work with these groups.

In contrast, dominant groups tend to be portrayed as having no culture, except for "civilization" [Pratt and Sokoloff, 2006]. Differences between cultures are, in this process, maximized, and the fact that the Western culture and the Christian religion actually promote values and customs that enforce patriarchal dominance and violence against women becomes obscured [Dasgupta, 1998; Volpp, 2006].

24.5.3 The Assumption That Culture Equates with Race

Most empirical studies on cultural differences, namely, prevalence studies, tend to assume the equivalence between culture and race, supposing that when they compare different ethnic groups they are in fact comparing different cultures [Kasturirangan et al., 2004]. This neglects the fact that each person develops a personal relation with the cultural inheritance of its ethnic group, and that the degree of identification and appropriation of that cultural heritage greatly depends on many other factors, such as the person's social class, resources, and interpersonal relationships outside that group. This can signify, for example, that a black, college graduate, professional woman can have more in common with her white colleagues than with the lifestyle, beliefs, and values of another black woman who lives in a ghetto and is unemployed.

24.5.4 The Assumption That Culture Is the
Only Cause for Violence

The intersection of culture with other problematic dimensions, such as racism, poverty, social isolation, and lack of access to community resources has already been pointed out. Therefore, there is the risk of confounding the causal role of culture with the impact of these other structural conditions, misattributing violence to culture [Kasturirangan et al., 2004; Malley-Morrison and Hines, 2007]. Thus, this hypervaluation of culture as *the* cause for violence can whitewash the role of other causal factors and contribute to the invisibility of structural disadvantage and inequality in our societies. Cross-cultural research has, as formerly explained, paradoxically reinforced the idea that structural conditions—such as financial autonomy of women, sanctions against violence, and shelter for victims—provide important protections from violent relationships.

This is not to say that culture does not matter. Cultural research, especially deep-oriented analysis of the way cultures are defined, perceived, appropriated, lived, and transformed by individuals and their communities, instead of mere comparisons between different ethnic or religious groups, is profoundly necessary in the field of wife abuse. But culture does not exist in a void. It is multiple, contradictory, changeable, and profoundly influenced by structural forces. Understanding this complex dance between structure and culture, as well as their transformations over time, is, in our perspective, the next main challenge for researchers in the area of wife abuse.

Acknowledgments

This study was conducted within the research project PTDC/PSI/65852/2006, financed by the Portuguese Foundation for Science and Technology.

References

Abney, V. 2002. Cultural competency in the field of child maltreatment. In *The APSAC handbook on child maltreatment,* ed. J. Myers, L. Berliner, J. Briere, C. Hendrix, C. Jenny, and T. Reid, 477–85. Thousand Oaks, CA: Sage.

Ahmad, F., S. Riaz, P. Barata, and D. Stewart. 2004. Patriarchal beliefs and perceptions of abuse among South Asian immigrant women. *Violence Against Women* 10:262–82.

Almeida, R. and K. Dolan-Delvecchio. 1999. Addressing culture in batterers' intervention: The Asian Indian community as an illustrative example. *Violence Against Women* 5:654–83.

Almosaed, N. 2004. Violence against women: A cross-cultural perspective. *Journal of Muslim Affairs* 24:67–88.

Anderson, S. A. and M. C. Schlossberg. 1999. Systems perspectives on battering: The importance of context and pattern. In *What causes men's violence against women?* ed. M. Harway and J. M. O'Neil, 137–52. Thousand Oaks, CA: Sage.

Archer, J. 2006. Cross-cultural differences in physical aggression between partners: A social-role analysis. *Personality and Social Psychology Review* 10:133–53.

Barash, D. P. and C. P. Webel. 2002. *Peace and conflict studies.* Thousand Oaks, CA: Sage.

Barnes, S. 1999. Theories of spouse abuse: Relevance to African Americans. *Issues in Mental Health Nursing* 20:357–71.

Belsky, J. 1993. Etiology of child maltreatment: A developmental–ecological approach. *Psychological Bulletin* 114:413–34.

Bent-Goodley, T. 2005. Culture and domestic violence: Transforming knowledge development. *Journal of Interpersonal Violence* 20:195–203.

Berns, N. 1999. My problem and how I solve it: Domestic violence in women's magazines. *The Sociological Quarterly* 40:85–108.

_____ 2001. Degendering the problem and gendering the blame: Political discourse on women and violence. *Gender and Society* 15:262–81.

Bowman, C. G. 2003. Domestic violence: Does the African context demand a different approach? *International Journal of Law and Psychiatry* 26:473–91.

Bronfenbrenner, U. 1979. *The ecology of human development: Experiments by nature and design.* Cambridge, MA: Harvard University Press.

Brownridge, D. A. 2006. Violence against women post-separation. *Aggression and Violent Behavior* 11:514–30.

Carll, E. K. 2003. News portrayal of violence and women: Implications for public policy. *American Behavioral Scientist* 46:1601–10.

Carlson, B. E. 2005. The most important things learned about violence and trauma in the past 20 years. *Journal of Interpersonal Violence* 20:119–26.

Carlson, B. E. and A. P. Worden. 2005. Attitudes and beliefs about domestic violence: Results of a public opinion survey: I. Definitions of domestic violence, criminal domestic violence, and prevalence. *Journal of Interpersonal Violence* 20:1197–218.

Chiu, M. Y. 2004. Why Chinese women do not seek help: A cultural perspective on the psychology of women. *Counseling Psychology Quarterly* 17:155–66.

Connell, R. W. 1987. *Gender and power.* Stanford, CA: Stanford University Press.

Counts, D., J. Brown, and J. Campbell. 1999. *To have and to hit: Cultural perspectives on wife beating.* Urbana: University of Illinois Press.

Crenshaw, K. 1994. Mapping the margins: Intersectionality, identity politics, and violence against women of color. In *The public nature of private violence*, ed. M. Fineman and R. Mykitiuk, 93–118. New York: Routledge.

Cribb, J. and R. Barnett. 1999. Being bashed: Western Samoan women's responses to domestic violence in Western Samoa and New Zealand. *Gender, Place and Culture* 6:49–65.

Crichton-Hill, Y. 2001. Challenging ethnocentric explanations of domestic violence: Let us decide, then value our decisions—A Samoan response. *Trauma, Violence, & Abuse* 2:203–14.

Dasgupta, S. D. 1998. Women's realities. Defining violence against women by immigration, race, and class. In *Issues in intimate violence*, ed. R. K. Bergen, 209–19. Thousand Oaks, CA: Sage.

Dell, P. F. 1989. Violence and the systemic view: The problem of power. *Family Process* 28:1–14.

Dias, A. R. and C. Machado. Forthcoming. Violência conjugal: Representações e significados no discurso mediático. *Psicologia* 22.

Dobash, R. E. and R. P. Dobash. 1980. *Violence against wives: A case against patriarchy.* Shepton Mallet: Open Books.

Dutton, D. G. 1995. *The domestic assault of women: Psychological and criminal justice perspectives.* Vancouver: University of British Columbia.

Edelson, M. G., A. Hokoda, and L. Ramos-Lira. 2007. Differences in effects of domestic violence between Latina and Non-Latina women. *Journal of Family Violence* 22:1–10.

Flake, D. F. and R. Forste. 2006. Fighting families: Family characteristics associated with domestic violence in five Latin American countries. *Journal of Family Violence* 21:19–29.

Foreman, S. and R. Dallos. 1993. Domestic violence. In *Social problems and the family*, ed. R. Dallos and E. McLaughlin, 7–46. London: Sage.

Gage, A. 2005. Women's experience of intimate partner violence. *Social Science & Medicine* 61:343–64.

Gamson, W. 1992. *Talking politics*. Cambridge: Cambridge University Press.

Garbarino, J. 1993. Childhood: What do we need to know? *Childhood* 1:3–10.

Garcia, L., E. L. Hurwitz, and J. F. Kraus. 2005. Acculturation and reported intimate partner violence among Latinas in Los Angeles. *Journal of Interpersonal Violence* 20:569–90.

Garcia-Moreno, C., H. Jansen, M. Ellsberg, L. Heise, and C. H. Watts. 2006. Prevalence of intimate partner violence: Findings from the WHO multi-country study on women's health and domestic violence. *The Lancet* 368:1260–69.

Gelles, R. J. 1997. *Intimate violence in families*. London: Sage.

Gelles, R. J. and M. A. Straus. 1979. Determinants of violence in the family: Toward a theoretical integration. In *Contemporary theories about the family*, vol. 1, ed. W. R. Burr, R. Hill, F. I. Nye, and I. L. Reiss, 549–81. New York: Free Press.

Gillum, T. 2008. The benefits of a culturally specific intimate partner violence intervention for African American survivors. *Violence Against Women* 14:917–43.

Go, V. F., S. C. Johnson, M. E. Bentley, et al. 2003. Crossing the threshold: Engendered definitions of socially acceptable domestic violence in Chennai, India. *Culture, Health & Sexuality* 5:393–408.

Goldner, V. 1999. The treatment of violence and victimization in intimate relationships. *Family Process* 37:263–86.

Grandin, E. and E. Lupri. 1997. Intimate violence in Canada and the United States: A cross-national comparison. *Journal of Family Violence* 12:417–43.

Greenspun, W. 2000. Embracing the controversy: A metasystemic approach to the treatment of domestic violence. In *Couples on the fault line*, ed. P. Papp, 154–77. New York: Guilford.

Hagemann-White, C. 2001. European research on the prevalence of violence against women. *Violence Against Women* 7:732–59.

Haj-Yahia, M. M. 2002. Beliefs of Jordanian women about wife-beating. *Psychology of Women Quarterly* 26:282–91.

Haj-Yahia, M. M. and A. Uysal. 2008. Beliefs about wife beating among medical students from Turkey. *Journal of Family Violence* 23:119–33.

Hassouneh-Phillips, D. 2001. American Muslim women's experiences of leaving abusive relationships. *Health Care for Women International* 22:415–32.

Hearn, J. 1996. Men's violence to known women: Historical, everyday and theoretical constructions by men. In *Violence and gender relations: Theories and interventions*, ed. B. Fawcett, B. Featherstone, J. Hearn, and C. Toft, 22–37. Thousand Oaks, CA: Sage.

Hoeffel, J. 2006. Deconstructing the cultural evidence debate. *University of Florida Journal of Law & Public Policy* 17:303–45.

Horne, S. 1999. Domestic violence in Russia. *American Psychologist* 54:55–61.

Horsburgh, B. 2006. Lifting the veil of secrecy: Domestic violence in the Jewish community. In *Domestic violence at the margins*, ed. N. J. Sokoloff and C. Pratt, 206–26. New Brunswick, NJ: Rutgers University Press.

Hyman, I., T. Forte, J. Du Mont, S. Romans, and M. M. Cohen. 2006. Help-seeking rates for intimate partner violence (IPV) among Canadian immigrant women. *Health Care for Women International* 27:682–94.

Jefferson, T. 1997. Masculinities and crime. In *The Oxford handbook of criminology*, ed. M. Maguire, R. Morgan and R. Reiner, 535–58. Oxford: Clarendon.

Kasturirangan, A. and E. Williams. 2003. Counseling Latina battered women: A qualitative study of the Latina perspective. *Journal of Multicultural Counseling and Development* 31:162–78.

Kasturirangan, A., S. Krishnan, and S. Riger. 2004. The impact of culture and minority status on women's experience of domestic violence. *Trauma, Violence & Abuse* 5:318–32.

Kim, J. Y. and K. Sung. 2000. Conjugal violence in Korean American families: A residue of the cultural tradition. *Journal of Family Violence* 15:331–45.

Kozu, J. 1999. Domestic violence in Japan. *American Psychologist* 54:50–55.

Kurz, D. 1998. Old problems and new directions in the study of violence against women. In *Issues in intimate violence*, ed. R. K. Bergen, 197–208. Thousand Oaks, CA: Sage.

Kwiatkowska, A. 1998. Gender stereotypes and beliefs about family violence in Poland. In *Multidisciplinary perspectives on family violence*, ed. R. Klein, 129–52. London: Routledge.

Latta, R. and L. Goodman. 2005. Considering the interplay of cultural context and service provision in intimate partner violence: The case of Haitian immigrant women. *Violence Against Women* 11:1441–64.

Lee, C., M. Oh, and A. Mountcastie. 1992. Indigenous models of helping in nonwestern countries: Implications for multicultural counselling. *Journal of Multicultural Counselling & Development* 20:3–10.

Lee, E. 2007. Domestic violence and risk factors among Korean immigrant women in the United States. *Journal of Family Violence* 22:141–49.

Lee, J., E. C. Pomeroy, and T. M. Bohman. 2007. Intimate partner violence and psychological health in a sample of Asian and Caucasian women: The roles of social support and coping. *Journal of Family Violence* 22:709–20.

Levesque, R. J. 2001. *Culture and family violence. Fostering change through human rights law*. Washington: American Psychological Association.

Levinson, D. 1989. *Family violence in cross-cultural perspective*. Newbury Park, CA: Sage.

Locsin, R. and M. Purnell. 2002. Intimate partner violence, culture-centrism, and nursing. *Holistic Nursing Practice* 16:1–4.

Machado, C. and A. R. Dias. 2008. Cultura e violência familiar: Uma revisão crítica da literatura. *Revista Brasileira de Informação Bibliográfica em Ciências Sociais* 64:43–74.

Machado, C., M. M. Gonçalves, M. Matos, and A. R. Dias. 2007. Child and partner maltreatment: Self-reported prevalence and attitudes in the North of Portugal. *Child Abuse and Neglect* 31:657–70.

Machado, C., A. Martins, A. Santos, M. Dias, C. Antunes, and A. Rato. 2005. Crenças e atitudes policiais sobre a violência conjugal. *Revista do CEJ* 3:293–303.

Malley-Morrison, K. (ed.). 2004. *International perspectives on family violence and abuse. A cognitive ecological approach*. Mahwah, NJ: Lawrence Erlbaum.

Malley-Morrison, K. and D. Hines. 2004. *Family violence in a cultural perspective*. Thousand Oaks, CA: Sage.

Malley-Morrison, K. and D. A. Hines. 2007. Attending to the role of race/ethnicity in family violence research. *Journal of Interpersonal Violence* 22:943–72.

Margolin, G., L. G. Sibner, and L. Gleberman. 1988. Wife battering. In *Handbook of marital violence*, ed. V. B. Van Hasselt, A. S. Bellack, R. L. Morrison, and M. Hersen, 89–118. New York: Plenum.

Marin, A. J. and N. F. Russo. 1999. Feminist perspectives on male violence against women: Critiquing O'Neil and Harway's model. In *What causes men's violence against women?* ed. M. Harway and J. M. O'Neil, 18–35. Thousand Oaks, CA: Sage.

Markowitz, F. E. 2001. Attitudes and family violence: Linking intergenerational and cultural theories. *Journal of Family Violence* 16:205–18.

McConaghy, J. S. and R. R. Cottone. 1999. The systemic view of violence: An ethical perspective. *Family Process* 37:51–63.

Mehrotra, M. 1999. The social construction of wife abuse experiences of Asian Indian women in the United States. *Violence Against Women* 5:619–40.

Menjívar, C. and O. Salcido. 2002. Immigrant women and domestic violence: Common experiences in different countries. *Gender & Society* 16:898–920.

Meyers, M. 1994. News of battering. *Journal of Communication* 44:47–63.

Michalski, J. H. 2004. Making social sense out of trends in intimate partner violence—The social structure of violence against women. *Violence Against Women* 10:652–75.

Narayanan, G. 2005. Theorizing police response to domestic violence in the Singaporean context: Police subculture revisited. *Journal of Criminal Justice* 33:429–39.

Nayak, M., C. Byrne, M. Martin, and A. Abraham. 2003. Attitudes toward violence against women: A cross-nation study. *Sex Roles* 49:333–42.

O'Keefe, M. 1997. Predictors of dating violence among high school students. *Journal of Interpersonal Violence* 12:546–68.

Parke, R. and N. Lewis. 1981. The family in context: A multilevel interactional analysis of child abuse. In *Parent-child interaction*, ed. R. Henderson, 169–204. New York: Academic Press.

Pratt, C. and N. J. Sokoloff. 2006. Introduction. In *Domestic violence at the margins*, ed. N. J. Sokoloff and C. Pratt, 15–23. New Brunswick, NJ: Rutgers University Press.

Romkens, R. and S. Mastenbroek. 1998. Budding happiness: Dynamics in relations of teenage girls who are abused by their boyfriends. In *Multidisciplinary perspectives on domestic violence*, ed. R. Klein, 58–75. London: Routledge.

Rotimi, A. 2007. Violence in the family: A preliminary investigation and overview of wife battering in Africa. *Journal of International Women's Studies* 9:234–52.

Sacco, V. 1995. Media constructions of crime. *Annals of the American Academy of Political and Social Science* 539:145–54.

Saraga, E. 1996. Dangerous places: The family as a site of crime. In *The problem of crime*, ed J. Muncie and E. McLaughlin, 183–226. London: Sage.

Schofield, K. 2004. Collisions of culture and crime: Media commodification of child sexual abuse. In *Cultural criminology unleashed*, ed. J. Ferrell, K. Hayward, W. Morrison, and M. Presdee, 121–31. London: Glasshouse.

Segal, U. A. 1999. Family violence: A focus on India. *Aggression and Violent Behavior* 4:213–31.

Shirwadkar, S. 2004. Canadian domestic violence policy and Indian immigrant women. *Violence Against Women* 10:860–79.

Sokoloff, N. J. and I. Dupont. 2006. Domestic violence: Examining the intersections of race, class, and gender—an introduction. In *Domestic violence at the margins*, ed. N. J. Sokoloff and C. Pratt, 1–13. New Brunswick, NJ: Rutgers University Press.

Stith, S. M., D. B. Smith, C. A. Penn, D. B. Ward, and D. Tritt. 2004. Intimate partner physical abuse perpetration and victimization risk factors: A meta-analytic review. *Aggression and Violent Behaviour* 10:65–98.

Sugarman, D. B. and S. L. Frankel. 1996. Patriarchal ideology and wife assault: A meta-analytic review. *Journal of Family Violence* 11:13–40.

Sumter, M. 2006. Domestic violence and diversity: A call for multicultural services. *Journal of Health and Human Services Administration* 29:173–90.

Tam, S. and C. Tang. 2005. Comparing wife abuse perceptions between Chinese police officers and social workers. *Journal of Family Violence* 20:29–38.

Tang, C. S. and B. P. Lay. 2008. A review of empirical literature on the prevalence and risk markers of male-on-female intimate partner violence in contemporary China, 1987–2006. *Aggression and Violent Behavior* 13:10–28.

Tang, C., D. Wong, and F. Cheung. 2002. Social construction of women as legitimate victims of violence in Chinese societies. *Violence Against Women* 8:968–96.

Taylor, B., M. Gambourg, M. Rivera, and D. Laureano. 2006. Constructing cultural competence: Perspectives of family therapists working with Latino families. *The American Journal of Family Therapy* 34:429–45.

Vandello, J. A. and D. Cohen. 2003. Male honor and female fidelity: Implicit cultural scripts that perpetuate domestic violence. *Journal of Personality and Social Psychology* 84:997–1010.

Volpp, L. 2006. Feminism versus multiculturalism. In *Domestic violence at the margins*, ed. N. J. Sokoloff and C. Pratt, 39–49. New Brunswick: Rutgers University Press.

Wolfgang, M. E. and F. Ferracuti. 1967. *The subculture of violence: Toward an integrated theory of criminology*. London: Travistock.

World Health Organization. 2002. *World report on violence and health*. Geneva: WHO.

Yick, A. 2007. Role of culture and context: Ethical issues in research with Asian Americans and immigrants in intimate violence. *Journal of Family Violence* 22:277–85.

Yllo, K. 1983. Using a feminist approach in quantitative research. In *The dark side of families: Current issues in family violence research*, ed. D. Finkelhor, R. Gelles, G. Hotaling, and M. Straus, 277–88. Beverly Hills, CA: Sage.

———. 2005. Through a feminist lens. Gender, diversity, and violence: Extending the feminist framework. In *Current controversies on family violence*, ed. D. Loseke, R. Gelles, and M. Cavanaugh, 2nd ed., 19–34. Thousand Oaks, CA: Sage.

Yoshihama, M. 2002. The definitional process of domestic violence in Japan: Generating official response through action-oriented research and international advocacy. *Violence Against Women* 8:339–66.

Yoshioka, M. R., L. Gilbert, N. El-Bassel, and M. Baig-Amin. 2003. Social support and disclosure of abuse: Comparing South Asian, African American, and Hispanic battered women. *Journal of Family Violence* 18:171–80.

The Idea of the Crime Victim as a Trojan Horse in the Swedish Social Services Act

25

CARINA LJUNGWALD

Contents

25.1 Introduction

Our philosophy is rooted in humanity—because we believe in people. That is why we put people before systems. We believe people can grow through personal effort, want to live independent lives and want to take responsibility for their actions. Our platform is based on the universal human right to freedom. Few things restrict people's freedom as much as the consequences of violence, drugs and criminality in society. We believe fighting crime is one [of] the most important public tasks in the effort to create a safe and secure society. It must be allocated the necessary resources.

So reads the introduction of "Nya Moderaterna* on Zero Tolerance for Crime," which explains the political agenda of the conservative

---

* Before the election, the Moderate Party was redesigned as the "Nya Moderaterna" (The New Moderates) symbolizing an ideological move toward the center.

liberal* political party Moderaterna [Moderaterna, 2006]. Moderaterna forms the governing majority of the Swedish government in the center-right coalition "Alliance for Sweden." The party leader of Moderaterna, Fredrik Reinfeldt, is the Swedish Prime Minister. The document was published shortly before the 2006 general election in which the social democratic government was defeated—remarkably, the Social Democratic Party had been in power for all but 9 years since 1932. Moderaterna uses the document to outline how crime should be fought; they suggest tougher sentencing and more stringent rules for deporting aliens. Drug testing of young people and covert wiretapping should be allowed. The document also recommends that the social services should no longer deal with youth offenders; the Prison and Probation Services should instead take over. Finally, the Moderate Party argues that crime victims should be treated with empathy and be given genuine, practical assistance. Assistants for crime victims should be on duty 24 hours a day at every police station in the country.

A political statement that actively promotes the interests of crime victims is a relatively new occurrence in Sweden. The word *brottsoffer* (crime victim)[†] first appeared in the Swedish language in 1970 [Österberg, 2002]. During the 1970s and early 1980s, there was little public interest in this group. The first two nongovernmental crime victim support centers opened in the early 1980s but had to shut down because of nonuse [Åkeström and Sahlin, 2001]. Until the mid-1980s, few motions (i.e., proposals tabled in the Swedish Parliament by one or more of its members) fell under the title *crime victim* [Tham, 2001a]. Since the mid-1980s, the concerns for crime victims have grown dramatically. Between 1989 and 1995, the number of crime victim support centers increased from 15 to 100 [Larsson and Stub, 1998]. In the late 1980s, the center-right opposition made several motions in support of crime victims; the Liberal Party was especially active [Tham, 2001a]. To date, as Tham [2001a] points out, all political parties, from left to right, have been unanimous in calling for increased support for crime victims. An indication of this consensus is that the Swedish H.M. Queen Silvia herself holds an honorary position in The Swedish Association of Victim Support. A member of the Royal Family can only be involved in politics where there is total political agreement [Tham, 2001a].

---

* Note that in Europe the term *liberal* refers to classical liberalism with an emphasis on free markets, limited government, laissez-faire economics, and individual freedom. This definition is not to be confused with the use of the term in the United States, where it often is associated with increased public spending and market regulation. Chambliss [2007:14] calls this ideology as liberalism in a "modern, welfare-state sense."

† *Brott* (crime) and *offer* (victim), on the other hand, a have long history in the Swedish language. *Brott* (crime) signals a deviation from rules and commands in society, whereas *offer* (victim) refers to someone who has suffered without guilt, to appraise a god or an enemy, or simply by a cruel accident [Österberg, 1997].

This chapter addresses a 2001 reform in the Swedish Social Services Act [SFS, 2001:452 SoL] that introduced crime victims as a target group [5:11 SoL]. It argues that the provisions on crime victims might only vaguely concern the problem they describe. Rather, this reform may symbolize a broader political trend, where the fundamental values of the Social Services Act, such as solidarity and equality, are losing their role as ideological influences. The crime victim provisions can be seen as part of an ideological makeover, where the Social Services Act increasingly embraces the core values of neoliberalism, such as free markets, limited government, and individual responsibility.

25.2 A Brief Overview of Crime Victim Legislation in Sweden

In Sweden, reforms intending to aid crime victims are often linked to the feminist movement's efforts to confront men's violence against women. Women have been the focus of crime victim policy and research in the past few decades. In 1971, the Swedish Minister of Justice appointed a commission of inquiry comprising seven men and one woman to review the Swedish legislation on sex crimes. The commission's report [SOU, 1976:9], presented 5 years later, represents a milestone in the history of crime victims in Sweden [Tham, 2001a]. The report emphasized decriminalization of certain sex crimes, recommended that incest between consenting adults be legalized, and specified that the victim's behavior before an alleged rape should be considered in court proceedings. The report provoked so much protest that none of its suggestions was adopted. However, the controversy made crime victims visible for the first time in the public debate in Sweden.

From the mid-1980s onward, various laws addressing crime victims have been enacted. Sweden ratified the European Convention on the compensation of victims of violent crimes in 1988. In the same year, the Act on Visiting Bans [SFS, 1988:688] and the Act on Counsel for the Injured Party [SFS, 1988:609] were passed. Under the provisions of the latter Act, crime victims may in some cases be represented by a legal adviser during the legal process. The 1994 Government Bill "Crime Victims in Focus" [Govt. Bill 1993/94:143] includes provisions designed to improve the situation for crime victims. For example, The Crime Victim Fund was established together with the Crime Victim Compensation and Support Authority. The Crime Victim Compensation and Support Authority is responsible for assessing state compensation and administering the Crime Victim Fund. It also acts as an expert center concerning the rights of crime victims. The Crime Victim Fund provides economic support for research, education, and information on crime victims, and is financed through a fee (of 54 euros) imposed on everyone convicted of a crime punishable by imprisonment. The fund generates approximately

2.7 million euros per year. Another important legislative landmark is the 1998 Government Bill "Kvinnofrid"* [Govt. Bill 1997/98:55]. The Bill proposed a new crime (gross violation of women's integrity), an extension of the crime of rape, a ban on the purchase of sexual services, and a clarification of the employer's responsibility for taking active measures to prevent sexual harassment at the workplace.

In 1996, the government initiated a special inquiry to review the measures taken for crime victims in the past 10 years. This inquiry produced a report published in 1998 titled *Crime Victims: What Has Been Done? What Should Be Done?* [SOU, 1998:40]. The Bill "Support to Crime Victims" [Govt. Bill 2001/01:79] presented 3 years later included proposals to improve support and information for crime victims. It also sought to extend the right to legal counsel for the injured party. In 2002, the Mediation Act [SFS, 2002:445] came into effect. The preparatory material defined mediation as the offender and crime victim coming together before an impartial mediator to talk about the crime [Govt. Bill 2001/02:126]. Starting in January 2008, the municipalities became responsible for ensuring that mediation is available when a crime has been committed by someone under the age of 21 [Govt. Bill 2005/06:165]. Another recent reform entitles criminal injuries compensation to children who have witnessed violence toward a person close to them [Govt. Bill 2006/07:166].

25.3 The Provisions on Crime Victims in the Social Services Act

In Sweden, as in many other countries, the recognition of crime victims has primarily been limited to reforms in the criminal justice system [Kirchhoff, 2005]. Policies and programs for crime victims are usually not seen as an integrated part of social policies, such as social security, employment, health services, education, and social care [Hill, 2006]. "Victims of Crime" is an area of concern for the Swedish Ministry of Justice, which supervises the Crime Victim Compensation and Support Authority [Justitiedepartementet, 2007]. In 1993, when the establishment of The Crime Victim Compensation and Support Authority was discussed in the Parliament, all political parties agreed that it was the state's responsibility to arrange *financial* support for crime victims. The issue of *social* support for this group was not even considered [Svensson, 2007]. During recent years, however, the crime victim has

---

* The English translation of the word *Kvinnofrid* has been vigorously discussed. Some examples of translations are "Women's Peace" and "Peace for Women." It has been intimated that the word is "too exclusive" to be translated and might be the third Swedish word, after *smörgåsbord* and *ombudsman*, to make an international career [K. Leander, personal communication, August 24, 2006].

emerged as an important focus of social welfare law and policy. Advocates for crime victims have highlighted how the so-called social rights of crime victims must be expanded. According to Victim Support Europe* [European Forum for Victim Services, 1998], free support services, staffed by volunteers and professionals, should be considered a basic right for all crime victims in Europe. In Sweden, Morgan Johansson,† the former Minister of Public Health and Social Services, worked actively in the area of women against violence.

In 2001, support for crime victims became a separate area of responsibility for the Swedish social services. The provisions, which are addressed in this chapter, can be found [5:11 SoL] in the Fifth Chapter of the Swedish Social Services Act, which regulates the social services goals for certain groups such as children and young people, elderly people, people with functional impairment, substance abusers, and people caring for relatives. Section 5:11 SoL was first incorporated in the Social Services Act in 1998 by the Government Bill "Kvinnofrid" [Govt. Bill 1997/98:55].‡ At that time, the Act only covered women who had been exposed to domestic violence. Since then, the section has been amended three times. The general provisions on crime victims were introduced in 2001 [Govt. Bill 2001/01:79]. In 2006, provisions concerning children who have witnessed violence or other abuse by or against a close adult were added [Govt. Bill 2005/06:166]. The most recent amendment was made in July 2007 [Govt. Bill 2006/07:38]. The wording was sharpened in the respect that the verb "should" was replaced by the more obligatory "shall" in the second and third paragraphs. Section 5:11 SoL now reads:

> The duties of the social welfare board include working for that those who are subjected to crime and those close to them receive support and help. The social welfare board shall especially consider that women who are or have been subjected to violence or other abuse by someone close to them may be in need of support and help to change their situation. The social welfare board shall also especially consider that children who have witnessed violence or other abuse by or against a close adult are victims of crime and may be in need of support and help.

According to the preparatory material for the legislation [Govt. Bill 1997/98:55; Govt. Bill 2000/01:79], the provisions were introduced in response to the lack of involvement by the social services in matters connected with

---

* Victim Support Europe is a network of nongovernmental organizations that provides community and court-based services for victims of crime. Victim Support Europe is in consultative status with the Council of Europe and the United Nations (UN).
† At a seminar in 2006, Morgan Johansson [M. Johansson, personal communication, June 20, 2006] declared that support and protection of women subjected to violence is a "natural" part of the welfare state and must be "considered a social right." He also argued that this issue "lands in the core of and must be dealt with within the welfare state." To be able to do this, Johansson mentioned legislation as crucial.
‡ For the legislative history of section 5:11 SoL, see Ljungwald and Hollander [2009].

the above-mentioned groups. As a result, section 5:11 SoL has raised high expectations for the social services, which are now regarded as among the most important resources for crime victims [Wergens, 2002; Lindgren, 2004].

There are, however, also criticisms of the reforms [5:11 SoL]. A recent study [Ljungwald and Hollander, 2008] shows that the legal guidance regarding crime victims in the Social Services Act is vague, indistinct, and contradictory. Additionally, section 5:11 SoL did not strengthen the rights of crime victims. All four Bills indicate that the provisions do not entail any actual legal change [Govt. Bill 1997/98:55; Govt. Bill 2000/01:79; Govt. Bill 2005/06:166; Govt. Bill 2006/07:38]. The most recent Bill [Govt. Bill 2006/07:38:11] declares that:

> The provisions exist only to demonstrate the obligations already incumbent on the social services according to other provisions in the Social Services Act.... Section 5:11 is not a provision about rights, and individuals are not granted supportive measures by it.

When the section was introduced in 1998 [Govt. Bill 1997/98:55 p. 128], the government claimed that because the reform did not involve legal changes, "the proposal would not result in any increased costs for the municipalities." The reform also does not seem to consider the interest and opinion of crime victims themselves. For example, women who have been exposed to violence show little willingness or inclination to approach the social services for assistance [Govt. Bill 1997/98:55]. Empirical studies also have shown that framework laws, such as the Social Services Act, are often ineffective in protecting vulnerable groups. This type of regulation has been criticized for not bringing significant improvement in the living conditions of various groups, including people with functional disabilities [Andenæs, 1992; Tuori, 1993].

Conclusions about the provisions on crime victims in the Social Services Act are consistent with international research that shows that reforms for crime victims are frequently contradictory and made without regard to the group's interest, opinions, or expressed needs [Fattah, 1992]. Many researchers claim that these reforms are "symbolic politics" and justify or divert attention from broader policies or trends [Fattah, 1992; Elias, 1993; Garland, 2001]. According to Fattah [1992], the reluctance of governments to go beyond symbolic gestures to improve the plight of crime victims is evident in the legislation of several countries. One recent example is victim compensation programs in Quebec, Canada, where crime victims have many rights on paper. Just like the provisions in the Social Services Act, however, very little supervision or enforcement mechanisms exist to ensure the law's application [Parent, 2006].

This research raises several important questions. If section 5:11 SoL did not change the social services' responsibility for crime victims, why was it incorporated in the Social Services Act? Was the intention to ensure that the needs of this group are met, or is this reform simply "clever advertising" or a "political placebo"? As a case of symbolic law and politics [Aubert, 1980], the provisions on crime victims in the Social Services Act [5:11 SoL] create the impression that a reform has occurred and that the rights of crime victims have been strengthened, when in reality there has been no significant change.

To investigate why this reform was enacted, it would be insufficient to describe the tangible purposes of the law. Such a description does not provide the history or the context. A law is also not always enacted to produce its prescribed effects, but rather because it symbolizes something important or embodies new ideals or values (Santesson-Wilson, 2003). In other words, the introduction of crime victims as a special target group in the Social Services Act [5:11 SoL] cannot be seen as an isolated event, but must be examined within the framework of broader social policy development. Considering the political and social context is essential to understand the origins of legal provisions.

25.4 Social Policy Trends

25.4.1 From Solidarity to Individual Responsibility?

Sweden has long been considered an archetypical social democratic welfare state, with an emphasis on values such as social solidarity, equality, and universality. The principle of solidarity,* which often refers to "unity" or "common responsibility," was essential when institutional social policy began to take form in the 1930s. The aim of the Swedish welfare state was to equalize the consequences of certain social risks, such as unemployment, disability, sickness, and aging. An adequate standard of living should be considered a social right of all citizens, partly without regard to previous performance and contribution [Esping-Andersen, 1990]. As pointed out by Ewald [2002], the logic of solidarity is not based on cause and fault but rather on distribution and risk. The critique of the social democratic tradition in Sweden has, nevertheless, been strong since the 1980s [Tham, 1995]. At that time, ideas associated with neoliberalism began to seriously enter the public debate [Boréus, 1997]. In addition, the economic crisis in the early 1990s posed severe tests on the rationale behind the Swedish welfare state. The recession ended more than 50 years of continuous expansion for the welfare sector [Bergmark, 2000]. Many of the cuts were inflicted by the social democratic government.

---

* For a discussion on solidarity and public welfare see Bergmark [2000].

In the past few decades, the rhetoric in the political realm, even under social democratic government, has shifted away from "solidarity" and "equality" and toward "individual responsibility," "privatization," and "efficiency." The arguments against the Swedish welfare state are often framed in terms of individual responsibility and freedom. Generous universal welfare programs are accused of fostering dependency, where people rely on state support rather than their own efforts [Schmidtz and Goodin, 1998].

Research does, however, show different and sometimes contradictory trends regarding the recent development of the Swedish welfare state, as well as that of other welfare states in other countries. The most debated issue concerns the relationship between neoliberalism, economic globalization, and welfare states. According to Olsen [2008], a distinction can be made between two principal research streams: "convergence theory" and "resilience theory." "Convergence theorists," on the one hand, argue that many welfare states in the developed world, such as Sweden, are undergoing a major transformation, where ideas of collective responsibility are increasingly undermined [Ewald, 2002; Gilbert, 2004]. Instead, ideas of workfare and individual responsibility are being spread throughout the world [Handler, 2008]. The shift in social policy is often portrayed as a convergence of welfare states toward a liberal and residual "U.S.-style" social policy under the spell of neoliberal globalization.* The belief is that economic liberalization in international and national economic systems has increased the power of those in capital markets, which can exert pressure on governments to make cuts in social spending and social legislation [Albert and Standing, 2000]. Gilbert [2004] describes the central tendencies in social policy as a silent transformation from "public provision to privatisation," from "protecting labour to promoting work," from "universal entitlement to selective targeting," and from "solidarity of citizenship to solidarity of membership." In line with "convergence theory," studies have sought to show that the Swedish welfare state is now losing its distinctiveness [Vahle Westerhäll, 2002]. A similar development has been observed in the other Nordic countries. As early as 1995, Midré argued that a moral dimension is gaining ground in Norwegian social policy, where individual responsibility is emphasized. According to Björk Eydal and Satka [2006], the long line of Nordic welfare policies, which emphasize structural prevention of social problems and shared social responsibilities, is now being challenged. Björk Eydal and Satka point out that in many cases politicians have adopted a new morality toward increased control of citizens who are

---

* Note that neoliberalism and globalization are not the same. Neoliberalism is often described as the driving ideology of globalization. Globalization is, however, not only an ideological project or solely an economic phenomenon. Steger [2005] underlines the complexity of the noneconomical dimensions of globalization and defines the concept as "a set of complex, sometimes, contradictory, social processes that are changing our current social condition based on the moderns system of independent nation-states" [Steger, 2005, s.13].

expected to be ever more responsible for themselves and their families than they were 20 years ago. Harrikari [2008] shows how the Finnish government's focus on expansive welfare and educational policy is shifting toward policing concern and fear.

"Resilience theorists," on the other hand, challenge claims of convergence and argue that economic globalization and neoliberalism have relatively small effects on welfare states such as Sweden [Taylor-Gooby, 2001; Bergh, 2004; Rothstein and Lindbom, 2004; Lindbom, 2007; Olsen, 2008]. According to this research stream, a transformation to a liberal and residual welfare state, like in the United States, is not likely to occur. It is widely accepted that social policy varies across nations and that "politics matters" as suggested early by researchers such as Gøsta Esping-Andersen and Walter Korpi. The role of social democracy and the working class in the development of welfare states has also been re-emphasized in more recent studies [Cousins, 2005]. In line with "resilience theory," studies have sought to show that despite the economic crisis in the early 1990s, the Swedish welfare state has maintained its distinctiveness. A few changes introduced in the 1990s were, according to Palme [2008], designed to diminish the welfare system but proved to be only minor disruptions. Some studies have even proved that the Swedish welfare state strengthened its distinctive characteristics in some areas during the 1990s [Kuhne, 2000; Montanari et al., 2007]. For example, in the 1990s, a larger portion of preschool children was granted child care than had been before [Bergmark, 2008a].

Finally, there are studies that show a balanced picture, accepting that the Swedish welfare state has moved in a liberal direction but that the original welfare model has not been altered in any significant way [Rothstein and Lindbom, 2004; Bergmark, 2008b; Olsen, 2008].

25.5 The Social Services Act: A Touchstone for Solidarity

The ideals constructed during the twentieth century clearly shaped Swedish social welfare legislation. The 1960s and 1970s were eras of extensive social reform. During this time, there was a strong belief in legal instrumentalism, which assumes that the law can be used to change and improve society. The way in which social assistance was organized, however, was long considered an anomaly of the Swedish welfare state [Sunesson et al., 1998]. The Central Organization of Social Work (CSA) retained liberal and philanthropic values from the turn of the century. There was a belief in that universal social policies would eventually eliminate the municipal poor relief (Wersäll, 2006).

The Social Services Act was adopted in 1982 after many years of extensive investigation. The expectations for change from previous patriarchal legislation were high [Holgersson, 2004]. A major reason for the Act's creation was to merge all legislation concerning social services administrated by the municipal government into one law [Åström, 1988]. The Social Services Act was designed as a framework for social goals with sections of substantive law. Framework laws are used in welfare reform because they can be easily adjusted for new political trends. Most of the legal provisions in these laws are open-ended rather than prescriptive, and they stipulate various benchmarks for the social services rather than establishing a set of rigid rules based on legal facts and consequences [Strömberg, 1981; Hollander, 1995; Warnling-Nerep, 1995; Hydén, 2000].

The Social Services Act came to reflect many of the ideals of the Swedish welfare state. It portrayed social and financial assistance as a right or an entitlement, rather than as alms or charity [Holgersson, 2004]. The preparatory material also opposed target- and symptom-oriented measures. The link between eligibility for social assistance and specific causes or situations, such as illness, age, or inability to work, was not compatible with the "holistic view" of social problems and individual needs that was to characterize the future of social work [Govt. Bill 1979/80:1]. Instead, "solidarity" became the foundation of the Social Services Act, according to which social and financial security should be ensured for everyone [Holgersson, 1988]. The Social Services Act declares that the social services shall, based on democracy and solidarity, promote people's economic and social security, equality of living conditions, and active participation in community life. According to the Act, the social services' activities shall also be based on people's self-determination and integrity [1:1 SoL]. All citizens shall be assured a reasonable standard of living* [4:1 SoL].

The tension between collective and individual responsibility has, however, always been visible in the Social Services Act. The fundamental conflict in the Act is between the notion that each person is entitled to receive a set minimum of the collective welfare and the notion that each individual is obligated to support him- or herself [Åström, 1988]. Social welfare law has always included clear requirements for seeking employment, and financial assistance from the social services has never been considered an unconditional right. The eligibility for welfare benefits is determined individually, based on means testing of applicants, and is considered to be the form of protection only when all other means of support have been exhausted [4:1 SoL]. This implies that individuals must first use all means at their disposal to fulfill their needs; individuals must first seek employment, or find out if the needs can be met by

---

* What is included in the financial assistance is specified in the Act. It shall be granted for reasonable expenses including food, clothing and footwear, play and leisure, disposable articles, health and hygiene, a daily newspaper, telephone costs, and a television licence. In addition, the right to financial assistance covers reasonable costs for housing, home electricity, commutes to and from work, home insurance and membership for trade unions, and funds for unemployment benefits [4:3 SoL].

sick leave, pension, or some other source. Although individual responsibility[*] is expressed in the Act [cf. 1:1 SoL] and has come more to the forefront in the past decade, research has shown that the legislation is primarily based on theories that attribute social problems to structural causes [Friis, 2005]. Also, the right to assistance [4:1 SoL] in the Social Services Act is still mainly tied to needs, rather than to previous contribution and performance. As stated by Arts and Gelissen [2001], social services were originally aimed at people who did not obtain sufficient resources based on their own efforts. The provision of social housing, unemployment benefits, and health protection was justified by the fact that people needed these resources.

There have been many movements to modify the Act to meet the demands of a free market economy. In 1998, under a social democratic government, there was a strong attempt [Govt. Bill 1996/97:124] to put the *individual's responsibility* in the spotlight, rather than the *individual's right to assistance*. Section 4:1 SoL, which stipulates an individual's right to assistance, was modified from "A person is entitled to assistance from the social services towards their livelihood and for their living in general, if this need cannot be provided for in any other way" to "Persons unable to provide for their needs or obtain provision for them in any other way are entitled to assistance from the social services towards their livelihood and for their living in general." Note how the word order was changed to place emphasis on individual responsibility. The change is of importance from a legal perspective, when the Act is to be interpreted. The reform also limited the right to appeal to the Country Administrative Court. The 1998 reform also included changes that were incongruous with this move toward individual responsibility, as it strengthened the individual's right to assistance by introducing a "national standard" (*riksnorm*) for basic living costs, such as food, clothing, and hygiene. The national norm is established each year by the government and is intended to guarantee minimum income maintenance.

When the Social Services Act was reformed in 2002 [Govt. Bill 2000/01:80], the right to appeal was reinstated. This was a return to the regulations before the amendments in 1998. The word order in section 4:1 SoL was, nevertheless, kept. The preparatory material also used the language of the Swedish welfare state, with an emphasis on social rights, public responsibility, a holistic view, a minimum standard of living, and the use of preventive measures. A recent publication concerning the Act from The National Board of Health and Welfare [Socialstyrelsen, 2002] includes headlines like "The Right to Assistance," "The Social Services' General Responsibility toward You," and "Social and Financial Security for Everyone."

In summary, the Social Services Act conflicts with liberalism because its main features are built on structural theories that clash with a strong belief

---

[*] There is a conflict regarding how the individual responsibility shall be interpreted in concrete situations. In case law, we can find examples of some of these conflicts.

in individual responsibility. The distribution of welfare according to need, as stipulated in the Act, is also a profoundly noncapitalist concept [MacGregor, 1999].

25.6 The Crime Victim as a Vessel for New Ideology

The main thesis of this chapter is that the provisions for crime victims [5:11 SoL] may be part of a normative reorientation in the Swedish Social Services Act, endangering its fundamental values, such as solidarity and equality. The provisions on crime victims appear benevolent, but they can, intentionally or unintentionally, delegitimize the Act's value system. International research has shown that reforms made in the name of crime victims are a way of blocking solidarity, enhancing neoliberal policy, and justifying measures of penal repression [Elias, 1993; Garland, 2001]. In the United States, the origin of the crime victim movement can be traced not only to the grassroots activism of the feminist movement but also to law-and-order policies of the U.S. Department of Justice [Weed, 1995]. In Sweden, there are also indications that the provisions on crime victims have been pushed substantially by policies promoted in the name of individual responsibility. One early example is in the Swedish budget proposal of 1992–1993 where the "crime victim" was portrayed as legitimizing the whole existence of the penal system [Andersson, 2002]. Another example is the political agenda "Nya Moderaterna on Zero Tolerance for Crime," cited in the introduction of this chapter, in which support to crime victims is included in a political package suggesting tougher sentencing, more stringent rules for deporting aliens, and a shift in interventions for young offenders from care and rehabilitation toward control and sanctions. When considering the development of Swedish social policy, the increasing fascination with crime victims since the mid-1980s raises some important questions. For example, even though most people affected by crime are poor and deprived, why has the image of the crime victim been divorced from welfare and structural explanations [Hacking, 1999]? Groups such as substance abusers, the homeless, and people with a criminal background are unquestionably the groups that are most affected by crime [SCB, 2004]. However, the conventional image of the crime victim is a "respectable" citizen, typically a middle-class woman and her children [Garland, 2001]. As early as the mid-1980s, Greenland [1987] pointed out that even though there is a close connection between poverty and child mortality, victim advocates have little or no interest in the ills caused to children by poverty and neglect. This has been confirmed by more recent studies, which show that most children who die from maltreatment are poor, and that poor parents are more likely than more financially advantaged parents to abuse or neglect their children [Rodriguez and Green, 1997; Azar, 2002]. Policies for crime victims, like compensation programs, often discriminate against the poor. For example, it is often useless for crime victims depending on financial assistance from the social services in Sweden to apply for criminal injuries compensation. The criminal injuries compensation will be considered an asset under the means test, reducing the assistance these individuals receive or even preventing them from receiving any additional financial assistance. For crime victims who depend on financial assistance from the social services, the idea of criminal injuries compensation as a remedy for psychological injuries, pain, or suffering is lost.

But, in what way can the concept "crime victim" reflect a new (or renewed) set of values and beliefs in how social problems are understood? The idea that the conceptualization of crime victims has been constructed as a part of liberalism (or now neoliberalism) is not new. At the first victimology symposium in 1973, Reiman [1973] observed that the definition of the crime victim incorporates liberal ideas,* such as individual responsibility and freedom. Thus, the core concept behind the crime victim is innocence. As a logical category, the crime victim relies on a fault-based distinction between the innocent and the guilty and the good and the bad [Christie, 1986]. An introduction of the former into the Social Services Act thereby introduces the latter. Moreover, the concept of blame has now penetrated the Act. As stated by one social worker in a recent study, "If you see yourself as a crime victim, you relieve yourself of guilt and put it … where it should be" [Ljungwald and Svensson, 2007:144]. To identify the crime victim is thereby a way to individualize and "agentify" social problems. The responsibility is passed on from the public to the individual, and structural analysis is replaced with moralism. In this way, a focus on crime victims can distract us from addressing economic inequalities. In other words, the idea of the crime victim places the fault for unfortunate conditions on "evil offenders," relieving society from any responsibility. This construction of demons is an essential strategy for avoiding an analysis of the structural foundations of victimization [Edelman, 2001]. It lets us all off the hook; we lose sight of how governments exert a sizable impact on social problems such as crime and poverty [Rank, 2004].

Normatively, the provisions on crime victims thereby seem to run counter to the fundamental values of the Social Services Act. If the Act is rooted in values based on solidarity, it is irrational to distinguish crime victims from

---

* In Sweden, advocacy for victims of crime can be traced to the Liberal Party. The first General Director of the Swedish Crime Victim Compensation and Support Authority was the Liberal Party politician Britta Bjelle. Before Bjelle was appointed General Director in 1994, a position she held for 10 years, she was a member of the Swedish parliament representing the Liberal Party (1985–1994). The Swedish Association for Victim Support also has a close collaboration with a study association (*Studieförbundet Vuxenskolan*), whose main interest organization is the Liberal Party. A search (June 2008) with the keyword *brottsoffer* (victim of crime) on the web page of the Liberal Party results in 1,148 hits. The same search results in 13 hits on the web page of the Left Party of Sweden.

others who need support [Fattah, 1992]. If we believe that crime is a social phenomenon and not only acts by individual offenders, then the boundary between victims of crime and the victims of disease, accidents, and poverty and the boundary between offenders and victims begin to disappear. From a solidarity perspective, society is a totality, and the good and bad of each individual depends on everyone else [Ewald, 2002]. Therefore, the logic of the Social Services Act assumes that victimization arises from structural causes, such as a lack of adequately paying jobs, affordable housing, or childcare. If the objective is to displace solidarity with neoliberalism, then introducing the concept of crime victim is an ideal vehicle. The justification of this shift requires a reconstruction of the "victim" and what (or now, whom) is to blame for "social problems." Ideas of freedom and individual responsibility do not correspond to the "victim" defined as a person suffering from societal injustice such as poverty. One of the cornerstones of neoliberal policy is that we can control our outcomes by being reasonable and responsible [Andersson, 2002]. In this way, the idea of the crime victim detaches the notion of the "victim" from structural explanations to individual responsibility. The idea of the crime victim also reconnects the link between contribution and benefits; from this perspective, innocent, law-abiding, and respectable citizens should receive special treatment. This conflicts with the right to assistance as it stands today in the Social Services Act, which is tied to needs and not to specific causes and situations [4:1 SoL]. In this way, the idea of the crime victim and neoliberal policy complements each other.

25.6.1 The Seductive Power of the Crime Victim Metaphor

Persuasive metaphors in statutory texts, such as the "crime victim," can give new meaning to an issue and make us accept analogies without further reflection or critical thinking [Ebbesson, 2008]. Thus, to change our way of thinking about welfare and social problems, we have to devise a new terminology. Alternatively, we can recycle and rephrase some words from the past. In the days of the New Poor Law and of workhouses and poorhouses, as pointed out by Schmidtz and Goodin [1998], character tests differentiated the deserving from the undeserving poor. The former were those who suffered their plight through no fault of their own, and the latter had only themselves to blame. The aim was to separate the deserving poor and subject them to a less harsh welfare regime, reserving the punitive regime for the undeserving poor [Schmidtz and Goodin, 1998]. Individual responsibility is the foundation for the distinction between the deserving and undeserving poor, just as it is the foundation for the distinction between the crime victim and the offender. Studies have shown that the rise of crime victims' rights has caused people to be divided into two categories: "victims," who are deserving of rights, and "offenders," who are undeserving of rights [Lomell, 2006].

It is an interesting finding that section 5:11 SoL has been amended three times since 1998 without the rights of crime victims being strengthened. Although the new provisions for victims of crime [5:11 SoL] do not create new rights for crime victims, they do encourage the adoption of a new identity. This may pave the way for more merit-oriented values and be a modest step toward changing the eligibility requirements for assistance, where the distribution of welfare reflects previous performance. By altering how social problems are viewed, the solutions for these problems will change. Thus, if we conceptualize social problems as a matter of individual rather than structural failures, then we are most likely less inclined to provide assistance. Across countries, there is a strong correlation between beliefs about the causes of poverty and the degree of resource redistribution [Alesina and Glaeser, 2007]. Additionally, the social services will be less responsible for preventing social problems such as crime and will only deal with the consequences of them, which implies protecting innocent victims [Wacquant, 2004]. The Swedish Crime Victim Fund does, for example, explicitly not grant money to projects with preventive purposes [Brottsoffermyndigheten, 2008].

A focus on crime victims also implies that it is not enough to be afflicted and in need to receive assistance; you must have been afflicted by *someone*. An individual responsibility orientation converts every transgression into a fault, which is the philosophical principle for apportioning liability [Ewald, 2002]. By this logic, the response is to provide compensation only to innocent victims and leave losses to those at fault [Simon, 2003]. One recent example of this development occurs in the book *Utsatta och sårbara brottsoffer* (*Afflicted and Vulnerable Victims of Crime*) [Lindgren, Hägglund, and Pettersson, 2003], where groups like women, the disabled, and the elderly struggle to present themselves not only as marginalized but also as victims of crime. If there is no one to blame for their problems, they do not have a right to anything [Ewald, 2002]. As Hacking [1999:133] points out:

> Don't bring up unpleasant topics like filth, danger, and the stench of urine in the halls, elevators that don't work, smashed glass everywhere, cancellations of food programs. Just tell us that your dad is abusing your little sister.

In this way, the classical boundary between the deserving and undeserving, which the Social Services Act was introduced to eliminate, is reinforced. You will have to prove yourself worthy to access welfare benefits, which may be denied to those who do not follow the social service demands of acceptable, responsible behavior.

The provisions on crime victims are not the only indication that the value system of the Social Services Act is being increasingly undermined. In recent years, the Act's provisions have become more focused on the social services' general responsibilities toward target groups of citizens, rather than the social rights of the individual [Ljungwald and Hollander, 2008]. Another example is a reform from 1997, in which family caretakers were introduced as a target group in the Social Services Act [SFS, 1997:313 SoL]. The provisions state that the social services should support people caring for relatives who are suffering from long-term illness, are elderly, or have functional impairments. The provisions could be interpreted as an extension of the values of solidarity and equality to include not only older people's needs but also family caretakers' needs. Another interpretation is that provisions to support family caretakers made it possible to save money during the economic recession because the provisions could increase family care and thereby decrease older people's need for public care services [Ulmanen, 2008]. In the Bill where these provisions were proposed to the Parliament, the government described support for family caretakers as a matter of saving money without expanding services because the proposal "concerns a voluntary commitment the costs are not assumed to rise" [Govt. Bill 1996/97:124, p. 165]. In other words, if the social services support relatives to care for older people or people with functional impairments, the social services do not have to give as much services to these people themselves. Thereby, trust in public responsibility can be undermined.

A governmental report from 2007 "From Social Assistance to Work" [SOU, 2007:2] proposes the introduction of so-called activity incentives for people who have received financial assistance for a period of 6 months under the Social Services Act. The report contends that it is important that society signals that it pays to work. According to the report, there are reasons to make exceptions for financial assistance acting as society's last-resort safety net; for example, if the result of these exceptions is reduced dependence on assistance and strengthened ties to the labor market. The report's proposals are, as far as possible, based on the individual person's opinion and view of changes needed to strengthen his or her links to the labor market. It is established that lasting change can only be achieved if it strengthens the individual's own motivation.

25.7 Addressing Social Policy Development with Qualitative Research

Identifying the introduction of the provisions on crime victims in the Social Service Act solely as the result of neoliberal logic is clearly an over-simplification. Distinctively Swedish national trends must be considered. After all, economic globalization and neoliberalism do not create the same effects everywhere. There are often several reasons for why a certain reform is enacted. It is important to underline that reforms intending to aid crime victims are linked to strategies to confront men's violence against women.

Men's violence against women has been a blind spot in the Swedish welfare state and Swedish welfare research, despite the belief that bodily safety and integrity is a basic condition for welfare [SOU, 2005:66].

The introduction of crime victims as a special target group in the Social Services Act also does not necessarily imply that values such as solidarity and equality are losing ground in Swedish social policy on the whole. Whether the Swedish welfare model has been altered is a much more complex question. Again, research has shown that the Swedish welfare state has been relatively resilient to economic globalization and neoliberalism. Values such as solidarity, universalism, and decommodification do remain strong in many areas, for example, in Swedish health care [Bergmark, 2008b]. In any case, the provision on crime victims in the Social Services Act can be *one* sign of a market-conforming trend in Swedish social policy. Thus, the support for different welfare programs varies greatly. Public support is stronger for welfare programs such as health care, education, pensions, and parental leave, whereas means-tested programs, such as social assistance from the social services, are less popular [Bergmark, 2000; Kahle, 2000; Rothstein and Lindbom, 2004]. Thus, change can be limited to some areas. As Rothstein and Lindbom [2004] point out, the Swedish welfare state is becoming more suited to the needs of the middle class than to the new working class consisting largely of immigrants and people with part-time jobs. Rothstein and Lindbom highlight that, although change is restricted, there is a clear trend from a universal model toward a more liberal model in a number of areas; for example, the share of means-tested expenditure has doubled in the past 3 decades. Also, both resilience theorists and convergence theorists tend to confine their focus on quantitative aspects of the "welfare state" with narrow economic indicators [Olsen, 2008]. Qualitative remodeling, such as the introduction of new concepts and ideals in social policy and social welfare law, may be overlooked. The welfare state can thus be attacked rhetorically. In the United States, under the Reagan administration, budget cuts and institutional restructuring were all justified and rationalized through a subtle shift in the existing welfare discourse [O'Connor, 1998]. Critical analyses of the language in different laws, such as the Social Services Act, are therefore important to understand the development of social policy.

To establish how the Swedish welfare state is responding to current pressures of economic globalization and neoliberalism it is also not sufficient to only study social policy development. The analysis also requires a close inspection of other areas such as crime policy, which often is in the forefront of change. The global spread of information about punishment during the past decade has, as highlighted by Cavadino and Dignan [2006], been significant; concepts such as "zero tolerance" have crossed the Atlantic with considerable speed. In Sweden, crime was not regarded as a political question until the 1960s, and, in 1970s, the government implemented several decriminalization policies, and the prison population was noticeably reduced [Tham, 2001b]. Today, the Swedish Prison and Probation Services (KV) are constructing more correctional facilities than any other agency in Europe. KV plans to create 2,287 new prison places by 2014 [Kriminalvården, 2008]. Crime policy is also closely linked to social policy; the deregulation of social security often goes hand in hand with tougher crime policy [Wacquant, 2001; Cavadino and Dignan, 2006]. Studies in the United States have shown that states that spend relatively little on welfare are likely to have higher imprisonment rates [Cavadino and Dignan, 2006]. In the 1980s, the Reagan administration redirected governmental policy away from the welfare expansion characteristics of the 1960s and 1970s; welfare programs were made more restrictive; benefit levels were reduced; and eligibility criteria were narrowed [O'Connor, 1998]. At the same time, Reagan declared that the 1980s would be the "decade of the crime victim" [Cole, 2007]. In 1994, 2 years before Clinton "ended welfare as we know it" [Clinton, 1996] in the "Personal Responsibility and Work Opportunity Responsibility Act" (PRWORA), the largest crime Bill in U.S. history, the Violent Crime Control and Law Enforcement Act (VCCLEA), was passed. Apart from expanding the federal death penalty and enhancing penalties for immigration-related crimes, the reform included extensive crime victim legislation, such as the Violence Against Women Act (VAWA). The Act also overturned a section of the Higher Education Act of 1965, which permitted prison inmates to receive a Pell Grant* for postsecondary education while incarcerated.

Research has also shown that structural explanations seem to be diminishing in favor of individualized explanations in other areas. In the media, categories such as "juvenile offenders" are now described as calculating superpredators [Estrada, 2001]. In a motion to the parliament in [2002/03:Ju375], panhandling is described as "vexatious behaviour," that should be criminalized. According to the former Mayor of Stockholm [2006–2008], a Moderaterna politician, the "threatening and studious begging a great problem" and that "there now are women who are afraid of riding the subway at night" [Situation Stockholm, 2007]. These descriptions reflect neoliberal values; thus, panhandlers are "free" actors in a market who can choose between legal and illegal behaviors [Tham, 1995]. These changing images of social problems create problems for social democratic ideas, a view that finds the cause of social problems on an individual level will not motivate a general social policy [Tham, 1995].

25.8 A Structural and Holistic Approach

In summary, the provisions on crime victims can be part of a trend, where ideals of solidarity and equality in the Social Services Act are replaced or

---

* The Pell Grant program is a federal grant program sponsored by the U.S. Department of Education.

complemented by neoliberal individualism. It is difficult to draw firm conclusions about the implementation of section 5:11 SoL because few empirical studies have been conducted. Some studies indicate, however, that the social services have not yet completely accepted the idea of the crime victim. A follow-up survey of the reform [5:11 SoL] shows that social workers within the social services know about the provisions about crime victims [Socialstyrelsen, 2004]. The reform has, however, not led to any major change in the activities of the social services. As one social worker says [Socialstyrelsen, 2004:16]: "We have considered the need of the individual both before and after the amendment."

In another recent study, Swedish social workers [Ljungwald and Svensson, 2007] express that an individual should not be entitled to support solely because he or she is categorized as a crime victim. The social workers claim that the social services should focus on individual needs rather than on fixed categories. Social workers also question the offender–victim dichotomy. They acknowledge the complexity of crime and the difficulty of making a distinction in real-life situations, where one party is clearly guilty and one party is innocent. Many people are on the both sides of the equation. In a study by Svensson [2006], a social worker claims that the provisions on victims of crime in the Social Services Act have not yet had any significance. According to the social worker, the social services work with anyone in need and do not distinguish between problems. The search for solutions is the same regardless of what the problem is, whether sexual abuse, substance abuse, a crisis after death, or another problem.

One explanation for the resistance of the social workers in these studies to target crime victims might be that their values are mainly based on solidarity. Social problems are perhaps principally conceptualized as a result of structural and not individual failings. Thus, targeting crime victims involves the establishment of blame. This implies that a social worker must not only assess needs but also determine guilt and innocence. How else can a social worker identify whether an individual is a crime victim? Social workers might not want to be involved in determining "right and wrong" and "good and bad." Social workers might not want to distinguish crime victims from offenders or confront and condemn the latter. Finally, social workers might want to focus on social relations rather than individual categories. Nevertheless, by placing the crime victims in the context of social work, a more complex understanding of issues regarding crime victims can be reached. A structural and holistic perspective can be one contribution.

How long will solidarity, equality, and social security remain the fundamental values of the Swedish Social Services Act? The question is still open. Considering how the Act has been redesigned lately, it is legitimate to doubt the future of these concepts. On the other hand, it might be possible to find a path where the Act's original goals can be preserved at the same time as the demands for recognition of categories, such as crime victims, are satisfied. Law is not always a rational unit of norms, but it can include many different values. Regardless, it is important to stop for a moment and to think about the main principles of social policy and where they are headed. In particular, one must consider policies concerning who will be defined as the weakest and poorest members of society, the worthy or unworthy, deserving or undeserving. How do we want to deal with social problems, and where do we place the responsibility for them? Who do we perceive as in need, and what is a just allocation of resources? Law can and should be challenged with these questions in mind. As Eriksson [1990] points out, if the law is nothing else than frozen politics, we have every right to question it. The Social Services Act has been changed many times and will be changed many more times. To answer the question of whether a crime victim perspective should be integrated in social work, there is no right or wrong answer. It all comes down to values.

References

Åkerström, M. and Sahlin, I. 2001. Inledning. In *Det motspänstiga offret*, ed. M. Åkerström, and I. Sahlin, 7–24. Lund: Studentlitteratur.

Albert, J. and Standing, G. 2000. Social dumping, catch-up or convergence? Europe in a comparative global context. *Journal of European Social Policy* 10(1):99–119.

Alesina, A. and Glaeser, E. L. 2007. *Fighting poverty in the US and Europe: A world of difference.* New York: Oxford University Press.

Andenæs, K. 1992. *Sosialomsorg i gode og onde dager.* Oslo: Tano

Andersson, R. 2002. Kriminalpolitikens väsen. Doctoral diss., Stockholm University.

Arts, W. and Gelissen, J. 2001. Welfare states, solidarity and justice principles. Does type really matter? *Acta Sociologia* 44:283–300.

Åström, K. 1988. *Socialtjänstlagstiftningen i politik och förvaltning: En studie av parallella normbildningsprocesser.* Studentlitteratur: Lund.

Aubert, V. 1980. *Inledning till rättssociologin.* Stockholm. Almqvist & Wiksell.

Azar, S. T. 2002. Parenting and maltreatment. In *Handbook of parenting:Vol. 4. Social conditions and applied parenting,* 2nd ed., ed. M. H. Bornstein. Mahwah, NJ: Lawrence Erlbaum.

Bergh, A. 2004. The universal welfare state: Theory and the case of Sweden. *Political Studies* 52(4):745–66.

Bergmark, Å. 2000. Solidarity in Swedish welfare—Standing the test of time? *Health Care Analysis* 8(4):395–411.

Bergmark, Å. 2008a. Welfare and the welfare state in Sweden: Trends during the turbulent 1990s. In *Sweden–Austria: Two roads to neutrality and a modern welfare state,* ed. Rathkolb, 107–128. Berlin: Lit Verlag.

Bergmark, Å. 2008b. Market reforms in Swedish health care: Normative reorientation and welfare state sustainability. *Journal of Medicine and Philosophy* 33(3):241–61.

Björk Eydal, G. and Satka, M. 2006. Social work and Nordic welfare policies for children—Present challenges in the light of the past. *European Journal of Social Work* 9(3):305–22.

Boréus, K. 1997. The shift to the right: Neo-Liberalism in argumentation and language in the Swedish public debate since 1969. *European Journal of Political Research* 31(3):257–86.

Brottsoffermyndigheten. 2008. *General information in English*. http://www.brott soffermyndigheten.se/default.asp?id=1345 (accessed July 10, 2008).

Cavadino, M. and Dignan, J. 2006. *Penal systems. A comparative approach*. London: Sage.

Chambliss, E. 2007. *When do facts persuade? Some thoughts on the market for empirical legal studies*. Paper presented at The Center for the Study of Law and Society CSLS Series, University of California, Berkeley, March 3, 2008. http:// www.law.berkeley.edu/centers/csls/CSLSspeakerseries/Chamblisspaper.doc (accessed July 10, 2008).

Christie, N. 1986. The ideal victim. In *From crime policy to victim policy*, ed. E. Fattah, 17–30. Basingstoke, UK: Macmillan.

Clinton, W. 1996. Text of President Clinton's announcement on welfare legislation, *The New York Times*, August 2, 1996. http://query.nytimes.com/gst/fullpage.ht ml?res=9407E1DC143FF932A3575BC0A960958260 (accessed July 10, 2008).

Cousins, M. 2005. *European welfare states*. London: Sage.

Ebbesson, J. 2008. Law power and language. Beware of metaphors. In *Law and Society. Scandinavian Studies in Law* 53:259–61.

Edelman, M. 2001. *The politics of misinformation*. New York: Cambridge University Press.

Elias, R. 1993. *Victims still: The political manipulation of crime victims*. Newbury Park, CA: Sage.

Eriksson, L. 1990. Rätten och moralen. *Retfærd, Nordisk juridisk tidsskrift* 13(48):4–13.

Esping-Andersen, G. 1990. *The three worlds of welfare capitalism*. Cambridge: Polity Press.

Estrada, F. 2001. Juvenile violence as a social problem. Trends, media attention and societal response. *British Journal of Criminology* 41(4):639–55.

European Forum for Victim Services. 1998. *The social rights of victims of crime*. London: European Forum for Victim Services.

Ewald, F. 2002. The return of Descartes's malicious demon: An outline of a philosophy of precaution. In *Embracing risk*, ed. T. Baker and J. Simon. Chicago: University of Chicago Press.

Fattah, E. 1992. Victims and victimology: The facts and the rhetoric. In *Towards a critical victimology*, ed. E. Fattah, 3–26. New York: St. Martin's.

Friis, E. 2005. Socialtjänstlagens värdesystem. En analys av dess praktiska innebörd i sociala utredningar om barn. *Retfaerd 111. Nordisk juridisk tidsskrift* 28(4):60–75.

Garland, D. 2001. *The culture of control. Crime and social order in contemporary society*. Chicago: University of Chicago Press.

Gilbert, N. 2004. *Transformation of the welfare state. The silent surrender of public responsibility*. New York: Oxford University Press.

Government Bill 2006/07:38. *Socialtjänstens stöd till våldsutsatta kvinnor*. Stockholm.

Government Bill 2006/07:63. *En anpassad försvarsunderrättelseverksamhet.* Stockholm.
Government Bill 2005/06:166. *Barn som bevittnat våld.* Stockholm.
Government Bill 2001/02:126. *Medling med anledning av brott.* Stockholm.
Government Bill 2000/01:80. *Ny socialtjänstlag m.m.* Stockholm.
Government Bill 2000/01:79. *Stöd till brottsoffer.* Stockholm.
Government Bill 1997/98:55. *Kvinnofrid.* Stockholm.
Government Bill 1996/97:124. *Ändring i socialtjänstlagen.* Stockholm.
Government Bill 1993/94:143. *Brottsoffer i Blickpunkten.* Stockholm.
Government Bill 1979/80:1. *Om socialtjänsten.* Stockholm.
Greenland, C. 1987. *Preventing CAN deaths: An international study of deaths due to child abuse and neglect.* London: Tavistock Publications.
Hacking, I. 1999. *The social construcion of what?* Cambridge, MA: Harvard University Press.
Handler, J. 2008. *The changing status of citizenship: The spread of workfare in the developed world.* Paper presented at The Center for the Study of Law and Society CSLS Series, University of California, Berkeley, March 3, 2008. http://www.law. berkeley.edu/centers/csls/CSLSspeakerseries/Paper-Handler.pdf (accessed July 10, 2008).
Harrikari, T. 2004. From welfare policy towards risk politics? In *Beyond the competent child, exploring contemporary childhoods in the nordic welfare societies,* ed. H. Brembeck, B. Johansson, and J. Kampmann. Roskilde: Roskilde University Press.
Hill, M. 2006. *Social policy in the modern world.* Malden: Blackwell.
Holgersson, L. 1988. *Socialtjänst en fråga om värderingar. En analys av socialvårdens värderingar från medeltiden fram till socialtjänstens lagar SoL, LVM, LVU samt LSPV.* Stockholm: Tidens Förlag.
Holgersson, L. 2004. *Socialpolitik och socialt arbete. Historia och idéer.* Stockholm: Nordstedts Juridik.
Hollander, 1995. *Rättighetslagstiftning i teori och praxis.* Justus: Uppsala.
Hydén, H. 2000. *Rättsregler: En introduktion till juridiken.* Studentlitteratur: Lund.
Justitiedepartementet. 2007. *Victims of crime,* August 24, 2007. http://www.sweden. gov.se/sb/d/2708/a/15164 (accessed July 10, 2008).
Kirchhoff, G. F. 2005. What is victimology? *Monograph series No. 1,* Tokiwa International Victimology Institute. Tokyo:Seibundo.
Kriminalvården. 2008. *Bygger mest i Europa.* http://www.kriminalvarden.se/ templates/KVV_InfopageGeneral____4127.aspx (accessed July 10, 2008).
Kuhne, S. 2000. The Scandinavian welfare state in the 1990s. *West European Politics* 23(2):209–28.
Larsson, E. and Stubb, L. 1998. *Handbok för stödpersoner.* Stockholm: Brottsofferjourenas Riksförbund.
Lindbom, A. 2007. Obfuscating retrenchment: Swedish welfare policy in the 1990s. *Journal of Public Policy* 27(2):129–50.
Lindgren, M. 2004. *Brottsoffret i rättsprocessen: Om ideala brottsoffer och goda myndigheter.* Stockholm: Jure.
Lindgren, M., B. Hägglund, and K-Å. Pettersson, 2003. *Utsatta och sårbara brottsoffer.* Stockholm: Jure.
Ljungwald, C. and Hollander, A. 2009. Victims of crime in the Swedish Social Services Act. *The International Review of Victimology* 15(3):299–326.

Ljungwald, C. and Svensson, K. 2007. Crime victims and the social services: Social workers' viewpoint. *Journal of Scandinavian Studies in Criminology and Crime Prevention* 8(2):138–56.

Lomell, H. M. 2006. Menneskerettigheter er vel og bra, men for hvem? Offeret eller gjerningsmannen? *Nordisk Tidsskrift for Menneskerettigheter* 24(1):59–74.

MacGregor, S. 1999. Welfare, neo-liberalism and new paternalism: Three ways for social policy in late capitalist societies. *Capital & Class* 67:91–118.

Midré, G. 1995. *Bot, bedring eller brød?* Oslo: Universitetsforlaget.

Moderaterna. 2006. *Nya Moderaterna on Zero Tolerance for Crime.* http://www.moderat.se/material/pdffiler/moderat_13605.pdf (accessed July 10, 2008).

Montanari, I., Nelson, K., and Palme J. 2007. Convergence pressures and responses: Recent social insurance developments in modern welfare states. *Comparative Sociology* 6(3):295–323.

Motion 2002/03:Ju375. *Bettleri.* Stockholm.

O'Connor, J. 1998. US social welfare policy: The Reagan record and legacy. *Journal of Social Policy* 27(1):37–61.

Olsen, G. M. 2008. Labour market policy in the United States, Canada and Sweden: Addressing the issue of convergence. *Social Policy & Administration* 42(4):323–41.

Österberg, E. 1997. Från part i målet till brottsoffer. Den oskyldiga människan och det moderna samhällets framväst. In *Tie tulkintaan*, ed. J. Kekkonen, 353–56. Porvoo: Söderström.

Österberg, E. 2002. Upptäckten av den oskyldiga människan. In *Offer för brott. Våldtäkt, incest och barnamord i Sveriges historia från reformationen till nutid,* ed. E. Bergenlöv, M. Lindstedt Cronberg, and E. Österberg, 9–24. Lund: Nordic Academic Press.

Palme, J. 2008. The Swedish model. In *Sweden–Austria: Two roads to neutrality and a modern welfare state,* ed. O. Rathkolb 69–76. Berlin: Lit Verlag.

Parent, G. 2006. *When crime pays. The politics of crime, law, and victim compensation in Quebec.* Paper presented at CPSA conference, June 1–3, Toronto.

Rank, M. 2005. *One nation. Unprivileged.* New York: Oxford University Press.

Reiman, J. 1973. Victims harm and justice. In *Victimology a new focus. Theoretical issues in victimology,* vol. 1, ed. I. Drapkin and E. Viano, 77–87. Lexington, MA: Lexington Books.

Rodriguez, C. and Green, G. 1997. Parenting stress and anger expression as predictors of child abuse potential. *Child Abuse and Neglect* 21(4):367–77.

Rothstein, B. and Lindbom, A. 2004. The mysterious survival of the Swedish welfare state. Paper presented at the American Political Science Association, September 2–5, Chicago.

Santesson-Wilson, P. 2003. Studier i symbolpolitik. Doctoral diss., Lund University.

SCB. 2004. *Offer för vålds—och egendomsbrott 1978–2002. Report nr. 88.* Stockholm: Statistiska centralbyrån.

Schmidtz, D. and Goodin, R. E. 1998. *Social welfare and individual responsibility.* New York: Cambridge University Press.

Simon, J. 2003. Wechsler's century and ours: Reforming criminal law in a time of shifting rationalities of government. Paper presented at The Center for the Study of Law and Society CSLS Series, University of California, Berkeley, September 8, 2003. http://repositories.cdlib.org/cgi/viewcontent.cgi?article=1032&context=csls (accessed July 10, 2008).

Situation Stockholm. 2007. *Hallå där.* http://www.situationsthlm.se/sv/Containers/ Halladar/Kristina-Axen-Ohlin/ (accessed January 17, 2009).

Socialstyrelsen. 2002. The Social Services Act (Socialtjänstlagen)—What are you rights after 1 July 2002? Socialstyrelsen. Stockholm. http://www.sos.se/fulltext/ 114/2002-114-9/2002-114-9.pdf (accessed July 10, 2008).

Socialstyrelsen. 2004. 5 kap. 11 SoL—en uppföljning av socialtjänstens arbete. Report. Stockholm: Socialstyrelsen.

SOU. 2007:2. *Från socialbidrag till arbete.* Stockholm.

SOU. 2005:66. Makt att forma samhället och sitt eget liv—jämställdhetspolitiken mot nya mål. Stockholm.

SOU. 1998:40. *Brottsoffer. Vad har gjorts? Vad bör göras?* Stockholm.

SOU. 1976:9. *Sexuella övergrepp: förslag till ny lydelse av brottsbalkens bestämmelser om sedlighetsbrott.* Stockholm.

Steger, M. 2005. Ideologies of globalization. *Journal of Political Ideologies* 10(1): 11–30.

Strömberg, S. 1981. *Rätt, rättskällor och rättstillämpning: En lärobok i allmän rättslära.* Norstedts: Stockholm.

Sunesson, S., Blomberg, S., Edebalk, P. G., Harrysson, L., Magnusson, J., Meeuwisse, A., Petersson, J., and Salonen, T. 1998. The flight from universalism. *European Journal of Social Work* 1(1):19–29.

Svensson, K. 2006. *Socialt arbete med brottsoffer. Sympati, empati och organisering.* Stockholm: Carlssons.

Svensson, K. 2007. Victim support in a changing welfare state. *Social Work and Society* 5(2). http://www.socwork.net/2007/2/articles/svensson (accessed July 10, 2008).

Taylor-Gooby, P. 2001. Sustaining state welfare in hard times: Who will foot the bill? *Journal of European Social Policy* 11(2):133–47.

Tham, H. 1995. From treatment to just deserts in a changing welfare state. In *Beware of punishment*, ed. A. Snare, 89–122. Oslo: Pax.

Tham, H. 2001a. Brottsoffrets uppkost och framtid. In *Det motspänstiga offret*, ed. M. Åkerström, and I. Sahlin, 27–45. Lund: Studentlitteratur.

Tham, H. 2001b. Law and order as a leftist project? The case of Sweden. *Punishment and Society* 3(3):409–26.

Tuori, K. 1993. Lagstiftningsstrategierna inom social—och hälsovården. *Retfærd (Nordisk juridisk tidskrift).* 62:5–18.

Ulmanen, P. 2008. Next of kin in Swedish elder care policy problem representations and outcomes. Paper presented at the conference Transforming Elderly Care at Local, National and Transnational Levels, June 26–28. Copenhagen.

Vahle Westerhäll, L. 2002. Den starka statens fall. En rättsvetenskaplig studie av svensk social trygghet 1950–2000. Stockholm: Norstedts Juridik.

Wacquant, L. 2001. The penalisation of poverty and the rise of neo-liberalism. *European Journal on Criminal Policy and Research* 9(4):401–12.

Wacquant, L. 2004. *Fattigdomens fängelser.* Eslöv: Symposion.

Warnling-Nerep, W. 1995. *Kommuners lag-och domstolstrots.* Juristförlaget: Stockholm.

Weed, F. J. 1995. *Certainty of justice. Reform in the crime victim movement.* New York: Aldine de Gruyter.

Wergens, A. 2002. *Ett viktimologiskt forskningsprogram.* Brottsoffermyndigheten: Umeå.

Conclusion

SHLOMO G. SHOHAM AND
PAUL KNEPPER

The *International Handbook of Victimology* is meant to be read alongside the *International Handbook of Criminology* [Shoham, Knepper, and Kett, 2010] and the *International Handbook of Penology and Criminal Justice* [Shoham, Beck, and Kett, 2008]. There are a number of chapters in these books relevant to the study of victimology.

The *International Handbook of Criminology* includes a chapter on victims and criminal justice by Edna Erez and Julian V. Roberts. They describe the role of the victim in the criminal justice system over time and report on relevant reforms within United States and other key common law jurisdictions. They present legislation recognizing the rights of victims at stages within proceedings and describe specific points of engagement of victims. Erez and Roberts devote particular attention to sentencing, which, as they point out, represents the apex of the system and the point at which victims' interests are the keenest. As a result of several developments, including the increase of restorative justice and therapeutic justice approaches, victims in common law jurisdictions have more input into the criminal justice process than was true decades ago. Research findings indicate that victims' rights can be helpful to victims desirous of participation in criminal justice, and the fact of their participation does not necessarily lead to problems limiting the efficiency of the system. However, victims' contribution, particularly at sentencing, continues to be met with resistance on the part of those within the system who believe otherwise. Victims will likely continue to become integrated in proceedings, although legal cultures will remain dominated by underlying values and ideologies that shape the nature of the integration.

Anthony E. Bottoms and Andrew Costello investigate the phenomenon of "repeat victimization," which refers to the same person or property being revictimized within a specified period. Analyses of this pattern have been drawn from victimization surveys and recorded crime information but have tended to examine short-term patterns (between 12 and 15 months). Using a unique data set from Sheffield, a city in the north of England, incorporating information about victims and offenders, they examined long-term trends in repeat victimization. Specifically, they examine patterns of domestic burglary repeat victimization over a period of some 9 years, distinguishing between short-term and long-term risk. They point to the need for more research in this area and suggest that policy implications are not simple. Although there is research to suggest that repeat victimization for household crime is concentrated in poor areas, the distinction that emerges between short- and long-term patterns of repeat victimization suggests that crime prevention should not automatically encourage the idea that households in the most deprived areas represent "long-term chronic" risk.

There are also chapters dealing with victims of sex crimes, domestic violence, and fear of crime. Joachim Obergfell-Fuchs focuses on perpetrators and victims of sex crimes. As he points out, there has been a great deal of media interest in sex crimes and in dealing with sex offenders across Europe and North America in recent years. The discussion examines the extent of sex crimes with a look at sources of statistical information, as well as patterns of offending, including sexual harassment in the workplace. Although sexual violence seems prevalent in modern societies, despite media reports to the contrary, the rate of sex crimes has decreased during the past century. The discussion also explains the challenges of dealing with sex crimes within the criminal law and reviews methods of dealing with sex offenders with a particular focus on the issue of recidivism. In some countries, the United States for example, the response has been to concentrate punishment on the offender by locking up offenders for a long time and to engage in public labeling to alert people to the potential for further crimes on release. There is criminological research to show that successful treatment of sex offenders is possible, although there remain considerable methodological limitations in the explanatory power of results so far.

Madelaine Adelman looks at domestic violence, specifically, anthropological studies of domestic violence. At the center of the anthropological approach to crime is the idea that meanings and manifestations of crime are constituted as part of the social construction of identity and power, and that claims for justice have been preshaped by cultural contexts and transformed by social actions in institutions such as courts. Understood in this way, anthropology has the potential to "inform, and perhaps transform" the understanding of crimes such as domestic violence. Adelman describes the anthropological approach and how anthropologists have studied domestic violence. She spotlights the most recent contributions to the study of domestic violence by anthropologists and gives examples of promising approaches. "Anthropological approaches," Adelman suggests, "can complement, as well as critique, extant studies of domestic violence by drawing scholarly and policy attention inquiries based on meaning and experience, historical and cultural context, comparison, and global connections."

Murray Lee considers the problem of "fear of crime." Fear of crime has attracted attention from criminologists since it was first "discovered" in the United States following implementation of the first wide-scale victimization surveys during the 1960s. Lee concentrates on whether socioeconomic disadvantage is correlated with fear of crime or is largely the result of methodological and conceptual devices used to study perceptions of crime. He proposes that "in wedding fear of crime to disadvantage and disorganization, we as researchers are missing or rendering invisible one of the principle drivers of fear of crime … that is the relative affluence and the conspicuous consumption that goes with it." If we perceive fear of crime as discursive, rather than a psychosocial quasi-objective phenomenon, the question of who fears crime, as well as who drives fear-of-crime discourse, becomes less clear but much more interesting.

The *International Handbook of Penology and Criminal Justice* includes a chapter dealing with reparation, compensation, and restitution. Charles F. Abel presents a detailed argument in support of his claim that reparation constitutes the only adequately explainable, and hence the best, form of punishment. Abel deploys ideas of a range of philosophers and social thinkers, from Habermas to Rawls, to build his argument. He spies a gap between offense and punishment and reviews a number of means for "leaping the gap." These are universal standards, traditional social standards, reflexive equilibrium, veils of ignorance, ideal speech, and money. He comes down in favor of money. Essentially, he finds that reparation, paid either as restitution or compensation, represents the most realistic, empirically informed, and unemotional sanction, aimed as satisfying the victim without humiliating the offender. Or as Abel puts it: "The only forms of punishment that can be explained satisfactorily are those that require reparation through a state-enforced transfer of money."

Ken Pease writes about victims and victimization. He argues that victim programs should foster an internal locus of control among victims, while remaining aware of the issue of victim blame. He emphasizes the need for prevention of repeat victimization and suggests some ways criminal justice efforts can be redirected toward this end. Pease rejects the view of victims as passive and fearful; he seeks to avoid simplistic depictions of offenders and victims. He points out that victims sometimes recognize their contribution to crime events, and this serves as an internal locus of control that should be so in some circumstances but not others. The progress toward practical victim support within a system that is otherwise hostile to victims must continue. The participation of victims in restorative justice schemes will require further evidence of benefit to be confidently advocated.

There are two chapters on restorative justice. In an extensive commentary on restorative justice, Lode Walgrave opens with a review of the history of restorative justice, its ancient and modern roots. He considers key concepts of harm, restoration, and justice and reviews different restorative justice practices commonly deployed in this field. These include victim support, victim–offender mediation, restorative conferencing, community service, and citizen boards. He also takes up the matter of restorative justice as a form of punishment; by examining its socioethical foundations, he makes a claim for its incorporation within criminal justice. He predicts that the future of restorative justice will be shaped not only by practical and scientific qualities of options but also more by the cultural and political environment in which these options will operate. To the extent that politicians favor repressive punishments, the chances for genuine restorative alternatives will be reduced. Walgrave expresses a measure of hope. "I have alluded to several scientific explorations of public attitudes that show results that are not at all unfavorable to restorative responses. Therefore, there is no reason to be too pessimistic about the future of restorative justice."

Mark S. Umbreit, Robert B. Coates, and Betty Vos give us an in-depth look at one of the most widely practiced forms of restorative justice, that of victim–offender mediation (VOM). Some 1,500 VOM programs in 17 countries have appeared in recent years, and there are about 50 empirical studies of them. Umbreit, Coates, and Vos explain what VOM is about, how it is carried out, and review evaluations of its effectiveness. VOM represents a restorative justice process with promise for repairing the harm of the criminal event, while holding criminal offenders accountable and allowing those affected by the crime to have a voice in its resolution. Their discussion includes findings concerning participation rates, participant satisfaction, diversion rates, recidivism, and costs of programs. They also comment on crimes of severe violence. They conclude that when practiced consistent with stated guidelines and values, VOM brings about positive results for victims, offenders, and members of the community.

References

Shoham, S. G., O. Beck, and M. Kett. 2008. *International handbook of penology and criminal justice.* Boca Raton, FL: Taylor & Francis.
Shoham, S. G., P. Knepper, and M. Kett. 2010. *International handbook of criminology.* Boca Raton, FL: Taylor & Francis.

Index

Milton Keynes UK
Ingram Content Group UK Ltd.
UKHW021936071024
449327UK00022B/1823